D1457909

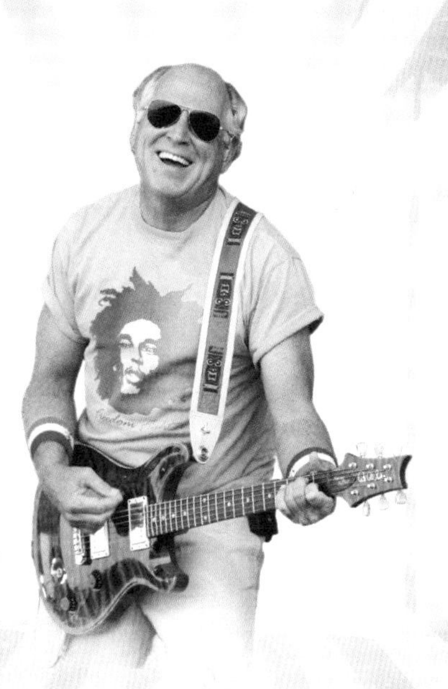

Microbiology
and Infectious Disease

Chapter 1

Structure and Function of the Microbial Cell

Marvin N. Schwalb

PERSPECTIVE

Cellular microorganisms are a heterogeneous group. Originally, those organisms were included which could not be seen with the naked eye. Early attempts at classification distributed these organisms between the plant and animal kingdoms. However, this proved unsatisfactory since several groups (e.g., photosynthetic protozoans and slime molds) could be placed in either (or neither) kingdom.

This led to the formation of a third kingdom for microorganisms, the Protista; this group consists of organisms with a relatively simple differentiation into cellular types and includes the bacteria, protozoa, slime molds, fungi, and algae. The designation Protista is a useful one. Its principal difficulty is the somewhat subjective nature of the description "relatively simple."

Modern techniques of electron microscopy and biochemistry have demonstrated that the Protista can be subdivided into two major groups on the basis of cell type. The two groups are the *prokaryotes* and the *eukaryotes.* As the names imply, there is a fundamental difference in the nuclei of these cell types. The eukaryotic cell has a "true" nucleus, with chromosomes

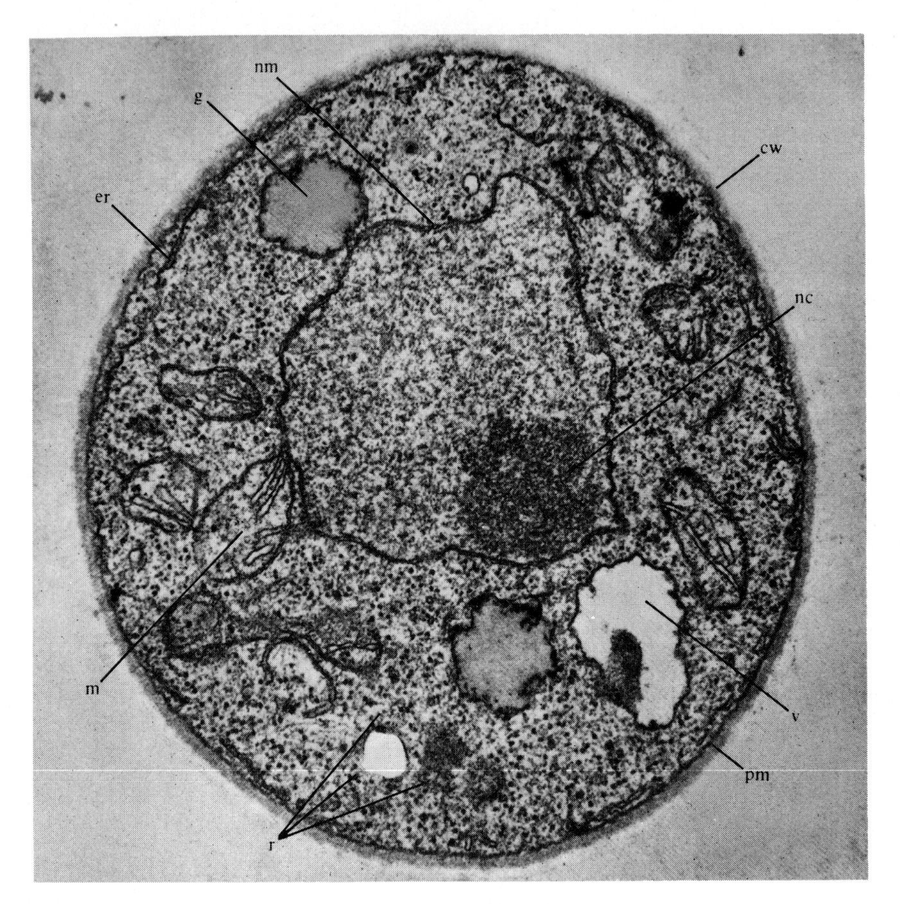

Figure 1-1 A eukaryotic cell, *Cryptococcus neoformans*, a pathogenic yeast showing cell wall (cw), plasma membrane (pm), a nucleus with nuclear membrane (nm) and a nucleolus (nc), mitochondria (m), ribosomes (r), endoplasmic reticulum (er), vacuole (v), and storage granule (g). × 30,000. *(From M. Edwards, M. Gordon, E. Lapa, and W. Ghiorse, J. Bacteriol., 94:766–777, 1967.)*

surrounded by a nuclear membrane. The prokaryotic cell lacks a nuclear membrane and highly structured chromosomes. As the following discussion will demonstrate, however, differences between these cell types are not limited to nuclear structure but are far more extensive (Figs. 1-1 and 1-2).

Prokaryotic Protista include the bacteria and blue-green algae. All other protists have a eukaryotic cell type.

THE EUKARYOTIC CELL

The basic feature of eukaryotic cells is the degree of compartmentalization of function associated with complex membranous structures. Electron micrographs reveal that most membranes consist of three layers, collectively referred to as a *unit membrane.* The membranes are composed of protein and lipid. In eukaryotic cells this lipid component includes sterols.

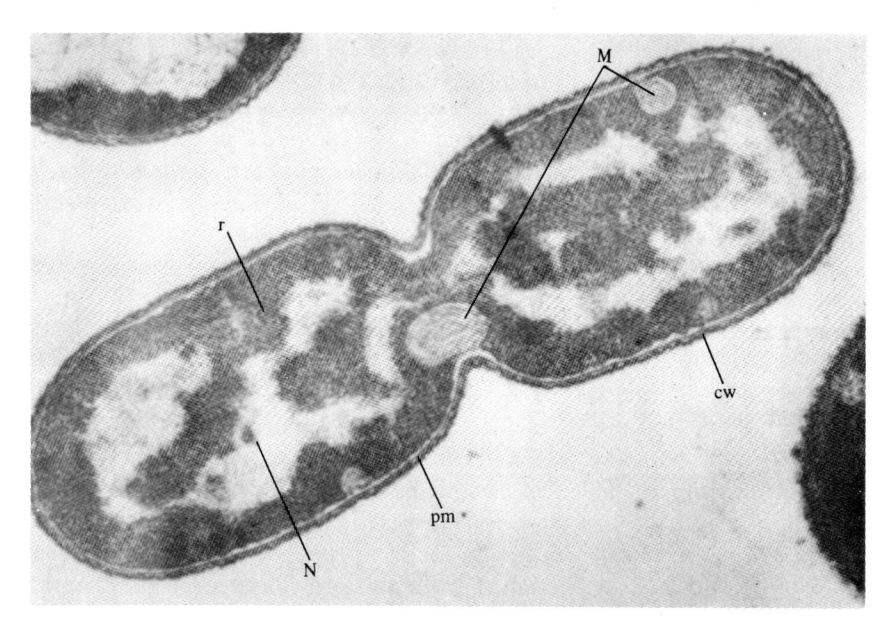

Figure 1-2 A prokaryotic cell, *Achromobacter,* a dividing gram-negative bacterium showing cell wall (cw), plasma membrane (pm), nuclear area (N), densely packed ribosomes (r), and mesosomes (M). × 42,000. *(From W. Wiebe and G. Chapman, J. Bacteriol., 95:1874–1886, 1968.)*

Containing the cell is the *plasma membrane,* which acts as a differentially permeable osmotic barrier between the cell proper and the surrounding environment, allowing the cell to maintain a different internal environment.

As already noted, the chromosomes of the eukaryotes are enclosed within a nuclear membrane. The nucleus, however, is not completely isolated from the cytoplasm, since pores are frequently found in the nuclear membrane, which itself is contiguous with cytoplasmic membranes.

The haploid genetic complement for eukaryotes is always greater than one. Each chromosome consists of folded strands of deoxyribonucleic acid (DNA) in association with histone, a basic protein. The histone is responsible for the folding of the DNA. It should be noted that each chromosome of a typical eukaryote contains at least several times the amount of DNA found in a prokaryotic chromosome.

In order to properly sort out the different chromosomes during various nuclear divisions (mitosis and meiosis), special structures called *spindle fibers* and *centrioles* are formed. The spindle fibers are composed of microtubules. The microtubules are about 200 Å in diameter and up to several microns in length and apparently operate in cytoplasmic functions involving movement. The centrioles are structurally similar to the basal bodies of flagella.

Also found within the nucleus are one or more nucleoli. These structures are involved in the formation of ribosomes.

The *endoplasmic reticulum* (ER) is a network of membranes found in the cytoplasm. The membranes are often covered with ribosomes, which appear as small dense granules. Such an

ER is called rough. Smooth ER does not have attached ribosomes. The ER may act in part to provide a physical continuum between the structural components of the eukaryotic cell.

Ribosomes in eukaryotes are relatively large, are composed of protein and ribonucleic acid (RNA), and function in protein synthesis. Their size and attachment to ER distinguish them from the ribosomes of prokaryotes.

In addition to ER, other membranous structures in the cytoplasm include vacuoles, the Golgi apparatus, and mitochondria. *Vacuoles* are surrounded by a single membrane and are usually used for storage. The *Golgi apparatus* is a complex of membranes which apparently functions in secretion. A number of eukaryotic protists lack a Golgi apparatus (e.g., ciliates).

Mitochondria consist of a double membrane with considerable internal folding, leading to the formation of cristae. The enzymes concerned with terminal oxidative respiration and the tricarboxylic acid (TCA) cycle are found in mitochondria. Evidence obtained principally from the fungi indicates that mitochondria possess their own DNA, distinct from nuclear DNA, and that this mitochondrial DNA codes some of the information needed for the genesis of the mitochondrion itself. A similar situation appears to occur in the formation of *plastids,* those structures which contain the pigments and some of the enzymes involved in photosynthesis in eukaryotes.

Motility in the eukaryotic protists is usually associated with flagella. A *flagellum* consists of an axial core composed of a ring of nine axial fibers surrounding two central fibers. The entire core is surrounded by a membrane which is continuous with the plasma or cell membrane. The core is attached to the basal body located in the cytoplasm. The basal body itself contains a ring of nine fibers, each composed of three subfibers. In some eukaryotes, motility is associated with *cilia,* which are structures similar to flagella but shorter.

Outside the plasma membrane in some species may be found a cell wall, which is responsible for maintaining the shape of the cell. The walls of fungi are composed primarily of simple linear and branched polymers of sugars, usually glucose but occasionally mannose, fructose, etc. Chitin (poly-β-1,4-N-acetylglucosamine) is also commonly found.

THE PROKARYOTIC CELL

The typical prokaryotic cell contains only two major membrane components: the plasma membrane, which contains the cell and acts as an osmotic barrier, and the *mesosome,* which is a convoluted membranous invagination extending into the cell proper. The mesosome is continuous with and probably represents an internal extension of the plasma membrane. Unlike eukaryotes, the membranes of prokaryotes usually do not contain sterols.

Attached to the mesosome, which provides increased surface area for the cell, are the cell's respiratory enzymes. Because mesosomes are often found at the site of septum formation, they may be responsible for distributing the DNA between daughter cells and thus are ultimately involved in cell division.

The *nucleus* or *nuclear area* of prokaryotes is the space occupied by the chromosome. The chromosome consists of a single closed circle of double-stranded DNA, tightly packed so that it occupies a discrete area.

There is no ER in prokaryotes. However, the cells are usually packed with ribosomes which are smaller than those in eukaryotes and which also function in protein synthesis.

Some prokaryotic cells contain cytoplasmic inclusions. These include granules of starch, glycogen, and volutin. The latter are metachromatic in that they appear red when stained with a basic blue dye, an effect associated with the presence of inorganic polyphosphate.

Flagella in prokaryotes consist of several

strands of protein called *flagellin* wound in a helix and covered with a sheath. They originate in the cytoplasm apparently from a basal body or granule. The arrangement of flagella is of taxonomic importance. Flagella may be polar (originating from one or both ends of the cell) or peritrichous (distributed over the entire surface of the organism).

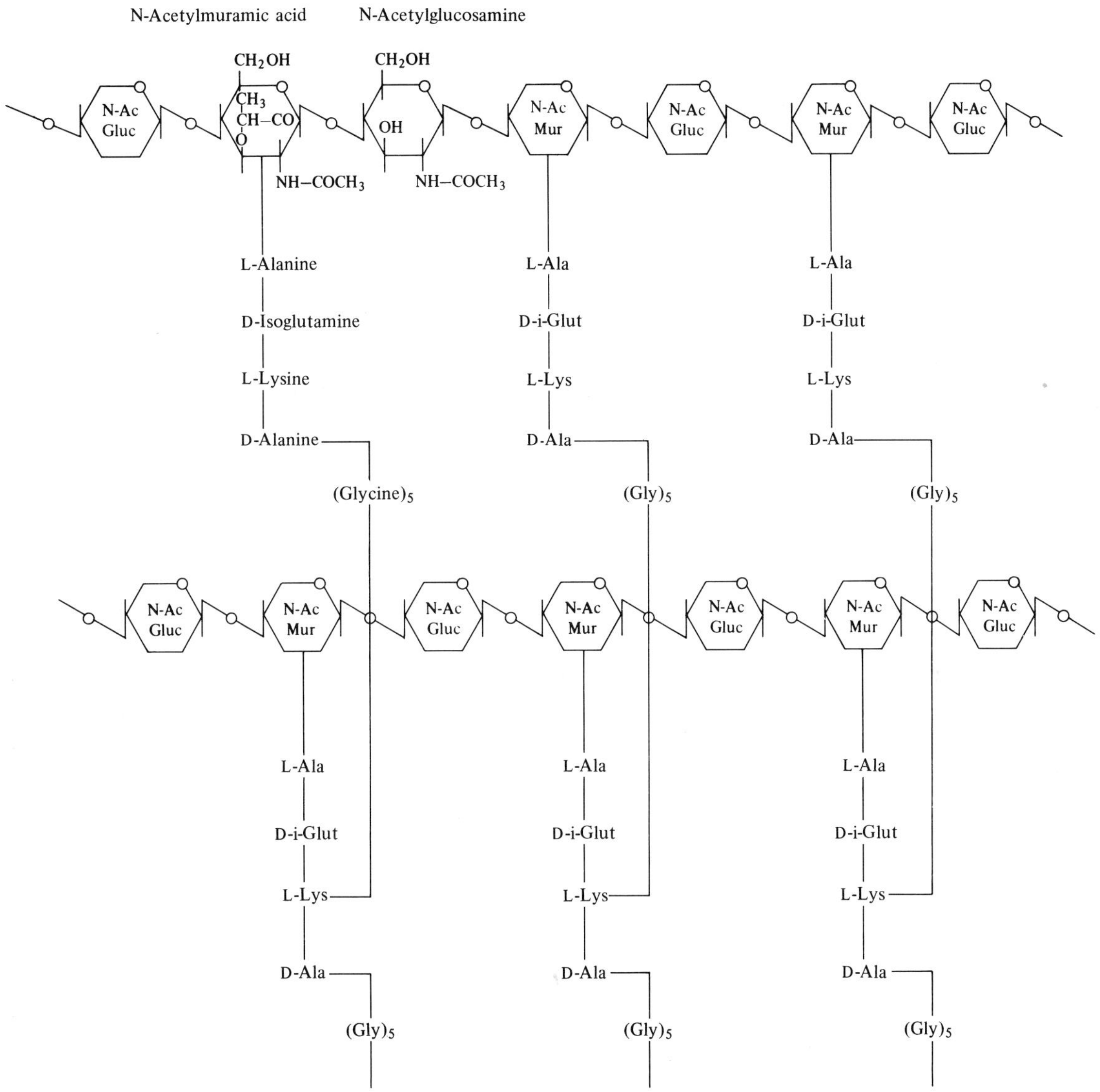

Figure 1-3 Structure of the glycopeptide of prokaryotic cell walls. Note the backbone of alternating units of N-acetylglucosamine (N-Ac Gluc) and N-acetylmuramic acid (N-Ac Mur). Attached to each muramic acid residue is a tetrapeptide. The layers are linked through glycine bridges between the D-alanines and L-lysines.

Almost all prokaryotes have a cell wall (exceptions are L-forms and mycoplasmas, see Chaps. 18 and 20). These walls are often very complex. The most universal component is the *glycopeptide* (mucopeptide or murein). The glycopeptide consists of two types of compounds: amino sugars and various amino acids. The structure is shown in Figure 1-3. The backbone is composed of alternating β-1,4- linked units of N-acetylglucosamine and N-acetylmuramic acid. To each muramic acid is attached a tetrapeptide of L-alanine, D-glutamic acid, L-lysine or *meso*-diaminopimelic acid, and D-alanine. Note the alternating arrangement of the *d*- and *l*- isomers. D-Amino acids are rarely found in nature outside prokaryotic cell walls. These layers are cross-linked to form a rigid wall structure. The cross-linking is accomplished by a peptide bridge which links the third amino acid of one layer with the fourth amino acid of the next layer. The resulting three-dimensional structure is diagramed in Figure 1-4.

In 1884 Gram discovered that bacteria could be divided into two classes on the basis of their ability to retain crystal violet dye fixed with iodine. *Gram-positive bacteria* are able to retain the dye after an attempt at decolorization by an organic solvent (alcohol or acetone). *Gram-negative bacteria* are decolorized by the same procedure but can be visualized by a pink counterstain. Under proper conditions the staining reaction is a constant feature of each species.

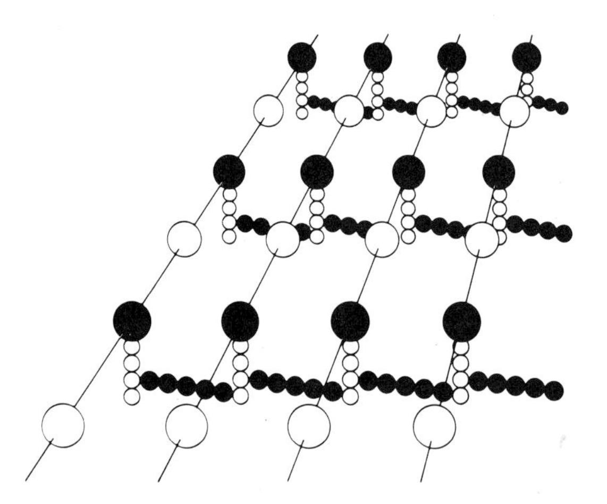

Figure 1-4 Structure of cell wall glycopeptide demonstrating how cross-linking by pentaglycine bridge builds layers of sugar tetrapeptide into a three-dimensional structure. ◯ = N-acetylglucosamine; ● = N-acetylmuramic acid; ○ = amino acids of tetrapeptide; • = glycines of pentaglycine bridge. *(From N. Sharon, Sci. Am., 220(5):92–96, 1969.)*

The Gram staining procedure was used empirically for many years. More recently, specific differences were discovered between gram-positive and gram-negative species. Gram-positive cells have a relatively thick glycopeptide layer. In addition, various polysaccharides and *teichoic acids* (polymers of glycerol or ribitol) may be present.

Gram-negative cell walls are more complex. The glycopeptide layer is thin and associated with a layer of *lipopolysaccharide* (LPS). The LPS is associated with a membrane-like structure located outside the glycopeptide layer. Also present in the outer "membrane" are protein and phospholipids.

LPS consists of a complex polysaccharide linked to a glucosamine-containing lipid known as lipid A. LPS apparently requires calcium ions for its stability and is therefore dissociated by metal chelating agents. Figure 1-5 gives the general structure of LPS. Note that attached to the outer core are repeating units of oligosaccharide composed of a wide variety of sugars whose particular sequence and conformational structure determine the unique features of the O antigens in the Enterobacteriaceae (Chap. 18).

LPS is responsible for the endotoxic effects of certain bacteria. When a bacterium with LPS enters the bloodstream, the LPS may cause a variety of clinical manifestations including fever, shock, and death (Chap. 5).

The enzyme *lysozyme*, which is found in saliva and tears, attacks the glycopeptide portion of the cell wall, hydrolyzing the polysaccharide backbone. The result is the removal of the wall in gram-positive species. In gram-negative cells, the LPS protects the glycopeptide. However, after removal of the LPS, lysozyme can hydrolyze gram-negative glycopeptide. When the glycopeptide is removed, the cell will lyse by bursting of the plasma membrane.

If the lysozyme acts on a gram-positive cell in a concentrated sugar solution, a *protoplast* will be formed. This consists of the plasma membrane and its contents. In gram-negative cells, the result will be a *spheroplast*, which differs from protoplasts in that some wall material apparently remains with the cell. The concentrated sugar solution provides sufficient osmotic tension to equalize the osmotic pressure within the plasma membrane and prevent bursting. When present, the cell wall prevents bursting in normal media. The cell wall is also responsible for cell shape, since protoplasts and spheroplasts are spherical regardless of the shape of the original cell.

Another agent which results in the formation of protoplasts and spheroplasts is the antibiotic *penicillin*. Penicillin acts *only* on growing cells by inhibiting the synthesis of new glycopeptide (see Chap. 4), thus resulting in defective walls. Again, if the medium is not at a high osmotic pressure, penicillin action results in cell lysis.

Typically protoplasts and spheroplasts are incapable of replication. However, occasionally such replication does take place. Then the replicating cells are known as L-forms. L-forms can also be isolated from normal and diseased patients (Chap. 18).

Under certain conditions L-forms, protoplasts, and spheroplasts can revert to microorganisms with intact cell walls. There has been much interest as well as speculation about the potential role that the revertants play in disease processes. In chronic bacteriuria and chronic pyelonephritis, for example, under conditions of increased toxicity and following chemotherapy, spheroplasts, protoplasts, and L-forms can be recovered from about 20 percent of the patients (Chap. 18). Another basic question involves the potential connection between stable L-forms and the mycoplasmas, a group of microorganisms distinguished by their lack of cell walls (see Chap. 20).

Outside the cell wall, some bacterial species

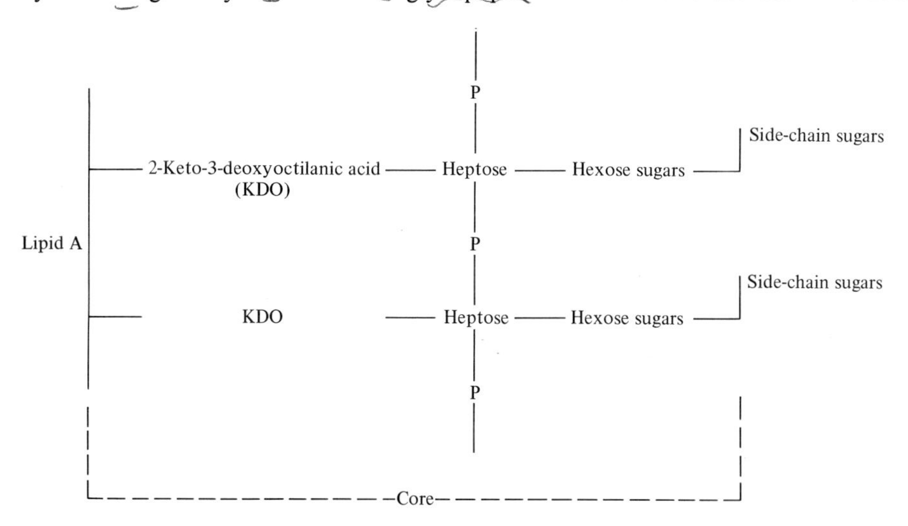

Figure 1-5 Lipopolysaccharide (LPS) of gram-negative walls. Only two units are shown. A large number of these units are covalently linked to form the LPS layer of the intact wall.

produce *capsules* and *slimes.* These may be thick, gelatinous, and relatively discrete (capsules) or comparatively thin and slimy (slimes). Most capsules are composed of polysaccharides and occasionally polypeptides. Some slimes are known to be complex, containing polysaccharides, polypeptides, and lipids.

Some gram-negative bacteria have straight rod-like projections passing from the cytoplasm through the cell wall called *pili.* Common pili are shorter and thinner than flagella and have no known function. Sex pili are longer than common pili and apparently function in bacterial conjugation (see Chap. 3).

Some species of gram-positive rods are capable of producing a resistant *endospore.* As the name implies, the endospore is found within the bacterial cell, generally one per cell. Therefore, endospores are not reproductive structures. On the other hand, endospores have survival value for the bacteria, since they are typically resistant to heat (100°C), desiccation, chemicals, and radiation.

The endospore is thick-walled and contains several layers of glycopeptide and protein. Formation of endospores involves a complex series of biochemical and cytological events including the synthesis of dipicolinic acid. This chemical and calcium both appear to be required for heat resistance.

A culture of potential spore-formers is induced to sporulate by suboptimal nutritional conditions (not actual starvation). Although some spores will germinate to form a vegetative cell when placed in nutrient medium, the germination of most endospores is readily facilitated by heat activation at 75°C, presumably because the heat breaks the natural dormancy of the endospores.

COMPARISON OF EUKARYOTIC AND PROKARYOTIC CELL STRUCTURE

The fundamental nature of the differences between eukaryotic and prokaryotic cells considered in the preceding discussion is summarized in Table 1-1. Obviously, structural differences reflect distinct metabolic pathways. For example, the glycopeptide of prokaryotic cell walls is constructed by a specific series of enzymatically catalyzed reactions. The structure and function of each enzyme are determined by the genetic information of the cell.

Table 1-1 Characteristics of Eukaryotic and Prokaryotic Cells

	Eukaryotes	Prokaryotes
Plasma membrane	+	+
Membrane sterols	+	− (usually)
Endoplasmic reticulum	+	−
Mitochondria, Golgi apparatus, plastids	+	−
Mesosome	−	+
Nuclear membrane	+	−
Mitotic apparatus	+	−
Haploid number of chromosomes	>1	1
Histone protein	+	−
Shape of chromosome	Linear	Circular
Ribosomes	80S	70S
Flagella	Complex	Simple
Cell wall glycopeptide	−	+

The description of prokaryotic and eukaryotic cell structure represents an attempt to provide an overall picture. There is, however, a great diversity of structures found in both groups of organisms, as will become evident in Chapter 2. Because the study of cell fine structure had to await development of the electron microscope and because relatively few prokaryotic species have been examined, considerable refinement in specific details applicable to one or another species can be expected.

GROWTH OF MICROORGANISMS

Every microorganism requires water, minerals, a source of energy, carbon, and nitrogen for growth. In addition, many microbes require amino acids, vitamins, and other complex metabolites which they are unable to synthesize.

Compounds are required as a source of chemical energy for biosynthetic processes *(anabolism).* The chemical energy is obtained during the enzymatic degradation of various carbon sources *(catabolism).*

Energy Sources

Many microorganisms obtain their chemical energy for biosynthesis through the breakdown of *preformed* organic compounds supplied exogenously (from outside the cell). Such organisms are called *heterotrophs.*

Some microorganisms can synthesize their own organic compounds by fixing CO_2, using nonorganic sources of energy for the fixation. These organisms are called *autotrophs.*

Photoautotrophs use light as the source of energy, and the CO_2 fixation process is called *photosynthesis.* Bacterial photosynthesis differs from the process in green eukaryotic plants in that water is not oxidized in bacteria. Instead, a variety of organic and inorganic compounds is used, such as H_2S, which yields elemental sulfur instead of oxygen.

A few microbial species can utilize the energy produced by the oxidation of inorganic compounds, such as ammonia, to fix CO_2. These are called *chemoautotrophs.*

Carbon Sources

In heterotrophs the carbon source is usually the same compound as the energy source. An extremely large number of organic compounds can serve as carbon sources for microorganisms. Individual species may be restricted to a few simple sugars, but other species may attack a variety of proteins, carbohydrates, fats, or lipids. In this way, microorganisms serve one of their principal ecological functions, the degradation of dead organic matter. Organisms which use dead organic material for growth are called *saprophytes.* Some microorganisms behave as *parasites,* using other living cells as a source of nutrients.

In autotrophs the primary carbon source is CO_2. Some autotrophic species, however, require a few other organic compounds. Even the organic compounds synthesized in autotrophs are subsequently degraded to provide energy for biosynthesis.

Nitrogen Sources

Many microorganisms obtain their cellular nitrogen from inorganic sources such as ammonium salts and nitrates. A number of bacteria and blue-green algae can fix nitrogen gas to form organic nitrogen. Other species can utilize or may even require organic nitrogen such as amino acids.

Minerals

Various other elements, usually supplied as inorganic salts, are required. Phosphorous, potassium, magnesium, sulfur, and iron are needed in relatively large quantities (10^{-3} to 10^{-4} M). Other so-called trace elements are needed in several hundred- to several thousandfold lower concentrations. These include manganese, calcium, copper, zinc, and cobalt. On the other hand, some species may require high concentrations of certain inorganic elements. For example, calcium is required in relatively large amounts by some algae, fungi, and bacteria.

Vitamins

These organic compounds, essential to enzyme function, are synthesized *de novo* by many microorganisms. However, other species require one or more vitamins supplied exogenously.

Other Growth Factors

Microorganisms differ widely in their ability to synthesize the compounds required for growth. For example, many organisms will grow on a medium of glucose, ammonium salt, inorganic salts, and water. These species have the capacity to synthesize the hundreds of compounds required for growth. On the other hand, some microorganisms require a medium with complex substances containing all the amino acids, vitamins, and other compounds whose specific requirement and function may not be known. This latter condition is more commonly found in parasites. Between these extremes, many intermediate conditions obtain. For example, in some species certain amino acids are required not only as a source of nitrogen but also because the organism cannot synthesize them.

Environmental Factors

Temperature As a group, microorganisms can grow over a wide variety of temperatures (about −5 to +80°C). However, most species are *mesophils,* growing optimally at about 24 to 40°C with an absolute range of about 10 to 45°C. Generally, the parasitic species grow best near the upper part of this range (32 to 42°C) and the saprophytes nearer the lower end. A few species are considered *thermophils* in that they have an optimum temperature range of 55 to 60°C. *Psychrophils,* on the other hand, grow best at temperatures below the optimum for mesophils.

pH Although there are exceptions at both ends of the scale, most microorganisms require a hydrogen-ion concentration between pH 2.3 and 9. The optimum range is usually between a slightly acid (pH 5) and a slightly basic (pH 7.5) environment.

Oxygen Concentration Many microorganisms are obligate *aerobes;* that is, they require molecular oxygen for growth. The oxygen is used as an electron acceptor during respiration. Other microorganisms are obligate *anaerobes,* being unable to grow in the presence of molecular oxygen. Facultative organisms can grow under aerobic or anaerobic conditions.

Light Light is obviously a requirement of photoautotrophic species.

Culture Media

In the laboratory, microorganisms can grow in either liquid or semisolid media. Solidification is usually brought about by adding 1.5 to 2 percent agar, although gelatin may be used in special cases.

A medium which contains all the specific nutritive requirements of the species being studied is referred to as a *defined* medium; that is, the chemical identity and quantity of its constituents are known.

The defined medium may also be the *minimal* medium for that species. A minimal medium is the simplest defined medium which will allow a given species to grow. Removal of any one of the constituents will prevent growth. Addition of other nutrients may improve growth, but they are not required.

When exposed to light and the atmosphere, some photoautotrophs will grow in a solution containing the proper inorganic salts. *Escherichia coli* will grow in the same medium if a carbon source such as glucose is added. *Neurospora crassa,* a filamentous fungus, will grow in the *E. coli* medium if biotin is added. These are minimal media for the respective species.

Any isolate of a particular species which can grow on the minimal medium for that species is called a *prototroph.* If, through a change in genetic constitution, an isolate cannot grow on the minimal medium but will grow on a medium *supplemented* with other nutrients, it is called an *auxotroph* (do not confuse with autotroph). This situation will be discussed further in Chapter 3. The supplement can be, for example, one or more of the following: amino acids, purines, pyrimidines, and vitamins. In other words, the auxotroph requires some nutrient in addition to those present in the minimal medium for its species.

The exact nutritive requirements of some microorganisms are unknown. These species require *complex* media containing undefined mixtures such as serum, protein hydrolysates, and yeast hydrolysates. This situation is particularly common in certain groups of pathogens. In essence, the minimal media for these species are unknown. Although the terms prototroph and auxotroph do not strictly apply to such species, the term auxotroph can be used for a strain which requires additional supplements.

Microorganisms grow either unicellularly or multicellularly. The former include most bacteria, yeasts, and protozoa, while filamentous fungi are an example of the latter. It should be noted that some species (dimorphic fungi) have different forms under different environmental conditions.

Measurement of Growth of Unicellular Organisms in Liquid Media

Total Number of Microorganisms (Living and Dead) The number of cells in a microbial population can be measured by counting a sample under the microscope using a counting chamber similar to a hemocytometer (blood counting chamber). This method is inconvenient when examining small organisms or large numbers of samples. Another method employs an electronic measurement of each cell as it passes through a small aperture. Perhaps the most convenient and widely used procedure is to determine the turbidity (cloudiness) of a suspension of cells with a photometer. In essence, the greater the number of microorganisms, the more turbid will be the suspension, and less light will reach the photocell.

Indirect measurements of the total number of cells can be made by removing the cells from suspension by centrifugation or filtration. The cells can then be dried and the dry weight determined. Assays can also be performed to examine the quantity of various cell constituents such as proteins, DNA, or nitrogen. Each of the above methods provides an indication of the number of cells present without regard to the physiological state of each cell; i.e., both living and dead cells are counted.

Number of Viable Cells Sometimes it is important to know how many cells in a culture are still capable of reproduction. As noted, the above methods measure living as well as dead cells. The usual method of counting viable cells is to make a suitable dilution of the culture and place the diluted sample on or in a semisolid medium which will support the growth of the cells. Each colony which arises is assumed to be the result of the growth of one living cell from the original culture. Thus, the functional definition of death is the inability to reproduce and not necessarily a cessation of metabolism.

Kinetics of Growth When a portion of a mature culture of bacteria is transferred to fresh medium, a typical growth curve (Fig. 1-6) is obtained. Four phases of growth can be recognized.

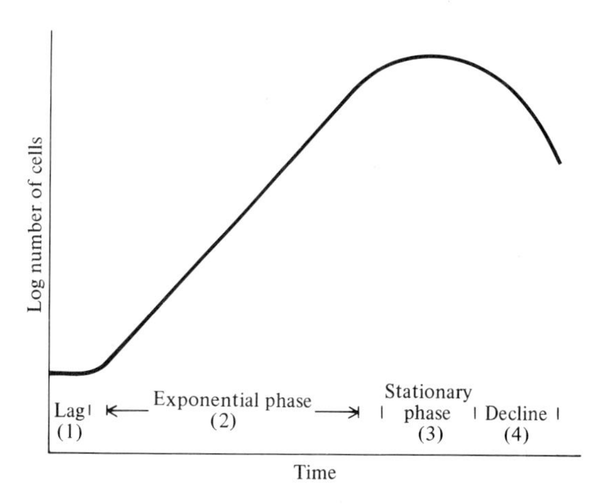

Figure 1-6 Growth curve of a unicellular microorganism.

1 *Lag phase.* The relatively short period of time required by the microorganism to adjust to the new environmental and/or nutritional conditions present in the fresh medium is known as the lag phase. The adjustment might be concerned with the synthesis of required enzymes and/or with an increase in size adequate for cell division to occur. During the lag phase, the cells are actively synthesizing new materials such as proteins, DNA, and cell wall polymers. Therefore, if one were to measure total protein rather than total cells, the lag may not be apparent.
2 *Log* or *exponential phase.* The time required for a population of unicellular organisms to double (doubling time) is a definite, constant period under a given set of conditions. For example, a population of *E. coli* cells in a nutrient broth at 30°C might double in number in about 20 min. At another temperature or in a different type of broth the doubling time might vary. In this example, if the initial inoculum was 1×10^5 cells per milliliter, then 20 min. later the population will contain 2×10^5 cells per milliliter. After an additional 20 min., the population will contain 4×10^5 cells per milliliter, and so on. From this example it is obvious that as the number of generations progresses arithmetically (1, 2, 3, 4 . . .), the number of cells progresses geometrically (1, 2, 4, 8, 16 . . .). In other words, the population increases exponentially and will appear as a straight line when plotted as a log function.
3 *Stationary phase.* The log phase cannot continue indefinitely. One or more factors act to stop the exponential growth of the cells. These factors include the exhaustion of the nutrient supply and the accumulation of toxic metabolic waste products. As a consequence, some cells fail to divide and eventually die. When the number of *viable* cells produced equals the number of cells dying, the growth curve levels off for a variable period of time before declining and is referred to as the stationary phase. Most of the cells are not growing at this time. When the total number of cells is assayed, however, the curve continues to rise, and the peak number of cells is reached at a later point in time, since only lysed cells will be lost to the count.
4 *Decline phase.* Eventually, the accumulation of toxic products will kill more cells than are produced. The result is a net loss of viable cells and, as lysis takes place, a loss in total cells. Again, the shape of the curve will depend on what parameter is measured.

The kinetics shown in Figure 1-6 depend in part on the nature of the inoculum. The kinetics given here are typical of the situation in which an inoculum from a stationary phase is transferred to a fresh medium. These kinetics will also be found when log phase cells are transferred to a medium with a different composition. However, when log phase cells are transferred to the same medium, no lag may occur, since the cells are already adapted to the medium.

METABOLISM

Metabolism is the sum of the chemical changes required for the growth of the cell. Catabolism is concerned with changes that involve the degradation of nutrients to obtain energy, whereas anabolism pertains to changes involved in the biosynthesis of cell components.

Most metabolic pathways are not strictly catabolic or anabolic. For example, during catabolism many of the intermediate compounds formed are used as precursors in biosynthesis. Such pathways can be termed *amphibolic.*

Although it may not always be specifically noted, almost every chemical change of living cells is catalyzed by an enzyme. Enzymes are proteins which may have a nonprotein component.

Many of the metabolic pathways in eukaryotic and prokaryotic cells are identical. Differences, of course, are observed in the synthesis of such components as cell walls. Since a cell is only the sum of its metabolic potential, there must be metabolic differences between even the most closely related organisms.

Sources of Chemical Energy

Although microorganisms as a group are capable of using a wide variety of natural products as energy sources, the degradation of glucose occupies a central position in most species.

The principal energy-yielding pathway of glucose degradation is the *Embden-Meyerhof glycolytic pathway* (Fig. 1-7). Here, each glucose is phosphorylated by two molecules of adenosine triphosphate (ATP) and eventually two 3-carbon compounds are produced. The 3-carbon

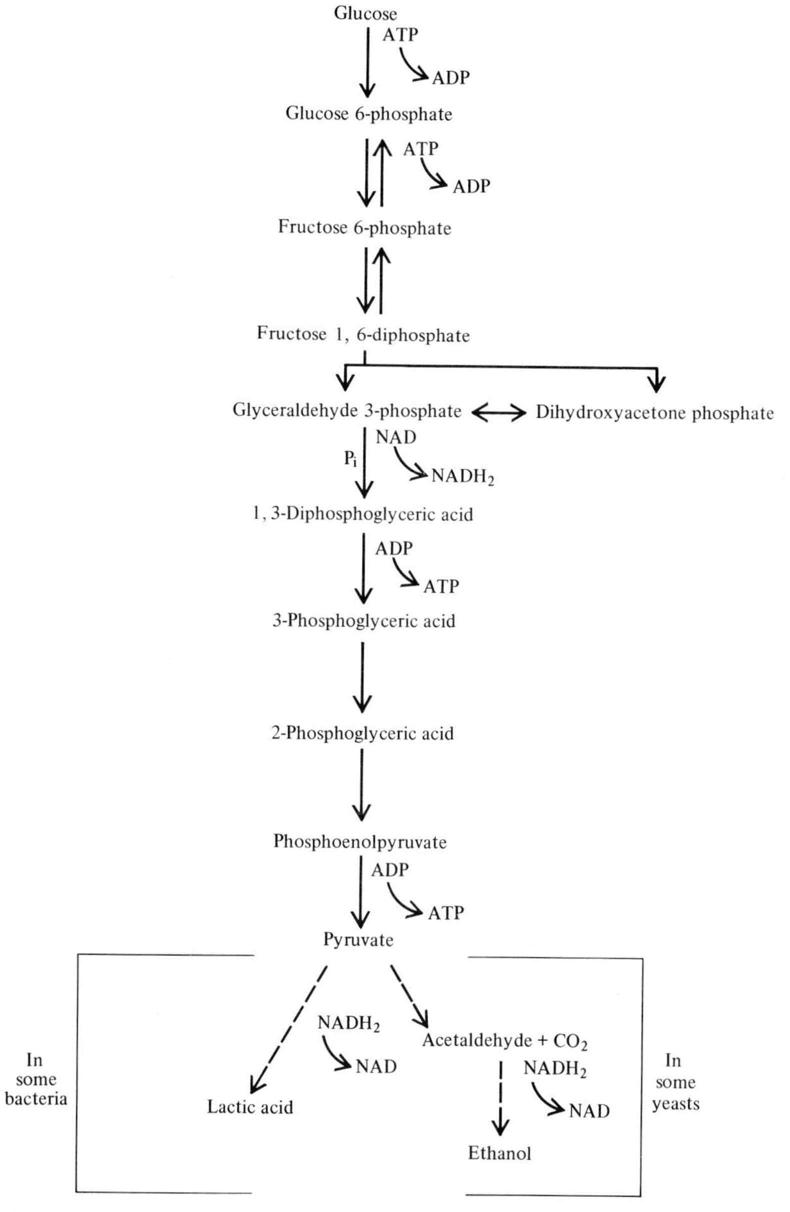

Figure 1-7 Glycolysis (Embden-Meyerhof pathway) showing two examples of fermentation. The fate of pyruvate in aerobic conditions is shown in Figure 1-8.

compounds are converted to pyruvate with the generation of two ATP's for each pyruvate formed or a net gain of two ATP's for each glucose molecule degraded to this point.

The fate of the pyruvate depends on the presence or absence of atmospheric oxygen. In addition to the pyruvate and ATP formed, glycolysis yields two molecules of reduced nicotinamide adenine dinucleotide (NADH). These hydrogens must be transferred to an acceptor in order to balance the reaction.

Under anaerobic conditions, an organic compound serves as the final hydrogen acceptor. The process of obtaining energy from an organic compound when another organic compound serves as the final hydrogen acceptor is called *fermentation.*

Several types of fermentation are known and are classified according to the products formed. Yeasts, for example, can undergo alcoholic fermentation. The pyruvate is converted to acetaldehyde, and CO_2 is released. The acetaldehyde is then reduced to ethyl alcohol by the NADH.

The fermentations found in bacteria include:

Type of fermentation	Products formed
Homolactic	Lactic acid
Heterolactic	Lactic acid, alcohol, formic or acetic acid
Propionic	Propionic acid
Butanediol	2-Pyruvate → acetylmethylcarbinol → 2,3-butanediol
Butyric	Butanol, acetone, isopropanol and others
Mixed acid	Formate, H_2, and CO_2

In addition to the Embden-Meyerhof glycolytic pathway, fermentation reactions may involve various other pathways. The exact products produced are often specific for the genus and/or species of microorganism and thus are of considerable taxonomic importance.

Under aerobic conditions the final hydrogen acceptor is molecular oxygen. This process is called *aerobic respiration.*

The aerobic oxidation of pyruvate is accomplished in several enzymatic steps. First, the 3-carbon pyruvate is oxidized to acetyl coenzyme A (acetyl CoA) and also yields a molecule of CO_2. The acetyl CoA condenses with a molecule of oxalacetate to form a 6-carbon citrate molecule. Then a series of reactions, including two which yield CO_2, result in the regeneration of oxalacetate. This cyclic degradation of acetyl CoA is called the *tricarboxylic acid (TCA) cycle* (Fig. 1-8).

Note from Figures 1-7 and 1-8 that glycolysis and the TCA cycle also yield NADH. In the presence of molecular oxygen the NADH is reoxidized by a series of electron transport reactions involving heme-proteins called cytochromes. The electrons flow from the NADH (regenerating NAD) and are finally transferred to oxygen with the formation of water. Some of the energy lost during the electron transfer is used to form ATP from adenosine diphosphate (ADP), a process which is designated *oxidative phosphorylation.*

Each $NADH^+$ oxidized yields 3 ATP molecules. Therefore, in aerobic respiration, as indicated in Figure 1-8, each molecule of glucose yields a net of 38 ATP molecules (40 ATP's generated, 2 used). In the fermentation to lactate only 2 ATP molecules are formed for each glucose molecule oxidized (4 ATP's generated, 2 used). The ATP is used as the principal source of energy for biosynthetic processes.

There are several alternate pathways of glucose catabolism. One of these, the *hexose monophosphate (pentose phosphate) pathway,* involves the formation of a 5-carbon sugar (pentose) which can be converted to sugars with different numbers of carbon atoms. The *Entner-Doudoroff pathway* involves the formation of 2-keto-3-deoxy-6-phosphogluconate which in turn is split to form pyruvate and glyceraldehyde 3-phosphate. The link between these pathways and glycolysis is shown in Figure 1-9.

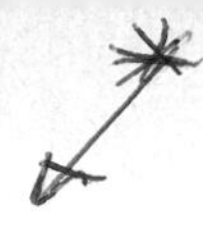

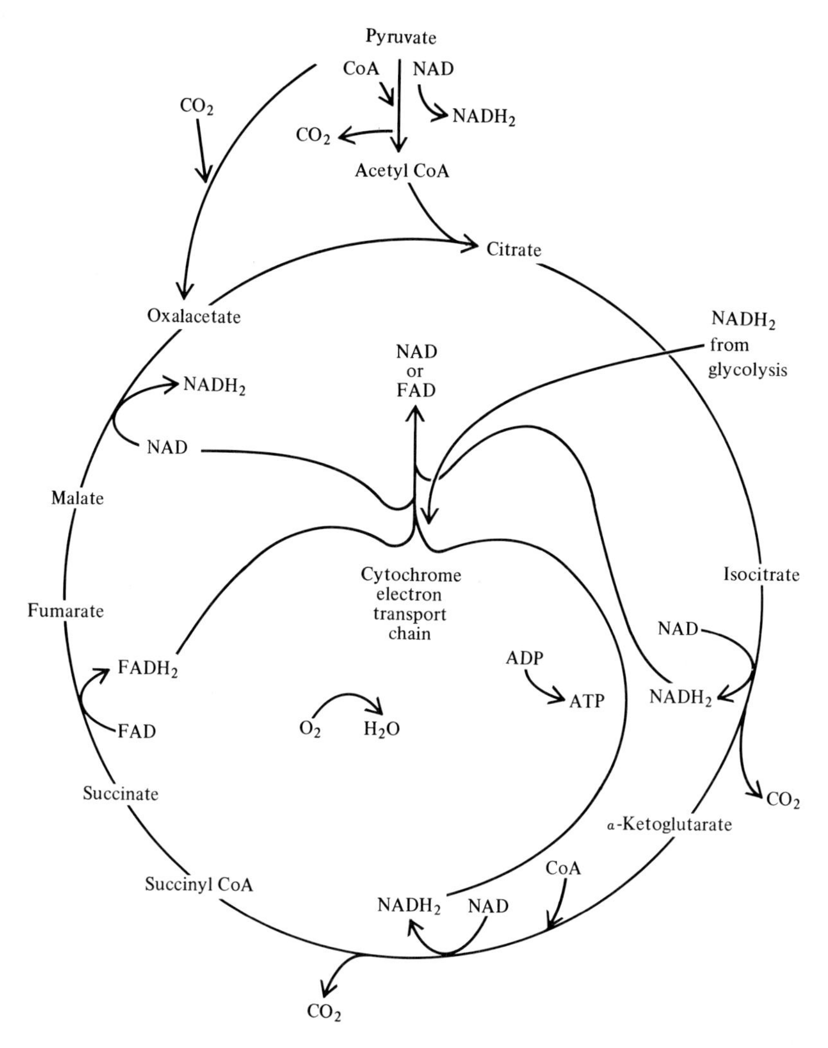

Figure 1-8 Tricarboxylic acid cycle and oxidative phosphorylation showing the fate of pyruvate under aerobic conditions.

Lipids

Acetate, through the acetyl CoA generated from pyruvate, is the principal source of carbon for fatty acid biosynthesis. Long chain fatty acids, typically C12 to C20, are formed by a step-wise condensation reaction. In addition, *Mycobacterium, Corynebacterium,* and *Nocardia* produce long chain α-branched, β-hydroxylated fatty acids (C60 to C88) called *mycolic acids* and a variety of related compounds.

Bacteria also produce phospholipids in which two carbons of a glycerol are linked to fatty acid residues and the third carbon is linked to a polyol, serine, or an ethanolamine through a phosphate bridge. The sterols of fungi are also synthesized from acetate.

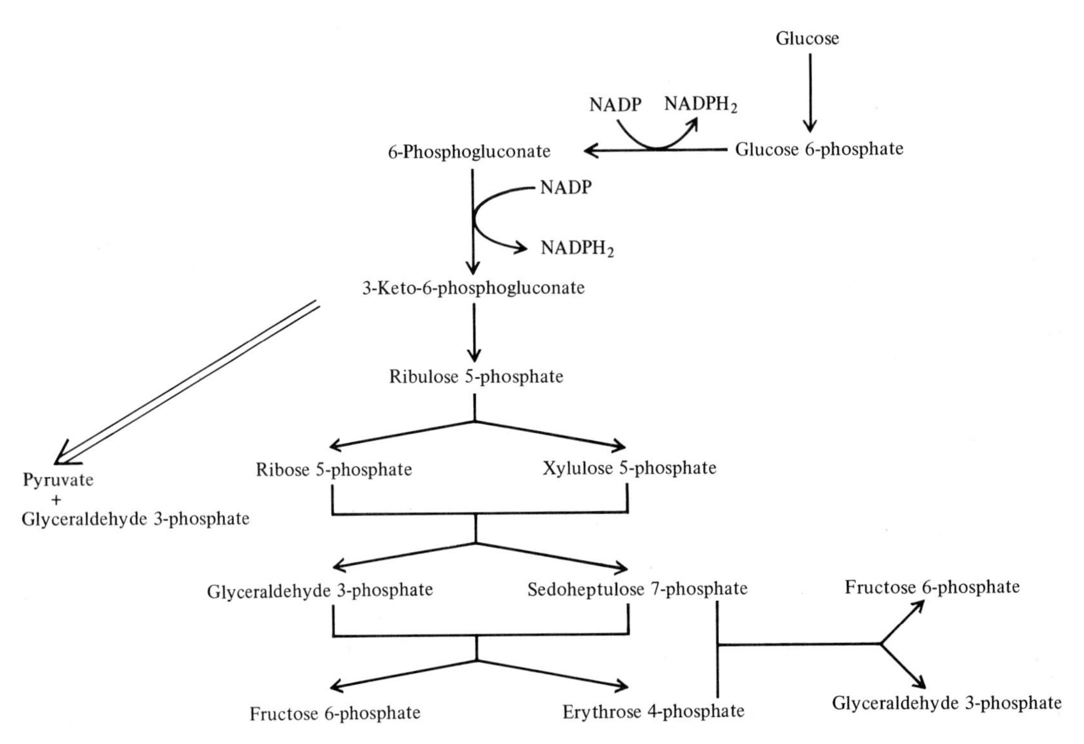

Figure 1-9 Hexose monophosphate and Entner-Douderoff (⇛) pathways. Note that both pathways yield a number of intermediates which are also found in glycolysis.

Amino Acids

The three principal sources of intermediates for the synthesis of amino acids are the Embden-Meyerhof glycolytic pathway, the hexose monophosphate pathway (HMP), and the TCA cycle. Note that in the case of the aromatic amino acids—tyrosine, phenylalanine, and tryptophan—both the HMP and the glycolytic pathway supply an essential part of the molecule (Fig. 1-10).

The use of TCA cycle intermediates, such as α-ketoglutarate and oxalacetate, results in an interruption of the cycle. The loss of intermediates is overcome by several carboxylation reactions which fix CO_2 with phosphoenolpyruvate or pyruvate to form the 4-carbon oxalacetate.

Nucleotides

Nucleotides, which are the precursors of nucleic acids, are composed of a base and a sugar phosphate. There are two types of nucleotide bases: purines and pyrimidines. The structures of some of the important nucleotides are given in Figure 1-11.

Both purine and pyrimidine nucleotides are synthesized from amino acids such as aspartate and glycine. Glutamine serves as a source of nitrogen, and the ribose phosphate is derived from the hexose monophosphate pathway.

In addition to nucleic acids, nucleotides are also used for storage and transfer of energy [ATP, uridine triphosphate (UTP), etc.]; for the activation and transfer reactions of sugars, some

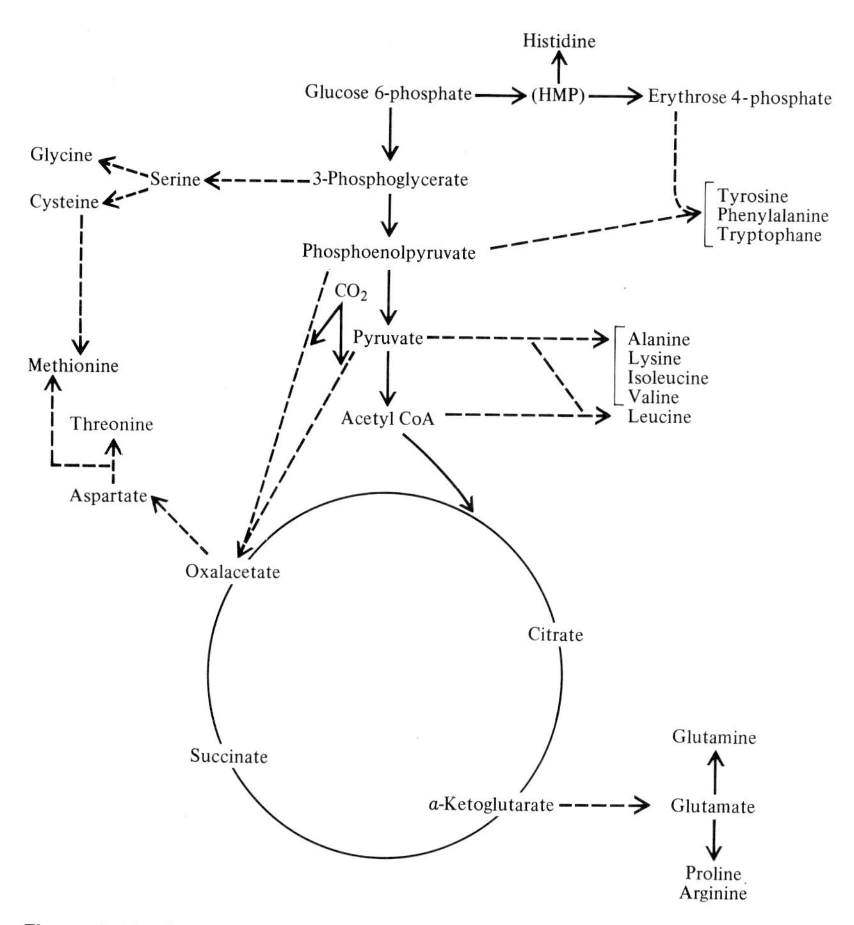

Figure 1-10 Origin of amino acids. Note the replenishment of the TCA cycle by CO_2 fixation.

amino acids, and polymers; and as structural components of some coenzymes (NAD, NADP, and coenzyme A).

Sugars

Upon entering the cell, monosaccharides are usually phosphorylated. The *sugar phosphates,* such as glucose 6-phosphate, can then enter the metabolic pathways discussed above. Most microorganisms can utilize glucose to produce all the other required monosaccharides either by enzymatic change to the glucose 6-phosphate itself or by changes in the sugar nucleotides. The latter are made from the sugar phosphates. The most common *sugar nucleotides* are of the uridine diphosphate (UDP) type. However, ADP, guanosine diphosphate (GDP), thymidine diphosphate (TDP), and cytidine diphosphate (CDP) sugars are also found.

In addition to facilitating sugar transformation, the nucleotide sugars are also involved in the synthesis of polysaccharides.

Some of the pathways of monosaccharide

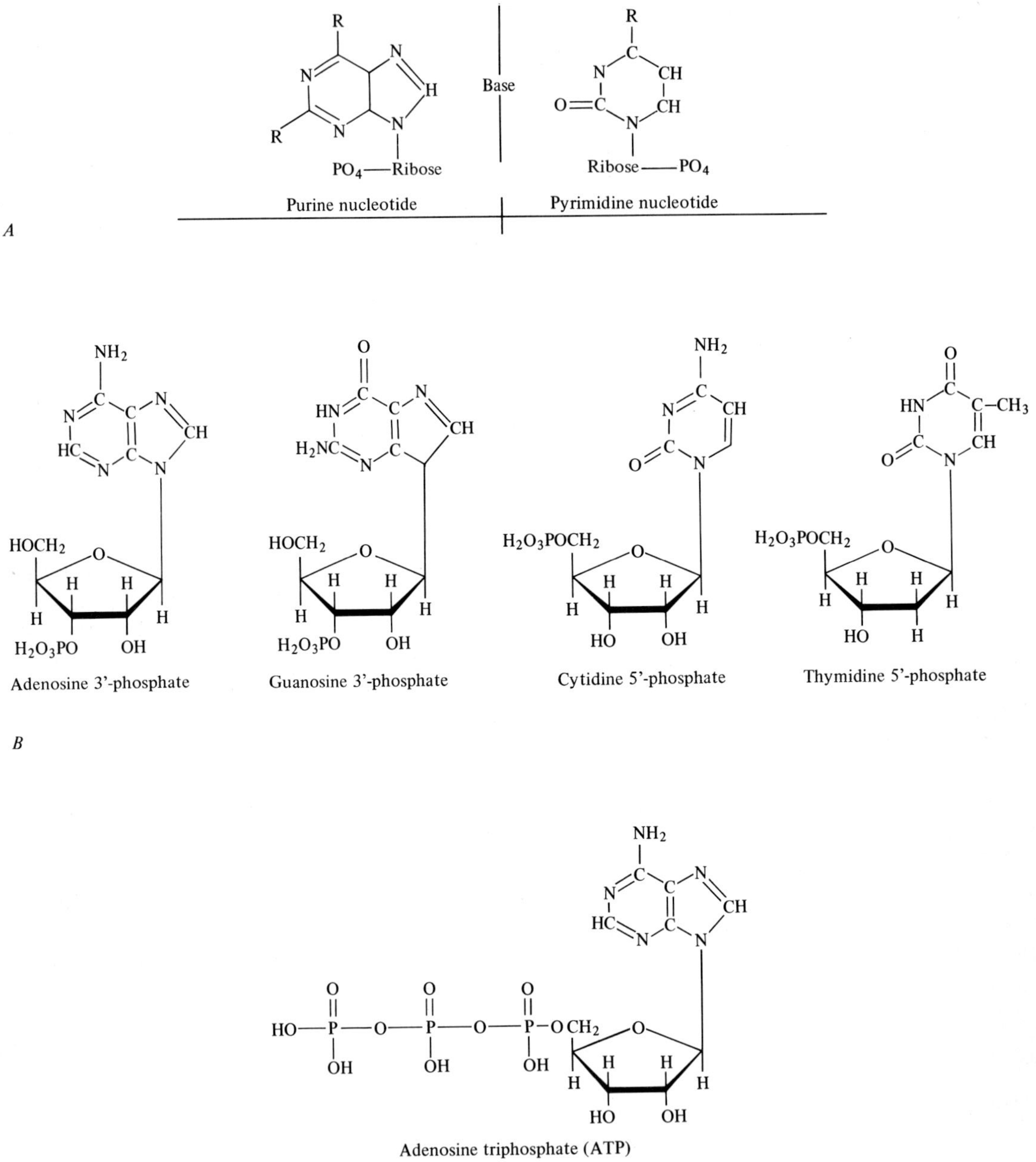

Base

PO4—Ribose

Ribose—PO4

Purine nucleotide | Pyrimidine nucleotide

A

Adenosine 3'-phosphate

Guanosine 3'-phosphate

Cytidine 5'-phosphate

Thymidine 5'-phosphate

B

Adenosine triphosphate (ATP)

Figure 1-11 Structure of some important nucleotides: *(A)* basic structure of purine and pyrimidine type nucleotides composed of the appropriate base and a ribose (or deoxyribose) phosphate; *(B)* the four nucleotides found in DNA; *(C)* adenosine triphosphate (ATP).

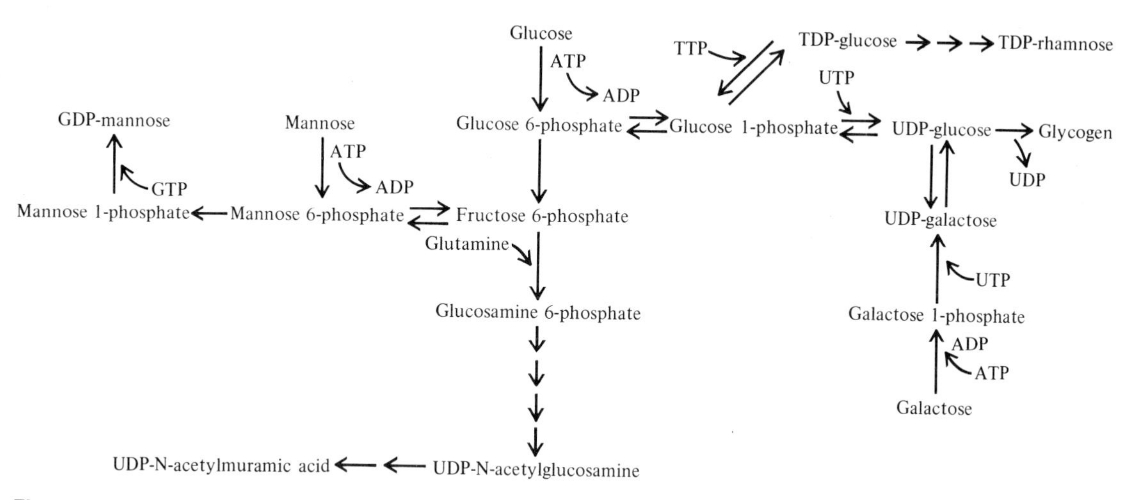

Figure 1-12 Some pathways of carbohydrate utilization and transformation.

synthesis and activation are shown in Figure 1-12. This figure also indicates how some sugars other than glucose can serve as sole carbon sources.

Biosynthesis of Macromolecules

Nucleic Acids DNA is composed of two polynucleotide strands in a helical configuration. The two strands are held together by the hydrogen bonding between the purine-pyrimidine pairs. The pairing is highly specific. Normally, adenine will pair with a thymine on the opposite strand and guanine will pair with cytosine. The sequence of these pairs is the genetic information of the microorganism.

The polymerization of the sugar phosphates (in this case, *deoxy*ribose) forms the backbone for each strand. During the replication of the DNA, the two strands separate and, using the preexisting strands as templates, two new strands are made by adding the appropriate complementary nucleotide to the growing strands, as illustrated in Figure 1-13. The result is two new double helices of DNA, each identical to the original and each containing one of the original strands. This is called *semiconservative replication.*

The RNA synthesized by the cell is *complementary* to the cell's DNA; that is, the specific order of *ribo*nucleotides in the RNA molecule is determined by the order of *deoxy*ribonucleotides of the DNA. Only one of the DNA strands is actually used as a template for RNA synthesis. The enzyme responsible for this transcription of DNA information to RNA information is called *DNA-dependent RNA polymerase.*

Three types of RNA are involved in protein synthesis: transfer RNA (tRNA), messenger RNA (mRNA), and ribosomal RNA (rRNA).

Proteins The sequence of the amino acids in proteins is determined by the order of nucleotides in a molecule of mRNA (Fig. 1-13). In this way, the cell's DNA indirectly determines the structure of each protein.

The protein consists of a chain of amino acids linked by peptide bonds between adjacent amino (NH_2^-) and carboxyl groups (COO^-). The amino acids are added to the growing peptide chain one at a time.

A molecule of mRNA associates with ribo-

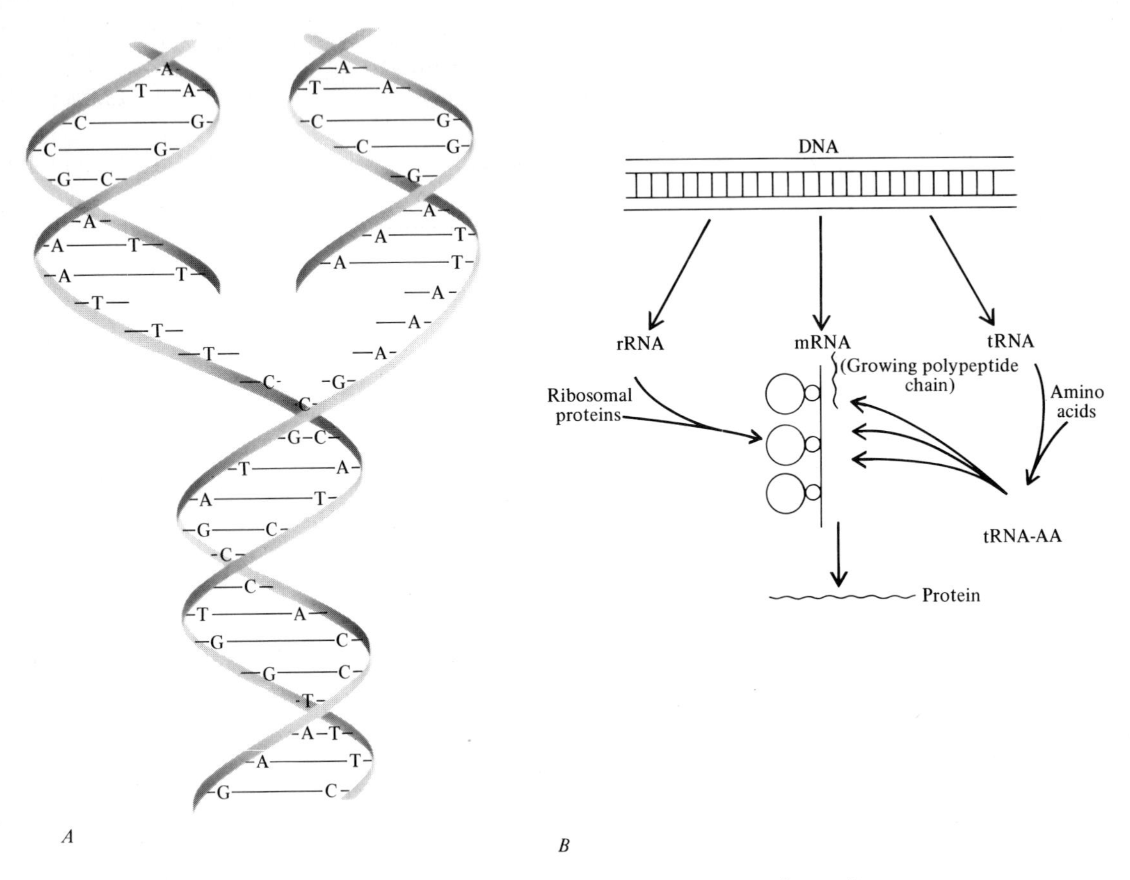

Figure 1-13 Biosynthesis of nucleic acids and proteins. *(A)* Semiconservative replication of DNA. Original duplex (shaded) unwinds, and two new complementary strands are synthesized using the original strands as a template. *(B)* Synthesis of RNA and proteins. The three types of RNA are coded by cellular DNA. The rRNA combines with ribosomal proteins to form functioning ribosomes. These associate with mRNA to form a polyribosomal complex. The mRNA codes the specific protein being synthesized. The tRNA recognizes the mRNA code and attaches the appropriate amino acids. When the peptide is complete, it is released.

somal particles. Then tRNA molecules, which carry the activated amino acids, recognize the three-nucleotide code of the mRNA *(codons)*, and the appropriate tRNA-amino acid molecule associates with the next available mRNA codon. The amino acid is then transferred to the growing polypeptide chain. The protein is released and proceeds to fold into a specific, functional three-dimensional molecule.

Cell Wall Components

Glycopeptide

1 Precursors. Figure 1-14 shows the pathway of glycopeptide synthesis. The five amino acids are added stepwise to the UDP-muramic acid. Note that there is one more amino acid than is found in the final polymer. The *d*- isomers of the amino acids are formed from the *l*- isomer by an enzyme called a *racemase*.

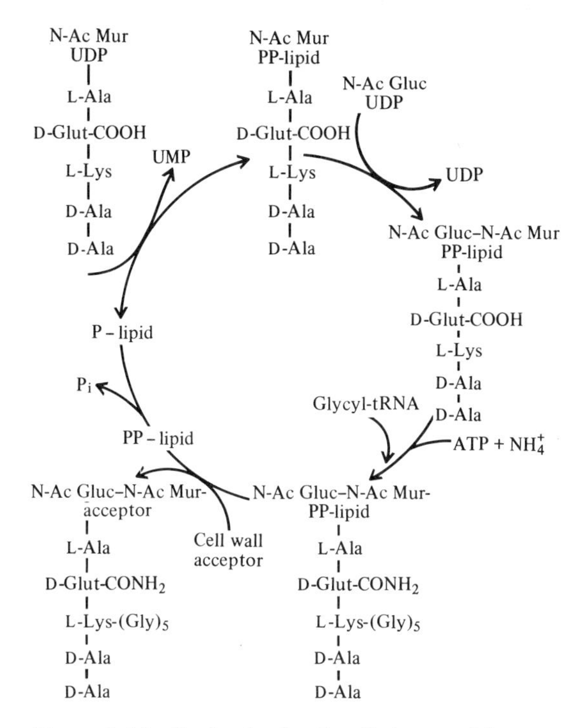

Figure 1-14 Synthesis of cell wall glycopeptide.

The *muramic acid pentapeptide* is then linked to a *lipid carrier.* This molecule now has the N-acetyl-glucosamine attached. Then, the pentapeptide which will form the cross-linking bridge is added (in this example, glycine) to the third amino acid.

2 Polymerization of precursors. The lipid-disaccharidepeptide molecule is then transferred to the glycopeptide of the wall. First, the disaccharide is attached to the polysaccharide portion of the glycopeptide with the release of the lipid. Then, the cross-linking occurs by a transpeptidation reaction. The latter results in the liberation of the terminal D-alanine.

Lipopolysaccharide The biosynthesis of LPS is not as well understood as that of glycopeptide. However, the involvement of nucleotide sugar precursors and the use of a lipid carrier in the transfer of the side chain to the core polysaccharide are known. This would suggest some similarity to the synthesis of glycopeptide.

Teichoic Acids CDP-glycerol and CDP-ribitol serve as the donors for the synthesis of polyglycerol phosphate and polyribitol phosphate respectively.

Fungal Walls Although the problem has not been extensively investigated in fungal cell walls, apparently UDP sugar derivatives act as precursor donors.

REGULATION

Feedback Inhibition The total activity of a metabolic pathway can be controlled at several levels. First, the activity is controlled by the amount of substrate available. Then, there is control of enzyme activity. In many pathways, the end product can interact with the first enzyme of the pathway reducing its activity. This process is called *feedback inhibition.*

Repression There can also be control over the *amount* of enzyme synthesized. In some anabolic pathways the end product can be responsible for shutting off the synthesis of the enzymes in that pathway. The end product interacts with a *repressor protein*, causing the activation of the repressor. The activated repressor then prevents the transcription of the genes coding for the enzymes of the pathway. This process is called *repression.*

Induction Induction involves the transcription and translation of genes which are normally repressed. This situation often occurs in catabolic pathways involved in the utilization of nutrients. When the nutrient is not present, the organism does not need the specific enzymes required to metabolize it. When the nutrient becomes available, it interacts with a repressor protein, causing inactivation of the repressor, thereby permitting the synthesis of the required enzyme *(induction)*. The time required for induction is often a part of the lag period observed for growth when cells are transferred to a different medium.

Induction and Repression: Similar Processes In repression, the repressor protein is usually inactive and is activated by a low-molecular-weight compound. With induction, the repressor protein is normally active and is deactivated by the low-molecular-weight compound. Induction is, therefore, also called *derepression.* Both processes are specific, requiring different repressor proteins for each pathway affected.

BIBLIOGRAPHY

Osborn, M. J.: "Structure and Biosynthesis of the Bacterial Cell Wall," *Annu. Rev. Biochem.,* 38:501–538, 1969.

Sokatch, J. R.: *Bacterial Physiology and Metabolism,* New York: Academic Press, Inc., 1969.

Stanier, R. Y., Douderoff, M., and Adelberg, E. A.: *The Microbial World,* 3d ed., Englewood Cliffs, N.J.: Prentice-Hall, Inc., 1970.

Chapter 2

Characteristics of Microorganisms and Other Infectious Agents

Pasquale F. Bartell, Marvin N. Schwalb, and Zigmund C. Kaminski

VIRUSES

Viruses are unique obligate intracellular parasites because they contain a single type of nucleic acid and because they replicate by separate synthesis and assembly of their components. In addition, some RNA and DNA viruses are *oncogenic* and can induce transformation and malignant changes in cells in vitro and in vivo, replicating the viral genome or a portion of the viral genome in synchrony with the host cell through countless generations.

Structure

Although they vary considerably in size (20 to 300 nm) and architecture (spherical, icosahedral, rectangular, complex, brick-shaped, and bullet-shaped), all viruses are composed of a single molecule of nucleic acid enclosed within a protein coat or capsid. The nucleic acid is either DNA or RNA, but not both, and may be single- or double-stranded. The outer protein coat *(capsid)* together with the nucleic acid forms the *nucleocapsid*. In more complex viruses (poxviruses, myxoviruses) the nucleic acid may be associated with an *internal protein*. The capsid is constructed of numerous structural subunits called *capsomeres*, which are formed by one or more polypeptides.

Many viruses (poxviruses, herpesviruses, myxoviruses, arboviruses) in addition to the nucleocapsid have a covering membrane called the *envelope,* or *peplos.* The envelope is composed of glycolipoproteins containing moieties that are specific for the virus *(proteins)* and the membranes of the host cell *(lipids).* In myxoviruses, for example, the final stage in maturation occurs at the surface of the plasma membrane through a budding process in which the membrane surrounds the nucleocapsid and two virus-specific proteins project as spikes through the envelope. The *hemagglutinin spike* is composed of structural subunits called *peplomeres* and is located in close proximity to a *neuraminidase spike.* When enveloped viruses are treated with lipid solvents (e.g., ether and chloroform), the infectivity of the virus is lost. Consequently, enveloped viruses are said to contain *essential lipid.*

Capsids are composed of repeating subunits (capsomeres) packed together symmetrically. *Icosahedral* and *helical symmetry* are recognized. An icosahedron has 20 triangular faces, each an equilateral triangle, and 12 corners. Virus particles *(virions)* with capsids conforming to this symmetry are called *icosahedral viruses.* In helical symmetry, capsid and nucleic acid are wound together in a helical structure.

Classification

Viruses can be grouped or classified in several categories according to size, shape, the host in which they replicate (bacteria, insects, plants, animals), the characteristics of their nucleic acid (type, strandedness, molecular weight), the symmetry of their nucleocapsid (icosahedral, helical, complex), the possession of an envelope containing essential lipid, and many other properties. The major concern of this text is with viruses that produce disease in man, conventionally included in the category of animal viruses. The simple classification included in Table 2-1 separates some of the human viruses into major groups on the basis of the type of nucleic acid, the symmetry of the nucleocapsid, and the presence or absence of an envelope. Bacterial viruses (phage) are considered in Chapter 3.

Cultivation

As obligate intracellular parasites, viruses require living cells in order to replicate. For many years viruses were propagated in the laboratory by infecting animals or embryonated eggs and, after an appropriate interval, harvesting the

Table 2-1 Some Characteristics of Viruses That Infect Man

Type	Nucleic acid strandedness	Virus group	Envelopes	Symmetry	Viruses included in group
DNA	Double	Poxvirus	+	Complex	Smallpox, alastrim, vaccinia, molluscum contagiosum, orf, milker's nodule
	Double	Herpesvirus	+	Icosahedral	Herpes simplex, varicella-zoster, cytomegalovirus, B virus, Epstein-Barr virus
	Double	Adenovirus	−	Icosahedral	Adenovirus
	Double	Papovavirus	−	Icosahedral	Papilloma (wart)
RNA	Single	Myxovirus	+	Helical	Influenza, parainfluenza, mumps, measles, respiratory syncytial
	Single	Arbovirus	+	Icosahedral	Eastern and western equine encephalitis, St. Louis encephalitis, California encephalitis, yellow fever, dengue
	Double	Reovirus	−	Icosahedral	Reoviruses
	Single	Picornavirus	−	Icosahedral	Enteroviruses (poliovirus, Coxsackie virus, echovirus), rhinovirus

progeny virus in particular organs or fluids. The development of *cell culture* methodology provided an effective means for analyzing the intricate details of virus-host cell interactions under quantitative conditions and gave a great impetus to the expansion of experimental and clinical virology. Application of the knowledge gained from studies of virus–cell culture interactions has led to the development and use of several important vaccines including poliomyelitis, measles, mumps, and rubella.

Cell Cultures

A suspension of single cells can be obtained by treating small pieces of tissue with a dilute solution of trypsin. When placed in a tube, flask, bottle, or petri dish and incubated after washing and resuspension in a suitable growth medium, the cells will attach to the flat surface and divide until a confluent *monolayer* or sheet of cells is formed. The growth medium usually consists of salts, glucose, amino acids, vitamins, and serum appropriately buffered with an atmosphere containing about 5 percent carbon dioxide. Antibiotics are also added to prevent the growth of bacterial contaminants. Some cell cultures can be passed serially by removing the cells from the surface with trypsin or the chelating agent ethylenediaminetetraacetic acid (EDTA), washing, resuspending in fresh medium, and seeding into new containers. Cell cultures derived from malignant tissues are particularly useful in studies of viral replication because they can be grown in suspension as well as in monolayers and because they can be cultured indefinitely as established cell lines.

Cytopathic Effects (CPE) in Cell Cultures

With most viruses, when a few virus particles replicate in cell monolayers, localized areas *(foci)* of cell damage and degeneration can be recognized with an ordinary light microscope. Progeny virus are released, the infection quickly spreads to other cells in the monolayer, and eventually the entire sheet of cells will be destroyed. At this point, the effects of viral replication are macroscopically visible, as the monolayer of cells can no longer be seen. Viruses that produce cellular damage of this type exert a *cytopathic effect* (CPE), and the virus is said to be *cytopathogenic.*

Plaque Assay

Based on the CPE of viruses and the reasonable assumption that a focus of infection is initiated by a single virus particle, a *plaque assay* was developed for the quantitation of viral preparations. In performing the assay, a virus suspension is added to a monolayer of cells long enough to allow the virions to attach to and infect the cells. The fluid medium is then replaced by nutrient agar that restricts the progeny virions to the original foci of infection. Only neighboring cells can be infected by progeny virus, and eventually plaques formed by the destruction of cells are visible. The plaques are sharply defined by adding neutral red, a vital dye that stains only living cells, producing clear plaques against a red background. Since each plaque counted originates from a single infectious virus particle, the infectivity titer of a viral suspension is expressed as plaque-forming units per milliliter (PFU/ml).

Hemadsorption

Some viruses fail to cause obvious CPE in cell monolayers but can be detected by other means. Parainfluenza viruses, for example, mature at the surface of the plasma membrane with hemagglutinin spikes projecting through the envelope of the virus. When red blood cells are added to the monolayer, foci of infection can be recognized because the red blood cells will adsorb to the hemagglutinin spikes on the virus particles *(hemadsorption).* In practice, infected monolayers are flooded with a suspension of red blood cells and washed. Areas where the red blood cells are fixed to the monolayer identify foci of viral proliferation.

Viral Hemagglutination

Many viruses including members of the adeno-, papova-, myxo-, arbo-, reo-, and picorna-groups agglutinate erythrocytes of various animal species *(viral hemagglutination).* Virus particles can adsorb to the surface of red blood cells, act as a bridge between adjacent red blood cells, and in this way build up an insoluble lattice which adheres to and completely covers the bottom surfaces of the test tube. In the absence of viral hemagglutinins, the red blood cells settle as a spherical pellet which covers but a small portion of the bottom of the tube.

The quantity of hemagglutinin in viral preparations can be assayed by mixing serial twofold dilutions of the virus with a standard suspension of red blood cells. The highest dilution of virus showing hemagglutination can be taken as the end point and thus provides a measure of the number of hemagglutinating units in the viral preparation. Since viral hemagglutination can be inhibited specifically by antibody, it forms the basis for a convenient and valuable *hemagglutinin inhibition test* which can be used for the detection of either a particular virus or a specific antiviral antibody.

In the case of myxoviruses, hemagglutination is a function of hemagglutinin spikes which project through the envelope of the virus particle and interact with *glycoprotein receptors* on the surface of red blood cells. After myxoviruses have adsorbed to the red blood cells, neuraminidase spikes can remove the N-acetylneuraminic acid from the glycoprotein, and the virus can eventually elute from the red blood cells. On the other hand, in the case of some poxviruses, the hemagglutinin is a soluble lipoprotein by-product of viral replication which cannot elute from red blood cells.

Viral Replication

Adsorption The attachment of viruses to cell membranes occurs at 0°C and appears to be a specific process that requires complementary chemical configurations. For example, myxoviruses adsorb by means of the hemagglutinin spike to a glycoprotein receptor on the cell membrane. Adsorption of poliovirus requires *cations* in order to combine with a specific protein or lipoprotein receptor on the cell membrane. Cells lacking the appropriate receptors cannot be infected with these viruses. On the other hand, in some cases, including poliovirus, the necessity for specific receptors can be circumvented and infection initiated by nucleic acid extracted from the virus particles in a phenomenon known as *transfection.*

Penetration Unlike phage or bacterial viruses (Chap. 3), viruses that infect man have no mechanism for injecting nucleic acid into the host cell. Instead, either the whole virus particle or a large part containing the viral genome is taken into the cell within phagocytic vacuoles. Penetration is a temperature-dependent process which, unlike adsorption, does not occur at 0°C.

Uncoating With most viruses that infect man, uncoating or release of viral nucleic acid is probably accomplished by the *lysosomal enzymes* of the host cell. For reasons that are not understood the viral nucleic acid escapes the hydrolytic action of lysosomal nucleases, is released into the cytoplasm, and either remains there or migrates to the nucleus.

Uncoating of vaccinia virus is a more complex process that involves two stages. In the first step, the outer coat is removed within the phagocytic vacuole by preexisting lysosomal enzymes and the inner core of the virus particle containing the internal protein and viral DNA is ejected into the cytoplasm. In the second stage, viral DNA is liberated from the internal protein by a virus-coded enzyme. The mRNA required for the synthesis of the uncoating enzyme is produced in the infected cell by a DNA-dependent RNA polymerase carried within the virion.

One-step Growth Curves As with phage (Chap. 3), the replication of viruses that infect man can be conveniently analyzed by the *one-step growth curve* which distinguishes between the *eclipse, latent,* and *rise periods.* Few human viruses, however, are released in a burst as phage is. Instead the viruses are frequently synthesized and released from the infected cell over a period of several hours. In addition, the time scale varies considerably. For example, the latent period in poliovirus may be 2 hr., but 14 hr. for adenovirus. The rise period may be completed within 6 hr. in poliovirus or may extend for 48 hr. with papovaviruses.

Synthesis of DNA Viruses

Since there are significant differences between the replication of DNA and RNA viruses, separate illustrative considerations are warranted. In the ensuing sections vaccinia virus has been selected as an example of DNA viral synthesis and poliovirus as an example of an RNA virus.

Vaccinia is the prototype of the poxvirus group, the largest and most complex of the viruses that infect man. The nucleic acid of vaccinia virus is a single molecule of double-stranded DNA with a molecular weight of 160 million. Even before the virus is fully uncoated, virus-directed mRNA is transcribed by a DNA-dependent RNA polymerase carried within the virion. The early protein synthesized by the viral mRNA is an uncoating enzyme required for the release of viral DNA, a process that occurs in the cytoplasm of the host cell.

Replication of vaccinia virus proceeds entirely within the cytoplasm of the infected cell. The uncoated viral DNA initiates replication by serving as the template for the synthesis of *virus-specific mRNA's.* The early transcribed viral mRNA's are small in size and are translated into early proteins of low molecular weight. Included in the resulting virus-specific early proteins are those concerned with the synthesis of viral DNA (thymidine kinase, viral DNA polymerase, deoxyribonuclease) and with the inhibition of cellular DNA, RNA, and protein synthesis. These early proteins appear approximately 1 hr. after infection, and the cellular ribosomes are utilized for their synthesis.

Synthesis of viral DNA commences 1.5 hr. after infection according to the semiconservative mode of replication (Chap. 3). Newly synthesized viral DNA enters a pool and is finally enclosed within the structural proteins during maturation of the virus at about 5 hr. after infection. Viral DNA formation requires one of the early proteins, *DNA polymerase.* Consequently, viral DNA synthesis will not occur in the presence of puromycin, which acts by preventing the formation of the virus-specific DNA polymerase.

Once viral DNA replication commences, late virus-specific mRNA's are formed and function as templates for the synthesis of regulatory and structural proteins. The late viral mRNA's and proteins are larger in size than their early counterparts.

Normally, synthesis of early virus-specific proteins such as thymidine kinase and DNA polymerase is stopped 4 to 5 hr. after infection. If, however, actinomycin D, which blocks DNA-dependent mRNA formation, is added 2 hr. after infection, synthesis of the early enzymes is not halted. Thus, it is apparent that early virus-specific mRNA's are stable and that a late viral mRNA codes for the synthesis of a virus-specific regulatory protein which is responsible for halting the synthesis of the early enzymes.

Although one of the structural viral proteins is translated from an early virus-specific mRNA and is formed throughout the replication cycle, the bulk of the structural proteins are coded for by late viral mRNA's. Synthesis of these latter proteins is evident 4 hr. after infection and increases rapidly over the next few hours. *Isatin-β-thiosemicarbazone* is a potent drug which selectively blocks translation of late virus-specific mRNA's and progeny virus formation without interfering with transcription of early and late viral mRNA's, translation of early proteins, or viral DNA replication.

In contrast with poxvirus replication which occurs exclusively in the cytoplasm, synthesis of progeny DNA by other DNA viruses (herpesvirus, adenovirus, papovavirus) occurs in the nucleus of the infected cell. Thus, virus-specific mRNA's are transcribed in the nucleus, migrate into the cytoplasm, and are translated on the ribosomes. The early virus-specific proteins return to the nucleus and are involved in progeny viral DNA synthesis. With the adenoviruses and papovaviruses, the capsid proteins that are translated on the ribosomes by late viral mRNA's migrate back to the nucleus where nucleocapsid formation occurs. While nucleocapsid formation of herpesvirus also is located in the nucleus, maturation occurs at nuclear or cytoplasmic membranes where the virus acquires its envelope.

Synthesis of RNA Viruses

Much insight has been gained into an understanding of RNA viral replication by a detailed analysis of poliovirus formation. In contrast with the large size of vaccinia virus, poliovirus is one of the smallest that infects man and the nucleic acid consists of a molecule of single-stranded RNA with a molecular weight of 2 million.

Poliovirus replication occurs entirely in the cytoplasm of infected cells. After uncoating, viral RNA attaches to host cell ribosomes and functions as a single polycistronic mRNA molecule that is translated into a single large protein. As infection progresses, the single large protein is cleaved into smaller fragments which are involved in the synthesis of viral RNA, in the inhibition of cellular RNA and protein synthesis, and in the formation of structural proteins.

Replication of viral RNA commences with the cleavage of a viral RNA-dependent RNA polymerase *(viral RNA synthetase)* fragment from the large protein. Shortly thereafter, other fragments are split off from the large protein and shut off cellular RNA and protein synthesis.

In the process of replicating progeny viral RNA, the parental viral RNA strand *(positive strand)* acts as a template for the synthesis of a complementary strand *(negative strand),* utilizing the viral RNA-dependent RNA polymerase. The resulting double-stranded RNA composed of a positive and a negative strand is known as the *replicative form* (RF). The negative strand then functions as the template for progeny positive strands which are transcribed, peeled off, and eventually incorporated within the capsid. The negative strand with progeny positive strands in various stages of completion is known as the *replicative intermediate* (RI). Obviously, the RI is the key to the replication of poliovirus, whereas the RF is probably only a transient form needed for the formation of RI.

Some of the progeny viral RNA (positive strands) function as mRNA for the synthesis of capsid proteins which are cleaved from the large protein. Thereafter, between 3 and 6 hr. the capsid proteins surround other positive progeny RNA strands, infectious particles are rapidly assembled and accumulated, and progeny virus is released in a *burst,* accompanied by lysis of the cell.

Through the use of inhibitors such as actinomycin D and bromodeoxyuridine (BUDR) the significant observation has been made that synthesis of poliovirus RNA and protein is independent of DNA. Actinomycin D can block

DNA-dependent mRNA formation, but is without effect on poliovirus replication. Similarly, the thymine analogue, bromodeoxyuridine, which is incorporated into DNA and results in nonfunctional DNA, fails to interfere with poliovirus synthesis. Consequently, poliovirus RNA has the capacity to specify and direct its own replication. On the other hand, if protein synthesis is inhibited by puromycin immediately after infection, replication of poliovirus RNA is prevented. Thus, it is apparent that a new virus-specific protein (viral RNA-dependent RNA polymerase) is required for initiation of poliovirus RNA synthesis.

In the replication of other RNA viruses, with appropriate modifications for double-stranded reoviruses, the RI presumably exerts a key role. However, in view of the emphasis given to the fact that poliovirus replication is independent of DNA, it is worth noting that some of the smaller myxoviruses (influenza) and the RNA animal tumor viruses are inhibited by actinomycin D, thus demonstrating their dependence on DNA. Myxoviruses and arboviruses mature at the surface of cell membranes where they acquire an envelope including the envelope proteins and are released by a budding process.

Synthesis of Interferon

Interferon is an antiviral protein produced as a by-product of cellular response to viral infection. Formation of interferon is stimulated not only by DNA and RNA viruses, but by exposure to any *foreign* material containing or leading to the synthesis of double-stranded nucleic acid including intracellular parasites (bacteria, rickettsiae, chlamydiae, viruses, protozoa, fungi) and synthetic polynucleotides, especially double-stranded polyribonucleotides such as poly-I:poly-C (polyinosinic:polycytidylic acids). In addition, *other polyanions* including bacterial endotoxins, polycarboxylic acid, and pyran copolymers can stimulate interferon synthesis. Finally, *any antigen* can cause *sensitized* thymus-dependent lymphocytes to release interferon, in which case interferon is but one of a number of agents collectively called *lymphokines* (Chap. 8) produced by the cells.

Depending upon the species in which it is formed, interferon has a molecular weight of 26,000 (human cells) or 38,000 (chick cells). Two properties which help to characterize interferon are that it is *species-specific,* but *not virus-specific.* For example, interferon produced by human cells will inhibit any virus capable of replication in human cells but will not prevent synthesis of the same viruses in mouse or chick cells. Conversely, mouse interferon will block the growth of a number of viruses in mouse cells but will not inhibit their replication in human or chick cells.

The fact that cellular genes code for the synthesis of interferon has been convincingly demonstrated by using actinomycin D in cells infected with poliovirus. Under such conditions synthesis of interferon is completely blocked, but poliovirus replication is unaffected. Since antinomycin D is known to prevent the formation of DNA-dependent mRNA (cellular mRNA) but not RNA-dependent mRNA (poliovirus mRNA), it is apparent that the formation of interferon (1) is coded for by the cellular genome and not the viral genome, and (2) requires transcription of a new cellular mRNA from cellular DNA. It is believed that under normal conditions cellular synthesis of interferon is repressed but that it is derepressed by viral infection.

At the molecular level, interferon has no direct effect upon viruses and is inactive in the cell in which it is produced. However, after release from appropriately stimulated cells, interferon can be taken up by and will protect normal cells of the same species against viral infection. Actually, interferon induces the synthesis of a cellular protein that prevents translation of viral mRNA's [translation inhibitory protein (TIP)], thereby interfering with viral replication. TIP is unique in its selective toxicity for viral mRNA's and in its lack of toxicity for cellular mRNA's. Since both interferon and TIP are proteins, their synthesis can be prevented by puromycin.

Much speculation has centered on the potential role exerted by interferon in the natural process of recovery from initial infection with viruses and other intracellular parasites. However, critical evaluation has revealed that interferon appears to be an innocent and secondary bystander to recovery which is mediated by other lymphokines (Chap. 8). On the other hand, strenuous and continuing efforts are being directed toward an assessment of the prophylactic value of interferon induction by poly-I:poly-C and other synthetic polyribonucleotides in the prevention of human virus disease, recognizing that interferon is virtually useless in therapy. Whatever the outcome, it appears that clinical use of interferon inducers will be restricted to selected situations and limited by temporal considerations.

Viruses and Cancer

Although viruses have been known to cause cancer in animals for more than 60 years, their potential etiological role in human cancer has generally been greeted with healthy skepticism. However, recently accumulated data at the molecular level have provided increasing support for presuming that viruses may cause cancer in man. On the other hand, the final evidence is not in, and the outcome remains in doubt.

As noted in Table 2-2, both DNA and RNA viruses can produce tumors or cancer in animals, persist in whole or in part in the tumor cells, form new antigens on the surface membrane of the tumor cells, and transform cells in vitro so that they induce tumors when injected into animals. Such viruses have been termed oncogenic, tumor, or transforming viruses. In contrast with viruses previously considered, oncogenic viruses transform the cells they infect into a state of unregulated growth (cancer), may or may not produce progeny virus, fail to produce a cytopathic effect, and replicate, in whole or in part, in synchrony with the cellular genome. In some respects the interaction of oncogenic viruses with their host cells is analogous to lysogeny (Chap. 3).

Included among the oncogenic DNA viruses are representatives of the pox-, herpes-, adeno-, and papova- groups. The oncogenic RNA leukoviruses comprise agents that induce leukemia, sarcoma, and carcinoma in birds, frogs, mice, hamsters, rats, rabbits, cats, monkeys, and marmosets. Leukoviruses are enveloped viruses with helical symmetry that are released by budding at the surface of cell membranes.

In Vitro Transformation As recorded in Table 2-2, both DNA and RNA oncogenic viruses

Table 2-2 Properties of Tumor Viruses

Property	RNA viruses	DNA viruses
Natural tumors in host of origin	+	+ or −
Persistence and synthesis of virus in tumor cells	+	usually −
Transplantation antigen (on surface of plasma membrane)	+	+
Tumor antigen (in nucleus)	−	+
Transformation of cells manifest by	+	+
New enzymes		
New antigens		
Higher rate of metabolism and division		
Altered morphology		
Loss of contact inhibition		
Oncogenicity		
Maturation by budding at surface membrane	+	−
Reverse transcriptase (RNA-directed DNA polymerase)	+	−

can transform the cells they infect in vitro. *Viral transformation* is manifest by the appearance of new enzymes, new transplantation antigens on the surface of the cell membrane, a higher rate of metabolism and division, altered morphology, loss of contact inhibition (continued membrane movement and division of cells upon contact with each other, resulting in the formation of densely packed, randomly arranged foci of rounded, refractile, transformed cells), and ability to induce tumors in animals (oncogenicity). The *transplantation antigens* appearing on the surface of transformed cells are coded for by the specific virus and will induce protection in animals against cells transformed by that virus.

Replication of DNA Tumor Viruses As is apparent from the information included in Table 2-2, DNA tumor viruses can transform the cells they infect without producing progeny virus, a fact that does not necessarily imply that the intact viral genome is missing from the transformed cells as noted below. In any event, it is obvious that at least a portion of the viral genome persists, is transcribed, and is replicated in synchrony with the host cell. Estimates vary, but perhaps 30 to 50 percent or less of the viral genome is expressed. Generally, the guanine-cytosine (G-C) content of oncogenic DNA viruses is 48 to 49 percent, a value similar to that of cellular DNA.

Transformed cells do not contain either capsid antigens or infectious viral DNA in a readily extractable form. On the other hand, transformed cells contain virus-specific transplantation antigen on the surface of the cell membrane, virus-specific tumor antigen in the nucleus, a small virus-specific mRNA which hybridizes with viral DNA, and a larger nuclear RNA capable of hybridizing with both viral DNA and cellular DNA.

Hybridization refers to the specific interaction between single-stranded DNA molecules to form double-stranded DNA or between single-stranded DNA and RNA molecules to form double-stranded DNA-RNA hybrids and is associated with complementary base pairing of the polynucleotide sequences. For example, mRNA can interact with a single strand of the DNA template from which it was transcribed to form an RNA-DNA hybrid molecule.

Experimentally, when double-stranded DNA is heated at 100°C the complementary purine-pyrimidine hydrogen bonds are ruptured and the DNA separates into single strands. If the heated solution is cooled slowly at room temperature, the complementary single polynucleotide strands recombine by homologous base sequences to form the original double-stranded DNA molecule. Similarly, single-stranded mRNA molecules bearing base sequences complementary to DNA will anneal to the separated single strands of DNA during slow cooling of the solution. The formation of such RNA-DNA hybrid molecules can be detected by radiolabeling of mRNA and counting the radioactivity retained on filters that permit free passage of single-stranded mRNA molecules.

These observations, together with the finding that intact SV_{40} virus (monkey papovavirus) can be recovered from transformed cells following fusion with untransformed cells induced by ultraviolet inactivated Sendai virus (a myxovirus), suggest that the entire viral genome may be integrated with cellular DNA in a state in which only some viral genes can be expressed in transformed cells. Unfortunately, the mechanism involved in this restriction is unknown, but the fact that at least some DNA tumor viruses contain a DNA polymerase may be pertinent.

Replication of RNA Tumor Viruses Unlike DNA tumor viruses, RNA tumor viruses produce progeny virus that is continuously released from cell membranes by budding without killing the transformed cells. The discovery in 1970 that RNA tumor viruses contained a *reverse transcriptase* (viral RNA-directed DNA polymerase) was not only an observation of great fundamental importance in molecular biology, but a finding that provided a vigorous and exciting impetus to cancer research and a mechanism for explaining how viral RNA genes can be incorporated into cellular DNA. Because of its potential significance for human medicine, the steps in the replication of RNA oncogenic viruses after the uncoating of viral RNA are tabulated below.

1 Viral RNA-viral DNA hybrids are made from a viral RNA template utilizing a reverse transcriptase (viral RNA-directed DNA polymerase) found in the virus particle along with single-stranded viral RNA.
2 Viral DNA-directed DNA polymerase activity, associated with the virus particle and possibly due to reverse transcriptase which can also use DNA as a template, converts the single strand of viral DNA in the hybrid into double-stranded viral DNA.
3 An *endonuclease,* brought in with the virus, cleaves the double-stranded viral DNA as it is synthesized and opens up the host cell DNA.
4 A *ligase* associated with the virus joins the free ends of the two DNA chains resulting in the integration of viral DNA into the host cell genome.
5 The integrated viral DNA transcribes viral RNA which is incorporated within progeny virus and virus-specific mRNA's required for the synthesis of virus-specific structural proteins.
6 Progeny virus particles containing single-stranded viral RNA, reverse transcriptase, polymerase activity, endonuclease, and ligase bud from cellular membranes, acquiring an envelope in the process. The synchronous replication of cellular and viral genomes continues indefinitely with the integrated viral genome being passed to each daughter cell. The infected cells are released from the regulatory mechanisms that normally control their multiplication and are transformed into neoplastic cells.

Viruses and Human Cancer Although the final evidence is not in and the outcome remains in doubt, the following observations with RNA oncogenic viruses may prove to be pertinent concerning the potential role of viruses in human cancer.

1 The cells of many leukemia patients contain a high-molecular-weight RNA associated with a reverse transcriptase that hybridizes with DNA copies of known RNA murine oncogenic viruses.
2 Normal chick and rat embryonic cells contain a reverse transcriptase whose RNA template is unrelated to that of any known avian or murine RNA virus, suggesting perhaps a role for the enzyme in differentiation.
3 An enzyme with the biochemical properties of reverse transcriptase has been purified from the circulating lymphocytes of acute leukemia patients.
4 Normal circulating human lymphocytes stimulated by mitogenic agents such as phytohemagglutinin (Chap. 8) have an enzyme that carries out DNA synthesis and is sensitive to ribonuclease but does not make DNA copies as do the enzymes from RNA tumor viruses and human leukemic cells.
5 Virus particles, closely resembling those associated with known RNA murine oncogenic viruses, have been detected in human milk from patients with breast cancer and from other human tumors.
6 RNA tumor viruses (avian and murine) can be induced by iododeoxyuridine (IUDR) and bromodeoxyuridine in an appreciable number of normal, supposedly virus-free cells and from tumors produced by chemical carcinogens.

To date the findings with DNA tumor viruses have been less promising. Tests designed to detect antibodies to virus-induced tumor antigens in the sera of cancer patients have yielded negative results. Efforts to recover virus-specific mRNA from human tumor tissues that would hybridize with herpes simplex, adeno-, and papovaviruses have failed. Attempts to isolate viruses from human cancer cells by fusion with normal susceptible cells in which the suspected DNA tumor viruses can replicate are continuing.

Special mention should be made concerning the potential role of the DNA containing herpes simplex viruses in human malignancies. Herpes simplex virus type 2 is venereally transmitted in man; serological studies reveal an association between infection with the virus and cervical carcinoma, and the virus can induce malignant transformation of hamster embryo cells. As yet, however, there is no strong evidence to suggest that herpes type 2 virus is etiologically responsible for human cervical carcinoma.

Another member of the herpes group, EB (Epstein-Barr) virus, is associated with Burkitt's lymphoma, a tumor found in children in Central Africa, and nasopharyngeal carcinoma in Chinese males in Southeast Asia. On the other hand, worldwide infection with EB virus is common, and the virus appears to be the cause of infectious mononucleosis. Recent findings show that EB virus can convert virus-free circulating leukocytes into virus-positive cells capable of continuous growth with some features of transformed cells. In addition, EB viral DNA has been detected by hybridization in virus-free biopsies of Burkitt's lymphoma and nasopharyngeal carcinoma. In animals the herpes group of viruses are associated with neurolymphoma, adenocarcinoma, and lymphomas in chickens, frogs, rabbits, monkeys, and marmosets; and an attenuated strain of Marek's virus can prevent neurolymphoma in chickens. Despite the accumulated data, however, the possibility remains that in man herpesviruses are merely contaminants present in but not etiologically involved in the cancers.

RICKETTSIAE

Rickettsiae are obligate intracellular parasites that reproduce by binary fission; contain DNA, RNA, ribosomes, and cell walls; appear as small, nonmotile coccobacilli resembling gram-negative bacteria; are sensitive to tetracyclines and chloramphenicol; and retain most of the major enzyme systems (Krebs cycle, electron transport, and protein, nucleic acid, and cell wall synthesis) but are unable to survive as free-living parasites because of the unusual permeability of their cytoplasmic membrane to nucleotides, coenzymes, and other essential cofactors. In effect, rickettsiae have lost many mechanisms for buffering themselves against unfavorable environments and are dependent on host cell *glutamate* (chief energy source), other substrates, cofactors, and a complex environment in which cellular integrity and function are maintained.

Structure and Chemistry

Rickettsiae are highly pleomorphic coccobacilli (usually 0.5 by 0.3 μm, occasionally up to 2 by 0.7 μm) appearing singly or in pairs, short chains, or filaments and are poorly stained by Gram's procedure, but they can be readily demonstrated with Giemsa's or Macchiavello's stains, in which case they are blue and red, respectively. As noted above, the cytoplasmic membrane is highly permeable. The cell wall contains mucopeptide, muramic acid, neutral fats, phospholipids, and diaminopimelic acid and is hydrolyzed by lysozyme, thus resembling gram-negative bacteria. An *endotoxin*, resembling that associated with the O antigen of gram-negative bacteria (Chap. 5), is present in the cell walls of rickettsiae and is lethal for mice within a few hours following intravenous inoculation. The antigenic structure of rickettsiae is associated with group-specific and species-specific antigens. In addition, most rickettsiae (those of rickettsialpox and Q fever excepted) share common cell wall antigens with *Proteus vulgaris*.

Metabolism

Apparently, intact rickettsiae are limited to oxidizing glutamate as their chief source of energy via the Krebs tricarboxylic acid cycle; they also have a functional cytochrome system capable of *oxidative phosphorylation* but are unable to utilize glucose or glucose 6-phosphate via the glycolytic pathway. Oxygen uptake confirmed by $^{14}CO_2$ production occurs with labeled α-ketoglutarate, succinate, fumarate, malate, and oxalacetate. Substantial evidence indicates that rickettsiae can form protein and lipids, probably in the absence of an endogenous pool of amino acids. Polyribonucleotides, but not the nucleoside triphosphate precursors, are also synthesized by rickettsiae. Although the contributions of the host cell to rickettsial replication are poorly understood, they are associated with the propensity of the rickettsiae to leak and the host cell to provide an adequate supply of adenosine triphosphate (ATP), nicotinamide adenine dinucleotide (NAD), and coenzyme A (CoA).

Aqueous suspensions of rickettsiae are highly unstable and quickly lose their biologic activities presumably because of the rapid leakage of essential metabolites. The inactivation can be prevented or even reversed by the addition of diphosphopyridine nucleotide (DPN), ATP, NAD, CoA, glutamate, and magnesium ions and may be slowed by the use of media high in potassium and low in sodium ions. It is not surprising, therefore, that rickettsiae are extremely labile to physical and chemical agents. However, *Coxiella burnetii,* the causative agent of Q fever, is resistant to drying and pasteurization at 60°C for 30 min., a pertinent observation in the consideration of its transmission to man.

Replication

Rickettsiae have been propagated in embryonated eggs and cell cultures. Growth is especially abundant in the yolk sac of chick embryos incubated at temperatures between 32 and 36°C, and most vaccines in current use have been prepared from infected yolk sacs. Critical to their perpetuation in nature and their transmission to man is the fact that rickettsiae multiply in the intestinal lining cells of arthropod vectors that have taken a blood meal from an infected host. In the case of ticks and mites, the infection is passed vertically from generation to generation by *transovarial transmission.*

Rickettsial penetration of susceptible cells is an active process involving phagocytosis and requiring divalent cations and viable and metabolically active parasites and hosts, even though growth of the organisms is enhanced during incubation at 32°C. Inside the cell the rickettsiae reproduce by transverse binary fission and appear to cause little initial damage, but eventually the cell becomes saturated with progeny parasites, bursts, and liberates the organisms. Most rickettsiae replicate in the cytoplasm, but *Rickettsia rickettsii,* the causative agent of Rocky Mountain spotted fever, grows in the nucleus as well. *C. burnetii* grows within membrane-lined cytoplasmic vacuoles.

Host-Parasite Interactions

Except for epidemic typhus, the microorganisms are natural parasites of arthropods and animals, rarely affecting their hosts adversely. Man is an accidental host, unimportant in maintaining the cycle, but infection is tantamount to disease and is usually severe, often lethal. In epidemic typhus in which man is the reservoir of infection and the human body louse is the arthropod vector, the parasitic interaction is precarious. The rickettsiae invariably induce a fatal disease in the louse within 2 weeks, and only rarely do recovered patients serve as a source of infection for the vector. On the other hand, in some patients recovered from epidemic typhus or Q fever, the rickettsiae may persist for 50 years or more.

Rickettsiae have a predilection for and multiply extensively in the endothelial cells lining the small blood vessels, leading to the appearance of vascular lesions which are most numerous in the skin, CNS, myocardium, kidneys, lungs, liver, and spleen. The basic lesion is an *endangitis* with perivascular infiltration with phagocytic cells which are predominantly mononuclear.

Concomitantly, the endangitis is responsible for the *rickettsemia* which is a regular feature of human infections (epidemic typhus, murine typhus, tick typhus, scrub typhus, rickettsialpox, and Q fever).

CHLAMYDIA (BEDSONIA)

Chlamydiae or bedsoniae are obligate intracellular parasites that reproduce by binary fission; contain DNA, RNA, ribosomes, and cell walls; appear as spherical bacterial forms 0.3 to 0.4 μm in diameter; are generally sensitive to the tetracyclines and chloramphenicol, with some members also being susceptible to sulfonamides and penicillin; and exhibit limited metabolic activity, catabolizing glucose by pathways independent of the cell and synthesizing folates and cell wall components; but they are unable to survive as free-living parasites because they have lost the capacity to generate energy (energy parasites). The chlamydiae show slight but definite homology of DNA with *Neisseria meningitidis,* the meningococcus.

Structure and Chemistry

Chlamydial cell walls contain mucopeptide and muramic acid and have a high lipid content composed of neutral fats and phospholipids, thereby resembling gram-negative bacteria. Antigens present in the cell wall exhibit both group-specific and species-specific characteristics. An endotoxin, similar to bacterial endotoxins, is found in the cell walls and is lethal for mice within a few hours following intravenous inoculation. For unknown reasons, the common amino acids arginine and histidine are missing from the proteins of these microorganisms.

Metabolism

The restricted biosynthetic capability of chlamydiae is unique among cellular organisms. Apart from oxidizing glucose to pentose and synthesizing folic acid, several amino acids including lysine, and probably a few other small molecules, the microorganisms lack endogenous enzymatic activity. Since the chlamydiae cannot obtain energy from glucose oxidation, they lack an energy generating system. Consequently, chlamydiae are totally dependent upon the host cell for the generation of ATP and thus are obligate intracellular energy parasites.

Replication

Chlamydiae have been propagated primarily in the yolk sac of embryonated eggs, growing best at 35°C, and have been adapted with some difficulty to growth in cell cultures. Within infected cells the microorganisms characteristically exhibit a typical bacterial growth curve associated with a developmental cycle.

Infection is initiated by adsorption of the microorganism in its typical infectious extracellular spherical form (0.3 to 0.4 μm) or *elementary body,* which consists of an electron-dense central body and a less dense peripheral mass. Adsorption is a slow process which may require up to 2 hr. The elementary body is then taken into the cytoplasm of the cell by a process resembling phagocytosis. Over the course of the next 8 to 10 hr., the dense internal mass of the elementary body is gradually reorganized into a large, highly granular, coarse-meshed, reticular *initial body* ten times the size of the elementary body. As the initial body divides, it forms a vacuole or vesicle without a cell wall from which elementary bodies with a rigid cell wall are derived approximately 20 hr. after infection. Synthesis within the vesicles containing the initial bodies continues until the cytoplasm of the host cell is literally filled with progeny elementary bodies and the cell bursts, releasing them. Generally, the developmental cycle and growth curve are completed in 24 to 48 hr.

Several stains can be used to detect elementary bodies, initial bodies, and *basophilic intracytoplasmic inclusions* composed of groups of initial bodies that take up most of the cytoplasmic space and may be imbedded in a glycogen matrix [trachoma and inclusion conjunctivitis (TRIC) agents]. With Giemsa's stain, elementary bodies are purple, initial bodies are blue, and cytoplasmic inclusions are purple. With acridine orange, elementary bodies rich in DNA stain green. Early in the developmental cycle initial bodies are rich in RNA and stain red, but later, when filled with elementary bodies, they stain green.

Host-Parasite Interactions

Chlamydiae pathogenic for man have a predilection for mucous membranes and typically have their reservoir either in birds (psittacosis-ornithosis) or in man [lymphogranuloma venereum (LGV) and the TRIC agents]. Man acquires infection by inhalation of dried secretions or excreta of infected birds or, in the case of the strictly human diseases, following venereal contact, direct contact with conjunctival lesions, or indirectly by contact with genital secretions in unchlorinated swimming pools or ponds (inclusion conjunctivitis). On rare occasions, man-to-man transmission of psittacosis-ornithosis agents has occurred by the respiratory route.

Subclinical infection is the rule and overt disease the exception in the natural hosts of these parasites. Upon recovery from infection, asymptomatic carriers are common, and the organisms may be shed for many months or years. In man, infection and disease are characterized by *prolonged latency* as evident in trachoma, inclusion conjunctivitis, LGV, and psittacosis; but acute disease is also the rule in psittacosis and in inclusion conjunctivitis of the newborn.

One of the hallmarks of infection with chlamydiae is the presence of large basophilic intracytoplasmic inclusions within infected cells. The extent of tissue involvement varies widely with the particular agent and in some cases the duration of the disease. Disease is limited to the conjunctival epithelium in inclusion conjunctivitis; seriously damages the cornea in trachoma; produces chronic regional lymphadenitis in LGV which may occasionally spread systemically to other tissues, including the CNS; and in psittacosis regularly involves the reticuloendothelial cells of the liver and spleen as well as the alveolar walls and interstitial tissues of the lung.

FUNGI

Fungi are heterotrophic, eukaryotic unicellular or multicellular organisms widely distributed in air, food, soil, plants, animals, and water. The individual organisms lack chlorophyll, have sterols in their plasma membranes, are surrounded by a cell wall, reproduce by spore formation, and are ubiquitously present in the environment as airborne spores. Included in the fungi are yeasts, molds, and mushrooms covering a wide range of sizes from microscopic to the giant mushrooms which may be several centimeters or more in diameter. In nature, fungi are principally saprophytic, although some species are parasitic. Fungi pathogenic for man are small in size (3 to 15 μm) and usually reproduce by means of asexual spores. Diseases caused by fungi are commonly termed *mycoses.*

Structure

Fungi have two basic cellular forms, yeast and hypha. *Yeasts* are spherical or ellipsoid unicellular organisms 3 to 6 μm in diameter, reproduce by budding or binary fission and form bacteria-like colonies on agar medium. The *hypha* is a tubular element (5 to 15 μm in diameter) which extends by apical growth and intercalary branching, resulting in a macroscopic cottony or woolly network of hyphae called a *mycelium.* The hyphae may have various types of partial *septa* or no septa at all. In the nonseptate hyphae there is no separation into individual cells, and the entire mycelium can be considered one cell.

Metabolism

Fungi as a group have metabolic activities generally conforming to the pattern discussed in Chapter 1. An important aspect of fungal metabolism is the variety of useful compounds generated by fungi, including alcoholic fermentations, fats, organic acids, and antibiotics. On the other hand, some fungi also produce potent toxins including the mushroom poisons, aflatoxins, and several hallucinogenic drugs. In addition, peptidases, collagenase, and elastase may be involved in the pathogenesis of superficial skin lesions caused by dermatophytes.

Replication

Asexual reproduction in hyphae takes place by the formation of spores. When spores are enclosed within a terminal swollen structure on a hyphal stalk (*sporangium*), they are known as *sporangiospores*. Spores which are borne externally by a budding-like process are called *conidia* and may be formed on simple or specialized aerial hyphae known as *conidiophores*. When spores are produced by hyphal fragmentation, they are called *arthrospores*. Sporangiospores, conidia, and arthrospores serve primarily to disseminate the fungi. Some fungi produce *chlamydospores*, which are thick-walled resting endospores formed within, on the end of, or on the side of hyphae.

Among the fungi there is a great diversity in asexual spores in terms of their size, shape, color, location, supporting structures, and method of development. The presence or absence of a mycelium, the type of mycelium, and the characteristics of the sexual stage of spore production, as well as the properties of asexual spores, all provide useful taxonomic criteria.

Many fungal species are capable of true sexual reproduction, which involves three steps: (1) fusion of the cytoplasm of two cells (*plasmogamy*), (2) fusion of two haploid nuclei from each cell (*karyogamy*), (3) reductive division (*meiosis*) of the diploid nucleus to restore the haploid condition. The products of meiosis are borne as spores, and fungi are classified in part according to the type of structure which bears the meiotic product.

Classification

Four classes of fungi are recognized.

1 *Phycomycetes*. The members of this class are relatively simple, usually nonseptate. Some are unicellular and motile. Mycelial forms may produce sporangiospores. Sexual reproduction in mycelial forms results in a *zygospore* which contains the haploid nuclei in a common cytoplasm.
2 *Ascomycetes*. Mycelial forms may produce conidia, arthrospores, or chlamydospores. Most yeasts are included in this class. Sexual spores develop in a sac-like cell called an *ascus*.
3 *Basidiomycetes*. Sexual spores (*basidiospores*), typically four in number, develop externally on a club-shaped cell called a *basidium*. Included in this class are the mushrooms, toadstools, rusts, and smuts. Poisonous species mistaken for mushrooms can cause serious intoxication in man, and the rusts and smuts produce great damage in cereal crops.
4 Imperfect fungi (*Deuteromycetes*). Since classification of fungi is primarily concerned with sexual reproduction, species with no known sexual or perfect stage are included together in a group called the imperfect fungi. Most of the molds, yeasts, yeast-like fungi, and dimorphic fungi pathogenic for man were originally classified as imperfect fungi. Subsequently, the perfect sexual stage was demonstrated for many human pathogens, most of which turned out to be Ascomycetes. However, because of common usage and the fact that laboratory diagnosis rests exclusively on the asexual (imperfect) stage, the human pathogens are still classified with the imperfect fungi.

Host-Parasite Interactions

A number of fungi, including several systemic pathogens of man, are capable of growing in both yeast and hyphal (*mold*) forms and are known as *dimorphic fungi.* The alteration in form can be brought about by several different environmental factors.

Temperature-dependent dimorphism is evident from the fact that the fungus is a mold at the normal temperature for growth of fungi in the laboratory (24°C), whereas it is a yeast at 37°C (*Blastomyces dermatitidis).*

Nutrition-dependent dimorphism occurs when the source of carbohydrate is varied. *Candida albicans* is a yeast when grown on glucose medium but develops hyphae on medium containing polysaccharides.

Nutrition-temperature-dependent dimorphism requires both a temperature of 37°C and complete nutritional supplements for the yeast phase of growth, as in *Histoplasma capsulatum.* Interestingly, a shift from the yeast to the mold phase requires only a lowering of the temperature.

Most of the dimorphic fungi pathogenic for man occur in the yeast form in host tissues. The principal exception is *C. albicans* which may show yeast, mycelial, or both forms in infected tissues.

In man, the portal of entry for airborne fungal spores is through minor skin abrasions or through the mucous membranes following inhalation or ingestion. The resulting infections may be localized to the skin (superficial mycoses), the mucous membranes (candidiasis), or the subcutaneous tissues with or without regional lymphadenopathy (sporotrichosis), or infection may be halted at the regional lymph nodes (histoplasmosis); in rare instances, infection is widely disseminated to the lungs, viscera, skeleton, CNS, or endocardium. Some infections are limited to the keratinized tissues, and these are caused by mycelial forms known as *dermatophytes.*

Many human pathogens including *Histoplasma, Coccidioides,* and *Candida* can survive, grow within, and be disseminated by phagocytes. Cryptococci have a thick mucopolysaccharide capsule and can grow in body fluids independent of phagocytes. On the whole, however, the regional lymph nodes form an effective barrier for limiting the spread of fungi, and untreated diseases characteristically pursue a chronic granulomatous course.

In addition, an increasing number of destructive or widely disseminated fungal infections in man are caused by fungi which are part of the normal endogenous flora. Most of these invasive infections occur in persons who have received antibiotics or immunosuppressive drugs, who have serious underlying disease (uncontrolled diabetes, autoimmune disease, cancer), or who have been subjected to trauma (mycotic keratitis, endocarditis in narcotic addicts). Included among the fungi commonly involved are *Candida, Aspergillus,* and *Geotrichum;* in *phycomycosis, Mucor, Rhizopus, Basidiobolus, Absidia,* and *Mortierella* are involved, and in *mycotic keratitis Aspergillus, Fusarium, Cephalosporium, Curvularia,* and *Penicillium* are involved.

Basically, fungi can produce disease in man by the invasion of living or keratinized tissues, following the ingestion of fungal toxins or by inducing *allergic alveolitis* following inhalation of airborne spores *(farmer's lung).* Delayed hypersensitivity is regularly present in most mycoses and probably is actively involved in the production of lesions in the superficial mycoses, but its role in the systemic or deep mycoses is obscure.

PROTOZOA

Protozoa are unicellular eukaryotic animals lacking cell walls, have simple or complex life cycles, usually reproduce asexually, are often motile, and are included with the Protista (Chapter 1). In nature, most protozoa are free-living forms (ameba, paramecium, vorticella) present in freshwater ponds containing an adequate food supply of microorganisms, principally bacteria. Other protozoa are obligate parasites requiring the host to compensate for biochemical and biophysical deficiencies. In this connection, it is interesting to note that *Ent-*

amoeba histolytica cannot be propagated in the intestinal tract of germ-free animals. A few protozoa are obligate intracellular parasites. The protozoa that infect man vary in size between a few micra and 100 μm and include amebas, flagellates, ciliates, and sporozoa as well as other microorganisms of undetermined status (toxoplasma, pneumocystis). In addition, many intestinal protozoa are part of the normal flora.

Structure

Depending on the stage in their life cycles, protozoa have the same or a different number of nuclei, may assume a variety of sizes and shapes, and may possess a battery of specialized structures. Protozoa contain between 1 and 24 nuclei. For a given parasite the number of nuclei may remain constant or may vary widely (1 to 24). Similarly, the size of a particular parasite may remain constant or increase tenfold or more. The shape of protozoa may be spherical, oval, rhomboidal, elliptical, fusiform, conical, pear-shaped, or crescent-shaped and may be maintained or may shift significantly during the different stages of development. Except for the sporozoa, protozoa are motile by means of pseudopodia, cilia, flagella, and undulating membranes, but they may become nonmotile at certain stages in their life cycles. In addition, the parasites may have oral and anal pores, macronuclei and micronuclei, and a thin or thick outer covering and may contain masses of chromatin, glycogen, and volutin granules, food and contractile vacuoles, or ingested erythrocytes. Identification of protozoa is based on the size and shape of the parasites and the possession and location of the specialized structures mentioned above.

Replication (Life Cycle)

With few exceptions, protozoa have at least two stages in their life cycles. In the intestinal ameba, flagellates, and ciliates, there is an active, motile *trophozoite* growing or feeding stage and an inactive, nonmotile resistant *cyst* stage. The trophozoite has a single nucleus; moves by means of pseudopodia, cilia or flagella, and undulating membranes; multiplies asexually by binary fission; and transforms into a cyst (encystation). In the process of *encystation*, the parasite often assumes a more spherical form, extrudes undigested food particles (occasionally erythrocytes), loses its organelles of locomotion, and secretes a cyst wall which protects the protozoa against adverse environmental influences. If nuclear division takes place within the cyst, it occurs without binary fission of the cyst. *Excystation* (release of trophozoites from the ingested cyst) occurs in the ileocecal region of the intestine under the influence of digestive enzymes.

The blood and tissue flagellates *(Leishmania* and *Trypanosoma)* are transmitted to man by *arthropod vectors* (sandflies, tsetse flies, triatomid bugs) and pass through two or four stages in their life cycle *(Leishmania, Leptomonas, Crithidia, Trypanosoma)*, having at least one stage in an arthropod and another stage in man. *Leishmania* are nonflagellate, obligate intracellular parasites of small size (2 to 4 μm × 1 to 2 μm) that replicate by binary fission and are present in leishmaniasis and in American trypanosomiasis (Chagas' disease). The other three stages are flagellates. *Crithidia* and *Trypanosoma* are 15 to 35 μm in length and a few micrometers in diameter with prominent undulating membranes and are found in the arthropod vectors of African and American trypanosomiasis and in cultures. Only the trypanosomal form is seen in human African trypanosomiasis, but the leishmanial form is also present in American trypanosomiasis. The leptomonad form is found in the arthropod vector and in cultures in leishmaniasis and appears to be a transitional form in American trypanosomiasis. The *Leptomonas* is shorter in length than the other flagellate forms, somewhat wider in diameter, and has a polar flagella but no undulating membrane. Culture of African trypanosomes is difficult, but leptomonad and trypanosomal forms can be readily grown on enriched blood agar medium at 23 to 28°C from patients with leishmaniasis and American trypanosomiasis respectively.

A complex sporozoan life cycle is illustrated by the malarial parasite which involves an alternation of sexual and asexual generations in anopheline mosquitoes and man. The sexual cycle *(sporogony)* is completed in the mosquito (the definitive, or final host), involves the formation of spores *(sporozoites)*, and requires 8 to 21 days. The asexual cycle *(schizogony)* occurs in man (the intermediate host), involves multiple fission, requires the formation of male and female gametocytes which initiate the sexual cycle within the mosquito, and is completed in 24 to 72 hr. (Chap. 25).

Metabolism

Except for the sporozoa, most protozoa can be cultured on artificial medium, but little is known concerning the metabolic activities of pathogenic forms because the parasites frequently show changes in morphology, antigenicity, and capacity to induce infection. Pathogenic amebas, for example, grow poorly in the absence of bacteria; this limits the evaluation of their metabolic activities. A few general observations, however, will illustrate some of the pertinent factors that may be involved in protozoan metabolism.

Intestinal protozoa grow best in an anaerobic environment under reduced oxygen tension in the presence of bacteria. Growth of the flagellate *Trichomonas vaginalis* in the vagina occurs only after the onset of puberty and may be influenced by hormones. Slender bloodstream trypanosomes metabolize glucose to pyruvate, and their terminal respiration involves a glycerophosphate oxidase system, but they lack pyruvate oxidase, a functional cytochrome system, and a TCA cycle. Cultured trypanosomes, on the other hand, have an active cytochrome system and a functional TCA cycle. Growth of malarial parasites within red blood cells utilizes hemoglobin as the primary source of amino acids, 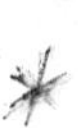 converts hemoglobin to a hematin-containing pigment, and is stimulated by high concentrations of glucose 6-phosphate dehydrogenase, hemoglobin A2, ATP, para-aminobenzoic acid, and methionine.

Host-Parasite Interactions

Several important diseases of man are caused by protozoa, including amebiasis, leishmaniasis, trypanosomiasis, and malaria. In addition, under appropriate conditions serious disease can be induced by *Toxoplasma, Pneumocystis,* and by *Naegleria* and *Hartmannella* species (amebic meningoencephalitis). In contrast, giardiasis, balantidiasis, and trichomoniasis are usually minor but annoying problems. Depending on the particular protozoa, the infection may be predominantly asymptomatic or may result in localized or systemic clinical manifestations which are in most cases chronically progressive.

Man may acquire infection by ingesting cysts (amebiasis, giardiasis, balantidiasis, toxoplasmosis), penetration of mucous membranes (amebic meningoencephalitis), from arthropod vectors (malaria, leishmaniasis, trypanosomiasis), venereally (trichomoniasis), in utero (toxoplasmosis), direct contact (cutaneous leishmaniasis), blood transfusion (malaria, trypanosomiasis, leishmaniasis), or by activation of normal flora by immunosuppressive drugs or agents (pneumonia due to *Pneumocystis carinii*).

HELMINTHS (WORMS)

General Characteristics

In addition to microorganisms (bacteria, viruses, rickettsiae, chlamydiae, fungi, protozoa), infectious disease in man can be caused by helminths (worms) and is often referred to as *infestation.* Helminths are metazoans, i.e., multicellular, macroscopic animals with digestive, excretory, reproductive, and nervous systems which may be lacking or primitive in some species. The pathogenic helminths vary in length from 1 cm to 10 meters and are usually much smaller in width (a few millimeters to a centimeter). The helminths are divided into the *roundworms, or nematodes,* and the *flatworms,* which include the *tapeworms (cestodes)* and the *flukes (trematodes).*

The nematodes are characterized by a cuticle-covered, unsegmented, bilaterally symmetrical body with pointed or rounded ends containing a body cavity with a digestive tract as well as excretory, nervous, and reproductive systems. The sexes are separate. Included among the nematodes that parasitize man are the *intestinal roundworms* (causing pinworm and whipworm disease, ascariasis, trichinosis, hookworm disease, and strongyloidiasis) and the *tissue roundworms* (causing filariasis, loiasis, onchocerciasis, dracontiasis, and cutaneous larva migrans).

The flatworms are more primitive than the roundworms; are flattened dorsoventrally; have no body cavity; possess only rudimentary alimentary, excretory, and nervous systems; and are hermaphroditic (except for the schistosomes) and often undergo asexual as well as sexual reproduction. Each segment of the hermaphroditic tapeworm has male and female reproductive organs. Included among the flatworms that parasitize man are the segmented tapeworms causing beef, pork, dwarf, and fish tapeworm infections, cysticercosis and echinococcosis (hydatid cyst), and the intestinal, lung, liver, and blood flukes.

Life Cycle and Host-Parasite Interactions

Most of the helminths have complex life cycles involving eggs, larval, and adult forms. Man can serve as the definitive host (i.e., has the adult sexual stage), intermediate host (i.e., has the larval stage), or both. Generally however, larval development occurs in the soil, in arthropod vectors, in mollusks (snails), in copepods (crustaceans), in fish, or in a variety of mammals. Important exceptions in which the larval stage causes disease in man include trichinosis and echinococcosis. In addition, clinical manifestations associated with larval development or migration can occur in cysticercosis, ascariasis, hookworm, and strongyloidiasis.

Man usually acquires infection following ingestion of eggs or larvae or penetration of the skin by larvae in the soil or through the bite of an arthropod. With few exceptions including trichinosis, echinocococcis, and filariasis, eggs or larvae are present in the intestinal contents of patients, and their characteristics are used to identify the helminth causing the disease. One outstanding feature of many helminth infections is their ability to survive for long periods (up to 25 years) within the host.

BIBLIOGRAPHY

Austwick, P. K.: "The Pathogenicity of Fungi," in H. Smith and J. H. Pearce (eds.), *Microbial Pathogenicity in Man and Animals,* Symposium 22, Cambridge: Cambridge University Press, 1972, pp. 251-268.

Darougar, S., Jones, B. R., Kinnison, J. R., Vaughan-Jackson, J. D. and Dunlop, E. M. C.: "Chlamydial Infection," *Br. J. Vener. Dis.,* 48:416-459, 1972.

Eiserling, F. A., and Dickson, R.: "Assembly of Viruses," *Annu. Rev. Biochem.,* 41:467-502, 1972.

Gershon, A., Cosio, L., and Brunell, P. A.: "Observations on the Growth of Varicella-Zoster Virus in Human Diploid Cells," *J. Gen. Virol.,* 18:21-31, 1973.

Hahon, N., Booth, J. A., and Eckert, H. L.: "Cell Attachment and Penetration by Influenza Virus," *Infect. Immun.,* 7:341-351, 1973.

Harding, H. B.: "The Bacteria-like Chlamydiae of Ornithosis and the Diseases They Cause," *CRC Crit. Rev. Clin. Lab. Sci.,* 1:451-470, 1970.

Howe, C., and Lee, L. T.: "Virus-Erythrocyte Interactions," *Adv. Virus Res.,* 17:1-50, 1972.

Joklik, W. K., and Zweerink, H. J.: "The Morphogenesis of Animal Viruses," *Annu. Rev. Genet.,* 5:297-360, 1971.

Kleinschmidt, W. J.: "Biochemistry of Interferon and Its Inducers," *Annu. Rev. Biochem.,* 41:517-542, 1972.

McAllister, R. M.: "Search for Oncogenes in Human Rhabdomyosarcoma Cells," *Prog. Immunobiol. Stand.,* 5:237-242, 1972.

Melnick, J. L.: "Classification of Animal Viruses, 1973," *Progr. Med. Virol.,* 15:380-384, 1973.

Merkow, L. P., and Slifkin, M. (eds.): "Oncogenic Adenoviruses," *Progr. Exp. Tumor Res.,* 18:1-293, 1973.

Newton, B. A.: "Protozoal Pathogenicity," in H. Smith and J. H. Pearce (eds.), *Microbial Pathogenicity in Man and Animals,* Symposium 22, Cambridge: Cambridge University Press, 1972, pp. 269-301.

Ormsbee, R. A.: "Rickettsial Diseases—A Public Health Problem?" *J. Infect. Dis.,* 127:325-327, 1973.

"Pathology Society Symposium. Herpesviruses and Cancer," *Fed. Proc.,* 31:1625-1674, 1972.

Rapp, F.: "Question: Do Herpesviruses Cause Cancer? Answer: Of Course They Do," *J. Natl. Cancer Inst.,* 50:825-832, 1973

Sugiyawa, T., Korant, B. D., and Lonberg-Hohn, K. K.: "RNA Virus Gene Expression and Its Control," *Annu. Rev. Microbiol.,* 26:467-502, 1972.

Sundquist, B., Everitt, E., and Philipson, L.: "Assembly of Adenoviruses," *J. Virol.,* 11:449-459, 1973.

"Symposium: Viral Infections in Gynecology and Obstetrics," *Clin. Obstet. Gynecol.,* 15:856-1023, 1972.

Temin, H. M., and Baltimore, D.: "RNA-directed DNA Synthesis and RNA Tumor Viruses," *Adv. Virus Res.,* 17:129-186, 1972.

Vogt, P. K.: "The Emerging Genetics of RNA Tumor Viruses," *J. Natl. Cancer Inst.,* 48: 3-9, 1972.

Wang, S. P., Kuo, C. C., and Grayston, J. T.: "A Simplified Method for Immunological Typing of Trachoma Inclusion Conjunctivitis-Lymphogranuloma Venereum Organisms," *Infect. Immun.,* 7:356-360, 1973.

Weiss, E., Newman, L. W., Grays, R., and Green, A. E.: "Metabolism of *Rickettsia typhi* and *Rickettsia akari* in Irradiated L Cells," *Infect. Immun.,* 6:50-61, 1972.

Wike, D. A., and Burgdorfer, W.: "Plaque Formation in Tissue Cultures by *Rickettsia rickettsi* Isolated Directly from Whole Blood and Tick Hemolymph," *Infect. Immun.,* 6:736-742, 1972.

Chapter 3

Microbial Genetics

Pasquale F. Bartell

EXPRESSION OF GENETIC INFORMATION

The structural and biologic characteristics of microbes are preserved through successive generations by hereditary mechanisms. Thus, daughter cells usually resemble the parents from which they are derived. It is important to recognize that it is not the characteristic itself which is transmitted through successive generations but rather the genetic information required to develop the characteristic under appropriate environmental conditions.

The Message Unit (Codon)

The genetic information of the bacterial cell is mainly contained in the chromosome in the form of a chemical code established by the sequence of nucleotides that make up the deoxyribonucleic acid (DNA). Each message unit, or codon, is represented by three neighboring nucleotides that specify a single amino acid. Thus, the linear sequence of nucleotides along the DNA molecule comprises the genes which code for specific polypeptide chains. Most DNA mol-

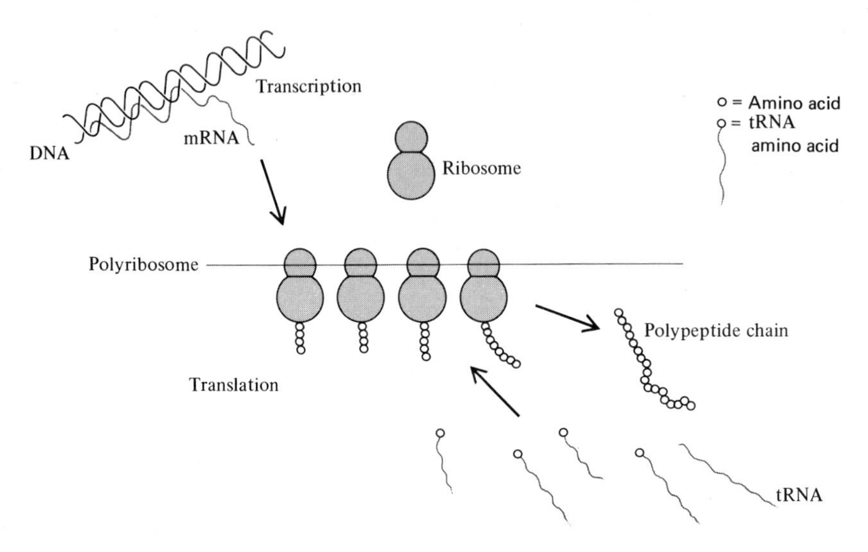

Figure 3-1 Stages involved in the production of functional polypeptides from genetic information contained in a DNA template.

ecules contain large numbers of genes, each of which contains hundreds to thousands of nucleotides.

Transcription

In order for the cell to make use of its genetic information, the information must first be transferred to messenger ribonucleic acid (mRNA) molecules. This is accomplished by the synthesis of RNA on a DNA template and involves the formation of a complementary sequence of RNA nucleotides by DNA-dependent RNA polymerase. This process is known as *transcription.*

Translation

The mRNA molecules then act as templates that determine the amino acid sequence of proteins by attaching to the cellular ribosomes and moving across them to bring successive codons into position for selecting the correct amino acid. This step is called *translation.* A given mRNA molecule generally is engaged simultaneously on many ribosomes which collectively are referred to as a *polyribosome.* During this process the individual amino acids do not attach to the mRNA templates but combine with, and are carried by, specific transfer RNA (tRNA) molecules. A given tRNA molecule is specific for a particular amino acid. The tRNA and its attached amino acid diffuse to the ribosomes on which the mRNA is attached, and the peptide bonds are formed. The protein chain then grows in a stepwise fashion (Fig. 3-1).

Templates

Thus, the flow of genetic information in the cell is from DNA to RNA which then serves as template for protein synthesis. This represents the *central dogma* of molecular genetics. Accordingly, DNA acts as its own template for self-replication and also acts as the template for synthesis of all cellular RNA.

However, there are two important exceptions to the central dogma which states that all cellular RNA is produced on a DNA template.

1 RNA can be produced on an RNA template. In the case of RNA viruses, viral RNA may act as its own template.
2 DNA can be produced on an RNA template. In the case of RNA oncogenic viruses, DNA can be made from an RNA template by means of a reverse transcriptase or RNA-directed DNA polymerase (Chap. 2).

Genotype

The assortment of genes that makes up the genetic apparatus of the cell establishes its *genotype*, which is the hereditary constitution of the cell that is replicated and passed on to the daughter cells. The genotype of a cell represents the full genetic potential of the cell which may or may not be expressed in a given environmental situation.

New bacterial genotypes can be established by a variety of different mechanisms. A new genotype can develop by a change or alteration of nucleotides in the genome of an organism as in mutation or by genetic recombination, a mechanism whereby genetic recombinants are formed through the exchange of genetic segments, by the transfer of extrachromosomal genetic determinants in which new genetic information is added to the existing genome of the bacterial cell, and by phage conversion. Through these mechanisms, microorganisms are endowed with a unique flexibility for survival under unfavorable environments and are provided with the opportunity to accumulate characteristics that enhance their ability to cause disease.

Since mutations are rare events, it is extremely unlikely that mutational events can affect more than one gene at a time in a single cell. Nonetheless, mutation is widespread, affects every known bacterium, and thus represents the major mechanism whereby new genotypes arise. In contrast, transformation and conjugation are known to occur in relatively few bacterial species and are of lesser significance in originating genotypes. However, conjugation is widely prevalent among the Enterobacteriaceae in the human intestinal tract, which provides an excellent environment for genetic interaction between pathogenic and nonpathogenic bacteria.

The wide dissemination of virulent and temperate phage among bacteria suggests that phage transfer of genetic information represents a major mechanism by which new genotypes arise. Genes may be transferred from one bacterium to another by transduction. In addition, phage genes may direct the synthesis of bacterial products (phage conversion).

Phenotype

In contrast with the genotype, the *phenotype* of a cell is established only by those characteristics that are observable. Thus, the phenotype depends upon the genotype but may vary according to which genes are expressed in a given environmental situation. For example, *Escherichia coli* carries the genetic information required for the synthesis of the enzyme beta-galactosidase. In a glucose medium this enzyme is not synthesized by the cell, but if the bacterium is placed in a medium containing lactose, the enzyme is synthesized. Thus, while the genotype of the organism remains unchanged, its phenotype varies depending upon the environment.

MUTATION

Genetic information carried by the cell is not to be considered *absolutely* stable. In rare instances, alterations in the sequence of nucleotides occur, and this is reflected by a corresponding change in the genotype of the cell. Subsequently, daughter cells inherit copies of the altered nucleotide sequence and also exhibit the changed parental phenotype. The change in phenotype is the very thing that makes a mutation recognizable. These heritable changes are called *mutations*.

Any component or characteristic of the cell is subject to mutation. If a vital function is involved, the mutation is lethal to the cell and is referred to as a *lethal mutation*.

In the study of microorganisms it is important to understand how they can become genetically modified. Mutations may provide the basis for changes in structural or metabolic characteristics that increase the organism's potential for survival. For example, mutations may involve alterations in such properties as virulence, resistance to antibiotics, and surface antigens which complicate the prevention and treatment of disease. Thus, from a practical point of view, genetic change has serious implications in man's effort to conquer disease.

Wild Type

A large population of cells is usually required to detect the rare mutant cell that is recognizable by some modification of its phenotype. For example, certain bacteria produce bright red colonies when grown on the surface of nutrient agar because of the synthesis of a red pigment. This is a phenotypic characteristic. Of the millions of cells that are derived from a single cell, all produce a red pigment. However, a rare mutant cell may emerge that cannot produce red pigment and gives rise to a white colony. In this case, the white mutant colony can easily be recognized and separated from the red pigment-producing wild-type colonies. Wild type is the term used to refer to the organism's characteristic form as found in nature.

Other bacteria produce capsules and as a consequence appear as shiny, moist colonies on the surface of nutrient agar. These are often referred to as *smooth colonies*. A mutational loss in ability to synthesize capsular polysaccharide results in production of a dull, granular *rough colony*. In each of the above examples, the mutants can be isolated by carefully touching the mutant colony with an inoculating needle and passing it to a fresh medium.

Auxotrophs and Prototrophs

A different class of mutants are those in which genetic alteration affects the production of biosynthetic enzymes. These mutants are then unable to synthesize nutrients that are essential for growth and are called nutritional mutants, or auxotrophs. Their deficiency can be demonstrated by the failure to grow in a minimal medium which is composed of glucose and simple salts (NH_4Cl, $MgSO_4$, KH_2PO_4, Na_2PO_4).

The parent or wild-type cell from which the auxotroph is derived is called a prototroph because it is able to synthesize the essential growth requirements from a minimal medium.

Isolation of Auxotrophs If the auxotrophic mutant is to survive, it must occur in a medium supplying the essential nutrient that it cannot produce. However, under this condition it is impossible to distinguish between the auxotroph and the parental prototroph. For this reason, special techniques are required for the isolation of auxotrophic mutants.

Replica Plating Technique (Lederberg and Lederberg) Probably the best technique that can be used for the isolation of auxotrophs is *replica plating*. Its key feature is the identical inoculation of agar plates, each containing different nutrients, in such a way as to preserve the relative positions of the bacterial colonies on the surface of the plates. This makes it possible to identify the nutritional requirements of particular colonies.

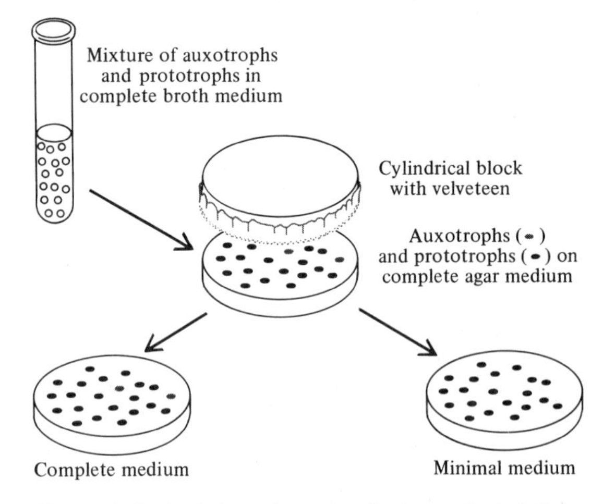

Figure 3-2 Isolation of auxotrophs by replica plating.

A mixture of auxotrophs and prototrophs is spread on the surface of an agar plate containing complete medium so as to obtain isolated colonies. After incubation, cylindrical blocks covered with velveteen are pressed on the surface of the agar plate so that the velveteen projections (like many inoculating needles clustered together) pick up a sample of each of the colonies. The velveteen block is then touched to the surface of two fresh agar plates, one composed of complete medium and the other of minimal medium. If care is taken to hold the block in the same position throughout the procedure, the imprints and growth of the colonies will be in the same position on all plates. Thus, it can be determined which colonies on the original plate are prototrophs and which are auxotrophs by comparing the position and growth of colonies on the plates containing complete or minimal medium (Fig. 3-2).

Penicillin Selection Technique Yet another technique useful for the isolation of auxotrophic mutants is *penicillin selection,* a procedure that takes advantage of the fact that penicillin kills multiplying bacteria but does not kill bacteria that are not multiplying.

In this procedure, the mixture of auxotrophs and prototrophs is sedimented by centrifugation, and the cells are washed and resuspended in a minimal medium containing penicillin. During incubation, the multiplying prototrophs are killed by the penicillin, but the nonmultiplying auxotrophs survive this treatment and are able to grow when placed on a complete medium after removal or effective dilution of the penicillin.

Antibiotic-resistant Mutants

In contrast to auxotrophic mutants, antibiotic-resistant mutants are quite easy to isolate. This is readily accomplished by placing a large population of bacteria, derived from a known antibiotic-sensitive cell, on the surface of a nutrient agar plate containing an inhibitory concentration of the antibiotic. The antibiotic-sensitive cells are inhibited and cannot grow under these conditions, but the resistant mutants survive and form colonies on the agar surface. The antibiotic employed in this procedure is referred to as the *selective agent,* since it selectively kills the sensitive bacteria in the population without interfering with the growth of resistant bacteria present in the culture prior to the addition of the antibiotic.

Gradient Plates By its construction, the *gradient plate* provides a series of antibiotic concentrations on a single plate and allows for the recognition of mutants which may differ in their degree of resistance (Fig. 3-3).

The gradient plate is prepared by pouring nutrient agar into a petri dish and allowing it to harden while the dish is in a slanted position. A mixture of nutrient agar and antibiotic is then

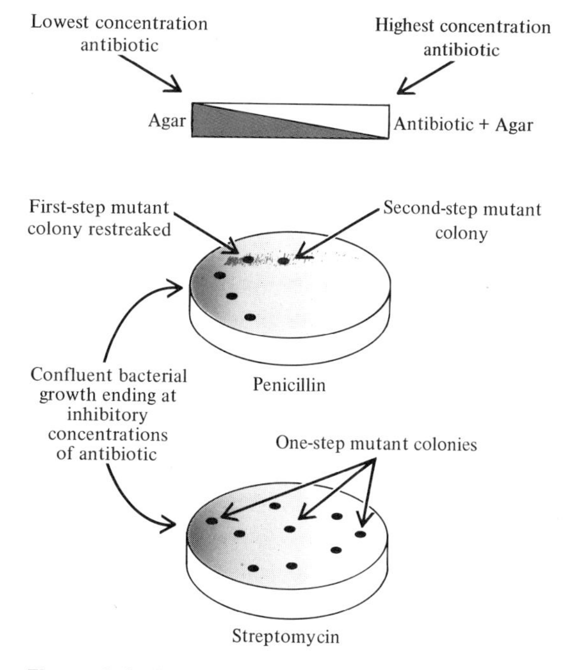

Figure 3-3 Demonstration of antibiotic resistance by gradient plating.

poured into the plate and allowed to harden while the plate is in a level position. The downward diffusion of antibiotic into the underlying agar provides a dilution of the antibiotic proportional to the thickness ratios of the agar layers from one side of the plate to the other.

Penicillin Resistance Pattern When a heavy inoculum of bacteria is placed on a gradient plate containing penicillin, confluent growth occurs on that area containing subinhibitory concentrations of penicillin. Immediately beyond this area, isolated colonies containing resistant mutants will develop. It is significant to note that the mutant colonies are not scattered over the plate, but are restricted to a localized area of agar containing a low concentration of penicillin. The bacteria found in the isolated colonies are quite uniform in their resistance to penicillin and are referred to as *first-step mutants.*

If the first-step mutants are streaked toward the area of higher penicillin concentrations and the plates reincubated, mutants resistant to slightly higher concentrations of penicillin grow and are called *second-step mutants.* By picking and culturing resistant mutants that emerge in gradually increasing concentrations of penicillin, mutants can be obtained that are resistant to successively higher concentrations of penicillin (Fig. 3-3).

On the other hand, if mutants resistant to low concentrations of penicillin are immediately placed in a medium containing high concentrations of penicillin, the resistant mutants will be killed. Thus, resistance to penicillin occurs in stepwise fashion, each sequential mutational event being a prerequisite for the next mutation, i.e., resistance to a slightly higher concentration of penicillin. Most of the commonly used antibiotics (the tetracycline drugs) show the same stepwise pattern of resistance as penicillin.

Streptomycin Resistance Pattern The emergence of streptomycin-resistant mutants is quite different from that of penicillin. When a large population of cells is placed on a gradient plate containing streptomycin, mutant colonies are scattered throughout the plate in areas of high as well as low concentrations of streptomycin. In addition, mutants can be isolated that prove to be *streptomycin-dependent,* streptomycin being a requirement for their growth.

Thus, mutants resistant to a wide range of concentrations of streptomycin can be isolated from large populations of cells in a single step and are called *one-step mutants* (Fig. 3-3).

Isonicotinylhydrazine (isoniazid) and sodium *p*-aminosalicylate (PAS) exhibit a similar one-step pattern of resistance.

Spontaneous Nature of Mutations

The decisive step in the recognition and isolation of antibiotic-resistant mutants is the application of a selective agent. The key problem, however, is whether the selective agent caused the mutation to occur, or the mutant cell existed prior to the application of the selective agent. This question can be answered in two ways: (1) indirectly, by fluctuation analysis, and (2) directly, by replica plating.

Fluctuation Test (Luria and Delbruck) The fluctuation test involves a statistical analysis of the variation in the number of mutants occurring in several independent cultures as contrasted with multiple samples taken from a single culture. The analysis provides evidence that mutants preexist in a given culture and are not caused by the selective agent employed for their recognition.

In order to perform the test, a young broth culture is diluted in fresh broth medium and divided into two equal aliquots. One aliquot is then subdivided equally into 50 test tubes, whereas the other aliquot is placed in a single flask. After incubation, the contents of each test tube are spread on the surface of an agar plate

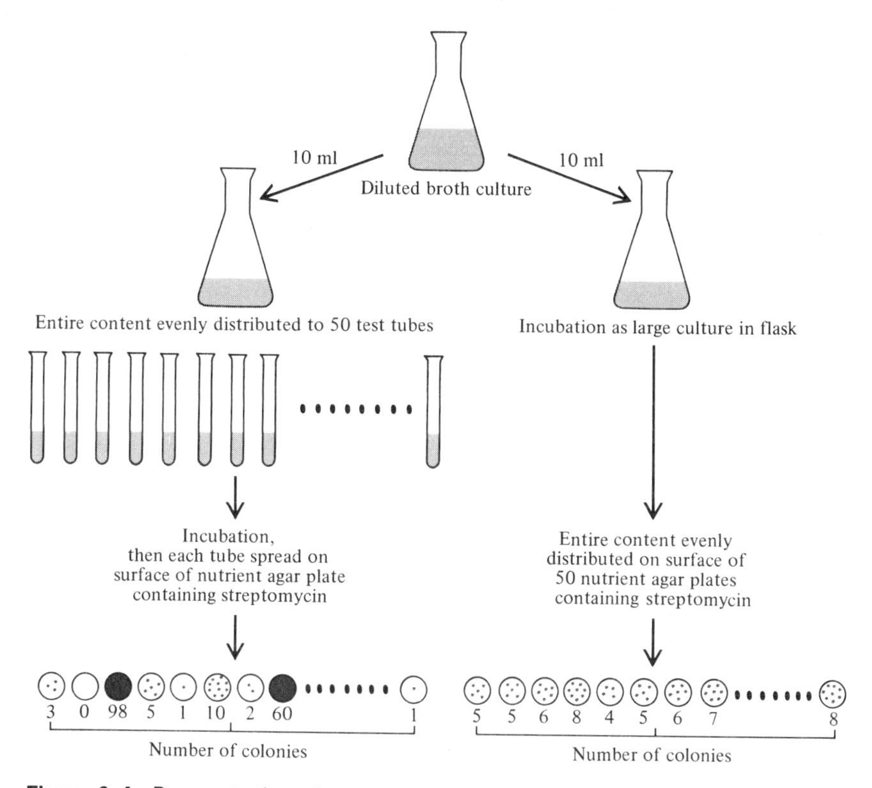

Figure 3-4 Demonstration of spontaneous mutation by fluctuation analysis.

containing streptomycin. Likewise, the entire content of the flask is evenly distributed over the surface of 50 agar plates containing streptomycin. The plates are incubated and the number and distribution of streptomycin-resistant colonies noted.

The results show that approximately the same number of streptomycin-resistant colonies grow on each of the 50 plates that are inoculated from the flask. On the other hand, plates receiving the contents of the individual test tubes show great variation in numbers of resistant colonies. Some plates contain no resistant colonies, while others contain widely varying numbers of resistant colonies (Fig. 3-4).

If the presence or application of the selective agent causes the mutation to resistance, similar numbers of mutants would be expected in all culture samples tested, test tubes or flasks. However, if the mutants occur as spontaneous chance events prior to exposure to the selective agent, great variation in the number of resistant mutants would be expected among the test tube cultures. The variation in the number of resistant mutants depends upon (1) whether or not mutation occurs in a particular test tube culture and (2) the time during incubation when the mutation appears. A large number of mutants indicates that the mutational event occurred early in the incubation period of the culture and was followed by the continued growth of the mutant cells.

The results of the fluctuation analysis indicate that resistant mutants do, in fact, occur as spontaneous, rare events and exist prior to the exposure to a selective agent.

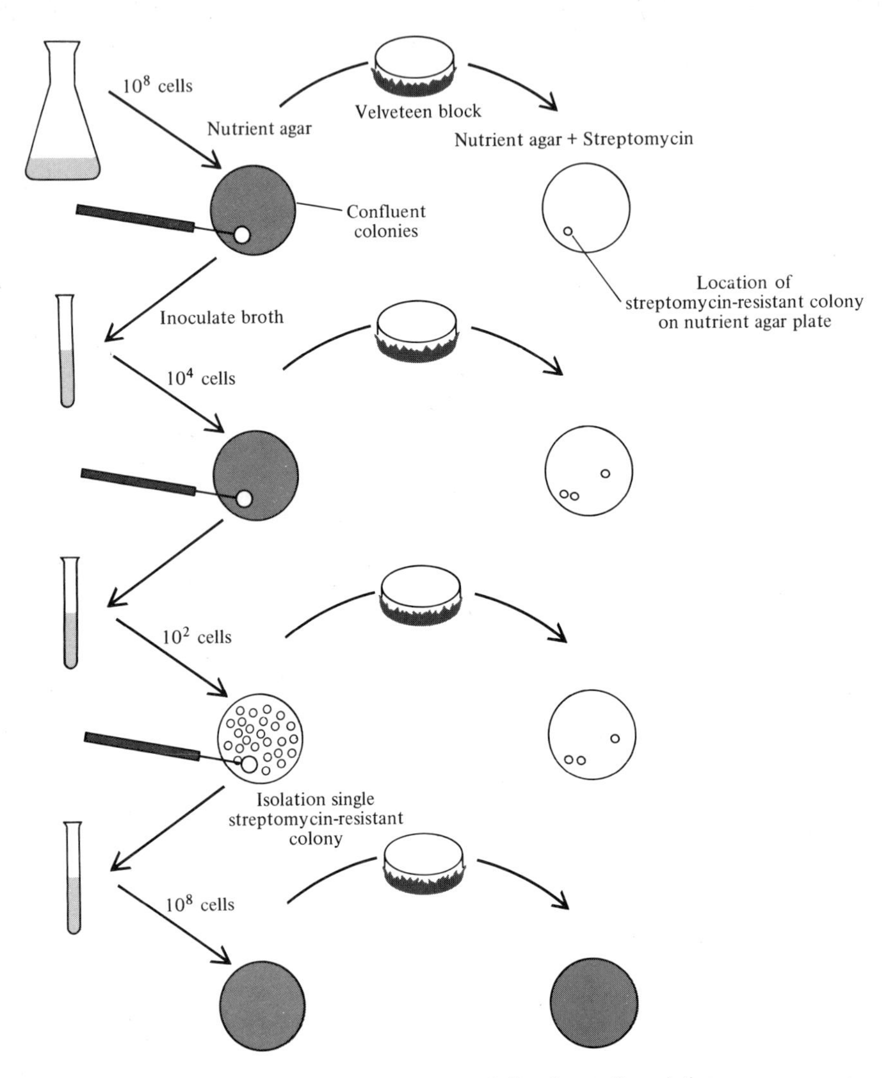

Figure 3-5 Demonstration of spontaneous mutation by replica plating.

Evidence Derived by Replica Plating The essential features of the Lederberg and Lederberg technique have been described previously. The procedure makes it possible (1) to identify streptomycin-resistant mutants in a population of cells that previously had not been exposed to streptomycin and (2) to obtain a pure culture of the streptomycin-resistant mutant in the complete absence of streptomycin as a selective agent. Thus, replica plating provides direct proof that mutations arise as random events in the absence of exposure to the selective agent.

The procedure involves growing a large population of bacterial cells on the surface of a nutrient agar plate. The presence of streptomycin-resistant mutants can be demonstrated by gently touching the bacterial growth with a velveteen-covered block and producing an identical impression of the colonies on a second nutrient agar plate containing streptomycin. In this way, the position of the streptomycin-resistant mutant colony, within the confluent growth of bacteria on the original nutrient agar plate, is identified. Then, from the nutrient agar plate, a sample of the resistant mutant colony is picked with a needle and inoculated into nutrient broth. At this point, it is impossible to pick only the resistant mutant because the bacterial growth is confluent and because sensitive cells are carried over into the broth along with the resistant mutants. Nonetheless, after growth the culture will contain a greater number of mutants. Consequently, the broth culture can be diluted prior to inoculation of the next pair of nutrient agar plates, a procedure designed to increase the probability of obtaining a clone of bacterial mutants. Serial repetition of the procedure eventually results in the isolation of discrete colonies of streptomycin-resistant mutants. Then, of course, one of the streptomycin-resistant colonies can be picked and grown as a pure culture without ever having been in contact with streptomycin (Fig. 3-5).

Types of Spontaneous Mutations

Mutations that arise under natural or under standard laboratory conditions in nutrient broth are called *spontaneous mutations.* The mechanism by which these mutations originate is not certain but may be influenced by a variety of factors such as heat, products of intermediary metabolism, radiation, or errors in DNA replication.

A spontaneous mutation can result from unstable shifts of hydrogen atoms on purine (guanine, adenine) and pyrimidine (cytosine, thymine) bases, resulting in codon changes. For example, if, during replication of DNA, the hydrogen atom at one position of adenine shifts to another position, then adenine will pair with cytosine instead of thymine. During the next round of DNA replication, cytosine pairs with its normal partner guanine, so that the original adenine-thymine (A-T) base pair is now replaced by the guanine-cytosine (G-C) pair and the code is permanently altered.

Point Mutations A change in a single base pair produces a *point mutation.* This may occur by (1) substitution of one base pair for another base pair, (2) insertion of an extra base pair, and (3) loss of a base pair (Fig. 3-6).

A point mutation may cause a relatively benign amino acid change, resulting in an altered protein that remains fully functional. This is called a *silent mutation.* On the other hand, a critical amino acid may be affected, resulting in a nonfunctional protein. If the protein is involved in a vital function, the result is a lethal mutation.

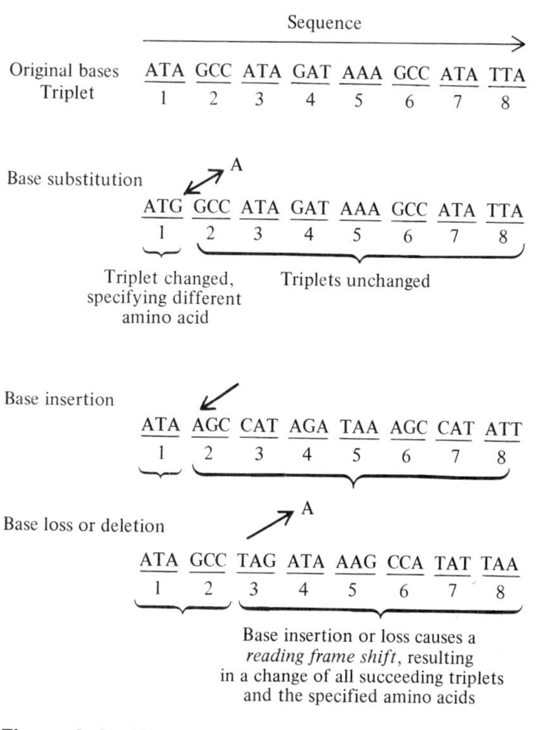

Figure 3-6 Alteration of nucleotides resulting in point mutations.

Point mutations associated with the insertion or the loss of a base pair produce *reading frame shifts,* or shifts in the sequence of bases being read. From the point of mutation the triplet composition differs from the original code. Whether or not the mutation is lethal depends on the length and nature of the garbled information.

Deletion Mutations Another class of mutation results from the elimination of genetic information from the chromosome and is called a *deletion mutation.* The segment of DNA deleted may involve a single base pair or thousands of base pairs.

Mutagens

Certain chemical and physical agents, called *mutagens,* or *mutagenic agents,* are known to induce mutations and increase the rate of mutation several thousandfold over the spontaneous rate occurring under natural conditions. These mutagens produce various chemical changes in DNA that can be analyzed and are, therefore, of great value in understanding the molecular aspects of mutation.

Base Analogues The base analogue 5-bromouracil resembles thymine. When the mutagen is present in the medium during growth and DNA replication, it is incorporated into the DNA molecule in place of thymine. The keto form of 5-bromouracil readily pairs with adenine but may undergo tautomerism to the enol form which more readily pairs with guanine instead of adenine. During the next round of replication, the guanine will pair with its normal partner cytosine on one of the DNA strands. Thus, mutation results from the substitution of a G-C pair for an A-T pair (Fig. 3-7).

The base analogue 2-aminopurine resembles adenine and may also bring about mutation by substitution when it pairs with cytosine, finally

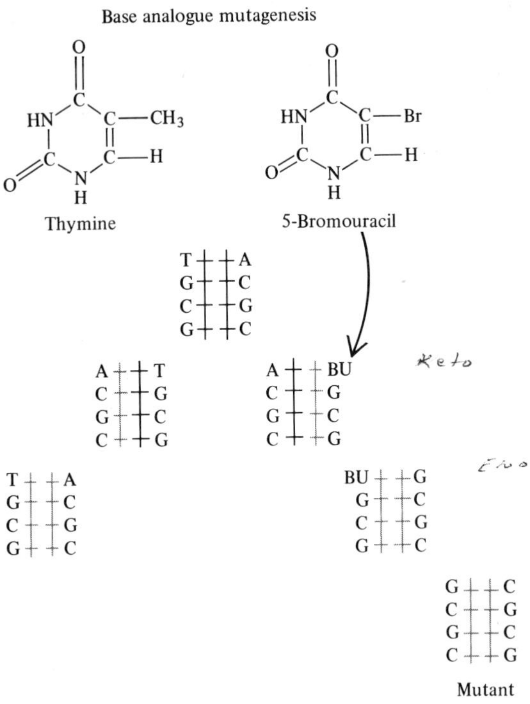

Base analogue mutagenesis

Thymine

5-Bromouracil

Mutant

Figure 3-7 Point mutation by base analogue (5-bromouracil) substitution.

substituting a G-C pair for the original A-T pair.

It should be noted that the base analogues are mutagenic only during DNA replication.

The base analogues provide examples of *transitional mutations (transitions)* in which one purine-pyrimidine base pair is replaced by another. For example, A-T is replaced by G-C or G-C by A-T in such a way that a purine in one strand is replaced by another purine, and a pyrimidine in the other strand is replaced by another pyrimidine.

In the case of *transversional mutations (transversions)* a purine-pyrimidine base pair is replaced by a pyrimidine-purine base pair, for example, A-T to C-G. Although transversions are known to occur, the mechanism is unknown, and no mutagens are known that selectively favor transversions.

Nitrous Acid Other mutagenic agents, including nitrous acid, act directly on nonreplicating DNA, altering the bases in such a way that they do not pair properly. For example, nitrous acid converts adenine to hypoxanthine by oxidative deamination. The hypoxanthine resembles guanine, and this causes the formation of a G-C pair in place of the original A-T pair. Nitrous acid may also react with cytosine and cause the formation of an A-T pair in place of G-C.

Several mutagens, including nitrous acid, may also react with both strands of the DNA molecule, producing cross-links. The cross-links prevent unwinding of the DNA, which is an essential part of DNA replication. The affected segment is therefore not replicated and is lost to the chromosome, resulting in a deletion mutation.

Ultraviolet Irradiation DNA bases strongly absorb radiations of wavelengths of 260 nm, leading to chemical alteration and point mutations. The best-known effect of ultraviolet irradiation on nucleotide bases is the dimerization of two adjacent thymine residues on the same DNA strand. Thymine dimers prevent normal replication of the DNA because no normal base can pair with them, resulting in mutation. It is believed that ultraviolet irradiation probably produces other changes in DNA, leading to mutations, but the mechanisms are not well understood.

Ionizing Radiations X-rays may produce mutations by chemically altering bases (point mutations) or by breaking the "backbone" of the DNA molecule by disrupting one or both strands (deletion mutations). Although not well understood, x-rays appear to produce excitation of chemical groups in the DNA, thereby creating highly reactive radicals in the surrounding water which lead to the hydration of thymine and the deamination of cytosine.

Acridine Dyes The acridine dyes can insert between two DNA bases and push them apart. During replication of DNA an extra base can be inserted where the acridine is located, thus lengthening the DNA by one base and shifting the reading frame from that point onward. On the other hand, the presence of acridine may prevent incorporation of a base that would otherwise have been inserted into the DNA, thus shortening the DNA by one base and also causing a shift of the reading frame.

Mutation Rates

Spontaneous mutations occur at relatively constant rates for a particular characteristic in a given bacterial strain. The mutation rate expresses the probability that a specific determinant in any one bacterium in the population will mutate during the generation time of the dividing bacteria. For example, in the *E. coli* gene governing the synthesis of histidine, a mutation rate of 1×10^{-6} for the mutation his^+ (prototroph) to his^- (auxotroph) means that when a population of 1×10^6 cells divides to form a population of 2×10^6 cells, *on the average,* one his^- mutant is formed. The mutation rate is for the histidine gene only and has no influence on the rate at which other genes in the same population of cells mutate.

The various characteristics of a given cell are subject to mutation at different frequencies. For example, in *E. coli* the mutation to histidine dependence ($his^+ \rightarrow his^-$) occurs at a rate of 1×10^{-6}, but the mutation to galactose dependence ($gal^+ \rightarrow gal^-$) takes place at a rate of 1×10^{-10}. Thus, the various genes in a cell mutate at rates characteristic for the particular gene.

Since mutations occur independently of each other, it is highly unlikely that any two mutations will occur in a single bacterium. The probability can be estimated as the product of the individual mutation rates. For example, consider that gene A has a mutation rate of 1×10^{-6} and gene B a rate of 1×10^{-9}. The probability of simultaneous mutation of both genes in the same bacterial cell is 1×10^{-15}.

Phenotypic Expression of Mutations

In considering the expression of mutation, it is important to keep in mind the fact that most bacteria contain two to four identical nuclei or chromosomes during the exponential phase of growth. In addition, bacterial cells are usually *haploid*, carrying only one representative of each genetic locus per chromosome.

Two kinds of mutation may be considered: (1) the mutation from prototrophy to auxotrophy (e.g., his$^+$ to his$^-$), or loss mutation which is the loss of a gene product, and (2) the mutation from auxotrophy to prototrophy (e.g., his$^-$ to his$^+$), or gain mutation which is the gain of a gene product.

The phenotypic expression of a mutation may be immediate or delayed in a quadrinucleated cell, depending upon the particular kind of mutation involved. In the case of a loss mutation occurring in a quadrinucleated his$^+$ cell, the mutation first occurs in just one nucleus or chromosome, and the cell becomes a *heterokaryon.* The mutated nucleus can no longer code for the synthesis of histidine (his$^-$), which is an essential nutrient for growth. However, the other nuclei are still capable of coding for the synthesis of histidine (his$^+$), and the essential nutrient is produced.

With ensuing nuclear replication and cellular division, two generations are required before the originally mutated cell becomes a *homokaryon*—i.e., contains identical his$^-$ nuclei—and the mutant clone is established. A *clone* is a population of genetically identical cells arising from a single cell following numerous divisions. The cell cannot synthesize histidine, and as soon as any carryover is exhausted, the cell ceases to grow unless histidine is supplied in the growth medium.

In the case of a loss mutation, a *segregation lag* of at least two generations is required before nuclear segregation reaches a degree sufficient to produce the homokaryon essential for the phenotypic expression of the loss mutation. Thus, there is a *phenotypic lag* of two generations (Fig. 3-8*A*).

In the case of a gain mutation, there is essentially no delay, or phenotypic lag, and the phenotypic expression may be considered immediate. For example, an auxotroph mutates to prototrophy; and, although only one chromosome of four is capable of coding for the synthesis of histidine, the cell receives its essential nutrient. However, as in the case of the loss mutation, a segregation lag of two generations is still required before the heterokaryon forms a homokaryon (Fig. 3-8*B*).

Back Mutations (Reversions)

Mutants may revert to the phenotype of the prototroph from which they originated by a process known as *back mutation,* or *reversion.* One way this can be accomplished is for another mutation to restore the altered nucleotide of the mutant to the original form *(true reversion).*

In addition, the phenotype may be restored by a mechanism that does not reestablish the original nucleotide. Instead of involving the same nucleotide region, *suppressor mutations* negate the effect of the first mutation and restore the original phenotype (Fig. 3-9).

Mechanisms by which suppressor mutations can exert their effect include (1) replacement of

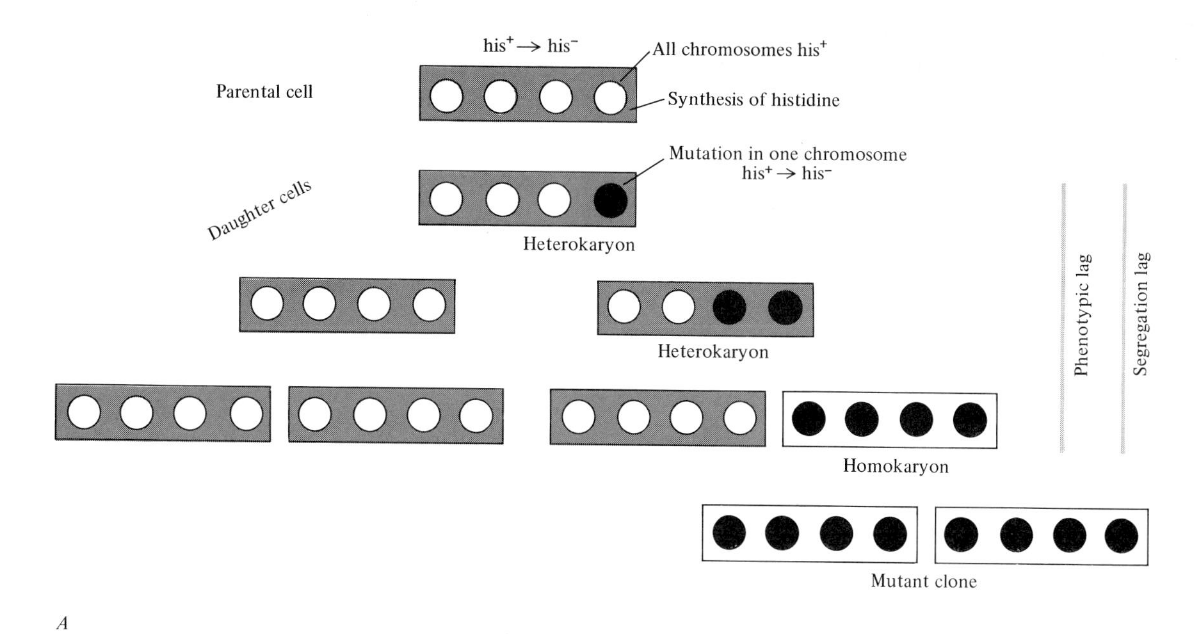

Figure 3-8 Expression of loss *(A)* or gain *(B)* mutations.

the altered codon with another that is less deleterious to protein function, (2) production of a reading frame shift in the opposite direction, and (3) a change in tRNA so that the proper amino acid for the synthesis of the functional enzyme is inadvertently provided. Thus, suppressor mutations act indirectly to abolish the effect of the original mutation. Rarely, however, is the product of the suppressor mutation as fully functional as that of a true reversion to the original prototroph.

GENETIC RECOMBINATION

In addition to mutation, a bacterium can become genetically modified by mechanisms involving the transfer of genetic material from one cell to another. In the process, only the recipient cell is genetically altered, becoming a cell that is genotypically different from either the donor or the recipient cell. Thus, a *recombinant* chromosome is formed from DNA derived from two different parental cells. This process is known as *genetic recombination* (Fig. 3-10).

On the basis of the available experimental data genetic recombination is believed to occur in the following manner. After entry into the recipient cell, a fragment of donor DNA aligns itself at a homologous area of the recipient chromosome, i.e., a region of the chromosome which has a similarity in base sequence with the donor fragment. Following the pairing of bases, the recombinant chromosome is formed as a consequence of chromosomal breakage and exchange of segments, a process that involves a complicated series of enzyme-mediated reactions including the hydrolysis, synthesis, and sealing of DNA. Since recombination affects only one nucleus in the multinucleated recipient cell, nuclear segregation of the heterokaryon must precede the formation of the homokaryotic recombinant. Bacterial recombination can be achieved by three processes which differ in the mechanism by which DNA is transferred from donor to recipient bacteria.

1 *Transformation* requires free DNA. Experimentally, DNA can be extracted from donor bacteria and mixed with viable recipient bacteria.
2 *Conjugation* involves the mating of bacteria during which DNA passes from donor to recipient bacteria through a conjugal tube.

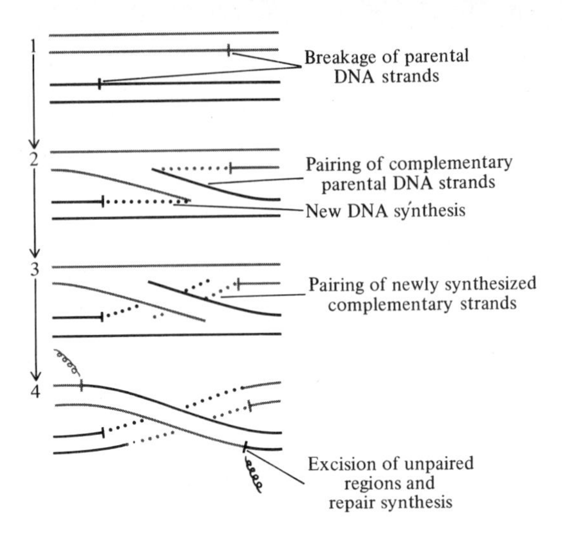

Figure 3-10 Possible sequence of events accounting for genetic recombination. (*Modified from H. L. K. Whitehouse, Nature, 199:1034–1040, 1963.*)

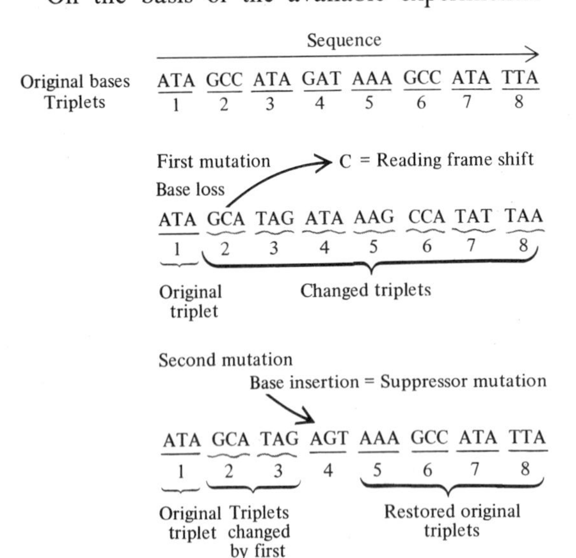

Figure 3-9 Partial restoration of genetic information by suppressor mutation.

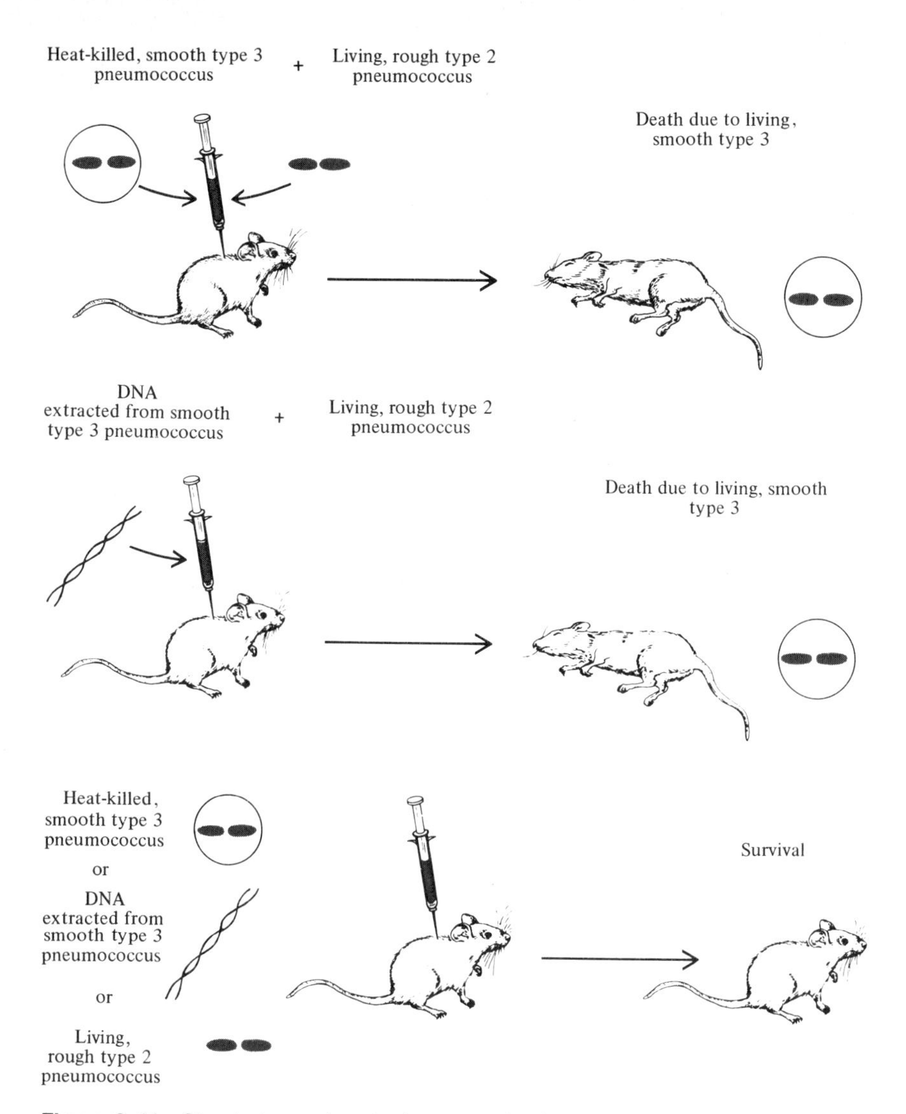

Figure 3-11 Classical experiments demonstrating bacterial transformation in mice.

3 *Transduction* refers to a process in which phage particles (bacterial viruses) carry fragments of bacterial DNA from a donor to a recipient cell.

BACTERIAL TRANSFORMATION

The Classical Experiments

Transformation has been observed to occur in a limited range of bacteria, principally in the genera *Diplococcus, Hemophilus, Bacillus, Streptococcus, Neisseria,* and *Rhizobium.* When viable bacteria take up DNA derived from a closely related donor, homokaryotic recombinants can arise following genetic recombination *(bacterial transformation).* The hereditary change which appears in the recipient is stable and can be readily passed on to the progeny.

The early experiments of Griffith, Avery, MacLeod, and McCarty which led to the discovery of bacterial transformation employed the pneumococcus *(D. pneumoniae)*. Virulent pneumococci possess a capsule and form smooth (S) colonies when grown on agar. Because of the chemical variation in the composition of the capsular polysaccharide, the pneumococcus exhibits many different antigenic types (e.g., type 1, type 2, type 3, etc.). The ability to produce a particular capsular polysaccharide is genetically determined, a property which may be lost as a consequence of mutation. Inability to synthesize capsular polysaccharide causes the pneumococcus to become avirulent and to grow as a dry, granular or rough (R) colony on agar.

Bacterial transformation can be demonstrated by injecting mice with a combination of viable rough pneumococci derived from smooth type 2 and with heat-killed pneumococci prepared from smooth type 3. Culture of the blood of dying mice yields only smooth type 3 pneumococci. Thus, the viable rough pneumococci derived from smooth type 2 are transformed to viable smooth type 3 pneumococci (Fig. 3-11).

In vitro extracted and purified DNA obtained from smooth type 3 pneumococci can transform viable rough pneumococci derived from smooth type 2, resulting in the formation of smooth virulent type 3 pneumococcal recombinants. The fact that all transforming activity is lost in the presence of deoxyribonuclease (DNase) proved for the first time that genetic information in the cell is contained in DNA.

Double Transformation

Although all genetic markers have an equal chance of being transferred by transformation, closely linked genes may be passed simultaneously. As a result of the fragmentation of the donor chromosome during the extraction procedure, adjacent genes are likely to be present on a single piece of transforming DNA. Consequently, if two genes are closely linked, double transformation is frequent. On the other hand, when two genes are located some distance from each other on the chromosome, they are found on different DNA fragments, and the probability of double transformation is much lower.

It is important to recognize that the linkage of two genetic markers on a single fragment of transforming DNA makes it possible for a cell to lose one function and gain another. Thus, a DNA donor fragment containing genetic markers for streptomycin resistance (str^R) and inability to ferment mannitol (mtl^-) yields str^R mtl^- recombinants when added to a streptomycin-sensitive (str^S) and mannitol-fermenting (mtl^+) recipient.

Uptake and Penetration of DNA

Much information concerning the initial events in transformation has been gained by growing donor bacteria in ^{32}P, thereby labeling the DNA. By following the labeled DNA, as well as genetic markers, it has been observed that the donor DNA fragments first are bound to and then penetrate into the recipient cell. Studies on transverse fragmentation of DNA indicate that transformation is dependent upon fragments with a molecular weight of at least 5×10^5 (presumably the minimum weight of a single gene).

Heating the DNA at 100°C results in separation of the two strands. If the DNA is then cooled rapidly, the two strands fail to reunite and are inactive in transformation experiments because the DNA is not taken up by recipient bacteria. However, if the heated DNA is cooled slowly, the strands reunite, are taken up, and transformation ensues. Thus, double-stranded DNA is necessary for uptake by recipient bacteria.

The frequency of transformation is generally proportional to the concentration of DNA employed, but at higher DNA concentrations a plateau is reached in which the number of transformed cells fails to increase. Penetration of donor DNA proceeds rapidly, as is noted by the effect of DNase on the process. Transforming activity of DNA is destroyed if DNase is present when donor DNA is mixed with recipient cells. On the other hand, if DNase is withheld for a few seconds after donor DNA makes contact with recipient cells, transformation occurs.

Eclipse Period

Shortly after penetration, the donor DNA fragment undergoes a change and can be shown to have lost its transforming activity if it is again extracted from the recipient cell. This is known as the *eclipse period* of bacterial transformation. Experiments with ^{32}P-labeled donor DNA indicate that only one strand is conserved in the recipient cell. The other strand appears to be broken down to low molecular weight products.

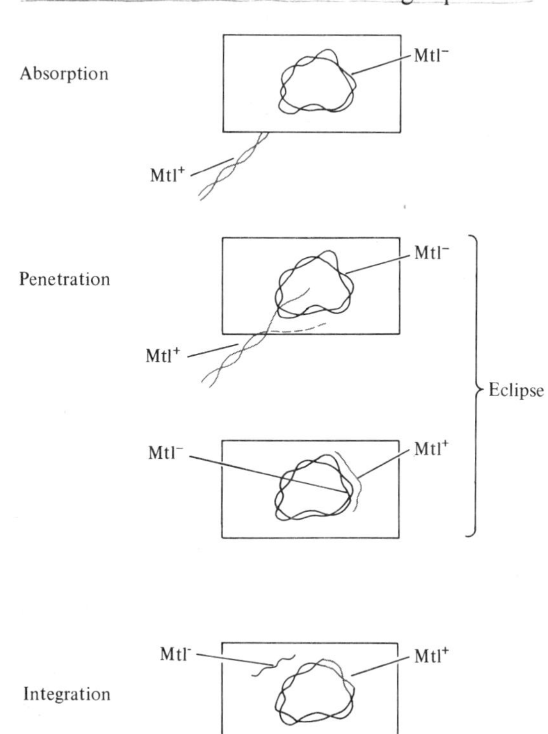

Figure 3-12 Sequence of events involved in bacterial transformation.

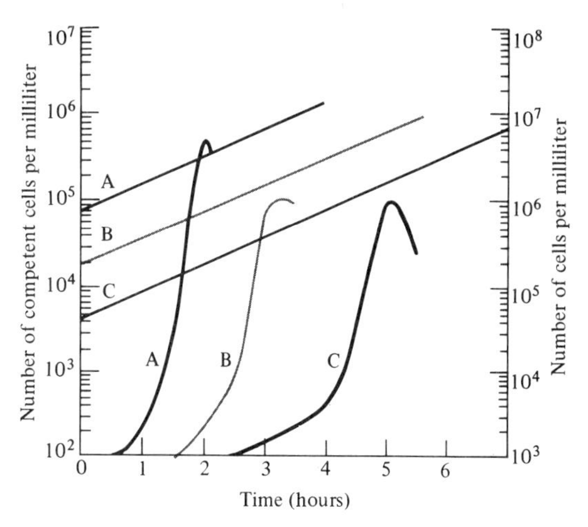

Figure 3-13 Relation of competence to cell concentration in bacterial transformation is illustrated. Three cultures of pneumococci *(A, B, C)* differ in their initial cell concentrations. The time required to reach peak competence (scale at left) varies approximately inversely with concentration (scale at right): the lower the concentration, the later the peak. *[A. Tomasz, Sci. Am., 220 (No. 1):38-44, 1969.]*

Subsequently, the surviving single strand of donor DNA is incorporated into the DNA of the recipient cell, is linked to other genes, and achieves potential transforming power (Fig. 3-12).

Competent Cells

A recipient cell that is able to take up donor DNA and undergo transformation is said to be a *competent cell.* Initially, in a freshly inoculated culture, the cells are incompetent. After growth of the culture, competence appears to be developed as a function of population density. Thus, when the cell concentration reaches a critical level, most of the cells suddenly become competent but almost as abruptly become incompetent (Fig. 3-13).

Competence Factor

Competent cultures produce a protein that can induce competence in incompetent cells *(competence factor).* The factor can be inactivated by proteolytic enzymes but not by RNase or DNase. The lack of competence early in the growth of a culture may be viewed as a period when the competence factor is in low concentration. When a sufficient concentration of the factor is attained, most of the cells become competent. The actual change produced by the factor that enables cells to absorb DNA remains unknown. However, an exclusive affinity for DNA is developed. Consequently, the change is believed to involve some modification of the cell surface in association with the development of receptor sites and/or increased permeability to large DNA molecules (Fig. 3-14).

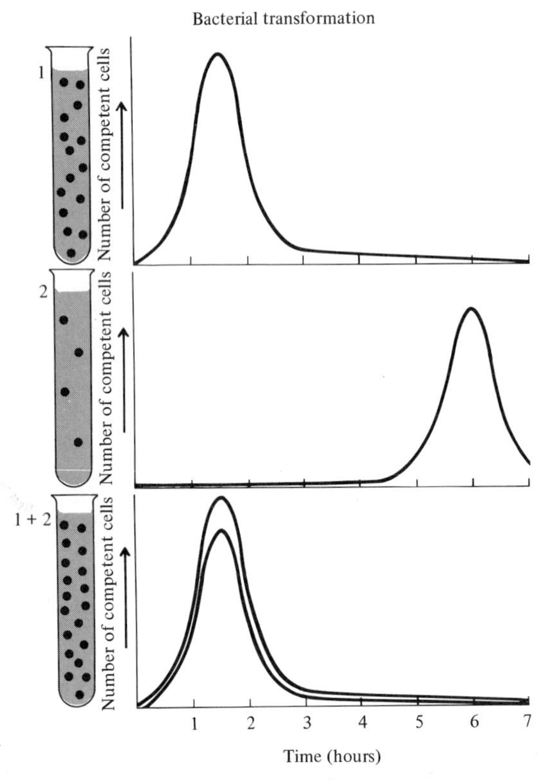

Figure 3-14 Induction of competence in low-concentration bacterial cultures. Induction of competence is demonstrated by growing two strains of pneumococci of different concentrations in control cultures (top and middle) and in a mixed culture (bottom). The graphs show, for each strain, the number of cells that are found to be competent for transformation. In the high-concentration culture (1) the degree of competence increases rapidly to a peak (top). The low-concentration culture (2), grown alone, takes a longer time to reach its peak of competence (middle). Yet, when the two strains are grown in the same tube, cells of the second strain "copy" the competence curve of the first strain (bottom). *[A. Tomasz, Sci. Am., 220 (No. 1):38–44, 1969.]*

CONJUGATION

A second mechanism whereby genetic information can be transferred from a donor to a recipient bacterium occurs through a mating process known as conjugation. Conjugation has been demonstrated in a limited number of bacteria, especially *E. coli,* and also *Salmonella, Shigella, Pseudomonas, Vibrio,* and *Streptomyces.*

The original experiments that demonstrated conjugation made use of doubly auxotrophic mutants of *E. coli* K 12 derived by successive treatment with a mutagenic agent. The auxotrophs differed from each other with respect to four genes, each concerned with a different growth factor requirement. One auxotroph (bio^- met^- pro^+ thr^+) required biotin and methionine as growth factors, while the other auxotroph (bio^+ met^+ pro^- thr^-) required proline and threonine as growth factors.

The two auxotrophs were mixed together in complete medium and incubated overnight. The culture was then centrifuged, washed free of the complete medium, and plated on minimal agar plates. The result was that prototrophic colonies (bio^+ met^+ pro^+ thr^+) appeared on the minimal agar, suggesting that genetic recombination had taken place (Fig. 3-15).

As controls, the auxotrophs were individually plated on minimal agar, and no prototrophic colonies were observed, indicating that simultaneous reversion of two genes did not occur.

The possibility of simultaneous reversion must be considered to be remote; if the mutation rate of bio^- to bio^+ is 1×10^{-7} and met^-

to met$^+$ is 1×10^{-7}, the simultaneous mutations would be likely to occur at a rate of 1×10^{-14}, the product of the individual mutation rates.

Cell Contact

Various experiments and observations have made it clear that the process of conjugation requires direct cell-to-cell contact.

In the famous "U-tube" experiment, one arm of the U tube was inoculated with one of the auxotrophs, and the other arm was inoculated with the other auxotroph. The arms were separated by a sintered glass filter having a pore size of 0.1 μm, thus preventing direct contact of the auxotrophs. However, the fluids of the two arms were passed freely from one arm to the other under pressure. Following incubation, prototrophic colonies failed to develop when samples from each arm were plated on minimal agar, indicating that mating and genetic recombination did not occur.

Sex Factor (F Factor)

Various experimental manipulations subsequently revealed that one of the auxotrophs functioned as the donor and the other as the recipient, thus implying *polarity,* or *one-way transfer,* of genetic material. The donor state is conferred on a bacterial cell by virtue of the presence of a *sex factor F,* originally called a fertility factor. Conventionally, donor cells are designated F$^+$, while recipient cells which cannot act as donors are F$^-$. Thus, F$^+$ × F$^-$ crosses are fertile, whereas F$^-$ × F$^-$ crosses are sterile. Under appropriate mating conditions, the F factor is transferred to F$^-$ cells at a high rate (1 per 10 parent cells), and in the process the F$^-$ cells become F$^+$, having received the sex factor (Fig. 3-16).

The sex factor has been characterized as an extrachromosomal genetic complex composed of circular DNA and capable of autonomous

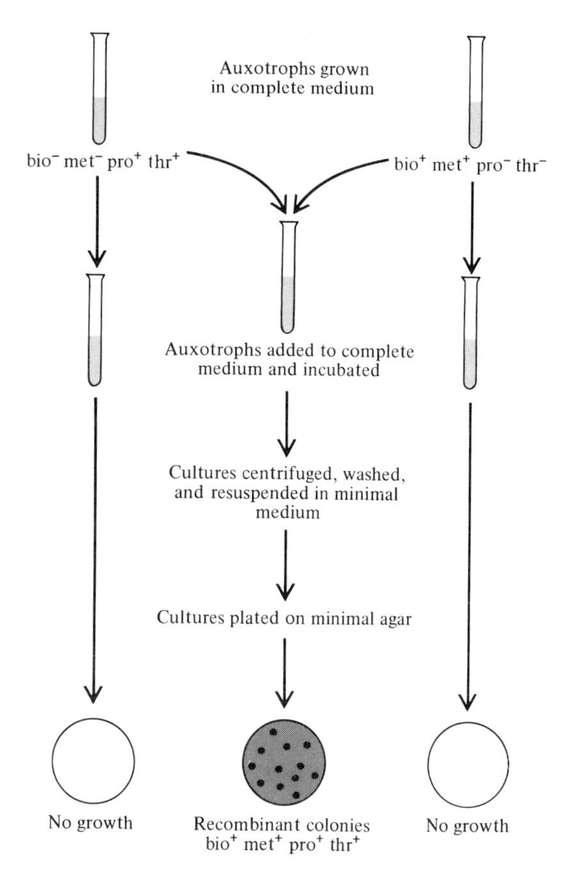

Figure 3-15 Conjugation of doubly auxotrophic mutants, yielding prototrophic recombinants.

replication. Its size is estimated to be approximately 2.5×10^5 base pairs. In addition to genes concerned with the regulation of its own replication, the sex factor possesses genes for the synthesis of *sex pili,* or *F pili,* to which male-specific, spherical RNA-containing phages and filamentous DNA-containing phages adsorb. The sex factor also carries genes that specify the synthesis of an antigenic surface component that may act to lower the negative electrical charge on the surface of the donor bacterium so that it can make intimate contact with recipient bacteria after random collision.

As a genetic structure, the sex factor is subject to mutation. In the case of spontaneous loss

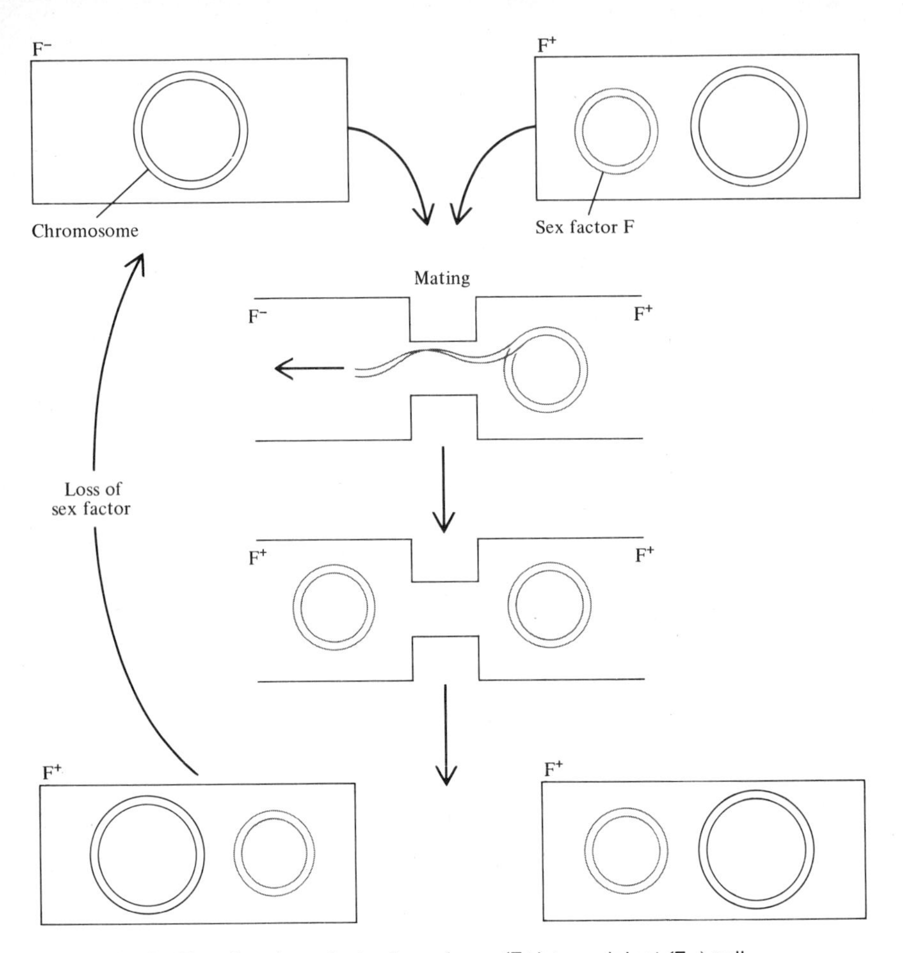

Figure 3-16 Transfer of sex factor from donor (F^+) to recipient (F^-) cell.

of the sex factor, the cell becomes F^- and ceases to have donor activity. In this F^- state, it can revert to F^+ only when it receives a sex factor from a donor F^+ cell (Fig. 3-16).

High Frequency of Recombination (Hfr) Donor State

When the F^+ sex factor leaves its extrachromosomal position and becomes integrated into the bacterial chromosome in the Hfr state, it acquires the potential for transmitting chromosomal genes to recipient cells during conjugation. The nucleotide sequences of the circular sex factor are homologous with specific base sequences on the circular bacterial chromosome. In the homologous regions, the sex factor and the chromosome adjoin, break open, and after reciprocal crossing-over, the sex factor is inserted into the bacterial chromosome, i.e., becomes integrated (Fig. 3-17).

Following integration, the sex factor is replicated in synchrony with the bacterial chromosome and retains the ability to establish conjugal tubes but loses the capacity to be transmitted to recipient cells independent of

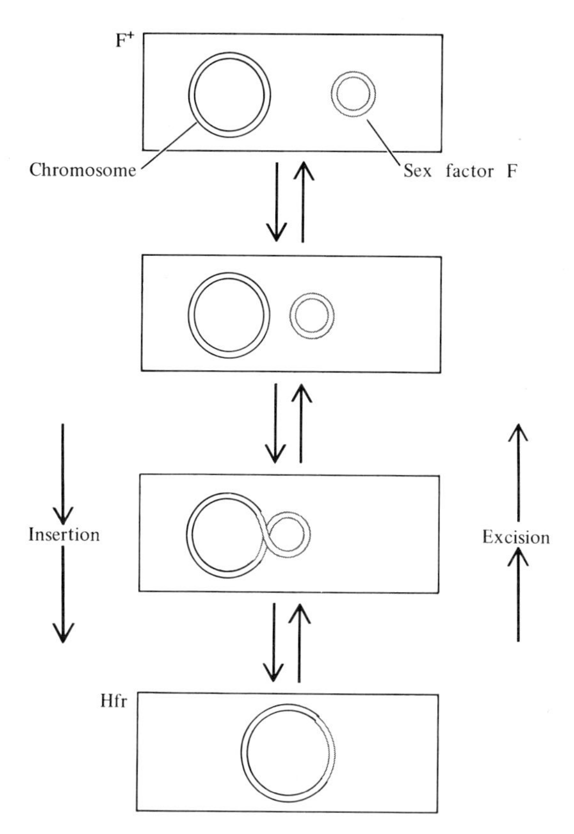

Figure 3–17 Origin of a high frequency recombination (Hfr) strain by integration of sex factor (F) into the chromosome.

other chromosomal genes. Nonetheless, the integrated sex factor (in the Hfr state) may leave the chromosome and reassume extrachromosomal autonomy (F^+).

After insertion of the sex factor into the bacterial chromosome, an F^+ bacterium is converted to a donor state that has a high frequency of recombination (Hfr). In contrast with F^+ donors, Hfr donors rarely transfer the sex factor to F^- recipients. However, the Hfr donor is more than 1,000 times as active as the F^+ donor in transferring chromosomal genes to recipient F^- cells. In fact, the observed low incidence of chromosomal gene transfer in $F^+ \times F^-$ crosses can be accounted for by a spontaneous shift to the integrated Hfr state in a few F^+ cells.

The Conjugal Tube

Whenever F^+ or Hfr donors are mating (conjugating) with appropriate recipients, electron photomicrographs reveal a connecting bridge or *conjugal tube* between donor and recipient. Electron microscopy has also established that donor bacteria possess a few specialized, hollow filamentous appendages called F pili, or sex pili. It is assumed that F pili serve as the conduit through which DNA passes from donor to recipient cell.

Hfr Transfer of Chromosomal Genes

The specific point at which an Hfr factor is inserted into the bacterial chromosome determines the sequence in which the bacterial genes will be transferred to recipient cells. For any given Hfr donor the sequence will remain constant. However, genetically distinct Hfr factors will integrate at locations on the chromosome where base homology exists, and consequently, the precise linear order in which the genes are transmitted will be different for the several Hfr donors.

Thus, there is a high frequency of recombination observed for those genes which are synthesized first and which represent the leading portion of the chromosome as it passes through the conjugal tube to the recipient cell. Since the Hfr factor is on the last portion of the chromosome to go through the conjugal tube and since random breakage of the fragile chromosome frequently occurs during conjugation, Hfr is rarely transferred to the recipient cell. Before Hfr transfer can be demonstrated, conjugation must continue for about 2 hr.

Transfer of the donor chromosome to the recipient cell is probably activated when the cells collide. At the point where the sex factor is located, circular donor DNA is attached to the

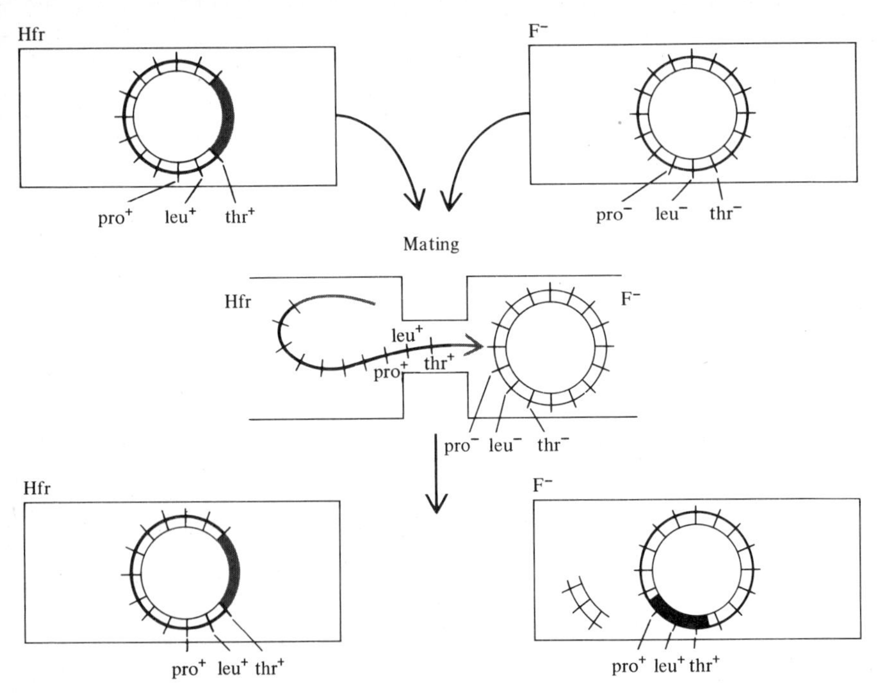

Figure 3-18 Chromosomal transfer from high frequency recombination (Hfr) donor strain to F^- recipient cell during conjugation.

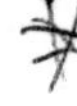

cell membrane. As replication of donor DNA proceeds, one of the daughter strands along with one of the parental strands is driven through the conjugal tube as double-stranded DNA into the F^- cell. The other daughter strand remains with the other parental strand in the donor cell (Figs. 3-18 and 3-19).

Interrupted Mating Experiments and Genetic Mapping

Mating bacteria are not firmly held together but can be separated easily by agitation with a mixer or Waring blender. Using the blender to separate mating bacteria at various time intervals, it was found that the longer the time between mating and agitation, the greater the number of donor genes that appeared in the F^- recombinant cell. For example, if agitation is delayed for 10 min. after mixing the donor and recipient bacteria, only gene A was transferred. At 14 min., genes A, B, and C were passed, and by 20 min., genes A, B, C, D, E, and F were conveyed.

Such interrupted mating experiments reveal that gene transfer occurs as an oriented process. A given Hfr strain always transfers its genes in a specific, linear order to the recipient cell. The method provides a mechanism for determining the order of the genes on a bacterial chromosome. If it is assumed that the chromosomal thread of genes moves at a constant rate into the recipient cell, then a genetic map can be constructed by using the time of entry as a measure of distance between the genes.

Circularity of the Bacterial Chromosome

A given Hfr strain always transfers its chromosomal genes in the same order, beginning with the same gene. Other Hfr strains transfer genes but differ in regard to the initial genes trans-

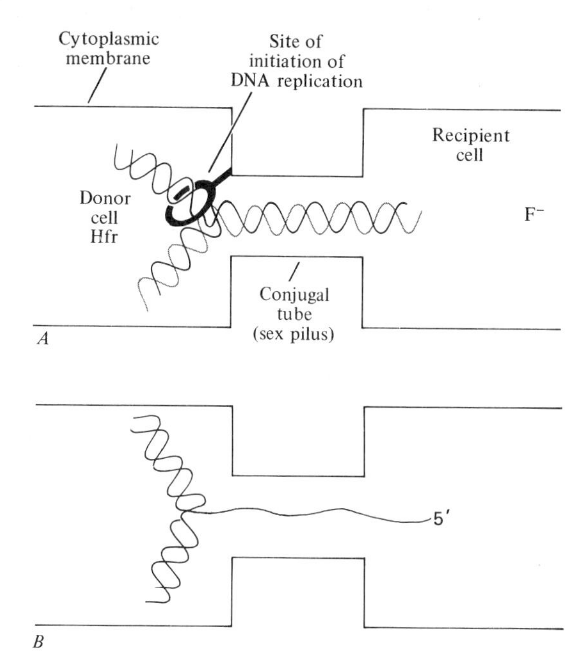

Figure 3-19 Possible mechanisms of DNA transfer during conjugation. *(A) (Modified from F. Jacob, S. Brenner, and F. Cuzin, Cold Spring Harbor Symp. Quant. Biol., 28:329-348, 1963.) (B) (J. D. Watson, Molecular Biology of the Gene, 2d ed. New York, W. A. Benjamin, Inc., 1970, p. 292.)*

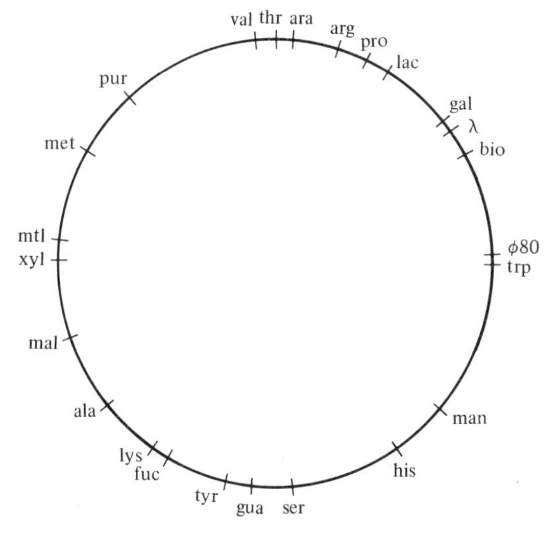

Figure 3-20 Abbreviated genetic map of an *E. coli* chromosome.

ferred, having their own characteristic pattern. Despite differences among a variety of Hfr donors, the position and linear relationship of one gene to another is always the same. For example, Hfr donor 1 may transfer genes in the order A B C D E, Hfr donor 2 transfers them in the order E D C B A, and Hfr donor 3 relays them as C B A E D. Thus, each Hfr donor behaves as though it is formed by the opening of a circular DNA molecule at a given point. Either end of the opened circle might serve as the initiation point for gene transfer, depending upon the particular Hfr strain. From these studies the concept of circularity of the bacterial chromosome evolved and was later confirmed by electron microscopic and autoradiographic studies (Fig. 3-20).

Sexduction (F-duction)

Occasionally, when the Hfr factor is excised from the bacterial chromosome, it takes along one or more of the adjacent genes and becomes an *F prime* (F′) cell. In this condition the circular F′ extrachromosomal complex (F^+ genes together with the companion chromosomal genes) replicates autonomously. Following conjugation with F^- recipients, the F′ complex, including the associated detached chromosomal genes, is transferred with great efficiency, a process known as *sexduction,* or *F-duction* (Fig. 3-21).

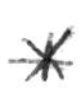

For example, one of the detached chromosomal markers that can be incorporated in an F′ complex is the gene for lactose fermentation (lac^+). When an F′ (lac^+) donor is crossed with an F^- (lac^-) cell, the recipient remains lac^- chromosomally, but the F′ (lac^+) complex replicates extrachromosomally. Thus, the recipient becomes a diploid (lac^+/lac^-) without undergoing genetic recombination. Because the lac^+ gene is dominant over its mutant allele (lac^-), the recipient cell ferments lactose.

Obviously, upon excision different Hfr factors will take along different genes, depending upon their precise points of attachment on the bacte-

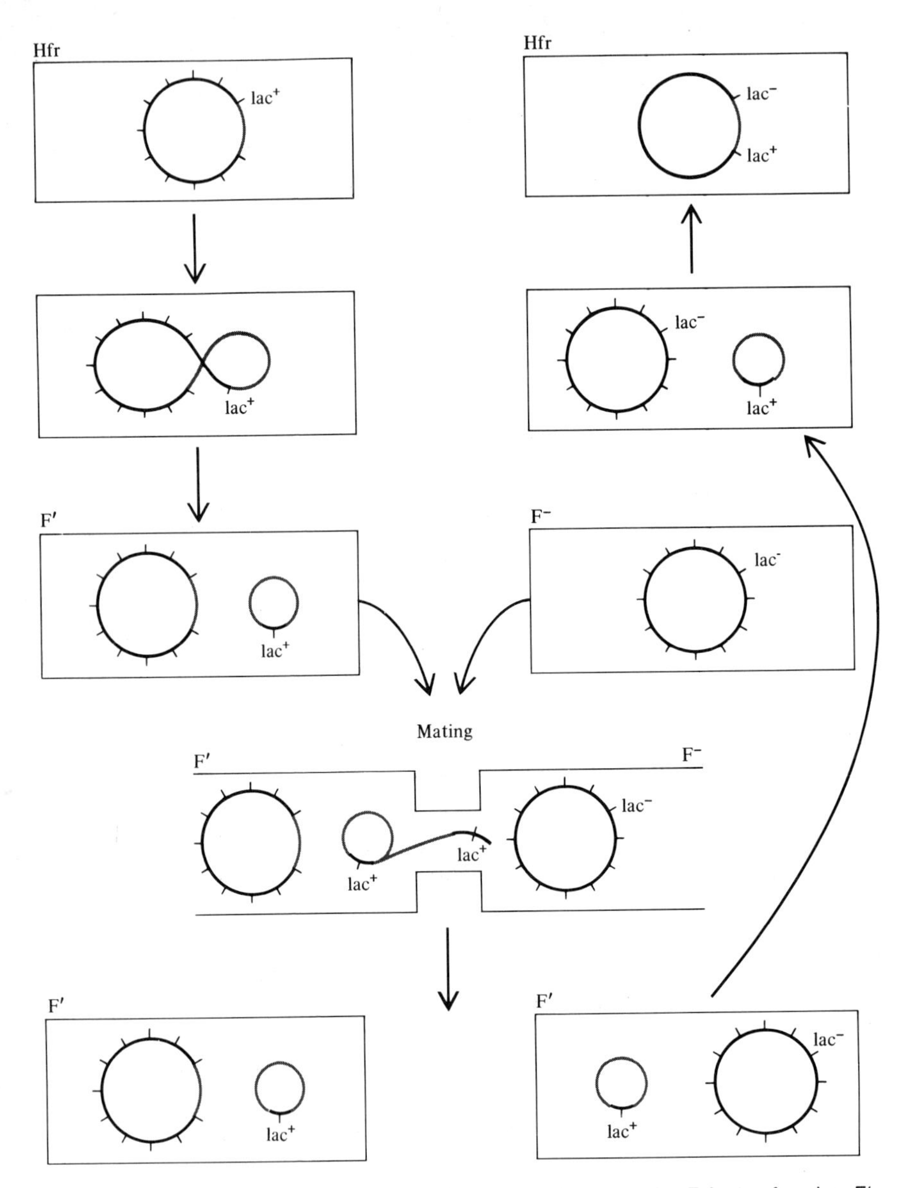

Figure 3-21 Excision of a chromosomal gene together with the F factor forming F′, and its subsequent transfer to a recipient cell (sexduction).

rial chromosome. The autonomous extrachromosomal F′ complex can return to the integrated condition. When this occurs, the F′ complex inserts at the homologous attachment site, the Hfr state is established, and the chromosome gains a gene or genes (Fig. 3-21).

Plasmids

There are a number of genetic elements, classically illustrated by the sex factor of *E. coli,* that can exist in alternate and mutually exclusive states. As autonomous extrachromosal complexes, for example, the F^+ or F' factors promote conjugation and are passed to F^- recipients with high frequency. In the integrated state, the Hfr factor replicates in synchrony with chromosomal genes, promotes conjugation, and provides an efficient mechanism for the transfer of the donor chromosome to F^- recipients.

In the past the term *episome* was used to designate genetic elements that can exist in alternate and mutually exclusive states in bacteria. Recently, however, the terminology has been revised, and the word *plasmid* is applied to define genetic material which can exist as an extrachromosomal complex capable of autonomous replication.

Plasmids may be grouped into those that are transferred by conjugation (sex factors, colicins and bacteriocins, resistance transfer factors) and those that have not been shown to be transferred by conjugation but can be transmitted by phage particles (penicillinase plasmids).

Colicin and Bacteriocin Factors *Colicins* are bactericidal proteins produced by and acting on other members of the family Enterobacteriaceae. Lethal proteins of a similar nature are produced by other bacteria (pyocin by *Pseudomonas aeruginosa* and megacin by *Bacillus megaterium*). Collectively, colicins, pyocins, and megacins are categorized as *bacteriocins.*

Colicins adsorb to specific receptors on the surface of sensitive bacteria. If the receptor sites are modified or lost, the bacteria become resistant to the specific colicin. In addition to host specificity, colicins differ in their diffusibility. Bacteria capable of producing colicins carry the col^+ determinant and are said to be *colicinogenic* or *bacteriocinogenic.* A single bacterium may carry several genetic determinants and consequently may produce several types of colicin. Bacteria possessing a specific col^+ determinant are immune to that colicin but are susceptible to other colicins.

The col^+ factors promote conjugation and are transferred to col^- cells by cellular contact. In some cases, col^+ cells can transfer large chromosomal segments to recipient cells, thus resembling Hfr donors.

Resistance Transfer Factor Of major clinical significance was the discovery that resistance to several antibiotics can be simultaneously acquired by sensitive bacteria. The initial observations of transmissible multiple resistance involved isolates of *Shigella* from cases of bacillary dysentery in Japan. Thereafter, multiple antibiotic resistance spread throughout the world and was found to involve all of the Enterobacteriaceae as well as other bacterial families. In some instances, increased virulence of bacteria has appeared to accompany transfer of drug resistance (Chap. 18).

The initial findings demonstrated that bacteria simultaneously became multiply resistant to sulphonamide, streptomycin, chloramphenicol, and tetracycline. Later it was recognized that the resistance could extend concomitantly to as many as eight antibiotics.

Transfer of multiple drug resistance requires cell contact. As with the F^+ and col^+ factors, the transfer involves conjugation. The sex factor present in the antibiotic-resistant donor cell is called *resistance transfer factor* (RTF). Apparently, the genetic determinants for antibiotic resistance *(r determinants)* either can be linked together in a circular arrangement with RTF (and together are called *R factor*) or can be separate from RTF, each of the genetic elements assuming a circular shape and replicating autonomously. Conjugal transfer of the genetic determinants for antibiotic resistance requires RTF. However, RTF can be transferred separately from donor to recipient cells in a similar fashion to the F^+ factor. In the latter case, the antibiotic-resistant genes continue to replicate in the donor, are phenotypically expressed, and may

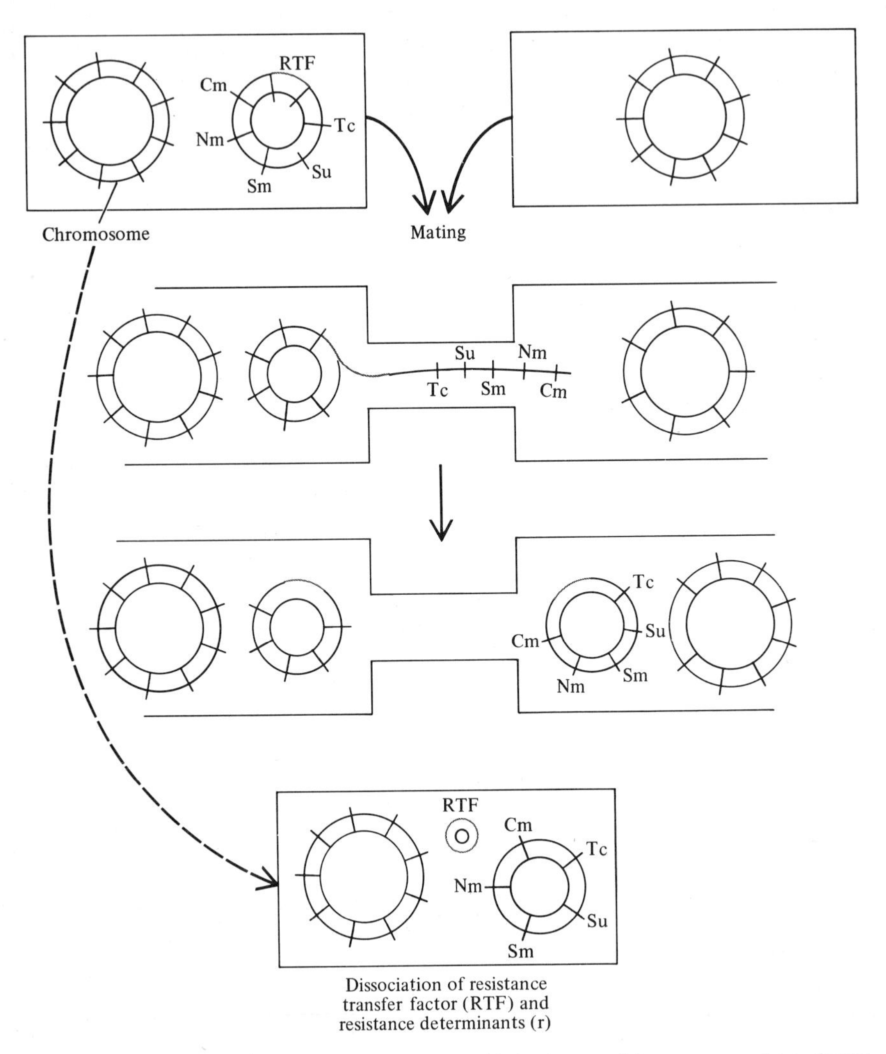

Figure 3-22 Transfer of R factor carrying multiple drug resistance genes from donor to recipient cell.

eventually be transferred to a recipient cell after linkage with an incoming RTF (Fig. 3-22).

Penicillinase Plasmids in Staphylococci Clinically, the resistance of *Staphylococcus aureus* to penicillin is due to the ability to produce penicillinase, an inducible enzyme that destroys the activity of penicillin by opening up the β-lactam ring.

The genetic determinant governing penicillinase synthesis in *S. aureus* is an *autonomously replicating plasmid* that lacks the genes required to establish conjugation and consequently cannot be transmitted by cell contact. However, the penicillinase plasmid can be transferred from bacteria possessing it to nonplasmid-containing bacteria through the intervention of phage particles.

Other genes are closely linked to the penicillinase locus, are an integral part of the plasmid, and often are transmitted with the penicillinase gene. Included in the plasmid are genes that determine resistance to mercuric ions and erythromycin. Penicillinase plasmids found to differ in various isolates of *S. aureus* are distinguished by the genetic determinants they carry as well as by the characteristics of the penicillinase produced.

PHAGE-MEDIATED RECOMBINATION (TRANSDUCTION)

As found in nature, bacteria interact with viruses designated *phage* or *bacteriophage.* There are two basic categories of phage: (1) virulent or lytic and (2) temperate or lysogenic. One or a few closely linked bacterial genes can be transferred by phage from one bacterium to a closely related bacterium which is susceptible to the same phage *(transduction).*

Both virulent and temperate phage can function as transducing agents. Consequently, essential features of the replication of virulent and temperate phage must be considered before an understanding of transduction can be achieved.

VIRULENT PHAGE AND THE LYTIC CYCLE

In infections with virulent phage, the virus diverts the metabolic machinery of the bacterial cell from its normal functions and directs the synthesis of hundreds of new phage particles which are released following lysis, or dissolution, of the bacterium. On the other hand, in infections with temperate phage, the viral genome persists, associates with, and replicates in synchrony with the bacterial chromosome without synthesizing new phage particles or causing the lysis of the bacterium.

Phage Structure

Electron photomicrographic techniques have demonstrated that phage may be spherical, rod-shaped, or filamentous and may possess a complex tail assembly. Notwithstanding their morphological appearance, however, all infectious phage particles are composed of an outer protein coat, or capsid, and an inner core of nucleic acid.

The most thoroughly studied phages are those of the T-even series, T2 and T4, that infect *E. coli.* As revealed by electron microscopy, these phages have a hexagonal head structure 1,000 Å long and 650 Å wide. Attached to the head is a tail approximately 1,000 Å long and 250Å wide. Near the point where the tail is attached to the head, a collar is present. The phage tail is a complex structure composed of an outer contractile sheath and an inner core 70 Å in diameter with a hollow cylinder or opening 25 Å in diameter. Proximally, the core opens into the head of the phage particle and distally has a hexagonal base plate from which project six short spikes and six long, thin tail fibers, 1,300 Å long and 20 Å wide (Fig. 3-23).

Phage Chemistry

Little information is available regarding the chemical and physical forces that mold the phage components together as an infective unit. Known phages are composed essentially of protein and nucleic acid. The polypeptides present in the capsid and in each of the components in the tail assembly are distinct.

When T-even phage particles are subjected to osmotic shock (by sudden transfer from high salt concentrations to distilled water), the DNA and internal proteins are released from the protein head. The empty hexagonal heads are called *ghosts.* Although phage ghosts cannot infect bacterial cells, they retain the ability to kill bacteria by a mechanism quite different from that of infectious phage.

The phage genome or hereditary material of the phage particle contains either DNA or RNA, but never both. As in bacteria and higher

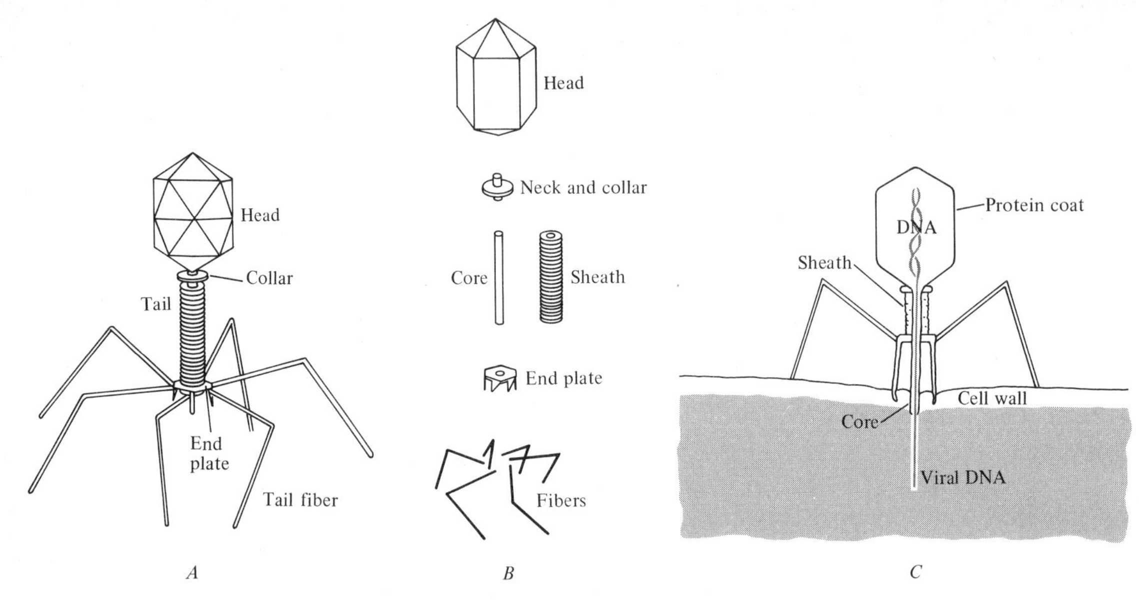

Figure 3-23 T4 bacterial virus is an assembly of protein components *(A)*. The head is a protein membrane, shaped like a kind of prolate icosahedron with 30 facets and filled with deoxyribonucleic acid (DNA). It is attached by a neck to a tail consisting of a hollow core surrounded by a contractile sheath and based on a spiked end plate to which six fibers are attached. The spikes and fibers affix the virus to a bacterial cell wall *(C)*. The sheath contracts, driving the core through the wall, and viral DNA enters the cell. [*W. B. Wood and R. S. Edgar, Sci. Am., 217 (No. 1):61–74, 1967.*] The individual components of T4 bacterial virus are shown in *B*. [*R. S. Edgar and R. H. Epstein, Sci. Am., 212 (No. 2): 70–78, 1965.*]

forms, the DNA of most phages is double-stranded (dsDNA), but some phages possess DNA in a single-stranded form (ssDNA). In other phages, the genome consists solely of single-stranded RNA (ssRNA).

The genome of T-even phages is double-stranded DNA. Unlike bacterial DNA, however, T-even phage DNA has a unique pyrimidine [5-hydroxymethylcytosine (HMC)] as a replacement for cytosine. Thus, it is possible to distinguish between the synthesis of bacterial and phage DNA in infected cells.

Phage Replication

Infection of bacteria with T-even phages terminates in lysis of the bacterial cells and the release of newly synthesized progeny phage. The lytic effect can be observed by simply mixing phage with a turbid broth culture of susceptible bacteria. During incubation, the turbidity of the mixture is measured at regular intervals of time. After approximately 20 to 24 min., there is a loss in the turbidity of the broth culture. In 30 to 34 min., the culture becomes clear, indicating that most of the bacteria are lysed by the infecting phage. Concomitant with the decrease in turbidity of the culture, newly produced phage particles are released (Fig. 3-24).

Plaques

Phage infection of susceptible bacteria *(indicator bacteria)* growing on the surface of a nutrient agar plate leads to the production of *plaques*, which are clear areas that represent foci of infection. In this procedure a dilute suspension of phage is added to 10^8 indicator bacteria, and

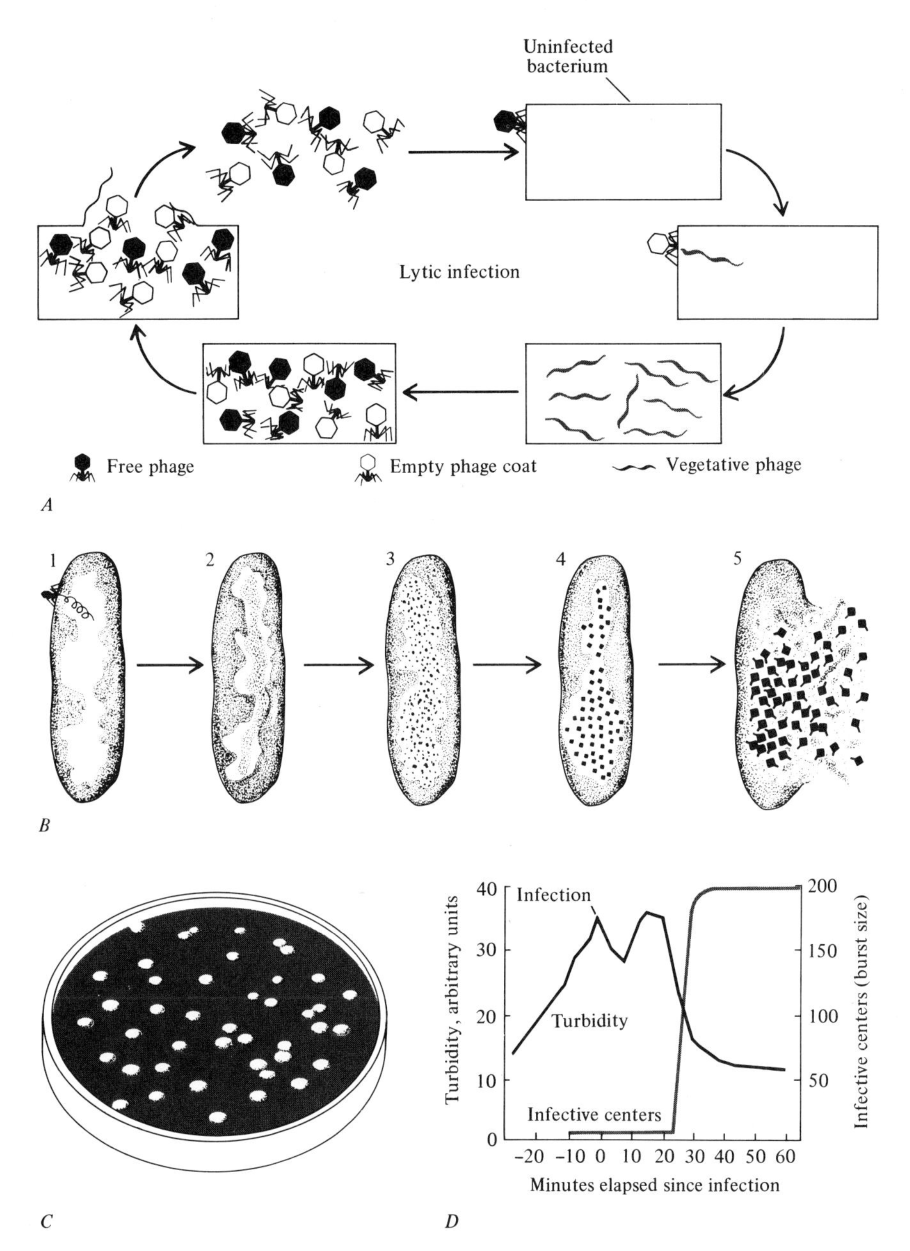

Figure 3-24 *(A)* Cycle of lytic infection. (*R. Y. Stanier, M. Doudoroff, and E. A. Adelberg, The Microbial World, 2d ed., Englewood Cliffs, N. J., Prentice-Hall, Inc., 1963, p. 200.*) *(B)* Viral infection begins when viral DNA enters a bacterium (1). Bacterial DNA is disrupted and viral DNA replicated (2). Synthesis of viral structural proteins (3) and their assembly into virus (4) continue until the cell bursts, releasing particles (5). [*W. B. Wood and R. S. Edgar, Sci. Am., 217 (No. 1):61–74, 1967.*] *(C)* A petri plate showing growth of a lawn of *E. coli* bacteria on which phage T2 has formed plaques, and (*D*) the turbidity and infective center content of an *E. coli* culture at various times after its infection with an average of five T4 phages per cell. (*G. S. Stent, Molecular Biology of Bacterial Viruses, San Francisco, W. H. Freeman & Co., 1963, pp. 41 and 79.*)

the mixture is spread over the surface of a nutrient agar plate and incubated. During incubation, phage infects the bacteria, replicates, and causes the lysis of the bacterial cells and the release of progeny phage. The progeny phage in turn infect neighboring bacteria, and the cycle is repeated several times. Eventually, a clear focus of infection, or plaque, is produced. Surrounding the plaque is the dense growth of uninfected bacteria called the *bacterial lawn*. The diameter of a plaque is usually 0.5 to 2.0 mm but can vary, depending upon the phage, the bacterium, and the conditions of plating (Fig. 3-24).

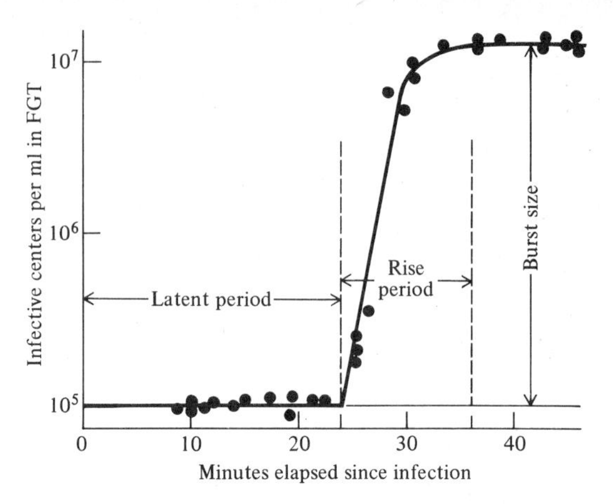

Figure 3-25 One-step growth curve of phage T4. *(G. S. Stent, Molecular Biology of Bacterial Viruses, San Francisco, W. H. Freeman & Co., 1963, p. 73; from A. H. Doermann, J. Bacteriol., 55:257-276, 1948.)*

Titration of Phage

Under appropriate conditions each plaque can be initiated by a single phage particle, thus providing a valuable quantitative tool. Consequently, the number of infective phage particles in a given sample can be determined by counting the number of plaques formed on a bacterial lawn and multiplying the number by the dilution of the phage suspension. For example, if 0.1 ml of a 10^{-6} dilution of a phage suspension produces an average of 100 plaques per plate, one would calculate a titer of 100×10^6 or 1.0×10^8 plaque-forming units (PFU) per 0.1 ml, or 1.0×10^9 PFU per milliliter.

One-step Growth Curve

When T-even phage is mixed with indicator bacteria, progeny phage is produced only after a certain period of time. This observation can be demonstrated in one-step growth experiments, the design of which is useful for studying phage multiplication (Fig. 3-25).

A dense suspension of indicator bacteria (5.0×10^8 per milliliter) in the exponential phase of growth is infected with one phage per bacterium. The mixture is incubated for 2 min. to allow the phage to adsorb to the bacterial cells and is then diluted 40-fold in broth containing specific antiserum to neutralize free phage that has not attached to the bacteria. The mixture is then diluted 250-fold in fresh growth medium in order to decrease the neutralizing capacity of the antiserum, and this dilution is called the first growth tube (FGT). Another tube is prepared containing a further 20-fold dilution of the FGT and is called the second growth tube (SGT). After incubation, samples from both tubes are periodically assayed for plaques on lawns of indicator bacteria.

Latent Period During the first 24 min. of infection the number of PFU remains constant *(latent period)*. After 24 min., the number of PFU in the culture rises rapidly until a plateau is reached about 10 min. later. Thereafter, there is no further increase in PFU. The interval during which PFU increase is the *rise period*. *Burst size* or average yield of progeny phage per infected bacterial cell is defined as the ratio of the final infective titer to the initial titer of phage-infected bacteria. The latent period thus represents the time between the initiation of infection and the commencement of lysis. During the rise period an increasing number of infected bacteria lyse, releasing progeny phage until a plateau is reached when all infected bacteria that are going to lyse have done so. Infection of residual uninfected bacteria does not occur because of the extremely high dilution imposed immediately after the initial infection. In effect, the dilution precludes contact between phage and bacteria (Fig. 3-25).

As a result, plaques produced from samples assayed during the latent period are derived from phage-infected bacteria that may contain numerous progeny phage particles. Nevertheless, the plating of each phage-infected bacterium before the end of the latent period yields a single plaque because progeny phage in a single cell are confined to a single focus of infection. After the latent period, lysis occurs, progeny phage are released into the medium, and each progeny phage forms an individual focus of infection on the lawn. The term *infective center* refers to the unit that produces a single plaque either from a single, free phage particle or from a phage-infected bacterium.

Eclipse Period In order to determine the events taking place inside phage-infected bacteria during the latent period, the cells are disrupted and their contents assayed for plaque-forming units. The data indicate that infective phage particles are not observed during the first 10 min. following infection. Thereafter, the titer of infective phage steadily increases. The interval between infection and the appearance of the first infectious intracellular phage particle is called the *eclipse period.* Thus, the eclipse period represents an interval during which the infected cell is synthesizing structural components that are subsequently assembled into infectious phage (Fig. 3-26).

The Lytic Cycle

Infection of a bacterial cell with a virulent T-even phage can be considered to occur in four stages: (1) adsorption of phage, (2) injection of phage nucleic acid, (3) synthesis and maturation of new phage particles, and (4) release of phage. These events constitute the *lytic cycle* of infection.

Adsorption of Phage Initial contact between phage and bacterial cell is the result of random collisions. Attachment and irreversible fixation of phage to the bacterial surface quickly ensues following interaction of phage tail fibers with bacterial receptor sites.

The presence of cations is essential for the irreversible fixation of phage to host cell, and certain phages (coliphage T4) require L-tryptophan as an *adsorption cofactor.* This amino acid acts to release the phage tail fibers from a fixed position on the surface of the tail sheath so that they can freely extend to engage the bacterial receptor sites.

Adsorption is highly specific and is believed to depend upon complementary chemical configuration on phage tail fibers and bacterial receptor sites. Thus, phage can adsorb only to bacteria that possess specific receptors. The variety of bacteria that a particular phage can adsorb to and infect constitutes the *host range* of

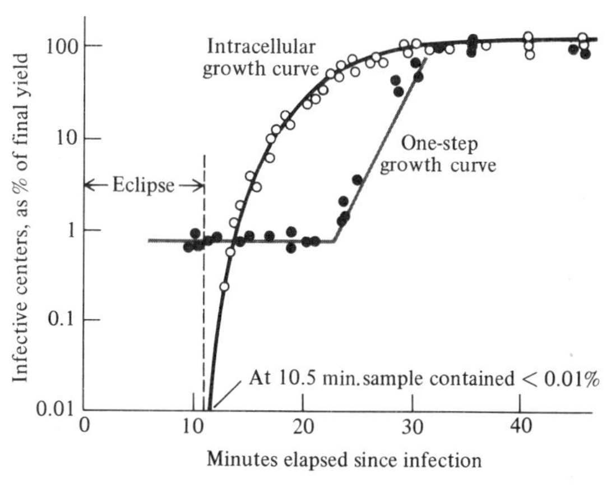

Figure 3-26 The intracellular growth curve of phage T4. (*G. S. Stent, Molecular Biology of Bacterial Viruses, San Francisco, W. H. Freeman & Co., 1963, p. 84.*)

the phage. Different phages have different host ranges. The chemical composition and structure of the receptors can be altered by mutation, causing a loss in capacity to absorb phage. Bacteria that lack specific receptors are said to be *resistant*.

The susceptibility of bacteria to different phages provides a method of identifying bacterial types within a species *(phage typing)*. The procedure involves the determination of which phages (in a battery of 15 to 20) can produce plaques on the lawn of a given bacterium. The group of phages to which a bacterium is susceptible is referred to as the phage type of the bacterium. For example, if the phages numbered 1, 3, and 5 produce plaques on the bacterial lawn, the phage type of the bacterium is 1/3/5. Bacteria having identical phage types are considered to be of common origin. From a practical viewpoint, this provides a powerful epidemiological tool in determining whether or not organisms isolated from various clinical sources have a common origin or line of transmission.

Most specific phage receptors are located in the bacterial cell wall. Purified receptors obtained from the cell wall can combine specifically with phage and prevent infection of indicator bacteria. In some T-even phages the receptor is a lipopolysaccharide, while in other phages it is a lipoprotein. Protoplasts (Chap. 1), devoid of cell wall components, cannot absorb phage and therefore will not be infected. However, if phage infection precedes the removal of the cell wall, protoplasts are fully capable of synthesizing phage.

In some bacteria phage receptors are present on sex pili or on flagella. For example, male-specific RNA phages of *E. coli* attach to the sex pili of donor cells. The spherical male-specific phage adsorbs to the sides of the pili, whereas the filamentous male-specific phage combines with the tip of the pili. Certain other phages adsorb to the flagella of indicator bacteria and subsequently slide along the flagella to the cell wall.

Data obtained from transformation experiments utilizing viral DNA or viral RNA extracted from the respective phage demonstrate that intact phage particles are not essential for infection. Phage nucleic acid alone can be taken up by competent bacteria and can initiate the lytic cycle of infection that leads to the synthesis and release of progeny viruses, a phenomenon known as transfection. Large (110×10^6 daltons) as well as small (1×10^6 daltons) phage nucleic acids have been used to infect spheroplasts. In addition to double-stranded DNA, single-stranded DNA and RNA have been effective in initiating phage infection.

Injection of Phage Nucleic Acid After T-even phage aligns tail-first to the cell wall of indicator bacteria, the tail sheath contracts, exposing the inner core, which penetrates the cell. In the process phage DNA is ejected from the head through the tail core into the bacterial cell *(injection of phage nucleic acid)*.

Penetration may be facilitated by *lysozyme*, an enzyme specified by a viral gene, associated with the tail structure of T-even phage and capable of hydrolyzing the rigid murein layer of the cell wall. Lysozyme may also act by releasing substances, possibly zinc, that trigger contraction of the sheath and ejection of phage DNA. However, the enzyme is not essential for penetration since mutants without lysozyme can inject phage DNA.

Contraction of the tail sheath is believed to resemble the contraction of muscle. At the time of DNA injection a small amount of adenosine triphosphate (ATP) on the phage tail is hydrolyzed to adenosine diphosphate (ADP) in the presence of Ca^{++}, presumably triggering the contraction of the sheath and the insertion of the core. Bacteria appear to play a passive role in the phage DNA injection process, since phage DNA can be injected into dead bacteria

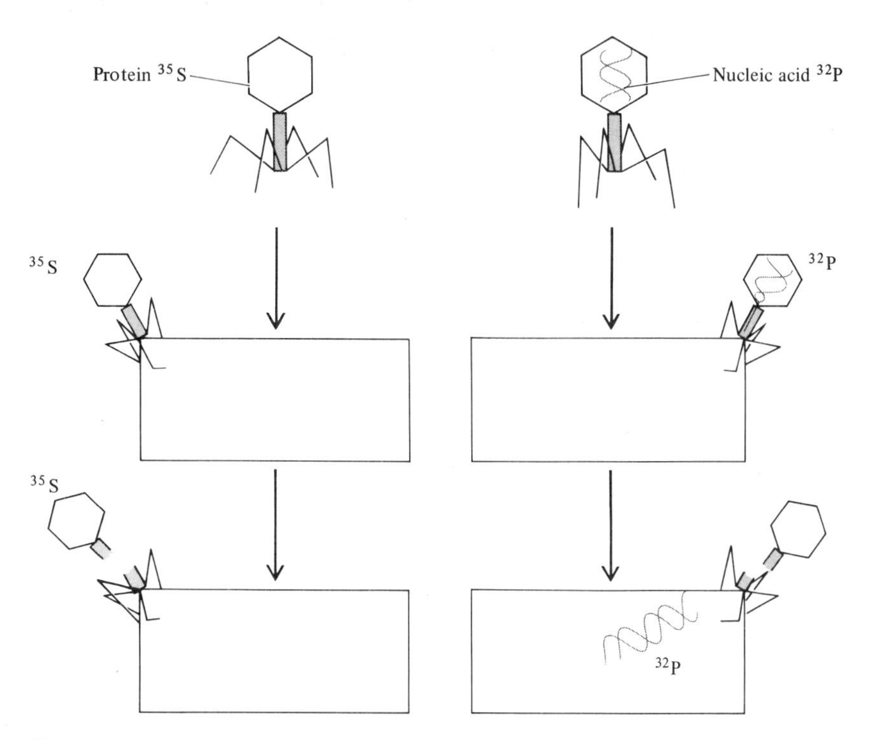

Figure 3-27 Classical blender experiment of Hershey and Chase demonstrating injection of phage DNA into the host bacterium and exclusion of phage protein coat.

and can be ejected upon contact with purified cell wall fragments.

Prior to the advent of refined electron microscopic and radioautographic techniques, the essential features of phage infection were demonstrated in the classical experiments of Hershey and Chase. The studies involved the radiolabeling of phage protein with ^{35}S and phage DNA with ^{32}P. After shearing off phage heads and tails from the cell wall with a Waring blender, analysis revealed that the ^{35}S label was found in the phage heads and tails, but that the ^{32}P label was associated with the bacteria and subsequently was present in the progeny phage. Thus, it was shown that phage DNA alone was essential for the production of progeny phage in indicator bacteria (Fig. 3-27).

Synthesis and Maturation of Phage Injected phage DNA supplies the cell with the genetic information required for the synthesis of progeny phage. Phage DNA, head proteins, tail proteins, and tail fibers are synthesized separately and are finally assembled into complete infectious particles (virions). The assembly of the various structural components into infectious phage is called *maturation*. In the process the metabolic machinery of the cell is diverted from producing structural bacterial components into new channels leading to the construction of phage components. Synthesis of progeny phage is partly achieved by the existing metabolic apparatus of the cell and partly by new phage-specific enzymes coded for by the injected phage genome. In addition, a few minutes after the onset of phage infection, synthesis of bacterial protein, DNA, and RNA ceases. Preexisting bacterial enzymes, however, may continue to function at their preinfection levels (Fig. 3-28).

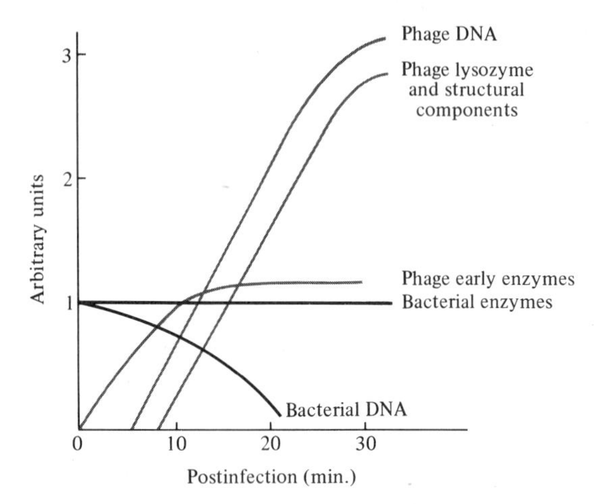

Figure 3-28 Sequence of biochemical events occurring in T4 infected *E. coli.* (*Modified from S. E. Luria and J. E. Darnell, General Virology, 2d ed., New York, John Wiley & Sons, 1967, p. 206.*)

Phage Messenger RNA's Viral synthesis commences when bacterial RNA polymerase produces several phage-specific messengers (phage mRNA's) using one strand of phage DNA as the template. Since phage mRNA's are transcribed in the presence of chloramphenicol, an antibiotic that inhibits protein synthesis, it is apparent that the RNA polymerase is a preexisting enzyme coded for by the bacterial genome.

Phage Proteins With the availability of phage mRNA's and the utilization of bacterial ribosomes, several new phage-specific proteins are synthesized and are classified as early or late.

Early proteins are primarily enzymes that are produced prior to the synthesis of phage DNA. Included among the early proteins are:

1 Enzymes required for phage DNA synthesis
2 Enzymes involved in the glucosylation of phage DNA
3 A DNase that hydrolyzes bacterial DNA
4 The internal head protein

Late proteins are produced during and after the synthesis of phage DNA. Included among the late proteins are the structural proteins that make up the head and tail of the phage and phage lysozyme.

Phage DNA In the synthesis of phage DNA, building blocks derived from parental phage DNA, hydrolyzed bacterial DNA, and the medium are utilized. Thus, there is established a pool of newly synthesized phage DNA. Replication of double-stranded phage DNA is semiconservative; that is, each strand serves as a template for and combines with a newly synthesized strand. In addition, replication is accompanied by breakage and rejoining of fragments to form intact DNA molecules. Accumulating evidence indicates that, rather than penetrating into the cytoplasm of the infected bacteria, parental phage DNA may remain bound to and initiate replication while attached to the inner surface of the plasma membrane.

Phage Maturation During replication when phage DNA and structural proteins are synthesized actively and separately and before the components are assembled into infectious phage, the terms *vegetative state* and *vegetative phage* are used to describe the process and the phage. During assembly, phage DNA is initially condensed into a compact polyhedron, presumably under the influence of the internal head protein. Then, phage DNA is "packaged" into the head protein which surrounds it, and finally the tail structure is added. The assembly of phage components into mature, infective phage is known as maturation.

Release of Phage Typically, the release of progeny phage from phage-infected bacteria accompanies lysis of the bacterial cell. In some cases, however, phage can leak out of infected bacteria in the absence of lysis.

Microscopically, phage-infected bacteria assume a spherical, swollen form immediately prior to lysis. In bacilli such as *E. coli,* intracellular phage replication weakens the cell wall, leading to a loss in rigidity and the assumption of a spherical shape; finally the cell wall is unable to resist the internal osmotic pressure. As a result, the bacteria explode, burst, or lyse, and mature phage is released.

Since phage lysozyme can break the β-1,4 glycosidic linkage between N-acetylmuramic acid and N-acetylglucosamine in the rigid murein layer of the cell wall, theoretically the enzyme can account for the destruction of the integrity of the cell wall and the release of progeny phage. Recent data, however, indicate that other substances present in phage-infected bacteria act on the cell membrane, permitting lysozyme to reach the murein layer. Thus, release of progeny phage is probably the result of several enzymes acting in concert.

Regulatory Mechanisms Associated with Phage Replication

The synthesis of early phage enzymes, phage DNA, and late proteins and the assembly and release of phage are sequential processes that appear to be subject to various regulatory mechanisms whose nature is not clearly understood. It is known, however, that there are two phage mRNA's operating, an early mRNA and a late mRNA. Synthesis of early proteins starts soon after infection and stops by the tenth minute after infection. Synthesis of phage DNA begins approximately 5 min. after infection, while the late structural proteins initially appear 7 min. after infection.

Phage DNA and late structural proteins continue to be synthesized throughout the lytic cycle, but synthesis of early proteins terminates at 10 min. after infection. In the presence of actinomycin D, however, synthesis of early proteins is not stopped. Presumably, the messenger required for regulating the production of early proteins is dependent upon the synthesis of progeny phage DNA which is prevented by actinomycin D. In the absence of actinomycin D, progeny phage DNA replicate and cause the transcription of a late phage-specific mRNA whose function involves the production of a regulatory protein that terminates the synthesis of early proteins.

Replication of Single-stranded DNA Phage

The replication of a single-stranded DNA phage, ϕ X174, is quite different from that of the double-stranded DNA phages. After the circular phage genome is injected, a double-stranded DNA replicative form (RF) is made by producing an outer *complementary (negative)* DNA strand on the single *positive* strand of phage DNA that was injected. Thus, the RF is composed of two complementary strands of DNA. The synthesis of the negative strand appears to be accomplished through the activity of a preexisting bacterial DNA polymerase.

Phage mRNA is produced by transcription of the outer or negative strand of the RF. In addition, the negative RF strand acts as a template for the synthesis of positive single strands of phage DNA that are incorporated within the structural protein of progeny phage prior to lysis of the bacterial cell.

It is significant to note that during replication of ϕ X174, bacterial macromolecular syntheses are not inhibited.

Replication of Single-stranded RNA Phage

Another variation in the pattern of phage replication is observed in the case of the lytic cycle produced by single-stranded RNA phage, such as f2 coliphage. After injection, the single positive strand of phage RNA serves two functions.

1 It acts as phage mRNA to specify the synthesis of RNA-dependent RNA polymerase and structural phage proteins.
2 It acts as the template for the replication of phage RNA through the production of a double-stranded RNA RF.

The negative strand of the RF, in turn, serves as the template for the synthesis of the single positive strands of phage RNA that become incorporated in progeny phage.

Abortive Infection (Host-induced Modification)

In some cases, injected phage DNA is enzymatically hydrolyzed, and infection of the cell is aborted. For example, a bacterial cell may be deficient in ability to synthesize uridine diphosphate glucose (UDPG). As a result, phage DNA cannot be glucosylated, a phenomenon termed *host-induced modification.* Phage-bearing unglucosylated DNA may be unable to infect certain other bacteria because the phage DNA is degraded by bacterial nucleases. Thus, a restriction is imposed on the infectious capacity of the phage. These observations have led to the suggestion that glucosylation may serve to stabilize phage DNA inside the bacterial cell. In other cases, failure to methylate phage DNA may result in degradation after injection. In addition to phage, the DNA of sex factor is also subject to host-induced modification and restriction.

Thus, host-induced modification represents a general phenomenon whereby an altered synthesis of DNA in one bacterium restricts the ability of the modified DNA to replicate in another bacterium. The primary significance of the phenomenon is that the bacterial environment can produce chemical changes in genetic material and modify its stability without altering the genetic code.

TEMPERATE PHAGE AND THE LYSOGENIC CYCLE

Instead of producing a lytic cycle, as does virulent phage after injection of phage DNA, the DNA of temperate phage persists, associates with, replicates in synchrony with the bacterial chromosome without synthesizing progeny phage or causing lysis of the bacterium, and is passed on through countless bacterial generations along with the bacterial genome. The stable relationship established between temperate phage DNA and the bacterial chromosome is termed *lysogeny*. The process by which phage DNA replicates in synchrony with the bacterial genome, each daughter cell receiving phage DNA, is known as the *lysogenic cycle.*

The Prophage State

When temperate phage DNA is integrated with the bacterial chromosome, the phage genome is termed *prophage.* Bacteria carrying temperate phage in the prophage state are said to be lysogenic. In nature, temperate phage is more prevalent than virulent phage. In fact, the prophage state represents almost the ultimate in parasitism, since phage and bacterial genomes replicate in synchrony and can coexist in equilibrium through many generations. The replication of prophage is controlled by bacterial regulatory mechanisms.

Nonetheless, the prophage state may confer new characteristics on lysogenic bacteria. For example, although the bacterial cell is not destroyed, it perpetuates the potential to be killed in a lytic cycle, hence the term lysogenic. The potential to be destroyed is genetically passed on to daughter bacteria cells in the form of prophage.

Often a single bacterium can carry two prophages and is termed *doubly lysogenic.* Occasionally, bacteria are found to carry more than two prophages and are *multiply lysogenic.*

Induction of Prophage

Prophage is not committed to an eternal existence as part of the bacterial chromosome. Under natural conditions of bacterial growth, prophage can become excised from the bacterial chromosome in a small proportion of cells, enter the vegetative state, direct the synthesis of progeny phage, and cause the lysis of the bacteria and the release of phage. This is known as *spontaneous induction.*

Whereas spontaneous induction is normally a rare event, all the bacteria in a lysogenic culture can be induced to shift to the lytic cycle following exposure to low doses of ultraviolet light, hydrogen peroxide, mitomycin C, and nitrogen mustard. Such physical and chemical agents can interrupt or slow down DNA synthesis, but the exact mechanism of induction is unknown.

Temperate Phage

As noted above, temperate phage has the potential to evoke either a lytic or lysogenic cycle. Consequently, upon infecting indicator bacteria, temperate phage will produce *turbid plaques.*

Shortly after temperate phage DNA is injected into indicator bacteria, there is a brief critical period when it is decided if phage DNA will be replicated in the vegetative or prophage state. Generally, the lysogenic cycle is favored at room temperature, while there is a shift to the lytic cycle at 37°C. In any event, if the early proteins associated with the lytic cycle are synthesized, the decision is irreversible. On the other hand, it will become evident from the ensuing discussion that if the prophage gene that specifies the synthesis of *repressor protein* becomes functional, then the lysogenic cycle is established.

Prophage Lambda (λ) and the Bacterial Chromosome

The close interaction of prophage with the bacterial chromosome is best demonstrated through bacterial mating experiments in which the distribution of lambda (λ) prophage among recombinants can be observed. Utilizing an Hfr *E. coli* K 12 donor that carries lambda prophage [*E. coli* K 12 (λ)], it can be shown that the prophage occupies a specific position on and acts as an integral part of the bacterial chromosome.

The pattern of prophage distribution among recombinant bacteria indicates that the prophage is linked to the gal gene (responsible for the fermentation of galactose). For example, when a nonlysogenic Hfr donor is crossed with a lysogenic recipient, the nonlysogenic character enters the zygote after the gal gene and before the tryptophan (trp) gene and segregates among recombinants like any other gene. In the same way, lambda prophages carrying different genetic markers in donor and recipient bacteria show that the prophage of the donor enters the zygote and segregates among the recombinants in the same way as the nonlysogenic character.

Integration of Lambda Prophage into the Bacterial Chromosome The chromosome of lambda is composed of double-stranded DNA and exists in the phage head as a linear molecule. At one end of the linear molecule one of the strands (A) is 20 base pairs longer than the other strand (B), while at the other end of the linear molecule, strand B is 20 base pairs longer than strand A. The base sequences in the 20 base-paired ends are complementary and provide the linear DNA molecule with the ability to form a circle by complementary base pairing.

A few minutes after injection into indicator bacteria, lambda DNA becomes circular. The circular phage DNA then pairs with the bacterial chromosome at a specific site, the attachment locus (att), which is present on both phage and bacterial genomes. Integration of lambda DNA into the bacterial chromosome subsequently occurs as reciprocal recombination following breakage, double crossing-over, and rejoining of phage and bacterial DNA. At least one phage gene (Int) product is required for the integration process (Fig. 3-29).

Excision of Lambda Prophage from the Bacterial Chromosome The integration process is completely reversible. At least two phage gene products, Int and Xis, are required for *excision,* a process in which prophage DNA "loops" out from the bacterial chromosome and reassumes a

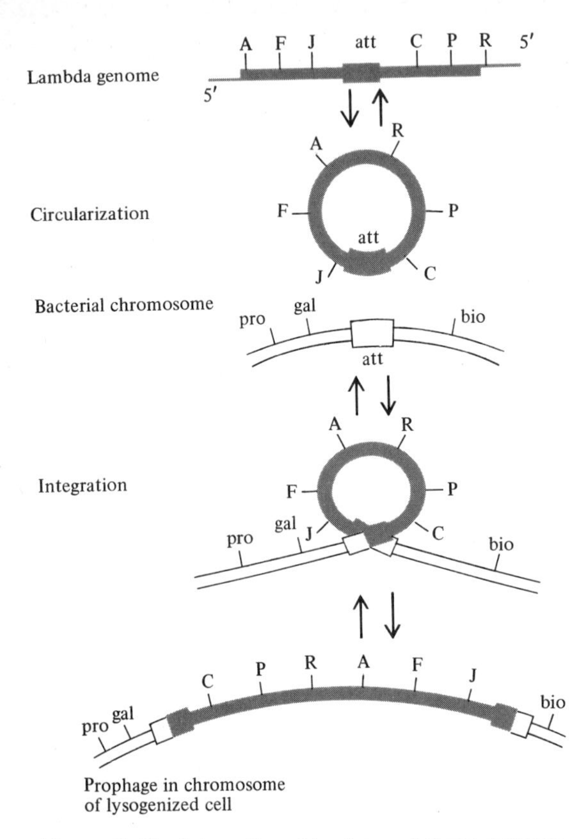

Figure 3-29 Integration of lambda coliphage genome into the host cell chromosome, resulting in resident prophage. (*Modified from E. R. Signer, Annu. Rev. Microbiol., 22:451–488, 1968.*)

circular structure. Initially, lambda DNA replicates in the circular form, but later the characteristic linear molecules are generated for inclusion into the phage head.

Zygotic Induction When lysogenic Hfr donors are mated with nonlysogenic recipients, few of the recombinants are found to be lysogenic. The reason for this is explained by the phenomenon called *zygotic induction.* In passage of the bacterial chromosome from the lysogenic Hfr donor to the nonlysogenic recipient, prophage is induced, i.e., excises from the bacterial chromosome and shifts into the lytic cycle (zygotic induction). Instead of lysogenic recombinants, the conjugation produces plaques.

On the other hand, if the recipient is lysogenic, zygotic induction does not take place. The lysogenic recipient is immune because it produces a cytoplasmic factor (repressor protein) that prevents vegetative replication of phage.

Repressor Protein Lysogeny depends on the synthesis of *repressor protein,* a gene product of prophage that prevents the expression of other prophage genes required for vegetative replication. In lambda prophage, repressor protein is a product of the C region of the phage genome. When lambda phage infects indicator bacteria, repressor protein is responsible for establishment and maintenance of the prophage state by acting on two sites of the phage genome, thereby preventing the synthesis of mRNA required for production of infective phage particles.

Repressor protein diffuses throughout the bacterial cell and endows it with a specific immunity to infection with other closely related phages. Thus, lysogenic bacteria are immune. Related phages can adsorb to and inject phage DNA into lysogenic bacteria, but repressor protein precludes synthesis of progeny phage particles. On the other hand, infection of lysogenic bacteria with unrelated phage can occur, since the injected phage DNA does not react with the repressor protein.

Study of C region mutants indicates that three genes (C_1, C_2, C_3) are involved in lysogeny. C_1 codes for the synthesis of the repressor protein, while C_2 and C_3 are ancillary genes required for the establishment, but not the maintenance, of the prophage state. The products of C_2 and C_3 are believed to transiently inhibit phage DNA synthesis, thus permitting an adequate accumulation of repressor protein.

Extrachromosomal Lysogeny Phage P1 represents a unique example of lysogeny because prophage does not integrate into the bacterial chromosome. The prophage remains extrachromosomal and replicates concomitantly with cellular division, maintaining one copy of the genome per cell. The extrachromosomal prophage also codes for repressor protein and can be induced to a lytic cycle.

Defective Prophage Mutations occur in prophage just as they do in any other nucleic acid that has genetic potential. The mutations, however, rarely interfere with replication of prophage. Usually, *defective prophage* is recognized by the inability to give rise to structurally intact, infective phage particles. Thus, prophage mutations can involve the synthesis of DNA, heads, tails, lysozyme, or the maturation process.

For example, if a mutation affects the maturation process, the lysogenic bacteria are still immune to infection with related phage, since synthesis of repressor protein is unaffected. When the lysogenic bacteria containing the defective prophage are induced by ultraviolet irradiation, vegetative replication will ensue and lysis of the bacteria will occur at the expected time, but intact, mature infective phage will not be released. Instead the lysate will contain unassembled phage DNA, head, tails, and lysozyme. Thus, the defective phage genome is capable of programming the individual phage components but cannot cause their assembly into infective phage.

Helper Phage The maturation of defective phage can be achieved with the assistance of *helper phage*. The procedure involves (1) *induction* of defective prophage by ultraviolet irradiation and (2) *superinfection* with a related helper phage. In addition to programming the synthesis of progeny helper phage, superinfecting phage DNA can supply the missing genetic information required for the maturation of intact defective phage particles. If superinfection is at-

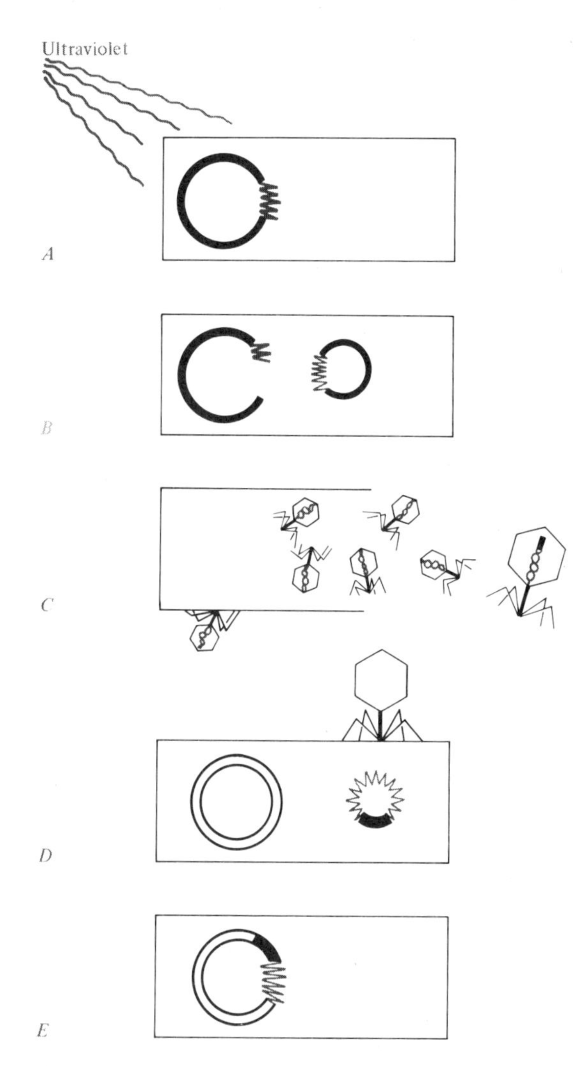

Figure 3-30 Restricted transduction requires induction of a lysogenic bacterium which carries a prophage in its chromosome *(A)*. During excision from the bacterial chromosome, some prophage genes (WWW) are exchanged for the adjoining bacterial gene (▬) *(B)*. An infective, but defective, transducing particle is produced when "helper" phage supplies the missing genes and their products *(C)*. The defective transducing particle (containing part phage genes and the bacterial gene) injects these genes into a recipient bacterial cell *(D)*, where the genes are inserted into the bacterial chromosome *(E)* as in lysogenization. The recipient cell now carries a defective prophage in its chromosome as well as a "new" bacterial gene. After induction, the cell in *(E)* can produce transducing particles only if a "helper" phage supplies the necessary phage genes.

tempted before induction, helper phage DNA will be prevented from functioning by repressor protein (Fig. 3-30).

TRANSDUCTION

Biologically, the significance of phage increased immensely when it was recognized that bacterial genes can be transferred by phage particles through a process known as *transduction*, or *phage-mediated recombination*. This mechanism of genetic exchange in bacteria is quite distinct from either transformation or conjugation. In contrast to conjugation, contact between bacterial cells is unnecessary, and unlike transformation, the presence of DNase has no effect.

Two types of transduction are recognized:

1 *General transduction* in which the phage may transfer any bacterial gene
2 *Restricted transduction* in which the phage may transfer only bacterial genes contiguous with the prophage position on the bacterial chromosome

Restricted Transduction

Restricted transduction can be demonstrated following the ultraviolet induction of lambda prophage carried by prototrophic, wild-type *E. coli* K 12 (λ), thereby producing progeny lambda phage. Auxotrophic, nonlysogenic *E. coli* K 12 are then infected with lambda phage and are plated on various selective media to determine which bacterial genes are transferred by phage from prototrophic to auxotrophic bacteria. The data indicate that only the gal^+ gene which is located next to the prophage on the bacterial chromosome is transferred to the lambda-infected gal^- auxotrophs. When plated on eosin-methylene blue-galactose medium, gal^+ transductants change the color of the indicator dye and appear as red colonies, while gal^- colonies are white because they cannot ferment galactose. The frequency of restricted transduction is such that only one in 10^6 lambda-infected cells acquires the gal^+ character (Fig. 3-31).

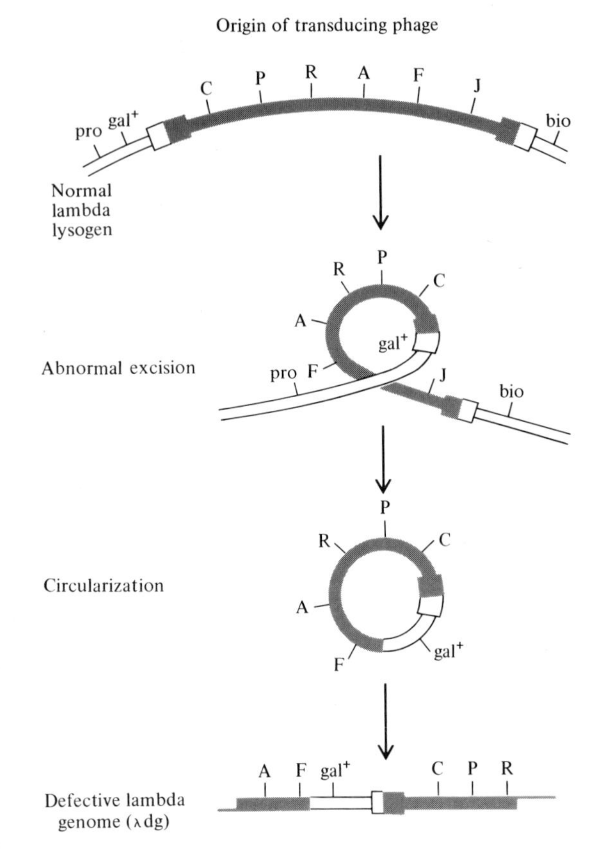

Figure 3-31 Origin of a defective lambda genome together with bacterial gene capable of causing restricted transduction. (*Modified from E. R. Signer, Annu. Rev. of Microbiol., 22:451–488, 1968.*)

Transductants Transductants acquiring the gal^+ gene of the prototrophic bacteria are unstable and revert to gal^- as seen by the segregation of gal^- daughter cells. This means that the gal^- gene persists and that the gal^+ gene is added to the transductant chromosome. In other words, the auxotrophic allele (gal^-) is not replaced by the transduced gene (gal^+) by genetic recombination. Thus, the transductant

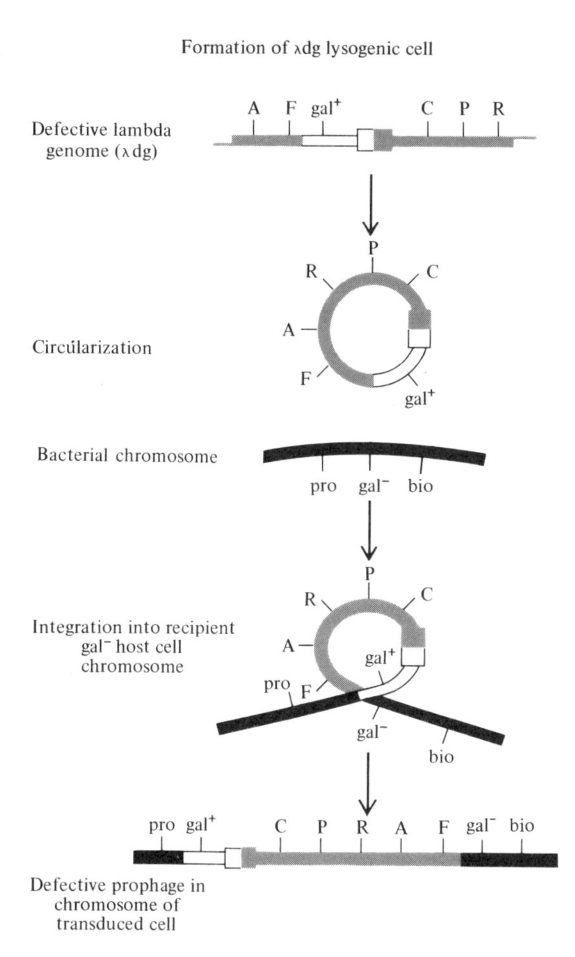

Figure 3-32 Integration of a defective lambda genome carrying a bacterial gene which results in restricted transduction. (*Modified from E. R. Signer, Annu. Rev. of Microbiol., 22:451–488, 1968.*)

chromosome is gal^-/gal^+, a partial diploid known as a *heterogenote* (Fig. 3-32).

Heterogenotes can carry defective prophage, are immune to infection by normal lambda phage, and lyse after a normal latent period following ultraviolet induction. However, intact phage particles are not released, and the lysate has no transducing activity.

Thus, the transducing agent is a defective phage particle that can lysogenize recipient bacteria but cannot produce intact progeny phage on induction. Defective gal^+-transducing lambda phage particles are designated by the symbol λdg. Therefore, the heterogenote chromosome is $gal^-/\lambda dg$ (or gal^-/gal^+ with respect to galactose fermentation).

High-frequency Transduction Heterogenotes yield intact, infective, transducing phage after ultraviolet induction only if they are lysogenized by normal lambda phage at the same time they acquire λdg; i.e., they are doubly lysogenized. Thus, when heterogenote chromosomes contain $\lambda/\lambda dg$ and gal^+/gal^-, normal lambda phage acts as helper phage after ultraviolet induction. Approximately half of the phage particles in the ultraviolet-induced lysates can transduce the gal^+ gene to gal^- bacteria. Such lysates contain phage that can cause *high-frequency transduction* (HFT) in contrast with the lysates that produce heterogenote transductants in low frequency (10^{-6}). Experimentally, HFT lysates are readily obtained by ultraviolet induction of heterogenotes carrying defective lambda phage followed by superinfection with normal lambda phage.

Formation of Defective Lambda Phage (λdg) On rare occasions, ultraviolet induction of *E. coli* K 12 (λ) gal^+ can lead to an error in excision and circularization of the phage genome. Some of the prophage genes remain on the chromosome, while the bacterial gal^+ gene moves off and forms a part of the excised circle that contains the bulk of the phage genes. Consequently, the portion of the phage genome that has separated from the bacterial chromosome is defective, since it lacks essential structural phage genes that make up as much as one-third of complete genome. Intact λdg phage, however, can be formed with the assistance of helper phage.

When gal^- bacteria are infected with λdg, the defective phage genome is integrated with the bacterial chromosome, yielding $gal^+/gal^-/\lambda dg$

heterogenotes. In the absence of helper phage, subsequent excision leads to the loss of λdg containing the gal$^+$ gene and accounts for the appearance of gal$^-$ segregants.

In doubly lysogenized bacteria, both normal λ and λdg circularize following excision from the bacterial chromosome. The presence of a normal vegetative λ genome provides the genetic information that codes for the structural proteins required to produce infective progeny phage particles, half of which contains the normal λ genome while the other half contains the λdg genome with the gal$^+$ bacterial gene.

In addition to transduction of gal$^+$ by defective λ, the bacterial gene coding for *biotin* synthesis, which is located at the other end of the integrated λ prophage, can become a part of defective λ by the same mechanism and is identified as λdb.

As noted earlier, incorporation of bacterial genes into the sex factor, F, by a similar mechanism yields F′ (lac$^+$) bacteria.

General Transduction

Either virulent or temperate phage can produce progeny phage that on rare occasions are capable of transducing any of the genes on the bacterial chromosome (general transduction). Experimentally, the phenomenon is readily demonstrated by infecting a large population of auxotrophic bacteria with phage that has been propagated in prototrophic bacteria. An overwhelming majority of the phage-infected auxotrophs will be either lysed or lysogenized by the phage and, in the latter case, will retain their auxotrophic character. However, a minuscule proportion will be neither lysed nor lysogenized but transduced to prototrophs following phage infection. The demonstration depends on plating a large number of phage-infected auxotrophs on agar plates deficient in a particular growth requirement. For example, on tryptophan(trp$^-$)-deficient media, only trp$^+$ transductants will form colonies.

Transducing Particles During the course of the lytic cycle the bacterial chromosome is fragmented. Rarely, a small piece of bacterial DNA may be packed into the head of the phage particle instead of phage DNA, thus producing a *transducing particle*. Since there are physical limits to the amount of nucleic acid that can be incorporated into the phage head, transducing

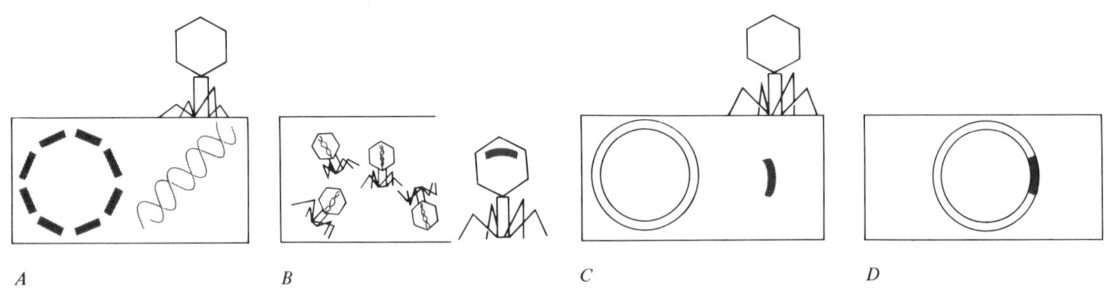

Figure 3-33 Generalized transduction requires infection of a bacterial cell by phage and fragmentation of the bacterial chromosome *(A)*. New phage particles are synthesized and sometimes bacterial genes (▬) are "packaged" by error into the head of the transducing phage particle *(B)*. Note absence of phage genes (∞∞) in the transducing phage particle, making it a defective phage particle. Subsequently, the transducing particle injects the bacterial genes it carries into another bacterial cell *(C)*, where the genes are incorporated into the bacterial chromosome by recombination *(D)*. This is known as *complete transduction*. More often, the injected genes do not undergo recombination and remain extrachromosomal. This is known as *abortive transduction*.

particles contain little, if any, phage DNA and therefore are defective phage particles.

When a transducing particle adsorbs to a bacterium, bacterial DNA is injected instead of phage DNA. The injected bacterial gene can undergo genetic recombination with its homologous allele on the chromosome of the bacterium. Since bacterial DNA is packed into the transducing particle on a random basis, any bacterial gene can be transferred to bacteria and may recombine with the bacterial chromosome. Consequently, the phenomenon is termed general transduction (Fig. 3-33).

Transduction of Linked Genes Even though limited in area, the phage head can accommodate approximately 2 percent of the total length of the bacterial chromosome. Thus, transducing particles can carry pairs of functionally unrelated but closely linked bacterial genes. Genetic markers that are not closely linked are not transduced together to a single bacterium.

Complete versus Abortive Transduction General transduction is complete when the transferred bacterial gene becomes part of the bacterial chromosome by genetic recombination. In most cases, however, the injected bacterial gene does not undergo genetic recombination, and the transduction is said to be *abortive.* The ratio of abortive to complete transduction is approximately 10 or 20 to 1. Both complete and abortive transduction can involve the transfer of a pair of functionally unrelated but closely linked genes.

In abortive transduction, the transduced gene remains extrachromosomal, fails to replicate, and is transmitted to only one of the daughter cells. The gene persists in this manner and is phenotypically expressed. The ultimate fate of the gene is not clear, but eventually it may undergo genetic recombination, be destroyed, or diluted out of the culture.

Minute Colonies Abortive transduction can be demonstrated by infecting a large population of auxotrophic bacteria with phage propagated on prototrophs. For example, if phage-infected his^- auxotrophs are plated on his^- medium and incubated, two types of colonies can be observed. Large colonies represent transductants that have genetically recombined the his^+ gene. Minute colonies develop because the his^+ gene has been transferred by the transducing particle but is not genetically recombined and is passed on to only one daughter cell. The transferred his^+ gene produces the enzyme required for the synthesis of histidine, but is rapidly diluted out with each succeeding bacterial division. The vast majority of bacteria within the colony do not have the his^+ gene, the supply of the enzyme quickly diminishes to the point where colonial growth ceases, and a minute colony results.

There is a simple procedure which will confirm that the minute colonies are due to abortive transduction. If large colonies are restreaked by rubbing the surface of the agar with a spreader, every bacterium in the colony, being nutritionally independent, yields a colony, and confluent growth results. When minute colonies are restreaked in the same manner, the number of minute colonies remains the same as before. Thus, each minute colony contains only a single bacterium that has the his^+ gene.

CONVERSION (PHAGE CONVERSION)

The intimate interaction between phage and bacterial genomes can be even more intriguing than that associated with transduction. In conversion, phage genes can direct the synthesis of important bacterial toxins and antigens without transferring bacterial genes. The phage-coded bacterial products are synthesized during either the lytic or lysogenic cycle and are not involved in the synthesis of progeny phage.

Nontoxigenic *Corynebacterium diphtheriae* are avirulent for man because they lack the genetic potential to synthesize diphtheria toxin (Chap. 13). Nontoxigenic bacteria, however, can be converted to the toxigenic virulent state following lysogenization with β phage. Actual production of diphtheria toxin occurs when β prophage is induced and the lytic cycle ensues. When toxigenic bacteria lose the ability to carry β prophage through mutation or recombination, concomitantly the potential to synthesize diphtheria toxin is lost and the bacteria become avirulent. However, virulent mutants of temperate β phage retain the capacity to direct the synthesis of diphtheria toxin during the lytic cycle.

Phage conversion is involved in the synthesis of somatic antigens in salmonellae (Chap. 18). For example, when salmonellae containing somatic O antigens 3 and 10 are lysogenized with phage ε^{15}, the bacteria produce O antigens 3 and 15 but not 10. The bacteria continue to synthesize O antigens 3 and 15 as long as prophage ε^{15} is present but will produce O antigens 3 and 10 if the prophage is lost. Similar interactions exist among other salmonellae and their phages. In one intriguing case, the production of O antigen 34 is dependent upon sequential expression of genes in phage ε^{15} and phage ε^{34} (double lysogeny).

Erythrogenic scarlatinal toxin associated with group A beta-hemolytic streptococci (Chap. 14) appears to be coded for by a phage gene. Following infection of nontoxigenic group A beta-hemolytic streptococci with temperate phage isolated from toxin-producing bacteria, the nontoxigenic bacteria acquire the capacity to synthesize the toxin.

Phage conversion also appears to be incriminated in the production of *α toxin* and *enterotoxin* in staphylococci (Chap. 14) and possibly certain somatic antigens in *Pseudomonas aeruginosa.*

Figure 3-34 A summary of the various factors involved in the transfer of bacterial genetic information by conjugation and bacteriophage.

Typical method of transfer	Factor	Normal location
Conjugation	F^+	Extrachromosomal
	Hfr	Chromosomal
	F′	Extrachromosomal
	Col	Extrachromosomal
	R	Extrachromosomal
	RTF	Extrachromosomal
	r determinants [RTF or F required for conjugal transfer]	Extrachromosomal
General transduction	Staphylococcal plasmid	Extrachromosomal
	Any bacterial gene	Chromosomal
Restricted transduction	Particular bacterial gene	Chromosomal

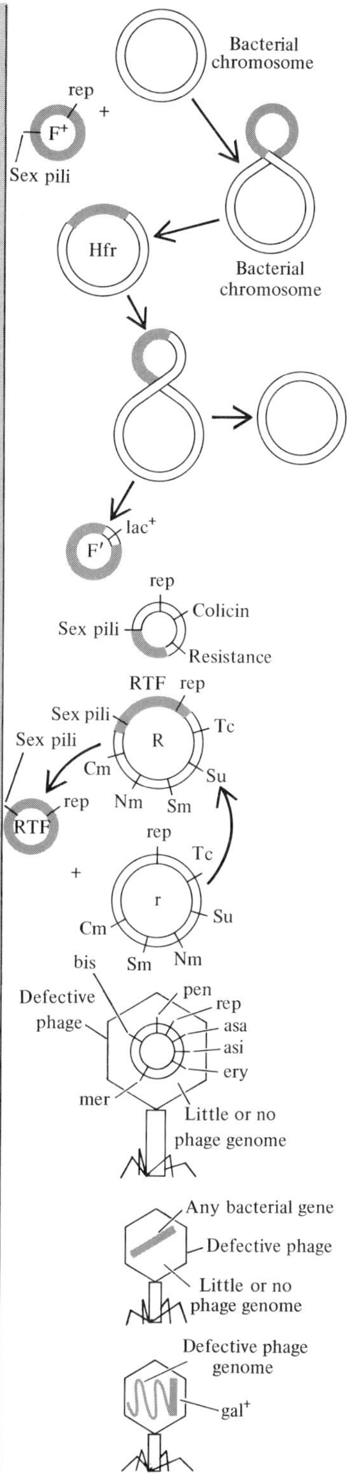

BIBLIOGRAPHY

Anderson, E. S., and Natkin, E.: "Transduction of Resistance Determinants and R Factors of the Δ Transfer Systems by Phage P1kc," *Mol. Gen. Genet.,* 114:261-265, 1972.

Clowes, R. C.: "Molecular Structure of Bacterial Plasmids," *Bacteriol. Rev.,* 36:361-405, 1972.

Downie, A. W.: "Pneumococcal Transformation. A Backward View," *J. Gen. Microbiol.,* 73:1-11, 1972.

Ebel-Tsipis, J., Botstein, D., and Fox, M. S.: "Generalized Transduction by Phage P22 in *Salmonella typhimurium:* I. Molecular Origin of Transducing DNA," *J. Mol. Biol.,* 71:433-448, 1972.

———, Fox, M. S., and Botstein, D.: "Generalized Transduction by Bacteriophage P22 in *Salmonella typhimurium:* II. Mechanism of Integration of Transducing DNA," *J. Mol. Biol.,* 71:449-469, 1972.

Echols, H.: "Developmental Pathways for the Temperate Phage: Lysis vs. Lysogeny," *Annu. Rev. Genet.,* 6:157-190, 1972.

Gill, D. M., Uchida, T., and Singer, R. A.: "Expression of Diphtheria Genes Carried by Integrated and Nonintegrated Phage Beta," *Virology,* 9:664-668, 1972.

Hayes, W.: *The Genetics of Bacteria and Their Viruses,* 2d ed., New York: John Wiley & Sons, Inc., 1968.

Hershey, A. D. (ed.): *The Bacteriophage Lambda,* New York: The Cold Spring Harbor Laboratory, 1971.

Kozak, M., and Nathans, D.: "Translation of the Genome of a Ribonucleic Acid Bacteriophage," *Bacteriol. Rev.,* 36:109-134, 1972.

Low, K. B.: "*Escherichia coli* K-12 F-prime Factors, Old and New," *Bacteriol. Rev.,* 36:587-607, 1972.

Meselson, M., Yuan, R., and Heywood, J.: "Restriction and Modification of DNA," *Annu. Rev. Biochem.,* 41:447-466, 1972.

Milliken, C. E., and Clowes, R. C.: "Molecular Structure of an R Factor, Its Component Drug Resistance Determinants and Transfer Factor," *J. Bacteriol.,* 113:1026-1033, 1973.

Notani, G. W.: "Regulation of Bacteriophage T4 Gene Expression," *J. Mol. Biol.,* 73:231-249, 1973.

Studier, F. W.: "Bacteriophage T7," *Science,* 176: 367-376, 1972.

Walker, E. M., and Pittard, J.: "Conjugation in *Escherichia coli:* Failure to Confirm the Transfer of Part of Sex Factor at the Leading End of the Donor Chromosome," *J. Bacteriol.,* 110:516-522, 1972.

Chapter 4

Mechanisms of Chemotherapy

Marvin N. Schwalb

PERSPECTIVE

Chemotherapy involves the application of chemicals to inhibit or kill a parasite within the host. The effectiveness of the chemotherapeutic agent depends upon the degree of *selective toxicity* which the agent exhibits; i.e., the agent must effectively kill or inhibit the parasite without causing serious damage to the host.

Suppression of microbial growth involves the interruption of some required metabolic function. In order to be selectively toxic, the chemotherapeutic agent must interact with a microbial function and/or structure which is either not present or substantially different in the host. Cell wall glycopeptide and ribosomes are examples of prokaryotic structures which are either not present or different in eukaryotic cells.

Eukaryotic parasites offer few metabolic targets distinct from their eukaryotic hosts. Therefore, most drugs which interrupt the function of eukaryotic parasites have significant effects upon the host. The result is that the number and variety of drugs effective against eukaryotic parasites is small compared to those useful against prokaryotes.

Selective toxicity is a relative, not an absolute, phenomenon. Many valuable chemotherapeutic agents do have side effects on host metabolism. Clinical use of a drug implies that the extent of host damage is tolerable in relation to the threat posed by the parasite.

Chemotherapeutic agents fall into two general classes on the basis of their origin: (1) natural products of microbes *(antibiotics)* and (2) *antimicrobial chemicals* synthesized in the laboratory. The distinction has lost its utility, however, since the natural product is frequently chemically modified in the laboratory. In common usage, the term *antibiotic* is often applied to any antimicrobial drug, regardless of its origin.

PHYSIOLOGY OF ANTIMICROBIAL ACTION

Static versus Cidal Effects

The activity of some chemotherapeutic agents leads to the irreversible inhibition of susceptible microbial cells. The result is cell death, and the effect is called *cidal.* Other drugs produce a cidal effect directly by *lysing* (dissolving) the cell.

Static drugs induce reversible inhibition of microbial growth, but upon dilution or removal of the drug, the cells can resume growth and reproduce. Static drugs are clinically effective because they limit the growth of the parasite, thereby enabling the host defense mechanisms to overcome the infection.

Physiological State of the Microbial Cell

Static and cidal effects are dependent in part upon the concentration of the drug and the growth of the susceptible microbe. Figure 4-1 illustrates the results of adding different drugs to a rapidly growing culture. A static drug such as sulfonamide causes a delayed cessation of bacterial growth because the bacteria must first use up the pool of folic acid whose synthesis the sulfonamide prevents. If the inhibited bacteria are washed and placed in a fresh medium without the drug, normal growth will resume.

Streptomycin is a cidal drug which does not cause rapid lysis of the bacteria. If, after a period of exposure to the drug, the cells are washed and placed in fresh medium, most of the bacteria fail to divide. Note, however, that contact with streptomycin eventually leads to a fall in the total cell count.

Penicillin is a cidal drug which causes cell death through lysis. Obviously, removing the drug would fail to alter the result, since the bacteria have been destroyed by the drug.

The cidal action of penicillin requires growing cells. If penicillin is added to bacteria in the stationary phase, lysis will not occur. Cidal action of streptomycin requires that the bacteria be actively metabolizing. A static drug may limit the activity of some cidal drugs. For example, when sulfonamide and penicillin are added together, there is an indirect inhibition of the activity of penicillin. The static drug (sulfonamide) stops bacterial growth. Under these conditions, the cidal drug (penicillin) is ineffective. When this type of combined therapy is applied clinically, the result achieved may be limited to the inhibition caused by the static drug. When the drug is diluted as a consequence of its distribution, metabolism, and excretion, renewed growth of the parasite may occur.

ANTIMICROBIAL SPECTRUM

If a drug can inhibit a number of gram-positive and gram-negative bacteria, it is said to have a *broad spectrum.* If a drug is active against a single bacterial group or only a few species, it is considered to have a *narrow spectrum.* Obviously, these are relative terms. Even within the confines of each spectrum, there is considerable species variation. For example, a drug may inhibit a number of gram-positive species, but the minimum inhibitory concentration for one organism can be 50 times that of the more sensitive species. Thus, it is often possible to inhibit a particular microorganism in the laboratory at a concentration that would be dangerous or impossible to achieve in vivo. These factors are taken into account in deciding what concentration of drug should be employed in performing the in vitro tests.

When a species is considered sensitive to a particular drug, this does not imply that every isolate of that species will be sensitive. Genetic differences among isolates can result in the recovery of populations of resistant bacteria from normally sensitive species. Since widespread administration of antimicrobial drugs has become a significant factor in the environment and evolution of microbes, changing patterns of antimicrobial spectra are frequently recorded. Consequently, the only way to determine the sensitivity of a microorganism to a particular drug is to isolate it from the patient and test it in vitro. As noted in Chapter 27, however, in some cases in vitro sensitivity is no guarantee that the drug will be effective in vivo, and conversely, failure to inhibit a microorganism in vitro does not imply that the drug is clinically useless.

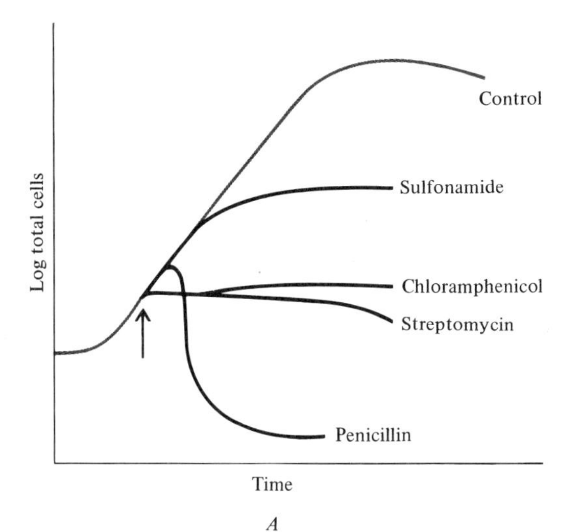

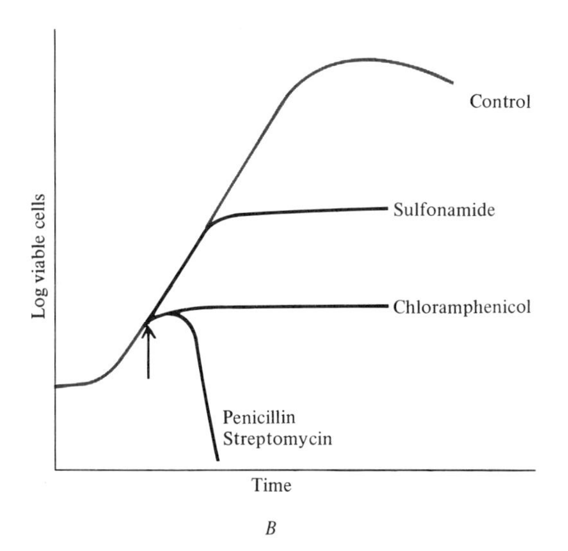

Figure 4-1 Effect of various drugs on the growth and viability of a susceptible organism. Drug added at arrow to log phase cells. *(A)* Effect on total number of cells. *(B)* Effect on cell viability. Sulfonamide and chloramphenicol are bacteriostatic. Penicillin and streptomycin are bactericidal.

MECHANISMS OF DRUG ACTION

Although many differences exist between a typical bacterial cell and a human liver cell, there are also many similarities. Because of this, the three principal areas of metabolism that present selective targets in prokaryotes are cell wall synthesis, ribosomal function, and vitamin synthesis. Human cells lack walls, have eukaryotic ribosomes, and by definition, do not synthesize vitamins. Selectively toxic compounds effective against other metabolic areas are rare, reflecting the many similarities between prokaryotic and eukaryotic organisms.

Competitive Inhibition

The precise mechanism of action of many antimicrobial drugs is not known; others, however, are understood in considerable detail. The following discussion will consider a number of antimicrobial drugs according to the area of metabolism they affect. There are several types of antimicrobial activity that are similar, regardless of the specific metabolic effect. One such activity is the *competitive inhibition* of enzyme function. In this case the drug is similar in structure to some essential metabolite, and competition occurs between them for the active site on the enzyme. The result is an apparent loss of enzyme activity, since the enzyme does not produce the required product when it is metabolizing the drug.

The inhibition of folic acid synthesis by sulfonamide is an example of competitive inhibition. Sulfonamide is structurally similar to para-aminobenzoic acid (PABA). The enzyme tetrahydropteroic acid synthetase (TASase) normally converts PABA to an essential precursor of folic acid. Sulfonamide competitively inhibits the TASase enzyme, producing a compound that cannot be made into folic acid. Thus, there is a reduction in the concentration of folic acid synthesized by the bacteria exposed to sulfonamide. There may also be secondary effects of feedback inhibition and/or repression by the sulfonamide products.

Competitive inhibition is a reversible effect, as is demonstrated by the fact that excessive quantities of PABA can overcome the inhibition produced by sulfonamide. Since there is no permanent binding by the drug, competitive inhibition often exerts a static effect.

Lethal Synthesis

Lethal synthesis involves the conversion of a drug by a microorganism to a toxic inhibitor. The original drug is not directly toxic but is metabolized by the organism to another related compound which is the active substance. Note that the original drug may cause competitive inhibition, but this is not the critical effect. Lethal synthesis can occur in the drug isoniazid, which is metabolized to an analogue of the hydrogen carriers NAD and NADP; at the same time, isoniazid is a competitive inhibitor of certain reactions involving pyridoxine. The lethal analogues cannot be applied directly to microbial cells because the microorganisms are usually impermeable to the metabolized drug (analogue).

Inhibitors of Cell Wall Synthesis

Cell wall glycopeptide is a unique prokaryotic component. Therefore, it is not surprising that a number of agents that inhibit the formation of glycopeptide are clinically effective. Glycopeptide synthesis can be inhibited at several points (Fig. 4-2). In general, the antibiotic causes an accumulation of cell wall precursors, such as sugar nucleotides.

Penicillins If the antibiotic penicillin is present when susceptible bacteria attempt to grow, functional cell walls will not be synthesized. The bacterial protoplasm continues to increase, and eventually the cell will burst its wall. In normal medium the consequence is cell death through lysis. In a medium of high osmotic tension, the action of penicillin results in the formation of protoplasts or spheroplasts. Penicillins inhibit the enzyme responsible for cross-linking between layers of glycopeptide. Penicillin has no effect on existing cell wall components and is only active against growing organisms.

The mold *Penicillium* produces a number of chemically different penicillins. Only two of these are of value in therapy. Penicillin G (benzyl penicillin) preparations are given intramuscularly. Penicillin V (phenoxymethyl penicillin) is resistant to acid decomposition and can therefore be given orally.

Isolates of *Penicillium* can also produce 6-aminopenicillanic acid, the so-called nucleus of penicillin-type molecules (Fig. 4-3). The nucleus can have numerous side chains added chemically to produce semisynthetic penicillins. More than 2,000 such compounds have been constructed, but only a few have proved to be of clinical value.

Semisynthetic Penicillins The semisynthetic penicillins possess one or more advantages over natural penicillins, including increased acid resistance, a broader antimicrobial spectrum, and resistance to penicillin-destroying enzymes (Fig. 4-3). Penicillinases are enzymes produced by staphylococci and some gram-negative enteric bacteria and are responsible for penicillin resistance in some members of these species. Examples of clinically useful semisynthetic penicillins include ampicillin, which is acid-resistant and has a broad microbial spectrum, and methicillin, which is resistant to penicillinase.

Although generally more cidal for gram-positive bacteria, penicillins as a group are broad-spectrum antibiotics. There are, however, considerable differences in activity among different

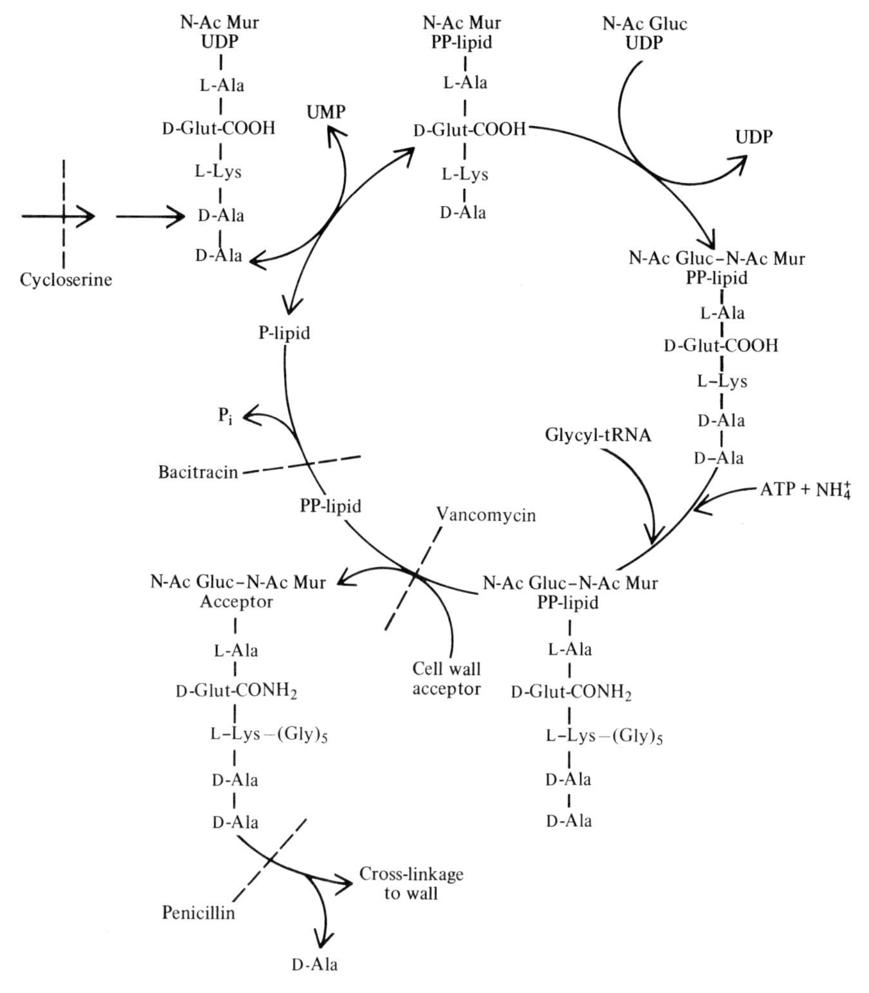

Figure 4-2 Inhibition of prokaryotic cell wall glycopeptide synthesis by various antibiotics.

penicillins, particularly toward some gram-negative bacteria. Ampicillin, for example, is several times more active than benzyl penicillin against a number of gram-negative bacteria. On the other hand, ampicillin may be less active than penicillin G in the treatment of infections caused by susceptible bacteria (Chap. 27).

Cephalosporins Cephalosporins are structurally similar to penicillin and apparently have a similar mode of action. The more potent and useful cephalosporins are semisynthetic forms, including cephalothin, which is injectable, and cephalexin, which is administered orally. The potential value of cephalosporins resides in their resistance to penicillinase, their broader spectrum of activity, and most important, the fact that they do not produce allergic reactions like those induced by penicillin.

Cycloserine Cycloserine interferes with the formation of the D-alanine-D-alanine portion of

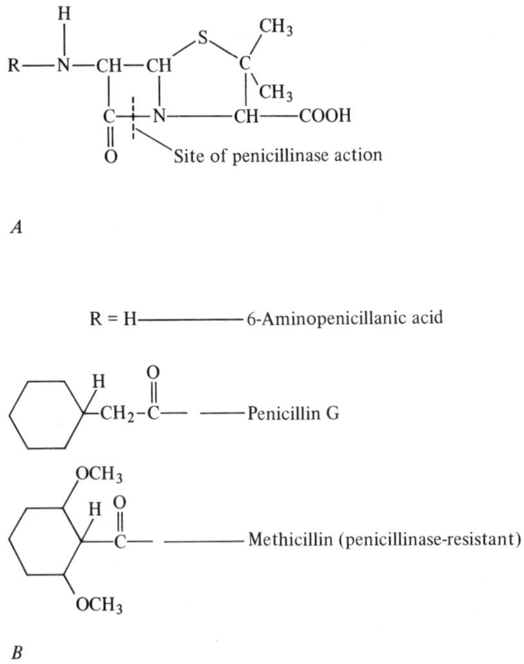

Site of penicillinase action

A

R = H —— 6-Aminopenicillanic acid

—— Penicillin G

—— Methicillin (penicillinase-resistant)

B

Figure 4-3 Structure of penicillins. *(A)* Basic penicillin molecule. *(B)* Various side chains.

the cell wall pentapeptide. Cycloserine is structurally similar to alanine and acts as an inhibitor of *alanine racemase* and the enzyme that produces D-alanine dipeptide, resulting in the accumulation of cell wall precursors and the formation of protoplasts. Cycloserine has a fairly wide spectrum of activity, but toxic side effects limit its use in therapy.

Bacitracin Bacitracin apparently interacts with the bacterial cell membrane to prevent the recycling of the lipid carrier that is involved in the transfer of structural cell wall units. Since bacitracin affects cell membranes, the protoplasts which are formed are inhibited. Bacitracin is active principally against gram-positive bacteria and is widely used in topical preparations in combination with other antibiotics (neomycin, polymyxin) to provide a broader spectrum of activity. High toxicity usually precludes systemic application.

Vancomycin Vancomycin is similar in function and spectrum to bacitracin. It interferes with the transfer of cell wall structural units from the lipid to the acceptor. Vancomycin is toxic but is still occasionally used in treating serious staphylococcal infections.

Inhibitors of Ribosomal Functions

The prokaryotic ribosome is smaller than the eukaryotic ribosome in both size and molecular weight. A number of different antibiotics act by binding to the prokaryotic ribosome, thereby interfering with protein synthesis.

Streptomycin, Neomycin, and Kanamycin (Aminoglycosides) The aminoglycosides have similar structures and modes of action, binding irreversibly to the smaller (30S) of the two ribosomal subunits. The result is miscoding of proteins so that nonfunctional peptides are produced. In addition, there is inhibition of peptide chain elongation.

Streptomycin causes a variety of secondary effects including inhibition of respiration and loss of membrane function. Although streptomycin is rapidly bactericidal, it does not cause immediate lysis (Fig. 4-1). Streptomycin is active against mycobacteria, gram-negative bacilli, and some staphylococci. Activity is reduced under acidic conditions. Resistance to streptomycin is a common phenomenon. Usually, streptomycin resistance is due to a mutation in the microbial cell which changes the structure of the 30S ribosomal subunit, thereby decreasing the ability of streptomycin to bind to the ribosome.

When streptomycin is added to a population of bacteria which contains a few resistant cells, the antibiotic acts as a selective agent for the resistant cells. The streptomycin rapidly kills off the sensitive bacteria and permits the resistant forms to proliferate, but does not cause the mutation. The selection of resistant bacteria is a serious problem in the case of streptomycin. Another mutation in the same gene causing resistance can result in streptomycin dependence. In this case, the mutation causes a damaging change in ribosomal structure which the binding of streptomycin partially corrects.

Neomycin and kanamycin are broad-spectrum antibiotics with strong activity on staphylococci and Enterobacteriaceae. Resistant mutants are less likely to be found with these antibiotics than with streptomycin.

Tetracyclines Tetracyclines also bind to the 30S ribosomal subunit, causing an inhibition of the function of tRNA. The effect is reversible, and the tetracyclines are bacteriostatic. Tetracyclines are broad-spectrum antibiotics which are active against a wide range of microorganisms including bacteria, rickettsiae, and chlamydiae. The activity of various tetracyclines is similar, and the appearance of resistant mutants is becoming a major problem.

Chloramphenicol Chloramphenicol is a bacteriostatic, broad-spectrum antibiotic that specifically binds to the larger 50S ribosomal subunit and inhibits protein synthesis. Chloramphenicol differs from the aminoglycosides and the tetracyclines in that it interferes with protein synthesis in eukaryotic cells, particularly in mitochondria and in rapidly proliferating cells. The latter action may be related to the toxicity of chloramphenicol in causing bone marrow aplasia as well as the gray syndrome in infants (see Chap. 27).

Erythromycin and Lincomycin Although erythromycin and lincomycin have distinctly different structures, they have similar modes of action and similar antimicrobial spectra. Both drugs inhibit protein synthesis by binding to the 50S ribosomal subunit and are active against a variety of gram-positive organisms and a few gram-negative species.

Intermediary Metabolism

The two most important inhibitors of intermediary metabolism (sulfonamides, isoniazid) have been discussed previously. Another competitive inhibitor of PABA is para-aminosalicylic acid (PAS). PAS is used with isoniazid or streptomycin in the treatment of tuberculosis to inhibit cells which might become resistant to the other two drugs.

Membrane Function

The polypeptide antibiotics polymyxin B and colistin cause damage to bacterial membranes, particularly in gram-negative species. The result is a loss of osmotic control, leading to leakage of bacterial components and ultimately in cell death. Polymyxins are quite toxic and are poorly absorbed from the intestinal tract. Consequently, these antibiotics are usually applied topically or are reserved for serious infections, such as *Pseudomonas,* that fail to respond to other antibiotics.

Inhibitors of Nucleic Acid

There are only two inhibitors of nucleic acid synthesis with sufficient selective toxicity to be of clinical value. *Nalidixic acid* specifically inhibits DNA synthesis without affecting RNA synthesis. The *rifamycins* are a group of antibiotics that inhibit DNA-dependent RNA polymerase activity, which is responsible for the synthesis of cellular RNA. Different rifamycins can inhibit the polymerase in prokaryotic and eukaryotic cells, or in both.

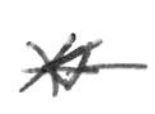

Several antibiotics, including actinomycin D and mitomycin, inhibit nucleic acid synthesis but are too toxic for general use. These agents have proved to be of great value in analyses of nucleic acid synthesis in viral replication, metabolic regulation, and development. Actinomycin D inhibits DNA-dependent RNA synthesis, and mitomycin inhibits DNA synthesis.

Antiviral Drugs

The intimate relationship of viral replication and host metabolism has hindered the development of antiviral drugs. Drugs such as 5-iodo-2-deoxyuridine inhibit viral DNA and are useful in the treatment of herpetic keratitis, but are too toxic for systemic administration. When given orally to smallpox contacts, N-methylthiosemicarbazone can reduce the incidence of the disease presumably by inhibiting the translation of late viral mRNA and thus preventing the formation of progeny virus. *Interferon* induces the synthesis of a cellular protein that prevents translation of viral mRNA's, but it appears to have limited therapeutic potential.

Antifungal Drugs

As is expected, because of their eukaryotic nature, fungi are susceptible to only a few drugs of a single type, the *polyenes.* The polyene antibiotics (amphotericin B and nystatin) affect the sterols of fungal cell membranes, causing permeability changes with resultant loss of vital cell constituents and, ultimately, cell death. Amphotericin B is the principal drug used in therapy of the systemic mycoses. Nystatin is useful in the treatment of cutaneous candidiasis.

Griseofulvin inhibits the DNA synthesis of mycelial fungi, causing an arrest in cell division, and is employed in therapy of superficial fungal infections *(dermatomycoses).* A variety of chemicals, including tolnaftate and gentian violet, is also used in the treatment of the dermatomycoses.

Antiprotozoal and Antihelminthic Drugs

Most of the drugs used to treat protozoal and helminthic disease are heavy metal poisons, including iodides, arsenicals, and antimony compounds. The agents are often general metabolic poisons and are frequently associated with serious side effects on the host. Examples include emetine hydrochloride for amebiasis and antimony potassium tartrate for helminths.

The mechanism of action of chloroquine on malarial parasites seems to be partly a function of its concentration in lysosomes. Within the malarial food vacuoles, chloroquine raises the pH, thereby reducing the digestion of hemoglobin by the parasite and preventing its growth.

RESISTANCE

Resistance to antimicrobial drugs is a property of the microbial cells. The genetic information for resistance is contained in the DNA of the microorganism. The information may be a normal part of the bacterial genome, in which case the species would be considered naturally resistant, or resistance can be acquired by either a mutation in a nuclear gene or the transfer of a plasmid bearing resistance information.

Resistance Due to Mutation

Resistance by mutation is a rare event in a population of cells, and the causes have been discussed in Chapter 3. When a bacterial cell resistant to a particular antibiotic appears, it passes the information for the resistance to its progeny and, in some cases, can transmit the resistance to other cells (via conjugation, transduction, transformation). In the absence of the selective agent (antibiotic) only a relatively small number of the population will possess the information. When the drug is applied to the bacterial culture, the large number of sensitive bacteria will be inhibited or killed. The resistant bacteria will continue to grow and will eventually represent the entire population.

The probability of finding a single microorganism with resistance to two or more antibiotics is extremely small (equal to the product of the frequency of each independent mutation). Note that this is not the same as finding two or more different bacteria which are each resistant to a different antibiotic, a probability equal to about two times the frequency of the independent events.

Resistance Due to Plasmids

In 1952, Japanese investigators discovered that *Shigella* bacteria recovered from a patient with dysentery were resistant to sulfonamide, streptomycin, and tetracycline. In 1955, the organisms were found to be resistant to chloramphenicol as well. In 1957, *Escherichia coli* were found to be multiply resistant to antibiotics when they were isolated during an epidemic of shigellosis. By 1966, about 75 percent of all shigellae isolated in Japan showed multiple resistance. At present, multiply resistant microorganisms are worldwide in distribution and are spreading to involve additional antibiotics and microorganisms, including typhoid bacilli.

The transmissible plasmid nature of multiple antibiotic resistance was confirmed by the following observations: (1) resistance is transferable with high frequency following conjugation regardless of the polarity of the F agent, and (2) resistance can be spontaneously lost by storage or treatment with acriflavine. The plasmid which carries the information for its conjugal transfer and resistance to antibiotics is called an *R factor*.

R factors can be transferred between many gram-negative bacteria including the Enterobacteriaceae *(Escherichia, Shigella, Salmonella, Klebsiella, Proteus, Enterobacter), Vibrio* species, and some species of *Pasteurella*. Resistance has been encountered to sulfonamides, streptomycin, tetracyclines, furazolidone, chloramphenicol, kanamycin, neomycin, and ampicillin. R factors carrying from one to eight different resistances have been detected and occur in various combinations.

The emergence of R factors may exert a significant effect on the ecology of pathogenic and nonpathogenic Enterobacteriaceae. Figure 4-4

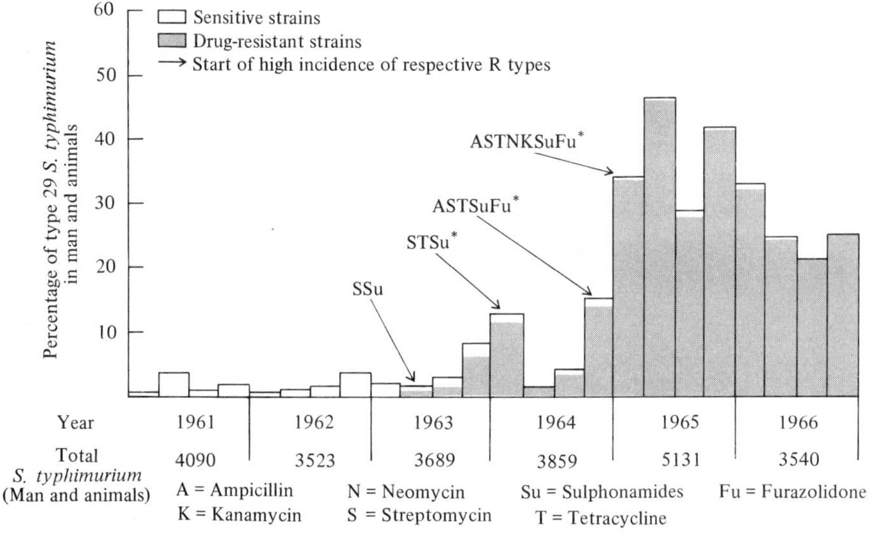

Figure 4-4 Changing pattern of microbial ecology and incidence of R factors in a natural population of *Salmonella typhimurium*. (*E. S. Anderson, Annu. Rev. Microbiol., 22:131–180, 1968.*)

shows the results of a study of the resistance pattern of *Salmonella typhimurium* phage type 29 in Great Britain. Before 1963, type 29 bacteria represented only a small percentage of the total isolates. In 1963, several R factor-containing bacteria were isolated for the first time. Since 1963, three changes have been observed: (1) a large number of type 29 isolates carry R factors, (2) as time progresses the R factors are carrying an increased number of resistances, and (3) the proportion of type 29 isolates among the total *S. typhimurium* population rose dramatically. Although it is not possible to ascertain from these data the exact nature of the R factors in the changing bacterial populations, clearly the findings are interrelated and interdependent. Since similar findings have been recorded from bacteria isolated from animals, the question of the role of animal sources in the selection and transmission of R factors to man requires study and evaluation. The transmissibility of R factors raises additional problems. For example, it is quite possible for members of the normal bacterial flora of the intestine to carry an R factor. If that person then is infected with an enteric pathogen lacking an R factor, the indigenous bacteria (i.e., *E. coli*) can transmit an R factor to the pathogen.

Differences between Resistance Due to Mutations and R Factors

The differences between resistance due to mutation and resistance carried by R factors include the following: (1) R factor resistance can be transferred to a population of cells without selection, (2) R factor resistance can be transferred between some species, (3) when one selective agent (drug) is applied, all resistances are selected for simultaneously, and (4) R factor resistance is currently limited to a few gram-negative bacterial species. It is important to note, however, that these species annually cause disease in millions of persons.

Mutations, on the other hand, occur in all microorganisms, are limited to a specific drug in a single mutational event, require selection by the specific drug, and rarely occur simultaneously in the same microorganism.

There has been considerable speculation concerning the origin of R factors. Essentially, the R factor consists of two components: (1) the genetic information for resistance and (2) the genetic information for conjugation, replication, and transfer. The latter function is similar to F factor activity. However, the mechanism of R factor resistance is often different from that for nuclear-coded resistance. For example, streptomycin resistance in R factors involves permeability changes and/or an inactivating enzyme. In contrast, changes in ribosomal structure are responsible for nuclear-coded streptomycin resistance. The detailed mechanisms are not known, but the evidence clearly indicates that R factors became much more widespread after the introduction of antimicrobial drugs.

Penicillinase activity in some staphylococci is coded for by a plasmid. Conjugation is absent in staphylococci, and the penicillinase plasmid cannot be transmitted by this mechanism, but it can be transferred by phage. Prevalence of penicillin-resistant (penicillinase-positive) staphylococci is probably the result of selection by the antibiotic of plasmid-bearing bacteria whose existence is known to antedate the clinical use of penicillin.

Molecular Mechanisms of Microbial Resistance to Antibiotics

Production of Enzymes Which Destroy or Modify the Drug The best-known example of this mechanism is penicillinase production. Penicillinase is a β-lactamase which hydrolyzes the lactam ring of penicillin (Fig. 4-3). *Penicillinacylase* (amidase) is a similar hydrolytic enzyme. The enzymes are produced by a number of bacteria, including staphylococci and gram-negative Enterobacteriaceae. In some species the enzyme is constitutive, and in other species it is induced by penicillin. As has been noted, there is a considerable difference in the sensitivity of penicillins to these enzymes.

There is also some evidence that some drugs can be modified by microbial enzymes through the addition of acetyl groups and can become therapeutically inactive. Apparently, some bacteria become resistant to chloramphenicol and kanamycin by this mechanism.

Altered Binding Affinity for the Drug Alteration of ribosomal structure to confer streptomycin resistance is an example of altered binding affinity. Another example occurs in some situations with sulfonamide-resistant bacteria in which the structure of the TASase enzyme is changed so that the enzyme has lower affinity for the sulfonamide molecule.

Changes in Cell Permeability Resistance to a number of different antimicrobial drugs occurs through alterations in the transport functions of the plasma membrane. The change is usually specific for a particular antibiotic and does not necessarily affect other drugs.

Changes in Metabolism Included in this category would be increased synthesis of a competitive precursor (i.e., PABA) or the development of alternate pathways of biosynthesis, bypassing the affected area of metabolism.

BIBLIOGRAPHY

Anderson, E. S.: "The Ecology of Transferable Drug Resistance in the Enterobacteria," *Annu. Rev. Microbiol.*, 22:131-180, 1968.

Garrod, L. P., and O'Grady, F.: *Antibiotic and Chemotherapy*, 3d ed., Edinburgh: E. & S. Livingstone, Ltd., 1971.

Mitsuhashi, S.: *Transferable Drug Resistance Factor R*, Baltimore, Md.: University Park Press, 1971.

Pestka, S.: "Inhibitors of Ribosome Function," *Annu. Rev. Biochem.*, 40:697-710, 1971.

Riva, S., and Luigi, G. S.: "Rifamycins: A General View," *Annu. Rev. Microbiol.*, 26:199-224, 1972.

Chapter 5

Factors That Determine Pathogenicity

Bernard A. Briody

PERSPECTIVE

Everyone recognizes that infectious disease is a fundamental accompaniment of human existence. On the other hand, the free-living microorganisms and helminths far outnumber the parasites, and they lead a saprophytic existence which rarely involves man. In addition, most parasites live in equilibrium with man as part of the normal flora of the skin, conjunctivae, nasopharynx, oral cavity, and intestinal and genitourinary tracts without invading tissues. In enunciating the requirements for successful parasitism, Theobald Smith emphasized that the parasite must (1) gain entrance to the host; (2) multiply and adapt to the host, preferably without causing serious harm; (3) exit from the host; and (4) be associated with an effective mechanism for transmission to a new host. In this context, infectious diseases represent unusual and aberrant forms of evolving parasitism in various stages of imbalance. Even in this frame of reference, subclinical infection rather than overt clinical disease is the rule. Nonetheless, it is imperative to consider those factors which enable a parasite to cause disease; i.e., one must determine the *pathogenicity*. The role of the host in influencing the outcome of interaction with the parasite is the major topic of Chapters 6 to 8 and 11. The other aspects of successful parasitism (entrance, exit, transmission) are included in Chapter 12.

PATHOGENETIC PATTERNS

Microorganisms, helminths, and their products are associated with a wide spectrum of pathogenetic patterns. When disease results following ingestion of microbial toxins, the term *intoxication* is applicable, since the organism is not involved as a parasite. When the parasite actually enters the host and produces disease, the term *infectious disease* is appropriate. *Disease* connotes the fact the the parasite causes an overt, clinically apparent alteration in function, structure, or both. However, most infections are subclinical (inapparent, asymptomatic), as determined by the fact that the parasites induce immunospecific responses in the host usually characterized by antibody (Chaps. 7, 8, and 11) or delayed hypersensitivity (Chaps. 8 and 11), or both in the absence of clinical manifestations.

Classically, the ability to cause disease (pathogenicity) and the degree of pathogenicity of a particular population of the parasite *(virulence)* are discussed in terms of toxigenicity and invasiveness. *Toxigenicity* refers to the ability of some pathogens (parasites able to produce disease in a susceptible host) to synthesize toxins *(exotoxins)* which are readily separable from the microbe and which usually appear in culture after lysis of bacterial cells. Microorganisms of exactly the same type but devoid of the ability to synthesize the toxin are nonpathogenic. For example, there are toxigenic (pathogenic) and nontoxigenic (nonpathogenic) diphtheria bacilli.

Despite exhaustive analysis, *endotoxins* defy definition. Their chemistry and location in microorganisms remains controversial, and components with similar biological properties occur in plant and animal tissues. For example, endotoxins are generally regarded as heat-stable *phospholipopolysaccharides* found principally at or near the cell surfaces of gram-negative bacteria, the bulk of the activity often being present in the cell wall. On the other hand, in some cases microbial components with endotoxic biological activity are secreted into the medium during growth of the bacteria (*Pseudomonas* slime polysaccharide). The current trend is to identify an endotoxin as a substance which induces a number of typical host responses, many of which involve injury to the cardiovascular system.

The traditional concept of *invasiveness* implies the capacity to produce a generalized infection in the host, i.e., the ability to enter host tissues, multiply there, and spread. Septicemic (overwhelming bloodstream invasion) anthrax and plague are cited as classical examples of invasiveness. Obviously, however, such situations represent the extreme form of unbalanced parasitism and are rarely encountered in clinical medicine.

While it has been recognized that there are degrees of invasiveness and toxigenicity and that a particular disease can result from a combination of the two, the concepts remain unrealistically vague in the light of accumulated data and are of limited value in understanding the sequential phenomena leading to the production of infectious disease (pathogenesis). In an effort to provide a more comprehensive insight into the many different ways in which a parasite can induce disease, pathogenetic patterns, factors, and mechanisms as well as their interactions and frequencies will be examined.

Intoxications

As indicated in Table 5-1, disease may result from intoxication following the ingestion of staphylococcal enterotoxins or of botulinus toxins (Chap. 13) or of fungal toxins, principally those produced by *Aspergillus* species (aflatoxins) and the mushrooms, especially *Amanita phalloides*. The consequences vary appreciably with the particular toxin. For example, the annual incidence of staphylococcal food poisoning in the United States may approach 1 million cases with few, if any, fatalities. Fungal intoxication and botulism annually account for far fewer cases (a few hundred and less than a hundred cases, respectively) but are associated with a fatal outcome in about half of the cases.

Table 5-1 Pathogenetic Patterns Associated with Parasites and Their Products

Pattern	Selected examples
Intoxication	Staphylococcal food poisoning, botulism, mushroom poisoning
Migration	Cutaneous larva migrans
Adherence	Fish tapeworm, trichuriasis, hookworm, many other helminthic diseases
Adherence and growth	Dermatomycoses, bacterial and giardial malabsorption
Adherence, growth, and toxin production	Diphtheria, cholera, diarrheal disease due to *Escherichia coli* and *Vibrio parahemolyticus*, scarlet fever
Adherence, penetration, and growth	Respiratory and gastrointestinal diseases caused by viruses, shigellosis, trachoma, inclusion conjunctivitis, salmonellosis, neonatal gonococcal conjunctivitis
Lymphatic spread	Tuberculosis, histoplasmosis, gonorrhea, chancroid, lymphogranuloma venereum, salmonellosis
Systemic distribution	Typhoid, hookworm disease, primary herpes simplex, poliomyelitis, Coxsackie disease, echovirus diseases, lymphocytic choriomeningitis, arbovirus diseases, anthrax, plague, tularemia, rickettsial diseases, psittacosis, viral hepatitis, bacterial meningitis, mumps, malaria, leishmaniasis, trypanosomiasis, schistosomiasis, syphilis, smallpox, varicella, rubella, measles, leptospirosis, relapsing fever, histoplasmosis, coccidioidomycosis

Mushroom poisoning *(A. phalloides)* is induced by heat-stable polypeptides which are rapidly bound to tissues and, after a latent period of 6 to 20 hr., lead to cellular destruction in liver, kidneys, muscle, and brain. Abdominal manifestations are succeeded by cardiovascular collapse, and signs of CNS involvement are common. Death ensues in 5 to 8 days in approximately half the cases; in the remainder, recovery is slow, and specific therapy is not available. Another mushroom *(A. muscaria)* synthesizes an alkaloid muscarine which stimulates the parasympathetic nervous system, inducing dyspnea, bradycardia, hypotension, signs of CNS involvement, and death within a few hours unless atropine is given until the manifestations are controlled, in which event complete recovery usually occurs in 24 hr.

Aflatoxins are a unique group of highly oxygenated, naturally occurring heterocyclic compounds of low molecular weight (300 to 350 range) produced by *Aspergillus* species. In accord with the distribution of the fungi, aflatoxins are found in a wide variety of edible materials including peanuts and peanut products, sweet potatoes, cassavas, rice, beans, coconuts, beer, milk, grains, cereals, and commercial animal feeds. While there is only suggestive evidence for a causal relationship between the ingestion of aflatoxins and the incidence of hepatotoxicity in man, including cirrhosis and cancerous conditions, these toxins have been shown to be responsible for pathologic hepatic conditions in cattle, pigs, poultry, and fish and, experimentally, have induced hepatotoxicity in primates. The precise mode of action is not known. Generally, however, aflatoxins resemble, but are not as potent as, actinomycin D in binding to DNA and blocking RNA synthesis. On the basis of studies in primates in which a high-protein diet countered the hepatotoxicity of aflatoxins, whereas a low-protein diet could not, it is suspected that kwashiorkor in children may enhance the carcinogenic potential of aflatoxins.

Migration

Clinical manifestations are occasionally associated with larval migration of various helminths. Disease may be the exclusive result of irritation produced by cutaneous migration of larvae of the dog and cat hookworms, producing an intense pruritis, or itching (creeping eruption). Cutaneous larva migrans occurs in the absence of replication of the parasite. Ground itch represents an early stage of cutaneous larval irritation in hookworm infection prior to the entry of the larvae into the circulation and involves intense itching and burning, followed by edema and erythema, papules, and vesicles. Transient pulmonary infiltration with eosinophilia (Loeffler's syndrome) may be observed as an incidental finding prior to localization of the parasite in a variety of helminth infections, including ascariasis, hookworm infection, trichinosis, strongyloidiasis, visceral larva migrans, and fasciolopsiasis. In visceral larva migrans, the larvae of the dog ascarid hatch from eggs in the small intestine and migrate into the liver, lungs, muscle, and brain, inciting granulomatous reactions with eosinophilia.

Adherence

The ability of a parasite to adhere or attach to the plasma membrane of tissue cells lining mucosal surfaces apparently represents an essential prerequisite for the overwhelming number of human pathogens. The evidence available strongly suggests that adherence is a highly specific process, the result of complementary chemical and conformational structures (receptors) on the surface of the parasite and the host cell plasma membrane. Similar receptors are involved in phage-bacteria interactions and in immunologic reactions.

The fundamental significance of adherence is that it provides a reasonable explanation for the localization of pathogens in selected tissue sites or represents the first step in a series of events which ultimately culminate in disease. For example, adenoviruses combine with conjunctival epithelial cells. In streptococcal pharyngitis the causative bacteria localize on the surface of epithelial cells in the pharynx because of the M protein. Other streptococci attach to oral membranes. Most of the respiratory viruses and pertussis bacteria attach to ciliated epithelial cells. Mycoplasma burrow into the crypts of the ciliated epithelial cells. Cholera organisms, shigellae, and salmonellae adhere to mucosal cells in the small intestine. Gonococci can attach to the columnar or transitional epithelium of the vagina until puberty and produce vulvovaginitis, but when this is replaced by stratified squamous epithelium after puberty they can no longer do so. The neurovirulence of poliovirus is a function of its ability to combine with receptors on the surface of neurones in the brainstem and spinal cord. Yeast, but not hyphal forms, of *Histoplasma* and *Blastomyces* can combine with tissue cells. Amebic and giardial trophozoites, but not cysts, can adhere to mucosal cells in the small intestine. Malarial sporozoites can attach to hepatic cells and merozoites to erythrocytes, whereas gametocytes are inert until taken up by anopheline mosquitoes. In a few cases specialized structures are involved in adherence (suction disks in giardial trophozoites, the scolex in tapeworms, the mouth parts of the hookworm, the posterior end in the species *Trypanosoma cruzi,* the anterior end in *Trichuris*).

Adherence alone is rarely, if ever, responsible for inducing disease. Perhaps the most primitive pathogenetic pattern is associated with a number of helminths that cause disease by their feeding habits. For example, in fish tapeworm, pathology is the result of attachment and preferential utilization of vitamin B_{12} which shuts off the host cell supply and leads to anemia.

There is no increase in the number of adult tapeworms as a consequence of attachment. In heavy infections with *Trichuris,* adherence to the plasma membranes of the mucosal cells in the small intestine permits the helminth to withdraw blood and cause anemia. As in the fish tapeworm, the number of adult worms is not increased, and the formation of eggs is of no consequence to the host, since they are simply passed out in the feces. While the earlier stages in pathogenesis are much more complicated, pathology in hookworm disease is largely dependent on the use of the host's blood as a source of nourishment following attachment of the worms to the mucosa of the small intestine.

Adherence and Growth

Except for the dermatophytes (superficial fungi) which are frequently encountered in the keratinized tissues of the body (skin, hair, nails), adherence and growth of the parasite is not a common pathogenetic pattern. Even among the dermatophytes, much of the tissue damage is apparently associated with delayed hypersensitivity to the fungi and their products. The malabsorption syndrome probably represents one of the few examples of adherence and growth causing disease. In this syndrome, bacterial growth on the mucosal epithelium of the small intestine blocks the absorption of vitamin B_{12}, and the giardial growth blocks the absorption of vitamin A and fats.

Adherence, Growth, and Toxin Production

The combination of adherence, growth, and toxin production determines the course of several diseases and is an integral element in the pathogenesis of other infections. In the case of diphtheria, the bacteria lodge on the epithelial surface of the nasopharynx, grow, and synthesize toxin. The toxin produces local tissue damage and, more important, is absorbed into the circulation and induces its specific effects (blocking polypeptide elongation factor, T2) in vital organs. In nonexudative diarrheal disease (cholera, traveler's disease, *Clostridium perfringens* infections), the causative agent adheres to the mucosal cells of the small intestine, grows, and synthesizes its specific enterotoxin which in turn induces the loss of fluid and electrolytes which constitutes the disease. In the process the intestinal mucosal cells remain intact. In the pathogenesis of scarlet fever, adherence, growth, and production of erythrogenic toxin are essential, but not exclusive, elements.

Adherence, Penetration, and Growth

It is estimated that approximately two-thirds of all infectious diseases in man, those involving the respiratory and gastrointestinal tracts, are the direct result of adherence, penetration, and growth of the parasite in the lining epithelial cells. As will be noted in Chapter 12, this pathogenetic pattern determines the short incubation period encountered in respiratory and gastrointestinal infections, invites serious secondary bacterial complications, severely handicaps efforts to develop effective vaccines (because the disease is over before an effective anamnestic antibody response can intervene), and illustrates the overriding significance of *secretory IgA antibody* in protection against most of the infectious diseases afflicting man.

The basic pathogenetic pattern is a localized infection in which the parasite adheres to, penetrates, grows within, and destroys mucosal epithelial cells. The most common causative agents are viruses, but a number of bacteria are also involved. Most clinical *Shigella* and *Salmonella* infections (e.g., exudative acute diarrheal disease) are classic examples of this pathogenetic pattern. Other epithelial surfaces are involved in trachoma, inclusion conjunctivitis, and gonorrhea (Fig. 5-1).

Lymphatic Spread

Following adherence, growth, penetration, and in some cases, toxin production, most parasites are promptly disposed of locally by infiltrating

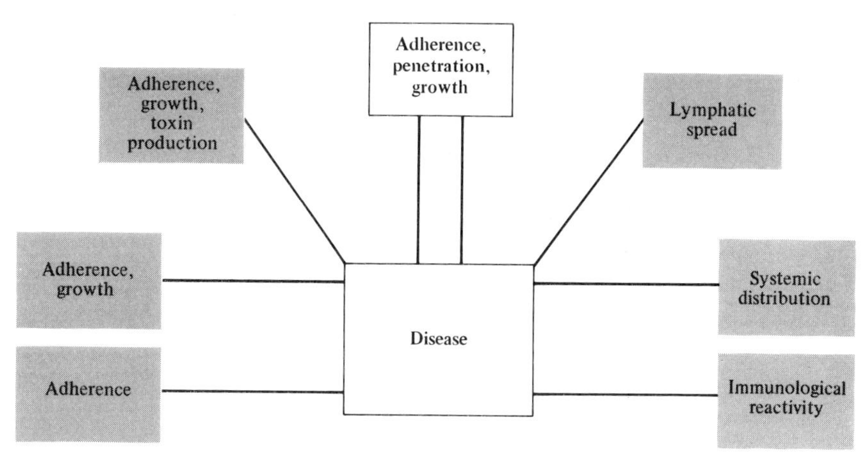

Figure 5-1 Pathogenetic patterns in infectious disease.

phagocytes or are eliminated by macrophages in the regional lymph nodes. In some cases, however, the pathogen can multiply to a limited degree within the lymph node. Classic examples of disease being halted after a period of growth within the regional lymph nodes include tuberculosis, histoplasmosis, gonorrhea, salmonellosis, and chancroid. In other cases, the pathogen may multiply extensively in the lymph nodes, as in lymphogranuloma venereum and African trypanosomiasis, or may destroy lymphocytes, as in measles and lepromatous leprosy.

Systemic Distribution

If the pathogen cannot be contained by the infiltrating phagocytes or within the regional lymph nodes, systemic distribution is the result. The consequences vary, depending upon the particular parasite. The presence of the pathogen in the blood may involve (1) a phase in pathogenesis of the disease, as in typhoid and hookworm infection; (2) a transient inconsequential episode without localized or systemic disease, as in the majority of infections associated with herpes simplex virus, polio-, Coxsackie, echo-, lymphocytic choriomeningitis, and the encephalitis (arbo-) viruses; (3) an overwhelming septicemia, as in anthrax, plague, gram-negative endotoxin shock, and the Waterhouse-Friedrichsen syndrome of circulatory collapse, shock, and bilateral hemorrhagic necrosis of the adrenals in meningococcemia and other bacterial septicemias; (4) disease of varying severity with localization in various tissues, as in metastatic staphylococcal abscesses, pneumococcal pneumonia and meningitis, gonococcal arthritis and meningitis, *Hemophilus* and meningococcal meningitis, bacterial endocarditis, cryptococcal and amebic meningitis, psittacosis, Q fever, typhus, paralytic poliomyelitis, viral encephalitis, yellow fever, viral hepatitis, rabies, mumps, amebic hepatitis, malaria, leishmaniasis, trypanosomiasis, and many helminthic diseases including schistosomiasis; or (5) extensive growth of the parasite in target tissues, followed by redistribution of the pathogen, as in typhoid, syphilis, the exanthemata (smallpox, varicella, rubella, measles), most rickettsial diseases, leptospirosis, relapsing fever, echovirus exanthemata, and in disseminated histoplasmosis and coccidioidomycosis.

PATHOGENETIC FACTORS

Genetic Structure

The genetic structure of parasites is ultimately responsible for their pathogenicity. A single gene may decide the issue, as in the case of pneumococcal polysaccharide, or a single chromosomal locus may determine the ability of *Shigella* bacteria to penetrate epithelial cells; but more commonly, pathogenicity is the result of the operation of multiple genes. Pathogenicity can be affected by mutation, transformation, transduction, conjugation, and conversion (see Chap. 3). Phage genes, rather than bacterial genes, are responsible for the pathogenicity of a number of bacteria because they can code for the synthesis of a number of toxins, including diphtheria, erythrogenic, and staphylococcal toxins, or because they direct the synthesis of new antigens, as in *Salmonella.* Ability to produce enterotoxin can be transmitted by conjugation in *Escherichia coli,* which thus will be able to induce traveler's disease.

The shift in yeast and hyphal forms among the dimorphic fungi and the various stages in the life cycle of malarial and helminthic parasites are intimately involved in pathogenicity and are unquestionably under genetic control.

In most cases, the genes exert their effects via surface structural components of the parasite itself or the surface conformation of the toxins produced by the pathogen. In the case of oncogenic viruses (see Chap. 2), on the other hand, the virus penetrates the cell, and viral DNA (in both DNA and RNA viruses) becomes integrated with the DNA of the host cell, leading to multiple changes in the cell including the appearance of new antigens and the unregulated growth of the cell. An analogous situation occurs when the genome of temperate phage integrates with the bacterial chromosome and induces multiple changes in bacteria (Chap. 3).

Surface Structure

The surface of human parasites is the key to their pathogenicity, virulence, and immunological reactivity (see Chaps. 7, 8, and 11). The chemical and conformational surface structure of parasites or their toxic products are responsible for (1) survival of the parasite or its toxic products prior to attachment, (2) adherence to susceptible host cells, (3) penetration of the susceptible target cells, and (4) the ability to resist phagocytosis, to survive within phagocytes, or to grow within phagocytes.

Staphylococcal enterotoxins, botulinus toxins, and fungal toxins are resistant to acid, bile salts, and enzymes and are therefore able to reach the mucosal cells of the small intestine. As a matter of fact, partial digestion of botulinus toxins by proteolytic enzymes leads to their dissociation into a greater number of toxic fragments. Enteric bacterial, viral, and protozoal pathogens are similarly resistant to acid, bile salts, and enzymes. For example, amebic cysts can traverse the upper gastrointestinal tract, the cyst wall disintegrates in the ileum, and eventually, trophozoites are released which can attach to the intestinal mucosa. Trophozoites, on the other hand, cannot induce infection following ingestion because they are inactivated before reaching the ileum. Viruses which are not generally considered enteric pathogens (poliovirus, Coxsackie virus, echovirus) are resistant to acid, bile salts, and enzymes and consequently are able to adhere, penetrate, grow locally, and thereafter induce systemic infection.

Since adherence and penetration are discussed above, the remaining comments concerning surface structures will deal with the resistance of pathogens to phagocytosis. At the most primitive level, phagocytosis may be precluded by the size of the parasite which, in the case of the helminths, may be billions of times as large as the phagocyte. At a more microscopic level, surface components of the pathogen may prevent phagocytosis. Included in this category would be the surface polysaccharides of pneumococci, meningococci, influenza bacilli, *Klebsiella,* and yeasts (cryptococci); the M protein of group A streptococci; and the glutamyl polypeptide of the anthrax bacillus. Within the phagocyte many parasites can survive or actually grow. Included in this group probably would be a number of protozoa, including *Leishmania, Trypanosoma, Toxoplasma,* and

Pneumocystis; typhoid, brucella, tubercle, and leprosy bacilli and gonococci, meningococci, and other bacteria; fungi such as *Histoplasma;* and viruses such as measles. In the case of tubercle bacilli, their ability to survive and grow within alveolar phagocytes is at least partly dependent on their surface lipopolysaccharides and mycolic acid which appear to prevent the discharge of lysosomal enzymes within the phagocytic vacuoles.

Toxins

The pathogenetic role of toxins in the production of human disease is clearly established in the intoxications associated with staphylococcal enterotoxins, botulinus toxins, and fungal toxins. In the presence of infection, toxins play a decisive role in diphtheria, tetanus, gas gangrene, and nonexudative acute diarrheal disease associated with enterotoxins produced by Microorganisms (*Vibrio cholerae, Escherichia coli,* and *Clostridium perfringens*) and at least an accessory role in anthrax, plague, brucellosis, and scarlet fever. Whether toxins are involved in other infectious diseases remains to be determined. Since more detailed discussions of the toxins and their mechanisms of action are included in Chapters 13, 14, and 18, their actions are summarized briefly in Table 5-2. In general, the toxins are proteins which have a specific effect on selected targets within particular cells.

Table 5-2 The Mode of Action of Toxins

Toxin	Mode of action
Botulinus	Inhibits release of acetylcholine at myoneural junction
Tetanus	Suppresses synaptic inhibition
Lecithinase (α-toxin) (gas gangrene)	Hydrolyzes lecithin in plasma membranes, but mechanism of lethal action is obscure
Diphtheria	Inhibits protein synthesis by inactivating T2 translocation factor required for elongation of polypeptide chains
Erythrogenic toxin (scarlatinal)	Increases permeability
Staphylococcal enterotoxin	Unknown, but may act directly on the intestinal mucosa
Choleragen	Activates adenyl cyclase in intestinal epithelial membrane, stimulating cAMP which in turn causes fluid and electrolyte loss
Other enterotoxins	*E. coli* and *C. perfringens* toxins have a choleragen-like activity
Anthrax	Increases permeability and causes fluid loss
Plague	Attacks cardiac myocardial membranes

Metabolites

There are many other metabolic products or metabolites synthesized by various microorganisms which may or may not be involved in the pathogenesis of disease but which are at least suspect. Included in this category are staphylococcal α-toxin and streptolysin S, which labilize lysosomal enzymes. Protein A of pathogenic staphylococci combines with the Fc fragment of 45 percent of IgG, results in aggregates of protein A and IgG which can fix complement and induce Arthus type reactions, and also has an antiphagocytic effect. A deoxycholate residue factor of pathogenic staphylococci inhibits neutrophilic chemotaxis and suppresses early inflammatory reactions. *Shigella* enterotoxin can cause fluid accumulation in ligated segments of the small intestine of animals, but its role in human shigellosis has yet to be delineated. A battery of peptidases, collagenase, and elastase may be involved in the pathogenesis of dermatomycoses, and toxins are suspected in disease induced by pertussis bacilli and mycoplasma. In hookworm disease, secretion of an anticoagulant facilitates the withdrawal of blood. In clostridial infections, collagenase and hyaluronidase may have accessory roles in the development of the disease.

Table 5-3 Biological Activities Ascribed to Endotoxins

Immunogenicity
Tolerance
Adjuvant activity
Protection against radiation
Fever and hypothermia
Leukopenia and leukocytosis
Granulocytopenia and granulocytosis
Depressed and enhanced resistance to pathogens
Depressed and enhanced clearance of particulate matter from the circulation
Release of lymphokines from sensitized thymus-dependent small lymphocytes
Increased glycolysis
Increased synthesis of corticosteroids
Inhibition of protein synthesis
Depressed or enhanced release of histamine, catecholamines, and anaphylatoxin
Increased and decreased permeability
Increased and decreased responsiveness to contractile effects of epinephrine
Depressed granulocytic diapedesis
Slowing of blood flow in microcirculation
Narrowing of effluent vessels
Dilation of arterioles and capillaries
Contraction of venules
Induction of type III Arthus' reactions
Cytotoxicity
Tumor-necrotizing activity
Depression of complement concentration in plasma
Circulatory collapse (hypotension and shock)
Labilization of lysosomes
Reactivity with leukocytes and platelets

Endotoxins

Perhaps no microbial components or products have generated as much confusion, controversy, and paradoxical findings as have endotoxins. Chemically, physically, and biologically, endotoxins represent diverse entities. Unfortunately, a critical review is beyond the scope of this text, and it is necessary to limit consideration to a listing of some of the activities ascribed to endotoxins (Table 5-3 and Fig. 5-2). Admittedly, definitive conclusions concerning the mode of action of endotoxins are not warranted. Generally, however, the most attractive hypothesis in the view of this author is that most, if not all, of the biological activities of endotoxins are compatible with immunologically mediated phenomena (Table 5-4 and Fig. 5-2).

Table 5-4 Responses Induced by Endotoxins Compatible with Immunological Phenomena

Antibody-mediated phenomena
Histological changes resembling allergic reactions, especially type III Arthus' reactions
Intensity parallel to antibody concentration
Poor responses in germ-free or antibody-deficient animals
Increased chemotaxis and granulocytosis
Depression of complement concentration in plasma
Inhibition by corticosteroids which stabilize lysosomes and inhibit neutrophilic chemotaxis
Labilization of lysosomes
Formation of thrombi in the microcirculation
Immune adherence
Aggregation of platelets
Anaphylatoxin formation
Release of histamine and catecholamines after perfusion of lungs with endotoxin in blood
Increased permeability
Hypotension and shock
Tolerance following a series of closely spaced injections of small doses
Biphasic fever curve
Primary reaction with leukocytes and platelets
Cell-mediated phenomena
Primary binding to sensitized thymus-dependent small lymphocytes
Release of lymphokines from sensitized thymus-dependent small lymphocytes
Inhibition by corticosteroids which stabilize lysosomes and inhibit macrophage infiltration
Depression of contact sensitivity to dinitrochlorobenzene

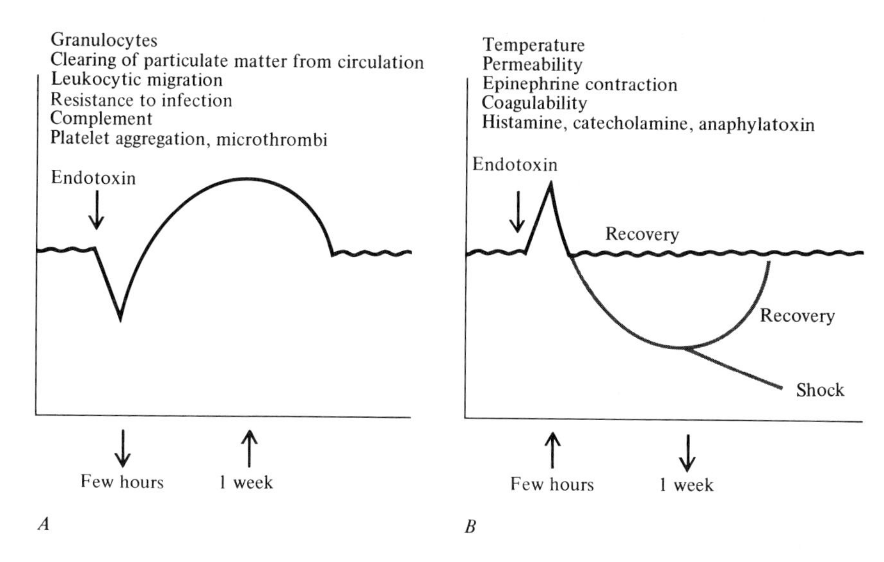

Figure 5-2 Selected biological activities of endotoxins. *A.* Following the injection of endotoxin, several parameters show a biphasic response. For example, there is an initial depression in the number of granulocytes, the clearing of particulate matter from the circulation, the migration of leukocytes, resistance to infection, plasma concentration of complement, aggregation of platelets, and formation of microthrombi which is quickly succeeded by an enhancement of each parameter and after a week or more by a return to preinjection levels. *B.* Other parameters show a variable response depending largely upon the concentration of endotoxin injected. For example, there may be an initial rise in temperature followed rapidly by a return to normal or succeeded quickly by a fall in temperature that persists for a week or more before returning to preinjection levels, or the hypothermia may be progressive and terminal. Similarly variable responses may ensue in the case of vascular permeability, epinephrine-induced contraction, coagulability, and the release of histamine, catecholamines, and anaphylatoxin.

Other Considerations

Many other factors influence the pathogenicity of parasites including the size of the parasite, its morphological form, the stage in the life cycle, the route by which it comes into contact with the host, and the dose. In many situations, the dose of the toxin or the parasite is inversely proportional to the incubation period and is directly proportional to the severity of the disease. For example, increasing the dose may convert a localized infection into a generalized or even fulminating infection. In helminthic infections, with the exception of cysticercosis, the hermaphroditic tapeworms, and strongyloidiasis in which autoinfection may occur, the dose of the parasite is absolutely proportional to the severity of the disease, since eggs or larvae do not mature and increase in number within the host.

PATHOGENETIC MECHANISMS

While the mechanisms whereby parasites induce disease are the proper subject for textbooks of pathology and pathophysiology, it is pertinent to indicate in this chapter the spectrum of effects that can lead to pathologic conditions and to reserve for subsequent chapters discussion of immunologically mediated diseases. As noted in Table 5-5, parasites can cause disease by irritation or migration, as in cutaneous larva migrans or onchocerciasis; can interfere with absorption of an essential metabolite (vitamin B_{12}), as in the case of malabsorption

Table 5-5 Pathogenetic Mechanisms

Mechanism	Selected examples
Migration	Cutaneous and visceral larva migrans, ascariasis, hookworm disease, strongyloidiasis, trichinosis, fasciolopsiasis, onchocerciasis
Malabsorption	Bacteria and *Giardia*
Utilization of vitamin B_{12}	Fish tapeworm
Withdrawal of blood	Hookworm disease
Mechanical blockage	Ascariasis, schistosomiasis, filariasis, candidiasis, aspergillosis, lymphogranuloma venereum, malaria
Interference with phagocytosis	Infections due to pneumococci, meningococci, group A streptococci, cryptococci, influenza, *Klebsiella,* and anthrax bacilli
Interference with phagocytic killing	Leishmaniasis, trypanosomiasis, typhoid, toxoplasmosis, pneumocystis pneumonia, brucellosis, tuberculosis, leprosy, measles, meningococcal meningitis, gonorrhea, histoplasmosis
Interference with vital functions	Diphtheria, tetanus, botulism, cholera, shigellosis, salmonellosis, rickettsial diseases, plague, anthrax
Intracellular growth and destruction of cells	Shigellosis, salmonellosis, leprosy, tuberculosis, typhoid, brucellosis, rickettsial diseases, chlamydial diseases, most viral diseases
Fusion of cell and viral membranes	Herpes simplex, varicella, measles, parainfluenza, respiratory syncytial disease
Genetic integration	Cancerous conditions induced by oncogenic viruses
Immunodepression	Measles, lepromatous leprosy, tuberculosis, syphilis, virus-induced cancer, lymphocytic choriomeningitis
Delayed hypersensitivity	Tuberculosis, leprosy, syphilis, dermatomycoses, systemic mycoses, protozoal and helminthic diseases
Immune complex disease	Potentially any infectious disease, pneumococcal lobar pneumonia

due to bacteria (Chap. 18); can preferentially utilize vitamin B_{12}, as in the case of the fish tapeworm, causing anemia and leading to megaloblastic anemia in 1 percent of the patients; or can produce anemia by sucking blood, as in hookworm disease. Many pathogens can produce pathology by mechanical blockage in the intestines (ascariasis), urinary tract (schistosomiasis), lymphatic system (filariasis), endocardium (fungi), glomeruli (fungi), lungs (*Aspergillus* and a number of helminths), and blood vessels (schistosomiasis and falciparum malaria).

As noted in Table 5-2, toxins induce a number of changes which interfere with essential functions, including the maintenance of fluid and electrolyte balance, the release of acetylcholine at myoneural junctions, synaptic inhibition, vascular permeability, protein synthesis, and the integrity of cardiac myocardial membranes.

In the case of most pathogens, tissue damage results from the attachment, penetration, and intracellular growth within mucosal epithelial cells. For example, influenza and other respiratory viruses destroy ciliated epithelial cells; shigellae and salmonellae damage mucosal cells of the small intestine; conjunctival epithelial cells are attacked in trachoma, inclusion conjunctivitis, and neonatal gonococcal conjunctivitis; and columnar epithelial cells in the genital tract are damaged in gonorrhea.

Other pathogenetic mechanisms include the fusion of viral and cell membranes leading to the formation of giant cells *(syncytia)* in herpes simplex, varicella, measles, parainfluenza, and respiratory syncytial viruses. The integration of viral nucleic acid with the cellular genome in infections with oncogenic viruses can lead to unregulated growth of cells in animals and may occur in man (Chap. 2). Finally, most infectious diseases exert a variety of effects on the immune responses of the host, ranging from antibody production to delayed hypersensitivity, the formation of immune complexes, autoimmune disease, and depression of cell-mediated immunity

(Chaps. 7, 8, 10, and 11). In most cases, it has been difficult to evaluate the role of immunological phenomena in the pathogenesis of infectious disease. The consensus is that immunological reactions are suspected of playing a more prominent role in chronic infections occurring in tuberculosis, leprosy, syphilis, dermatomycoses, systemic mycoses, and protozoal and helminthic diseases. Increasing interest is evident in those diseases accompanied by depressed cell-mediated immunity as in measles, lepromatous leprosy, tuberculosis, syphilis, lymphocytic choriomeningitis, and experimentally, in virus-induced cancers.

BIBLIOGRAPHY

Carpenter, C. C. J.: "Cholera and Other Enterotoxin-related Diarrheal Diseases," *J. Infect. Dis.,* 126: 551-564, 1972.

Cluff, L. E.: "Effects of Endotoxins on Susceptibility to Infections," *J. Infect. Dis.,* 122:205-215, 1970.

Diamond, R. D., and Bennett, J. E.: "Growth of *Cryptococcus neoformans* within Human Macrophages in Vitro," *Infect. Immun.,* 7:231-236, 1973.

Ellen, R. P., and Gibbons, R. J.: "M Protein-associated Adherence of *Streptococcus pyogenes* to Epithelial Surfaces: A Prerequisite for Virulence," *Infect. Immun.,* 5:826-830, 1972.

Frost, A. J., Smith, H., Witt, K., and Keppie, J.: "The Chemical Basis of the Virulence of *Brucella abortus* in Bovine Phagocytes," *Br. J. Exp. Pathol.,* 53:587-596, 1972.

Gemski, P., Jr., Sheahan, D. G., Washington, O., and Formal, S. B.: "Virulence of *Shigella flexneri* Hybrids Expressing *Escherichia coli* Somatic Antigens," *Infect. Immun.,* 6:104-111, 1972.

Jones, T. C., and Hirsch, J. G.: "The Interaction between *Toxoplasma gondii* and Mammalian Cells: II. The Absence of Lysosomal Fusion with Phagocytic Vacuoles Containing Live Parasites," *J. Exp. Med.,* 136:1173-1194, 1972.

Kadis, S., Montie, T. C., and Ajl, S. J. (eds.): *Microbial Toxins, vol. 2A: Bacterial Protein Toxins,* New York: Academic Press, Inc., 1971.

Kordová, N., Hoogstraten, J., and Wilt, J. C.: "Lysosomes and the Toxicity of Rickettsiales: IV. Ultrastructural Studies of Macrophages Infected with a Cytopathic L Cell-grown *C. psittaci* 6BC Strain," *Can. J. Microbiol.,* 19:315-320, 1973.

Newsome, T. W., and Eurenius, K.: "Suppression of Granulocyte and Platelet Production by *Pseudomonas* Burn Wound Infection," *Surg. Gynecol. Obstet.,* 136:375-379, 1973.

Nowotny, A.: "Molecular Aspects of Endotoxic Reactions," *Bacteriol. Rev.,* 33:72-98, 1969.

Polk, H. C., and Miles, A. A.: "The Decisive Period in the Primary Infection of Muscle by *Escherichia coli,*" *Br. J. Exp. Pathol.,* 54:99-109, 1973.

Smith, H.: "Mechanisms of Virus Pathogenicity," *Bacteriol. Rev.,* 36:291-310, 1972.

Swanson, J.: "Studies on Gonococcus Infection: IV. Pili: Their Role in Attachment of Gonococci to Tissue Culture Cells," *J. Exp. Med.,* 137:571-589, 1973.

Tacker, J. R., Farhi, F., and Bulmer, G. S.: "Intracellular Fate of *Cryptococcus neoformans,*" *Infect. Immun.,* 6:162-167, 1972.

Ward, M. E., and Watt, P. J.: "Adherence of *Neisseria gonorrhoeae* to Urethral Mucosal Cells: An Electron-microscopic Study of Human Gonorrhea," *J. Infect. Dis.,* 126:601-605, 1972.

Chapter 6

Structural and Functional Integrity of the Host

Bernard A. Briody

PERSPECTIVE

Emphasis was given in the preceding chapter to the overwhelming frequency with which infectious disease is the consequence of adherence, penetration, and growth of pathogens within mucosal epithelial cells. Nonetheless, the mucous membranes together with the skin constitute the major barrier that maintains the structural and functional integrity of the host. Paradoxically, too, the mucous membranes of the conjunctivae, nasopharynx, oral cavity, and portions of the gastrointestinal and urogenital tracts and the skin support an abundant growth of parasites which (1) operate to hold down the growth of certain pathogens and (2) exert their pathogenic potential when the integrity of the mucous membranes and skin is compromised. The inflammatory response represents a second level of defense against infectious disease and is adequate to contain the challenge in the vast majority of cases. However, when essential elements of the inflammatory response are missing or impaired, the balance is shifted sharply in favor of the parasite. If developmental, genetic, or functional defects affect a vital organ, tissue, or barrier (bone marrow, thymus, CNS, heart, kidney; cardiopulmonary, cardiovascular, cardiorenal systems; blood-brain, blood-placenta, blood-skin barriers) in the third phase of defense, the prognosis is grave. Within this context, it is appropriate to examine briefly some of the factors that maintain the natural resistance of the host, to illustrate ways in which the resistance is depressed, and whenever possible, to indicate the underlying mechanisms involved.

ROLE OF THE NORMAL MICROBIAL FLORA

The two primary mechanisms whereby the indigenous microbial flora interferes with the establishment and growth of respiratory and enteric pathogens apparently are based on the ability of the flora to (1) attach to the mucosal epithelium of the upper respiratory tract, oral cavity, and small intestine, or (2) stimulate active peristalsis in the small intestine. Exhaustion of nutrients and the elaboration of inhibitory metabolic products by the normal microbial flora probably represent secondary phenomena.

The foregoing conclusions derive from several lines of evidence. For example, prior attachment of or colonization with coagulase-negative (nonpathogenic) staphylococci interferes with the establishment and growth of coagulase-positive (pathogenic) staphylococci on the skin, nasopharynx, and umbilicus of newborns and is known to reduce the incidence of staphylococcal disease in neonates and their mothers in the hospital environment.

The viridans group of streptococci can inhibit the growth and/or prevent the establishment of group A streptococci, staphylococci, meningococci, gram-negative Enterobacteriaceae, and probably *Candida albicans.* The extent to which group A streptococci are antagonized reflects the qualitative composition of viridans streptococci present in different individuals. After parenteral administration of large doses of penicillin (20 million units or more daily for a week), viridans streptococci are suppressed, and there is a marked numerical predominance (overgrowth) of gram-negative Enterobacteriaceae normally present in small numbers. Serious, often lethal, superinfection may follow such overgrowth. On the other hand, oral treatment with low doses of penicillin prior to administration of the large doses is effective in (1) selecting antibiotic-resistant viridans streptococci which persist throughout the observation period and (2) protecting the individual from overgrowth with Enterobacteriaceae.

Experimental and clinical observations, employing a variety of pathogens and antibiotics and involving spontaneous and induced depression of small intestinal motility in germ-free and conventional animals and in human volunteers and patients, support the conclusion that the protective effect of the normal flora of the small intestine against enteric pathogens is primarily a function of its ability to stimulate peristaltic emptying of the luminal contents. Ligation, opium treatment, and antibiotics dramatically increase the susceptibility of animals to salmonellosis, shigellosis, and cholera. Germ-free animals are much more susceptible to a variety of enteric pathogens than are conventional animals. A single dose of oral neomycin or streptomycin in man strikingly enhances the ability of typhoid bacilli to cause disease, and enteric diseases (blind-loop syndrome, jejunal diverticulosis, strictures, and fistulas) lead to bacterial overgrowth and malabsorption. The common mode of action of these diverse phenomena appears to be due to direct or indirect depression of small bowel motility.

A few examples will illustrate the magnitude of the effect that can be achieved. Germ-free guinea pigs succumb to oral challenge with *Shigella* in 12 to 36 hr. whereas conventional animals are resistant. However, if *Escherichia coli* are introduced orally 1 week preceding the *Shigella* challenge in germ-free animals, the guinea pigs experience neither illness nor death. In a study in germ-free and conventional mice, the viable counts 24 hr. after intragastric challenge with *Salmonella typhimurium* were 8.6×10^9 and 3.0×10^3, respectively.

In conventional guinea pigs production of experimental shigellosis or cholera requires ligation or opium-induced reduction of intestinal motility. In a study in guinea pigs, *S. typhimurium* in a challenge dose of 10^2 induced focal granulomatous lesions and death in opium-treated animals, whereas a dose of 10^8 organisms was required to produce the same effect in conventional animals.

A single dose of streptomycin in conventional mice causes a 10,000-fold reduction in the number of *S. typhimurium* required to kill the animals. In man, a single oral dose of neomycin or streptomycin regularly leads to disease following ingestion of 10^3 typhoid bacilli, a dose that cannot infect controls. Even a dose of 10^5 organisms in controls produces disease in only 27 percent of those challenged. Presumably, the destruction of the normal flora of the small intestine by the antibiotic results in decreased peristalsis, unimpeded multiplication of the pathogen, and/or its subsequent penetration and multiplication within the mucosal epithelium. In contrast, the peristaltic action of the small intestine of untreated individuals represents an effective protective mechanism, since the organisms are transported rapidly into the large intestine where their pathogenic potential cannot be expressed, probably for many reasons, including inability to adhere to mucosal cells, dilution with the large volume of intestinal contents, and the presence of inhibitory substances. The primary event, however, involves the peristaltic emptying of the luminal contents of the small intestine.

INTEGRITY OF THE SKIN AND MUCOUS MEMBRANES

The Skin

The most convincing evidence of the significance of the skin as a major protective mechanism against infectious disease derives from the consequences of injury. The precipitating insult may appear inconsequential, as in the case of an inapparent or minor abrasion, frequent soaking in water, perspiration, irritation, obesity friction, eczema, or exposure to sunlight. On the other hand, the trauma may be extensive, as in the case of burns, puncture wounds, combat or surgical wounds, or lodgement of foreign bodies, or may reflect inhibition of the inflammatory response. The predominant organisms involved are members of the normal microbial flora, especially the gram-negative enteric bacilli and staphylococci and, to a lesser extent, organisms of *Candida* and *Aspergillus* and of actinomycetes. Soil saprophytes including tetanus and gas gangrene bacilli, nocardia, and streptomycetes may contaminate wounds and produce minor or fatal disease. In addition, a considerable number of pathogens including group A streptococci and the causative agents of cutaneous diphtheria, brucellosis, leptospirosis, listeriosis, melioidosis, glanders, rat-bite fever, relapsing fever, sporotrichosis, blastomycosis, paracoccidioidomycosis, chromomycosis, cryptococcosis, rabies, B virus disease, molluscum contagiosum, cat-scratch fever, milkers' nodules, and the numerous bacterial, viral, rickettsial, and protozoal diseases transmitted by arthropod vectors enter the host and produce disease when the integrity of the skin is compromised.

A few examples will illustrate the wide range of effects associated with infectious agents that enter the body following injury to the skin. Cutaneous candidiasis, caused by a member of the normal flora of the skin *(Candida albicans)*, is an occupational disease of bartenders, housewives, and fruit packers whose hands are macerated by frequent soakings in water. Dermatomycoses seem to prevail in areas of the skin subjected to perspiration, moisture, irritation, or obesity friction. Surgical wounds and burns create a favorable environment for the growth of gram-negative enteric bacilli and staphylococci which constitute the vast majority of the causative agents. In burned patients, infections with *Pseudomonas* and staphylococci involve a grave prognosis. In susceptible persons who are suffering from eczema, infection with herpes simplex or vaccinia viruses leads to generalized disease which often terminates fatally. The importance of acidosis as a factor predisposing the diabetic to serious staphylococcal infections of the skin is supported by studies which indicate that a pronounced impairment of the granulocytic inflammatory response is attributed to acidosis alone.

Such a diverse group of compromising situations varying widely in the degree of injury and the ability of the parasite to grow progressively in the injured tissues precludes a single explanation and mechanism of action. In some cases, the altered environment favors the growth of the parasite as in cutaneous candidiasis and dermatomycoses. In other cases, access to the internal environment together with calcium ions in the soil and a lowered oxidation-reduction potential consequent to injury provides a suitable milieu for the germination of spores and the production of tetanus or gas gangrene. The presence of foreign bodies (sutures, for example) greatly reduces the number of bacteria required to produce infection, and interestingly enough, removal of the sutures is followed by resolution of the infection. In diabetics and others with impaired inflammatory and/or immunological responses, growth of the parasite tends to be unimpeded and progressive. With respect to pathogens, the injury provides the mechanism for bringing the organism into direct contact with susceptible cells which are inaccessible in the absence of injury. Thereafter, the disease follows one of the pathogenetic patterns outlined in the preceding chapter.

The Mucous Membranes

The integrity of the mucous membranes is most frequently abrogated as a consequence of viral and bacterial infection with pathogenic microorganisms, especially those that damage the upper respiratory tract. The result can be pneumonia (see Chaps. 14 and 20), acute otitis media or conjunctivitis (see Chap. 19), or meningitis (see Chap. 24) in which the causative agents are primarily members of the normal flora or the carrier state (staphylococci, pneumococci, meningococci, *Hemophilus* species). In addition, group A streptococci are occasionally involved.

The basic lesions are associated with interference with the mucociliary, secretory, and mechanical functions of the mucosal epithelium. Influenza virus, for example, destroys the ciliated epithelial cells of the trachea and bronchi, thus providing easy access to the lower respiratory tract for staphylococci, pneumococci, and other bacteria. No doubt, excess secretion (rhinitis) facilitates the passage of bacteria to the lower respiratory tract. In addition, there is hyperemia, edema, and thickening of the cuboidal epithelial mucosa lining the cavity of the middle ear, neutrophils migrate through the mucosa, and the cavity is filled with purulent fluid. With closure of the lumen of the eustachian tube, the exudate accumulates under pressure, leading to acute otitis media and, occasionally, to more serious consequences, including meningitis. A similar obstruction associated with the inflammatory exudate leads to acute bacterial conjunctivitis following a viral infection of the upper respiratory tract. In this connection, it is interesting to note that allergic rhinitis often precedes acute bacterial conjunctivitis.

Interference with the microbial flora of the oropharynx or intestinal tract by antibiotics leads to the destruction of the normally protective microorganisms and/or intestinal hypomotility with consequent overgrowth by *Candida*, staphylococci, gram-negative enteric bacilli, and *Giardia* which are resistant to the antibiotics employed. The consequences may be oral or intestinal candidiasis, staphylococcal pseudomembranous enterocolitis, pneumonia caused by staphylococci or gram-negative enteric bacilli, or the malabsorption syndrome.

Under other injurious situations—such as those caused by chemical irritants (alcohol, phenol, and environmental pollutants including excessive smoking and strong mouthwashes), mechanical irritants (dental extractions or ill-fitting dentures), physical damage (surgery, radiation, and perforation), and obstruction (urologic abnormalities)—or under conditions that favor the growth of organisms normally present in small numbers (riboflavin deficiency and pregnancy), members of the indigenous flora can induce trivial, self-limiting, or fatal disease.

A few examples will illustrate the range of effects which can occur when the integrity of the mucous membranes is subverted along these lines. Candidiasis is associated with strong mouthwashes, excessive smoking, ill-fitting dentures, and pregnancy. In pregnancy, the presence of excess sugar and glycogen-like compounds in blood, urine, and vaginal secretions favors the growth of *Candida* organisms. Actinomycosis is often preceded by dental extractions. Urinary tract infections (see Chap. 18) are greatly facilitated by any obstruction to the flow of urine and are caused predominantly by the gram-negative Enterobacteriaceae. Physical damage due to radiation and traumatic or spontaneous (peptic ulcer or ruptured appendix) perforation of the gastrointestinal tract is regularly accompanied by peritonitis and septicemia caused primarily by members of the indigenous gram-negative flora and occasionally by gram-positive members of the normal flora, including staphylococci, streptococci, and *Clostridium perfringens.*

THE INFLAMMATORY RESPONSE

The Early Critical Phase

The inflammatory response of the tissues to injury induced by foreign materials (microbes, microbial antigens, other antigens, and haptens) constitutes the essential subject matter of this text. The emphasis is directed toward the development and release of pharmacologically active mediators as a consequence of either antigen-antibody reactions *(humoral immunity)* or the interaction of antigens with specifically sensitized thymus-dependent small lymphocytes *(cell-mediated immunity)* and the cellular elements involved in these phenomena. Although the detailed analysis of the spectrum of acute and chronic inflammation is beyond the scope of this text, perhaps an outline of the initial phases of the response of the host to injury is appropriately mentioned in this chapter.

As noted in Figures 6-1 and 6-2, a biphasic increase in vascular permeability, a variable response of the circulating leukocytes, an exudation of fluid and leukocytes, and an accumulation of infiltrating cells *(induration)* are often associated with localized inflammation. The altered permeability is generally restricted to a small portion of the microcirculatory system, es-

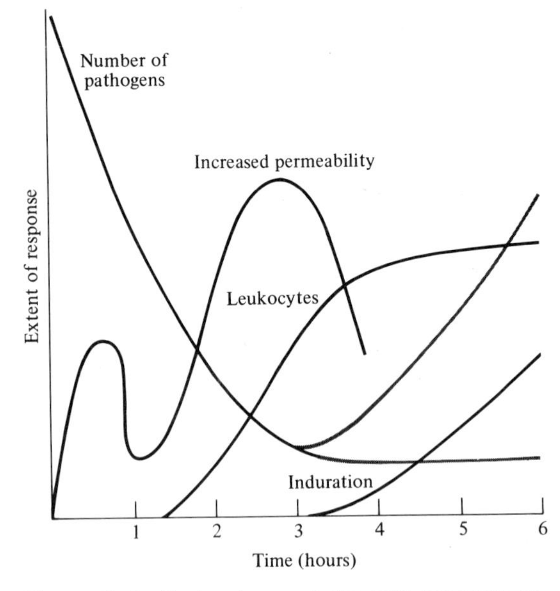

Figure 6-1 Early phase of the inflammatory response. [*A. A. Miles, "The Acute Reactions of Injury as an Antimicrobial Defense," in L. Thomas, J. W. Uhr, and L. Grand (eds.), International Symposium on Injury, Inflammation and Immunity, Baltimore, Williams & Wilkins, 1964.*]

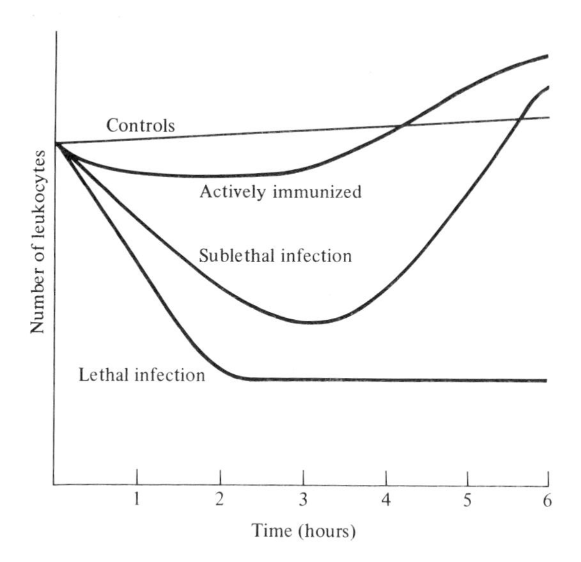

Figure 6-2 The early leukocyte response in *Pseudomonas* infection. *(Courtesy of J. W. Sensakovic and P. F. Bartell.)*

pecially the small venules, and is the earliest manifestation of inflammation. The mediators of enhanced permeability probably include histamine and, later on, slow-reacting substance A and plasma kinins (Chap. 8). An increasing number of neutrophils marginate along the walls of the venules and traverse the intervening tissue by sticking and crawling between the vascular endothelial cells *(diapedesis)*. Thereafter, the cellular pattern of the response varies with the pathogen and the tissue under attack. In many acute infections (staphylococci, for example) the exudation of neutrophils continues; whereas in chronic infections (tuberculosis) the influx of neutrophils ceases, and macrophages begin to accumulate in the injured area. As indicated in the preceding chapter, the subsequent course of events is partly determined by the response of the parasites to phagocytosis either before or after penetration and replication of the parasite in tissue cells. Sequentially, the specific immune responses are later episodes that involve lymphocytes, plasma cells, and macrophages (Chaps. 7 and 8).

If the pathogen is injected intravenously, the outcome is parasite- and dose-dependent, but usually involves rapid clearance of the pathogen from the blood by endothelial cells in the blood and lymph. The clearance may be a terminal event in which the parasite is eliminated, or the pathogen may survive, replicate, and reappear in the tissues and blood of the host to produce disease.

Phagocytes

With the influx of leukocytes into the localized area of inflammation, attempts at phagocytosis commence. The principal cells involved are the short-lived (about 10 hr.) neutrophils and the longer-lived (months to years) macrophages that comprise the emigrating blood monocytes which soon become indistinguishable in appearance and function from the local tissue macrophages that also participate in the inflammatory response. In addition to phagocytizing microorganisms, the macrophages can engulf neutrophils, tissue debris, and particulate matter, transport the material to the regional lymph nodes, and process antigens for lymphocytes. Both neutrophils and macrophages possess membrane-bound granules (lysosomes) which bud from the Golgi apparatus and contain numerous digestive enzymes (acid hydrolases) capable of degrading various macromolecules and microorganisms at an acid pH. Peroxidase, antibacterial cationic peptides, alkaline phosphatases, lysozyme, and lactoferrin (an iron-binding protein with antibacterial properties) are also present in neutrophils.

Neutrophils enter the bloodstream from the bone marrow and are continuously replenished. The blood pool comprises about 6×10^{11} cells, half of which are marginated and half of which are circulating at any given time. After a half-life of 6 to 7 hr. in the circulation, the neutrophils migrate into the tissues by diapedesis and subsequently disappear from the tissue pool at the rate of about 10^{11} cells daily, mostly through the mucous membranes. The bone marrow contains a large reserve pool of mature neutrophils (3×10^{12}) which can be rapidly delivered in times of need.

Monocytes are derived from the bone marrow but are not backed up by a large reserve pool of mature monocytes. Before moving into the tissues by diapedesis, the monocytes circulate on the average for about 32 hr. Within the tissues the monocytes mature and function as skin, alveolar, and peritoneal macrophages and as Kupffer cells and are continuously replenished from the marrow-derived blood monocytes. Tissue macrophages have a long life span and ordinarily do not synthesize DNA or divide, but significantly can be stimulated to do so under the influence of *lymphokines.* Mature macrophages include cells that wander in tissue and body spaces (alveolar, peritoneal, and skin macrophages and histiocytes) and endothelial cells in the blood and lymph (Kupffer cells and splenic and lymph node macrophages).

Nonimmune Phagocytosis

The exudation of fluid and leukocytes in the early phase of inflammation may increase or decrease the probability of contact between parasite and phagocyte. The phagocyte can respond with directed locomotion (chemotaxis) toward the parasite and can trap the parasite against tissue surfaces (surface phagocytosis). Later, when the number of phagocytes in the exudate is increased or when fibrin is deposited, the parasites can be pinned between adjacent phagocytes or engulfed in the network of fibrin. On the other hand, the exudation of fluid and increased lymphatic drainage can facilitate the transport of the pathogen to the regional lymph node and thence to the blood and tissues (Chap. 5). With many parasites there is much evidence to indicate that the eventual outcome of the infection is determined by the critical events occurring within the first few hours, especially by the effect of the parasite on the neutrophil and the activity and efficiency of phagocytosis (Figs. 6-1 and 6-2).

Surface phagocytosis requires energy derived primarily from glycolysis or occasionally from oxidative metabolism. After contact, the phagocyte sends out microprojections of the plasma membrane to encircle the parasite; they then fuse with one another, enclosing the microbe in a pouch which is evaginated into the cytoplasm where it becomes a *phagocytic vacuole.* Within 5 to 10 min. the lysosomal granules coalesce with the phagocytic vacuole and discharge their contents, usually killing the trapped parasites within 30 to 60 min. Phagocytosis is generally a highly efficient mechanism for destroying pathogens. Even those parasites that contain surface components that tend to prevent phagocytosis are promptly killed after ingestion. On the other hand, as noted in Chapter 5, there are a number of pathogens that can prevent lysosomal fusion with the phagocytic vacuoles containing living parasites. As a result, the parasite can survive, grow within, and destroy the cell.

Immune Phagocytosis

On their surface membranes, neutrophils and macrophages possess Fc receptor sites which have a weak affinity for IgG antibody *(cytophilic antibody)* and receptor sites for the C3 component of complement. When the surface antigen of a parasite combines with IgG antibody, conformational changes are induced in the structure of the Fc fragment which enable the immune complex (antigen-antibody) to (1) bind complement and (2) exhibit an enhanced affinity for the Fc receptor site on the phagocyte. Antibodies with this function are termed *immune opsonins* because they exponentially increase the rate of phagocytosis in the presence of complement or, in some cases (encapsulated type 3 pneumococci), permit phagocytosis to occur.

SELECTED FACTORS THAT LOWER HOST RESISTANCE

As indicated in Table 6-1, there are many factors that can depress the resistance of the host to parasites. In the preceding sections, the role of the normal microbial flora, the integrity of the skin and mucous membranes, and the effectiveness of the inflammatory response in preventing infectious disease are stressed. A more serious, but less frequent, cause of decreased resistance, involves developmental, functional, or genetic defects in vital tissues, organs, and barriers. Of the factors listed in Table 6-1, it is evident that in most cases multiple mechanisms are involved.

In terms of frequency, the resistance of the host is lowered by (1) injury, (2) malnutrition, (3) antibiotics, (4) corticosteroids and other immunosuppressive drugs, and (5) lymphoreticular malignancy and other forms of cancer. In most cases, the resulting disease is caused by parasites which are part of the normal flora. The majority of organisms isolated as the causative agents of conjunctivitis, acute otitis media, pneumonia, wound infections, urinary tract infections, bacteremia, and endocarditis are members of the normal flora, and many cases of meningitis are induced by the resident population of parasites. In addition, the same factors can operate to convert a subclinical or minor infection by a pathogen into a more serious or fatal disease. Group A streptococci, tuberculosis, varicella, zoster, measles, herpes simplex, salmonellosis, and amebiasis could be cited as illustrative examples.

Injury that predisposes to infectious disease may be the consequence of a preceding viral or bacterial infection (acute otitis media, conjunctivitis, pneumonia), congenital anomalies (urinary tract infections, malabsorption, bacteremia, meningitis), instrumentation (urinary tract infections), allergic rhinitis (conjunctivitis), perforation (peritonitis), surgery (wound infections), obstruction (urinary tract infections, pulmonary infections, glandular infections), diabetes (skin infections, urinary tract infections, rhinoorbitalcerebral form of phycomycosis), immunosuppression caused by viruses and bacteria (almost any type of infection), cancer (almost any type of infection), cystic fibrosis (pulmonary infections), and mucopolysaccharidosis (pulmonary infections). The diverse nature and site of the injury is reflected in a variety of underlying mechanisms including loss of integrity of the skin and mucous membranes, localization of infection in the damaged tissue (brain, heart), reduction in the number of neutrophils (neutropenia), and depression of cell-mediated immunity.

The mechanism responsible for lowering the resistance of the host often influences the type of organism involved in the subsequent infection. For example, when antibiotics are used the resulting disease is associated with antibiotic-resistant members of the normal flora (staphylococci, gram-negative enteric bacilli, *Candida* organisms). In chronic granulomatous disease of childhood, the neutrophilic lysosomes can dispose of catalase-negative parasites (streptococci, pneumococci, meningococci, influenza bacilli) but cannot kill the catalase-positive organisms (staphylococci, *Enterobacter, Escherichia, Serratia, Candida, Aspergillus, Nocardia*). Defects in the C3, C4, and C5 components of complement are associated with an inability to dispose of gram-negative enteric bacilli and staphylococci. Agammaglobulinemic individuals can effectively eliminate intracellular parasites (viruses, protozoa, fungi, rickettsiae, chlamydiae, tubercle bacilli) but cannot destroy pyogenic bacteria (staphylococci, streptococci, pneumococci, me-

Table 6-1 Selected Factors That Lower Host Resistance

Factor	Mechanisms
Antibiotics	Remove protective parasites of normal flora; depress small intestinal motility; permit overgrowth of normal microbial flora
Injury	Provides direct access to susceptible tissues for the normal microbial flora of the skin and mucous membranes, for pathogens, or for saprophytes; permits overgrowth of normal microbial flora; causes excess secretion or more viscid secretion; induces stasis or obstruction to flow of tears, saliva, acid, bile, urine, blood, or air; depresses intestinal motility; facilitates localization; causes neutropenia; inhibits discharge of lysosomal enzymes; inhibits diapedesis; depresses cell-mediated immunity
Age	Less efficient antibody production and cell-mediated immunity at extremes of age; lower concentrations of C3, C4, and C5 components of complement during first 3 months of life, depressing complement-mediated immune reactions; receipt of maternal antibodies across the placenta which may predispose to more serious disease of the lower respiratory tract by a specific virus; increased permeability of connective tissue in infants facilitating dissemination of parasites; availability of susceptible vaginal epithelium prior to puberty permitting gonococcal vulvovaginitis
Pregnancy	Greater stasis of urine which predisposes to urinary tract infections
Malnutrition	Depresses intestinal motility; facilitates microbial overgrowth; causes neutropenia
Immunological deficiency	Prevents antibody formation, cell-mediated immunity, or both and may involve B cells, T cells, and/or stem cells
Complement defects	Depress or prevent normal elimination of parasites through complement-mediated reactions
Agranulocytosis	Causes lack of phagocytosis by neutrophils
Altered lysosomes	Inability of neutrophils and macrophages to kill ingested parasites which may be general (Chediak-Higashi giant lysosome syndrome) or may be limited to catalase-positive organisms (chronic granulomatous disease of childhood)
Aplastic anemia	Causes neutropenia
Lymphoreticular cancer	Causes neutropenia; depresses cell-mediated immunity
Multiple myeloma	Impairs antibody production; increases rate of immunoglobulin metabolism; depresses cell-mediated immunity
Immunosuppression	Impairs cell-mediated immunity; depresses diapedesis; causes neutropenia

ningococci, influenza bacilli). Individuals with cell-mediated defects in immunity, whether genetically inherited or acquired during the course of other diseases, are unable to destroy intracellular parasites and experience progressive disease following immunization with attenuated organisms (*Mycobacterium bovis,* vaccinia virus), following natural infection (varicella, measles), after activation of latent infections (herpes simplex, zoster, cytomegalovirus, pneumocystis), or after overgrowth of the normal flora *(Candida).* Individuals with combined humoral and cell-mediated defects are unduly susceptible to almost any infectious agent.

BIBLIOGRAPHY

Adam, M., Morgan, O., Persand, C., and Gibbs, W. N.: "Hyperinfection Syndrome with *Strongyloides stercoralis* in Malignant Lymphoma," *Br. Med. J.,* 1:264-266, 1973.

Baehner, R. L.: "Disorders of Leukocytes Leading to Recurrent Infection," *Pediatr. Clin. North Am.,* 19:935-956, 1972.

Barton, A. D., and Lourenço, R. V.: "Bronchial Secretions and Mucociliary Clearance," *Arch. Intern. Med.,* 131:140-144, 1973.

Braun, W., and Ungar, J.: *Host Resistance, "Nonspecific" Factors Influencing: A Reexamination,* Basel: S. Karger, 1973.

Carey, R. M., Kimball, A. C., Armstrong, D., and Lieberman, P. H.: "Toxoplasmosis: Clinical Experiences in a Cancer Hospital," *Am. J. Med.,* 54:30-38, 1973.

Cline, M. J.: "A New White Cell Test Which Measures Individual Phagocyte Function in a Mixed Leukocyte Population: I. A Neutrophil Defect in Acute Myelocytic Leukemia," *J. Lab. Clin. Med.,* 81:311-316, 1973.

Edelson, P. J., Stites, D. P., Gold, S., and Fudenberg, H. H.: "Disorders of Neutrophil Function: Defects in the Early Stages of the Phagocytic Process," *Clin. Exp. Immunol.,* 13:21-28, 1973.

Finkel, A., and Dent, P. B.: "Abnormalities in Lymphocyte Proliferation in Classical and Atypical Measles Infection," *Cell Immunol.,* 6:41-48, 1973.

Flavell, S. G.: "Advances in Treatment No. 9: Acute Bronchitis, Chronic Bronchitis and Bronchiectasis," *Br. J. Clin. Pract.,* 27:9-12, 1973.

Freter, R., and Abrams, G.D.: "Function of Various Intestinal Bacteria in Converting Germfree Mice to the Normal State," *Infect. Immun.,* 6:119-133, 1972.

Giannella, R. A., Broitman, S. A., and Zamcheck, N.: "Influence of Gastric Acidity on Bacterial and Parasitic Enteric Infections: A Perspective," *Ann. Intern. Med.,* 78:271-276, 1973.

Hamon, C. B., and Klebanoff, S. J.: "A Peroxidase-mediated, *Streptococcus mitis*-dependent Antimicrobial System in Saliva," *J. Exp. Med.,* 137:438-450, 1973.

Jaffe, H. J., and Katz, S.: "Current Ideas about Bronchiectasis," *Am. Fam. Physician,* 7:68-76, 1973.

Klastersky, J., and Weerts, D.: "Recent Experience with Bacteremia in Patients Presenting Cancer," *Eur. J. Cancer,* 9:69-76, 1973.

Meyer, R. D., Young, L. S., Armstrong, D., and Yu, B.: "Aspergillosis Complicating Neoplastic Disease," *Am. J. Med.,* 54:6-15, 1973.

Miles, A. A., Miles, E. M., and Burke, J.: "The Value and Duration of Defence Reactions of the Skin to the Primary Lodgement of Bacteria," *Br. J. Exp. Pathol.,* 38:79-96, 1957.

Moncrief, J. A.: "Burns," *N. Engl. J. Med.,* 288:444-454, 1973.

Reller, I. B., MacGregor, R. R., and Beaty, H. N.: "Bactericidal Antibody after Colonization with *Neisseria meningitidis,*" *J. Infect. Dis.,* 127:56-62, 1973.

Sant'Agnese, P. A.: "Cystic Fibrosis (Mucoviscidosis)," *Am. Fam. Physician,* 7:102-111, 1973.

Savage, D. C.: "Survival on Mucosal Epithelia, Epithelial Penetration and Growth in Tissues of Pathogenic Bacteria," in H. Smith and J. H. Pearce (eds.), *Microbial Pathogenicity in Man and Animals,* New York: Cambridge University Press, 1972.

Smith, M. J., Browne, F., and Slungaard, A.: "The Impaired Responsiveness of Chronic Lymphatic Leukemia Lymphocytes to Allogeneic Lymphocytes," *Blood,* 41:505-509, 1973.

Sprunt, K., Leidy, G. A., and Redman, W.: "Prevention of Bacterial Overgrowth," *J. Infect. Dis.,* 123: 1-10, 1971.

Valdimarsson, H., Higgs, J., Wells, R. S., Yamamura, M., Hobbs, J. R., and Holt, P. L. J.: "Immune Abnormalities Associated with Chronic Mucocutaneous Candidiasis," *Cell. Immunol.,* 6:348-361, 1973.

Williams, R. C., Jr., and Fudenberg, H. H. (eds.): *Phagocytic Mechanisms in Health and Disease,* New York: Intercontinental Medical Book Corporation, 1972.

Zigmond, S. H., and Hirsch, J. G.: "Leukocyte Locomotion and Chemotaxis: New Methods for Evaluation, and Demonstration of a Cell-derived Chemotactic Factor," *J. Exp. Med.,* 137:387-410, 1973.

Chapter 7

Antigens and Antibodies

Bernard A. Briody and Arthur E. Krikszens

Perspective
Properties of Antigens
Characteristics of Antibodies
Factors Influencing Antibody Production
Antigen-Antibody Interaction
The Precipitin Reaction
Bacterial Agglutination
Complement and Complement Fixation
The Coombs' Test

PERSPECTIVE

Immunology is a broad subject that deals with the responses of the host following contact with antigens. Major immunological responses include the formation of antibodies (*humoral* immunity) and *cell-mediated* immunity. Under appropriate circumstances each category of immunological response may be involved in protection against infectious agents or in the production of cellular and tissue damage.

At the cellular level immunological response is primarily a function of small lymphocytes which are often referred to as immunologically competent cells. Current evidence suggests that there are two populations of small lymphocytes: (1) short-lived, gut-dependent small lymphocytes associated with antibody production and (2) long-lived, thymus-dependent small lymphocytes associated with delayed hypersensitivity reactions. After exposure to antigen, gut-dependent small lymphocytes transform and differentiate into plasma cells, which in turn synthesize and secrete antibody. After primary contact with antigen, thymus-dependent small lymphocytes transform into blast cells, replicate as blast cells, and revert to sensitized lymphocytes. When they, in turn, are exposed to the same antigen, the sensitized lymphocytes release a number of different lymphokines, which are soluble molecules which exert diverse biological effects on nonsensitized, thymus-dependent lymphocytes, macrophages, and other target cells. Although the end result of antigen-induced lymphokine release always involves cellular damage, if the target cell is supporting intracellular multiplication of a microorganism, protection against the infectious agent may be achieved.

A third category of reaction to antigenic stimulation involves the induction of a specific state of immunological unresponsiveness, or tolerance. The tolerant state develops either as a result of natural exposure to one's own antigens during fetal life *(self-recognition)* or may be induced in prenatal or postnatal life under conditions which favor direct contact of the antigen with small lymphocytes and persistence of the antigen, while limiting the ability of the lymphocytes to transform, differentiate, and replicate *(acquired tolerance).*

An antigen is usually a substance of high molecular weight provided with a surface composed of a number of specific determinant groups of small size. When the determinant groups on the antigen are foreign to the host, they may stimulate the production of complementary antibody molecules. An antibody has two (or polymers of two) identical combining sites that react specifically with a particular determinant group on the surface of the antigen. The interaction of antigen with antibody is extremely sensitive and may be used to detect as little as 0.001 μg of antibody nitrogen.

In this chapter emphasis will be placed on the requirements for antigenicity, the characteristics of antibodies, the factors that influence the production of antibodies, the features of antigen-antibody interaction, the methods for detecting and measuring antigens and antibodies, and the role of antibodies in protection against infectious diseases.

PROPERTIES OF ANTIGENS

Foreignness

A potentially antigenic material must contain determinant groups on its surface that are foreign to the viable, immunologically competent cells of the host. In man immunological competence develops by about the third month of gestation. Prior to this, the fetus becomes tolerant to antigens contained in its own tissues. Failure to produce antibodies against one's own antigens has been designated as tolerance or self-recognition. Once developed, tolerance normally persists throughout the life of the individual.

Presumably, the principle of self-recognition, or tolerance, has broad biological significance. As noted in Chapter 11, if an individual produces an immunological response against his own tissue antigens, the result is immunological crippling or suicide.

Chemical Nature

Functional Antigens Most naturally occurring *immunogens* (complete antigens) are proteins or polysaccharides that can induce the formation of antibodies by themselves. Data based on genetic coding for proteins suggest that different microorganisms may contain from as few as 10 to more than 1,000 distinct antigens.

Synthetic polypeptides representing random polymers of two or more L-amino acids have been shown to be functional antigens. On the other hand, polymers of D-amino acids are devoid of antigenicity.

Haptenic Antigens There are numerous reactive chemicals *(haptens)* which are not antigenic unless combined with carrier proteins. Such haptenic, or incomplete, antigens include simple chemicals of low molecular weight, such as tartaric acid, arsanilic acid, aniline dyes, drugs, and *p*-aminophenol glucosides, as well as nucleic acids and lipids of high molecular weight. Note that by definition haptens are not immunogens.

One important feature of the immunogenic response to *hapten-protein conjugates* is the formation of antibody that can combine specifically with the hapten.

Molecular Weight

Molecular weight is an important factor in determining whether a given material will be antigenic. As noted above, most naturally occurring antigens are proteins and polysaccharides. Frequently, these substances have a high molecular weight (40,000 to 1,000,000) and are powerful antigens. Materials of lower molecular weight often are weakly antigenic. On the other hand, it has been shown that the polypeptide pancreatic hormone glucagon and synthetic polypeptides with a molecular weight of 3,000 to 5,000 may also be antigenic.

As an approximation, and within certain limits, it can be expected that the larger the molecule, the greater the antigenicity. Presumably, this finding is partly related to the fact that, in general, the number of determinant groups on the antigen is proportional to the molecular weight and to the greater chance that an active antigenic fragment containing the determinant group will make effective contact with an immunologically competent cell before it is excreted.

Metabolizability

When most labeled soluble protein antigens of low or high molecular weight are injected intravenously into an immunologically competent host, most of the antigen is rapidly excreted in the urine; 50 percent of the label is excreted in 1 hr., and 70 percent in 24 hr. The antigenic material found in the urine is quite heterogeneous with respect to physical properties, and much of it is associated with RNA. The rapid breakdown of the antigen probably results from extracellular digestion by proteolytic enzymes in the circulation and intracellular digestion by circulating granulocytes and by macrophages lining sinusoids.

These observations indicate that most of the antigen apparently plays no part in the subsequent production of antibody and that the antigen is quickly digested into fragments of smaller but variable size. Other data, to be reviewed below, provide ample evidence that antigenic molecules are degraded by the host into fragments of appropriate size that contain a specific determinant group against which antibody is produced. Phagocytosis and the phagocytic enzymes appear to play an essential role in the processing of antigenic information for the immunologically competent cells.

In this connection, it is notable that proteins, polysaccharides, and synthetic polypeptides that cannot be metabolized by the host are not immunogenic. An illustrative example is the failure of synthetic polypeptides consisting of D-amino acids to be metabolized by the host and the concomitant inability to induce antibody formation. This finding is to be contrasted with the metabolizability and antigenicity of synthetic polypeptides consisting of L-amino acids.

Specificity

Structurally and functionally, the concept of a number of different active sites on the surface of the antigen molecule is fundamental to an understanding of antigenic specificity. Antibody molecules are produced against selected localized areas on the antigenic surface, not against the entire surface area of the antigen. Antibody molecules do not react randomly with portions of the antigenic surface, but combine specifically with the selected localized area that directed their synthesis. Each different active site or each selected localized area on the surface of the antigen that directs the synthesis of specific antibody molecules that combine with that site and no other site is known as a determinant group, an antigenic determinant, or an antigenic site.

When the determinant group is artificially introduced and is covalently linked into the surface structure of a protein, it is termed a hapten. The molecule into which the hapten is incorporated is referred to as a carrier.

Determinant Groups

Valence The number of determinant groups on the surface of an antigen is known as the valence. Antigens are multivalent; they usually contain 5 to 10 determinant groups per molecule but may have 200 or more. In general, the valence of an antigen is proportional to its molecular weight.

In some antigens, the determinant groups are not present in equal concentration. One determinant group might be present as a repeating unit on the surface of a virus particle, a capsular polysaccharide, or a red blood cell. Another determinant group may involve only the terminal sugar residue of a polysaccharide.

As discussed below, the valence of an antigen has important implications in terms of antigen-antibody interaction and the heterogeneity of any particular population of antibody molecules.

Size There is every reason to believe that the size of the determinant group has a well-defined upper limit which is equivalent to the antibody combining site. Several independent studies indicate that the determinant groups on proteins consist of penta- or hexapeptides. With polysaccharides, the determinant group probably has a maximum size equivalent to a hexasaccharide. These findings reveal that the determinant group has a length of around 25 to 35 Å in its most extended form and a molecular weight between 400 and 1,000.

The lower limit for the size of a determinant group on proteins probably involves a tetrapeptide, while on polysaccharide antigens a trisaccharide is involved.

Immunodominant Groups

Within the determinant group a particular amino acid or sugar residue often makes a predominant contribution to the binding affinity of the determinant group for antibody. The residue within the determinant group that shows this preferentially high affinity is termed the *immunodominant group.*

Examples of immunodominant groups include not only the terminal amino acid of peptides and the terminal nonreducing ends of hexasaccharides, but also any of the residues in the interior of the determinant group. An interior residue may exert its dominant role directly, as does the terminal group, or it may function indirectly by maintaining a particular shape, or conformation, among the adjacent residues in the determinant group. Although much remains to be learned about the mechanism of immunodominance, it is known that it increases the heterogeneity of antibody molecules that can be formed to a single determinant group. In addition, it may prove to be an important factor in understanding cross-reactions among antigens.

Monovalent Haptens

As noted above, a hapten is a determinant group that can be artificially introduced by covalent linkage into the surface structure of carrier proteins. Although a hapten cannot by itself induce the formation of antibody, it combines with antibody produced against the hapten-protein conjugate but does not form a precipitate. However, the hapten can prevent precipitation of the hapten-protein conjugate by antibody. This reaction, known as *hapten inhibition*, has formed the basis for establishing the nature of determinant groups in natural antigens as well as in hapten-protein conjugates. In addition to conferring a new antigenic specificity, a hapten frequently masks the antigenic specificity of the carrier protein.

Landsteiner and others showed that haptens could be conjugated by a diazo or a peptide linkage to free amino groups on a protein. If, for example, arsanilic acid is coupled to a number of antigenically unrelated carrier proteins and antibody is prepared against each, the specificity of the antibody is directed primarily against the arsanilic acid. This was evident when it was shown that any one of the protein–arsanilic acid conjugates formed a precipitate with antibody produced against any of the conjugates. The carrier protein, on the other hand, often failed to react or reacted poorly with antibody prepared against the specific carrier-hapten complex. In addition, the serum proteins of the animal to be immunized can also be used as the carrier, since they become antigenic by virtue of the attached hapten groups.

Perhaps one of the most striking illustrations of the chemical basis of antigenic specificity is associated with the findings of Landsteiner with the dextro- (*d*-), levo- (*l*-) and *meso*- isomers of tartaric acid. After diazotization of the tartaric acid isomers to carrier proteins, antisera were prepared in rabbits. The specificity of the antibodies produced was dependent upon the particular isomer that was coupled to the carrier. For example, the *d*- isomer–protein conjugate formed a precipitate with antibody against the *d*- isomer–protein conjugate, but failed to precipitate with antibodies against the *l*- or the *meso* isomer–protein conjugates.

d-Tartaric acid	*l*-Tartaric acid	*meso*-Tartaric acid
COOH	COOH	COOH
HCOH	HOCH	HCOH
HOCH	HCOH	HCOH
COOH	COOH	COOH

Apart from their fundamental contribution to an understanding of antigenic specificity, including cross-reactions between apparently unrelated antigens that have chemically identical determinant groups, haptens are important in clinical medicine. Numerous reactive haptens to which man is naturally or artificially exposed may conjugate with epidermal or plasma proteins, thus forming a functional antigen by virtue of the attached hapten groups. In this category are various metals (nickel, mercury, chromium), solvents (Formalin, picric acid, benzene), aniline dyes, plant products (poison ivy, sumac, oak), and drugs (aspirin, sulfonamides, penicillin, quinine). In addition to antibody production, the hapten–protein conjugates may sensitize the body in a number of ways. Subsequent contact with the hapten may lead to reactions of immediate or delayed hypersensitivity (Chap. 8) or autoimmune disease (Chap. 11).

Summary

An immunogen or functional antigen is usually a high molecular weight protein or polysaccharide with numerous specific determinant groups scattered over the surface. After introduction, an antigen (or, in the case of a microorganism, many distinct antigens) is usually metabolized by the host into smaller fragments often associated with RNA and presumably containing one of the determinant groups. Most of these digested fragments are rapidly excreted. An immunological response will ensue if the fragments that remain (1) contain determinant groups that are foreign to the host or (2) make effective contact with immunologically competent small lymphocytes. In some cases, the antigen may make direct contact with the lymphocyte, thus avoiding macrophage processing, or it may require the collaboration of T cells.

In this chapter, the immunological response under consideration is the formation of antibody molecules that have two (or polymers of two) identical combining sites that react specifically with a particular determinant group. Thus, the concept of antigenic specificity is a function of the determinant group and not of the antigenic molecule per se.

Certain determinant groups, or haptens, can combine with epidermal or plasma proteins of a host, mask the antigenicity of the host protein, confer a new antigenic specificity, and induce the formation of antibody or other immunological responses.

CHARACTERISTICS OF ANTIBODIES

Nomenclature of Human Immunoglobulins

Definition Immunoglobulins are proteins of animal origin endowed with known antibody activity and certain other proteins related by chemical structure and hence antigenic specificity. The related proteins include Bence Jones, myeloma, and macroglobulinemia proteins; cryoglobulins; and naturally occurring subunits of the immunoglobulins.

Immunoglobulins are not restricted to the plasma but may be found in other body fluids and tissues including lymph, urine, spinal fluid, saliva, tears, bile, intestinal and nasal secretions, lymph nodes, spleen, and bone marrow.

Classes Currently there are five classes of human immunoglobulins known to possess antibody activity. They have many differing physicochemical properties such as electrophoretic mobility, sedimentation coefficient, diffusion coefficient, carbohydrate content, and amino acid sequences. Regardless of its class, each antibody molecule is composed of two identical light polypeptide chains and two identical heavy polypeptide chains (or a polymer of the two light and two heavy chains) and can react specifically with the same determinant group on the antigen.

Terminology is based on the identification of the polypeptide chains which by complementation make up the immunoglobulin molecule. Provision is made for abbreviated notations to designate the major classes of immunoglobulins and their component polypeptide chains.

Based on differences associated with the heavy polypeptide chains, immunoglobulins have been separated into classes with the following symbols: IgM, IgA, IgG, IgD, and IgE. Each class of immunoglobulin has two (or multiples of two) identical heavy chains present in the molecule. The heavy chains are designated by a Greek letter corresponding to the Roman capital letters used for the immunoglobulin classes: μ, α, γ, δ, and ε.

Types The light polypeptide chains are the subunits known to be common to IgM, IgA, IgG, IgD, and IgE. Two types of light chains are recognized as occurring in man. The symbols for the types of molecules identified by the properties of light chains are K and L, and Greek letters kappa (κ) and lambda (λ) are used for the corresponding chains. A given antibody molecule contains either two κ or two λ chains (or multiples of two), but not one of each type.

Subclasses, Subgroups, and Subtypes The polypeptide chains of immunoglobulins consist of two well-defined regions. The variable (NH_2)

region has been so designated because of the diversity of its amino acid sequences, whereas the constant (COOH) region is relatively invariable in molecules of the same class and type. In light chains the constant and variable parts are approximately equal in length, but in heavy chains the constant region is almost three times as long as the variable region.

Differences involving small genetic changes in the constant region of heavy chains of a given particular light chain group are called subgroups and are designated by Roman numerals. As illustrated below, in human κ-chain groups three discrete sets of amino acid sequences have been recognized, and in human λ chains five sets of sequences have been recognized to date. Subgroups are identified as I, II, III, etc., in order of their frequency of occurrence. Subtypes represent the variable subgroup with its associated constant region.

Light chain	Light chain subgroup	Light chain subtype	Formulas for an IgG molecule with gamma 1 heavy chains
κ	$V_{\kappa I}$	$V_{\kappa I}C_{\kappa}$	$[(V_{\kappa I}C_{\kappa})\ (V_{\gamma}C_{\gamma 1})]_2$
κ	$V_{\kappa II}$	$V_{\kappa II}C_{\kappa}$	$[(V_{\kappa II}C_{\kappa})\ (V_{\gamma}C_{\gamma 1})]_2$
κ	$V_{\kappa III}$	$V_{\kappa III}C_{\kappa}$	$[(V_{\kappa III}C_{\kappa})\ (V_{\gamma}C_{\gamma 1})]_2$
λ	$V_{\lambda I}$	$V_{\lambda I}C_{\lambda}$	$[(V_{\lambda I}C_{\lambda})\ (V_{\gamma}C_{\gamma 1})]_2$
λ	$V_{\lambda II}$	$V_{\lambda II}C_{\lambda}$	$[(V_{\lambda II}C_{\lambda})\ (V_{\gamma}C_{\gamma 1})]_2$
λ	$V_{\lambda III}$	$V_{\lambda III}C_{\lambda}$	$[(V_{\lambda III}C_{\lambda})\ (V_{\gamma}C_{\gamma 1})]_2$
λ	$V_{\lambda IV}$	$V_{\lambda IV}C_{\lambda}$	$[(V_{\lambda IV}C_{\lambda})\ (V_{\gamma}C_{\gamma 1})]_2$
λ	$V_{\lambda V}$	$V_{\lambda V}C_{\lambda}$	$[(V_{\lambda V}C_{\lambda})\ (V_{\gamma}C_{\gamma 1})]_2$

Note: V = the variable region of a kappa or lambda light chain or the variable region of the gamma heavy chain; C = the constant region of a kappa or lambda light chain or the constant region of the gamma heavy chain.

class are used as a basis for separating immunoglobulins into subclasses. To date, subclasses have been identified in IgM, IgA, and IgG. As illustrated below, subclasses associated with IgG differ in terms of the frequency of their occurrence, biological properties (ability to bind complement), and genetic markers (allotypes).

Heavy chain subgroups, sets of variable region sequences in heavy chains analogous to those in light chains, have been recognized recently. However, heavy chain subgroups are independent of the class of the chain which is determined by the sequence of the constant region, whereas κ light chain subgroups are restricted to κ chains and λ subgroups to λ chains. For example, the variable region of the μ heavy chain of a particular subgroup may show a

Heavy chain subclass	Percent of total molecules	Ability to bind complement	Gm allotypes observed*
Gamma 1	70	+	1, 2, 4, 17, 22
Gamma 2	18	−	24
Gamma 3	8	+	3, 5, 6, 13, 14, 15, 16, 21
Gamma 4	3	−	—

* Gm allotypes are genetically controlled determinant groups located on the heavy chain of IgG that vary from individual to individual.

Changes in the variable regions of a light chain of given type are used as a basis for defining groups. Subdivisions distinguished within a

Table 7-1 Concentration and Metabolism of Some Human Immunoglobulins*

Class	Plasma concentration (mg/100 ml)	Percent in plasma	Synthesis: mg/kg body weight per day	Synthesis: moles/unit time or molecules/unit time	Half-life (days)
G	800–1680	78.0	28	20	15
A	140–420	16.6	8–10	4	5–6
M	50–190	5.0	5–8	1	5–6
D	0.3–40	0.4			3
E	0.0001–0.0007				

* The values given are designed to represent general approximations and will vary among individuals and in the same individual at different times.

greater identity in amino acid sequence with the variable region of a γ heavy chain than it does with the variable regions of other μ chain subgroups. To date the heavy chain subgroups have not been assigned Roman numerals to indicate their relative frequency of occurrence.

Abnormal structural analogues *(paraproteins)* are found in the sera of many persons. The myeloma proteins have both light and heavy chains and are structurally similar to either IgM, IgA, IgG, IgD, or IgE. They are classified M, A, G, D, or E on the basis of their antigenic similarity to the heavy chains of IgM, IgA, IgG, IgD, or IgE. The percentage of *monoclonal gammopathies* (myelomas) formed by each immunoglobulin class is roughly proportional to the percentage of the immunoglobulin class found in normal plasma (Table 7-1). Other paraproteins are composed only of light chains as in Bence Jones proteins or may occasionally contain only heavy chains as in some forms of heavy chain disease.

Concentration, Metabolism, and Distribution

Failure to find immunoglobulins in most germ-free animals has led to the belief that all immunoglobulins found in serum represent specific antibody. The total concentration of immunoglobulins (i.e., all proteins recognized by antibody to IgG) in normal adult human plasma is approximately 1.26 Gm percent, or 1,260 mg/100 ml.

At the risk of oversimplification, it is necessary to introduce certain data concerning the average distribution of antibody among the various classes of immunoglobulins and to indicate some features of their metabolism. It is important, however, to emphasize that the concentration and the physicochemical properties of antibody depend on the nature of the antigen, the site, stage, and intensity of the immunization response, the species, age, and genetic constitution of the recipient, and other factors that will be considered in the section on antibody production.

IgG is the predominant class of antibody found in human plasma, the steady-state concentration being about five times as high as IgA and fifteen times as high as IgM (Table 7-1). The combined concentration of IgD and IgE is usually less than 1 percent of the total immunoglobulin content.

A more dynamic reflection of the metabolism is indicated by the rate of synthesis of the immunoglobulins in terms of milligrams per kilogram of body weight per day, the number of molecules synthesized per unit time, and their catabolism, or half-life (measured in days). Regulation of the catabolic rate is a function of the Fc fragment of the heavy chains. The predominant steady-state concentration of IgG is thus a composite of both a more rapid rate of synthesis and a longer half-life than IgM and IgA. On a weight basis, the rate of synthesis of IgM and IgA is about one-fourth that of IgG. However, expressed in terms of the molecules synthesized per unit time, only 1 molecule of IgM is synthesized for every 4 molecules of IgA and for every 20 molecules of IgG. Since the half-life of IgG is about three times as long as IgA and IgM, the absolute rate of synthesis of IgG is twice that of IgA and seven times that of IgM. The shortest half-life of any of the immunoglobulins is associated with IgD. It is probable that IgE will be found to have the lowest rate of synthesis and catabolism of any of the immunoglobulins.

Except for IgG, immunoglobulins are catabolized at a constant rate irrespective of their concentration in the blood. IgG is unique in that the catabolic rate increases with the IgG concentration in the blood. Thus, the half-life of IgG will be much shorter in IgG myeloma patients in whom the blood concentration of IgG is markedly elevated, and these patients are liable to show antibody-deficiency syndromes following antigenic stimulation. Even though IgG antibody is synthesized at the normal rate, its absolute concentration in the blood will fall precipitously because it has a greatly reduced half-life.

IgG is distributed approximately equally between the intravascular and extravascular compartments. About half of the IgG in the plasma passes into the interstitial fluids daily and is replaced at the same time by an equal amount passing into the plasma from the interstitial fluids via the lymphatics. The distribution of IgE is generally similar to IgG, but the majority of the total body IgM and IgD, perhaps 80 percent, is found in the plasma. It is important to note that IgE can remain firmly bound to the surface of tissue cells for several weeks, a finding of paramount importance in atopic allergic reactions occurring in man.

Concerning the distribution of IgA, it is necessary to distinguish between circulating IgA and secretory IgA. Small lymphocytes destined to transform and differentiate into plasma cells synthesizing IgA are predominantly and strategically located in the interstices of the salivary glands and in the submucosa at all interfaces between the internal and external environments. After their synthesis by the plasma cells, monomeric units of IgA may move into the general circulation (circulating IgA), or the monomeric units may pass through the epithelial cells lining the mucous membranes, forming dimers and acquiring a secretory piece in the process (secretory IgA). Thus, there is a mechanism for selectively concentrating IgA in saliva, tears, nasal mucus, tracheobronchial washings, and gastrointestinal, genital, urinary, and mammary secretions. The attachment of the secretory piece, a glycoprotein with a molecular weight of 50,000, confers on IgA an increased resistance to digestion by proteolytic enzymes. Following antigenic stimulation of mucous membranes, secretory IgA production can occur in the absence of demonstrable circulating IgA.

Physicochemical Properties

Electrophoretic Mobility Plasma proteins can be separated into four main groups on the basis of their mobilities in an electric field. In decreasing order of their electrophoretic mobility these have been designated as albumin and the α-, β-, and γ-globulins. Through the application of more sophisticated procedures, such as starch gel electrophoresis and immunoelectrophoresis, human plasma can be resolved into more than 30 distinct antigenic proteins.

Table 7-2 Electrophoretic Mobilities of Immunoglobulins

Immunoglobulins	Electrophoretic mobility (cm²/volt/sec × 10⁵)
IgG	−0.6 to +3.0
IgM	+2.0
IgA	+1.2 to +3.6
IgD	⋝ −1.9
IgE	⋝ −1.9

The immunoglobulins show a broad range of mobility which extends over the electrophoretic regions designated α-, β-, and γ-globulins (Table 7-2). The widest range of electrophoretic mobility is observed with IgG, which migrates with the faster-moving α- and β-globulins as well as with the γ-globulins. IgM, IgA, and IgE show a somewhat narrower range and generally migrate with the β-globulins and the fast-moving γ-globulins. Without question, however, the bulk of antibody is localized in the fraction that migrates with the γ-globulins.

Sedimentation Constant (S_{20} or S) Various techniques of ultracentrifugation have been applied to whole serum and to isolated serum components. Antibody activity has been found to be associated with slow- and fast-sedimenting fractions having coefficients of 7S and 19S, and with fractions having intermediate sedimentation coefficients. Generally, IgG, IgD, and IgE have coefficients of 7S, IgM has a value of 19S, and IgA values range between 7S and 14S, depending upon the state of polymerization.

Molecular Weight The molecular weight of antibody varies from approximately 150,000 to 900,000. IgG has a molecular weight of 150,000, IgM a weight of 900,000, and IgA a weight of 150,000 to 400,000, depending upon its state of polymerization. The molecular weights of IgD and IgE are approximately 200,000.

Size and Shape As shown below data based on low-angle x-ray scattering and visualization by electron microscopy in antigen-antibody complexes indicate that IgG is a slender, asymmetrical, tight Y-shaped molecule with antigen-binding (Fab) sites located on the two arms, which are flexibly hinged to each other near the point where they are attached to the base (Fc). After combining with two molecules of the antigen, the two arms of the antibody molecule open to a variable degree, including full extension to a T shape. In this way, antibody molecules form bridges between antigen molecules, thus building a large, complex, insoluble lattice. The overall length of the antibody molecule in its extended T shape is approximately 230 Å.

Even when most of the base (Fc) is digested away with pepsin, antibody molecules retain the capacity to extend their arms $F(ab)_2$ after contact with molecules of the antigen, forming bridges which are built into an insoluble lattice. After removal of the Fc fragment, however, antibody molecules do lose other important biological properties, including the potential ability to bind complement, to release anaphylatoxin, to cross the placenta, and to attach firmly to tissue cells.

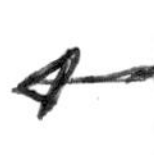

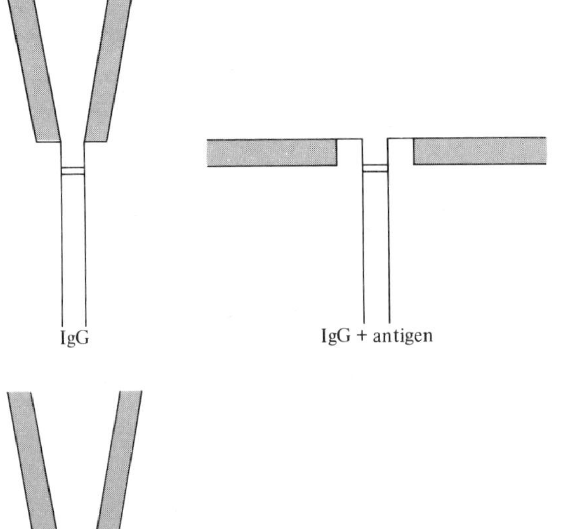

Although IgM is a much larger molecule than IgG, its structure is basically similar to other immunoglobulins. IgM is a polymer composed of 5 units, each of which contains two heavy and two light polypeptide chains, The Fc portions of alternate heavy chains are linked with sulfhydryl bonds so as to produce a central, shallow cylindrical portion and five radiating pairs of arms. Thus, the overall structure of IgM appears to be spherical.

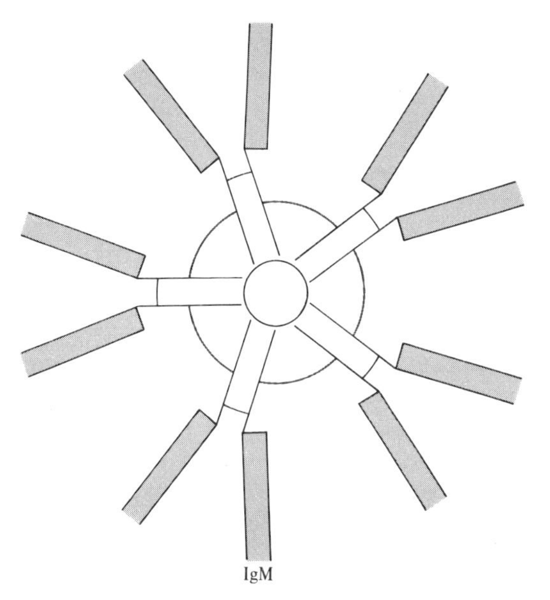
IgM

Circulating IgA, despite having two combining sites on each molecule which can bind two molecules of antigen, fails to extend to a T shape. The heavy chains of IgA are held together by an additional disulphide bond which keeps the antigen-binding sites close together and impedes the formation of a complex lattice. Secretory IgA and myeloma IgA polymers are similarly restricted. An analogous situation may occur with IgD and IgE, which also cannot form insoluble lattices with antigen.

Chemical Components Chemically, antibody molecules are glycoproteins which contain 2 to 14 percent carbohydrate and 86 to 98 percent amino acids. IgG has a low carbohydrate content, usually 2 percent but in a few rare cases as high as 6 percent. The other immunoglobulins have a high carbohydrate content of 10 to 14 percent. Most of the carbohydrate is located on the Fc fragment of heavy chains. The significance of the carbohydrate is uncertain, but it may be involved in the secretion of antibody from plasma cells or in maintaining the conformational structure of the heavy chains which are involved in the fixation of complement and in the firm binding of antibody to the surface of tissue cells.

Structural and Functional Components

The Basic Units Previous discussion has indicated that antibody molecules are composed of light and heavy polypeptide chains, that the light chains contain determinant groups that are common to all antibody molecules, and that the heavy chains carry unique determinant groups that separate immunoglobulins into five classes. Antibodies contain two light and two heavy chains or polymers of these. A given antibody molecule contains either two κ or two λ light chains (or polymers of these), but not one of each type.

The usual population of antibody molecules produced in response to immunization with an antigen contains a predominance of K to L molecules in the ratio of 2 to 1. However, the ratio of K to L molecules in purified antibodies varies widely among individuals and sometimes diverges markedly from the normal K to L ratio of 2 to 1.

Antihapten antibodies frequently are more homogeneous than antiprotein antibodies in their light chain patterns. For example, antidinitrophenol antibodies show an excess of K molecules above the normal 2 to 1 ratio irrespective of the protein carrier, degree of conjugation of the hapten, or stage of immunization. On the other hand, anti-pipsyl (para-iodobenzenesulfonyl chloride) antibodies contain a higher proportion of L molecules than is found in the usual population. In some individual cases, 70 percent of the molecules may contain λ light chains. In an antibody population with a marked divergence from the normal K to L ratio, the synthesis of light chains is not linked to a particular class of immunoglobulin, since an equivalent ratio is found in the different classes of immunoglobulin.

Fragments The term *antibody fragment* is reserved for portions of the molecule that are obtained as a result of cleavage of peptide bonds. Proteolytic enzymes produce heterogeneous groups of fragments which can be distinguished by immunological and chemical properties. It will prove most useful from a structural and functional approach to name the fragments and to explore their interrelationships. As will be emphasized later, the designation of these fragments does not imply their homogeneity.

Fragment	Produced by digestion with
$F(ab)_2$ (antigen binding)*	Pepsin
Fab (antigen binding)	Papain
Fc (crystallizable)	Papain
Fd (heavy chain portion of Fab fragment)	Papain

* 5S antibody is a synonym for the F(ab)2 fragment.

Diagrammatic Representation of the Structure of IgG Each molecule of IgG is composed of four polypeptide chains. Two κ or λ light chains have molecular weights of approximately 25,000, and the two heavy chains have molecular weights of approximately 50,000. The light and heavy chains differ in their primary structure (amino acid sequence) and in their determinant groups. The polypeptide chains are held together primarily with disulfide bonds which link the light chains to the heavy chains and the heavy chains to each other (Fig. 7-1).

Under appropriate reducing conditions papain hydrolyzes IgG into three fragments which are roughly equivalent in molecular weight. The Fc fragment contains the COOH-terminal portion of the heavy chains which are held together by two disulfide bonds, and the two Fab fragments each contain a complete light chain and the NH_2-terminal portion of one of the heavy chains linked together by single disulfide bonds. Each Fab fragment has one of the antibody-combining sites on the intact IgG molecule, while the Fc fragment is devoid of antibody activity. On reduction and alkylation an Fab fragment yields a light chain and the NH_2-terminal portion of the heavy chain (the Fd fragment).

If pepsin at pH 5 is used to digest IgG, a fragment $F(ab)_2$, with a molecular weight of approximately 100,000 and a sedimentation constant of 5 is obtained, together with smaller peptides. Since the $F(ab)_2$ fragment will precipitate with antigen, it has also been referred to as 5S antibody. Reduction with thiol or mercapto-

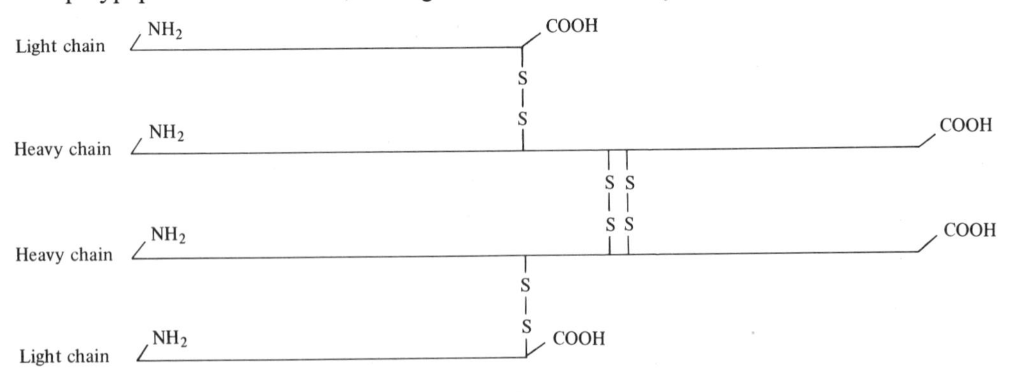

Figure 7-1 Structure of human IgG.

ethanol splits the $F(ab)_2$ fragment into two Fab fragments. On oxidation the Fab fragments can recombine to form the $F(ab)_2$ fragment.

The Fab fragments obtained from IgG are not homogeneous, since some will contain κ chains and others will have λ chains. Intact K molecules of IgG as well as Fab fragments prepared from K molecules are more positively charged and have a faster electrophoretic mobility than L molecules and Fab fragments of L molecules.

The Structure of Immunoglobulins Other than IgG IgM is a polymer of 5 units, each composed of two light and two heavy chains. When IgM is reduced by mercaptoethanol, it readily dissociates into monomers with a sedimentation coefficient of 7S. In accordance with these findings, IgM is generally considered to have 10 combining sites. For unknown reasons, however, the monomers are devoid of agglutinating or precipitating activity.

IgD, IgE, and circulating IgA are monomers and, like IgG, contain two light and two heavy polypeptide chains, two antigen-binding sites, and one Fc fragment per molecule. The heavy chains of IgD and IgE have a greater molecular weight than those of IgG. Secretory IgA is a dimer plus a glycoprotein secretory piece which increases the resistance of the molecule to proteolytic enzymes. IgA myeloma proteins usually occur in plasma as polymers which contain 2, 3, 4, or more monomers. Like IgM, polymers of IgA revert to monomeric 7S units on gentle treatment with reagents which break disulfide bonds.

Specificity

The fundamental property of an antibody molecule is its ability to react specifically with an antigen. The specific reactivity of antibody is a function of selected localized areas, combining sites, or antigen-binding sites on the surface of the antibody molecule which have a structure that is complementary to a particular determinant group on the surface of the antigen. Two or more identical combining sites are present on each antibody molecule. The available data indicate that the combining sites are localized to amino acid residues 95 to 99 on the NH_2-terminal portion of the heavy and light chains that make up the Fab fragments. Heavy chains apparently make a greater contribution to the antigen-binding sites than do the light chains. To a limited extent, Fd fragments of heavy chains can combine with antigen, whereas light chains cannot. The light chains, however, greatly increase the firmness of the binding with antigen, presumably by maintaining a conformational structure more complementary to the antigen.

Accordingly, variation in the primary amino acid sequence of the NH_2-terminal portion of light and heavy chains would account for the formation of antibodies of different specificities. Consequently, each individual must have a mechanism for synthesizing antibody molecules of many different primary structures.

Combining Sites

Valence The number of combining sites on the surface of an antibody molecule is referred to as the valence. Except for IgM and sometimes for IgA, most antibody molecules are divalent. IgM is multivalent and has 10 combining sites. Although IgA is generally divalent, it may polymerize, in which case it may have a valence of 4, 6, or 8.

The fact that antibody is at least divalent has important implications in terms of antigen-antibody interaction, since it may act to form a bridge between two antigen molecules.

Size Estimates of the size of the combining sites on antibody molecules are based primarily on studies of hapten inhibition by peptides or saccharides. In these experiments it was found that the smallest determinant groups that combine with antibody to cause maximal inhibition of precipitation of the antigen consist of penta- or hexapeptides in the case of protein antigens and hexasaccharides in the case of polysaccharide antigens. Since a further increase in the number of amino acid residues in the peptide or sugar residues in the saccharide does not enhance hapten inhibition, it may be assumed that five or six amino acid or sugar residues represent the approximate size of an antibody-combining site. Expressed in dimensions this represents a size of 25 to 35 Å and a molecular weight between 400 and 1,000. In this connection, it is interesting to note that independent measurements based on x-ray diffraction and electron microscopy indicate that antibody molecules have a width of approximately 40 Å and a depth of 19 Å.

These findings indicate that the two combining sites on IgG comprise about 1 percent of the molecule. Thus, it is not surprising that no convincing differences in overall amino acid composition have been found between antibodies induced in the same species by different antigens or by the same antigen in different hosts.

Antibodies as Antigens

For a variety of theoretical and practical reasons that will become evident as the discussion proceeds, it is appropriate to consider antibodies as proteins that can function as antigens. Many of the determinant groups on intact antibody molecules are localized in the COOH-terminal ends of the light and heavy polypeptide chains. As noted earlier, all proteins recognized by antibody to the light chains of IgG are classed as immunoglobulins. Variability in the peptides that form the COOH-terminal portion of the κ and λ light chains is an important and unique characteristic of immunoglobulins. In addition, it is probably related to the specificity of antibodies, since it increases the range of configurations that immunoglobulins can assume. Much greater diversity is introduced into the structure of antibodies by the heavy polypeptide chains which are antigenically distinct in each of the five classes of immunoglobulins.

Among human immunoglobulins there are other genetically controlled determinant groups that vary from individual to individual; these groups are known as allotypes. InV 1, 2, and 3 allotypes are found on light κ chains and presumably are present on all antibody molecules containing κ chains. The genes controlling the InV determinants are codominant alleles and are independent of those that control the Oz^+ and Oz^- allotypes on λ light chains or the Gm determinants on heavy chains of IgG.

Molecular heterogeneity is marked within the IgG class of immunoglobulins. Four heavy chains have been differentiated on the basis of specific antisera prepared in rabbits or primates. Most individuals contain all four types of molecules which have been designated as the gamma 1, 2, 3, and 4 subgroups. In addition, there are the different, genetically controlled Gm determinant groups that vary among individuals. Precise information concerning the allelic state of the various genes controlling the Gm allotypes is lacking, but there are more than 20 such determinants.

As illustrated earlier, there is some association of Gm determinants with the molecular subgroups of IgG.

Apart from their contribution to immunology, the Gm determinants provide a useful tool for anthropologists and population geneticists. Certain determinants, for example, are usually inherited together in Caucasians, but not in non-Caucasians.

Heterogeneity in Affinity of Antibody Molecules One of the principal sources of heterogeneity is the affinity of antibody molecules. *Affinity*, or *average affinity constant* (K), is a term used to describe the equilibrium for the reaction between an antigen-binding site on the antibody and the determinant group on the antigen. K

can be measured with precision by employing the technique of equilibrium dialysis to assay the strength of binding between antibody and monovalent hapten. In this system, K is equal to the reciprocal of the concentration of free hapten at equilibrium when half the antibody sites are bound with the hapten. The available data demonstrate that different antisera consist of populations of antibody molecules with a range of K values for a specific antigenic determinant which may vary as much as 10,000-fold. When these observations are extended to include the multivalent character of immunogens, it is apparent that affinity is probably the major factor in the heterogeneity of antibody molecules.

Homogeneous Immunoglobulins

Because of their remarkable molecular homogeneity, the chemical and immunological analysis of Bence Jones, myeloma, and Fc proteins has contributed greatly to an understanding of the structure and inheritance of antibodies. These homogeneous immunoglobulins have provided a ready source of most of the component units found in antibody molecules.

Although Bence Jones proteins show many different patterns, in a given individual each one is homogeneous with respect to its light chain and InV or Oz allotype and is totally deficient in heavy chain material. Thus, the formation of free Bence Jones protein represents asynchronous synthesis, more light chains being formed than heavy chains. Bence Jones proteins usually consist of light chain dimers (molecular weight of approximately 50,000), but occasionally these proteins may occur as monomers or as polymers with more than two monomeric units.

Similarly, in some forms of heavy chain disease, Fc proteins may be excreted in large quanity in the urine or serum as a result of excess synthesis of heavy chains. The name Fc protein is used because Fc fragments, rather than isolated heavy chains or dimers of heavy chains, are found. Homogeneity of Fc protein is indicated by their association with a particular molecular subgroup of IgG and a specific Gm allotype.

Myeloma proteins contain only one type of light chain, one type of heavy chain, one Gm allotype, and one InV or Oz allotype. Different myeloma proteins show many different patterns but each one is homogeneous with respect to its polypeptide chains and its allotypes.

Summary

An antibody is one of a group of high molecular weight proteins with two (or polymers of two) identical combining sites that react specifically with and have a structure that is complementary to a particular determinant group on an antigen. The combining sites comprise about 1 percent of the antibody, are localized in the area comprising amino acid positions 95 to 99 from the NH_2-terminal of the heavy and light polypeptide chains, and form a bridge between two antigen molecules.

There are five classes of human immunoglobulins that are known to possess antibody activity: IgM, IgA, IgG, IgD, and IgE. The classes differ in their concentration, metabolism, distribution, physicochemical properties, and structure. Within a particular class of immunoglobulins, marked molecular heterogeneity is apparent. In addition, there are genetically controlled determinant groups on antibody molecules (allotypes) that vary from individual to individual. Despite the remarkable diversity of antibody molecules, however, all share the fundamental property of reacting specifically with the same determinant group on the antigen that stimulated their formation.

FACTORS INFLUENCING ANTIBODY PRODUCTION

General Considerations

Introduction of an antigen into an immunologically competent host may initiate a sequence of events that results in the production of a population of antibody molecules, each of which is stereospecific for a particular determinant group on the surface of the antigen. The quantitative relationships are such that more than 100,000 antibody molecules are usually synthesized for each antigen molecule introduced.

Antibody is produced almost entirely as a result of *de novo* synthesis from amino acids by plasma cells and their precursors. Studies with labeled amino acids reveal that labeled antibody is secreted by these cells within 20 min. and is not stored intracellularly to any appreciable extent.

In an effort to delineate some of the factors that are known to affect the kinetics of antibody formation, many of the parameters will be considered independently. It must be emphasized, however, that antibody formation is a dynamic rather than a static process and that it represents a special problem in protein synthesis, many facets of which are poorly understood.

At the risk of oversimplification, in order to permit convenient consideration, the ensuing discussion will be restricted to the synthesis of 19S and 7S antibody. While 19S is generally equated with IgM, it must be admitted that there is some evidence based on studies in germ-free animals to suggest that some 19S antibody may actually be IgG. At the same time, while 7S antibody is often used synonymously with IgG, it is known that IgA, IgD, and IgE may have a sedimentation value of 7S. On the other hand, it is generally agreed that in man 19S is predominantly IgM, and 7S is predominantly IgG.

The Fate of Injected Antigens

Primary Contact The fate of antigens can be assayed quantitatively and conveniently following their initial introduction by the intravenous route. A variety of particulate antigens including viruses, sheep red blood cells, and bacterial flagella are removed from the circulation in two phases. The first is the *nonimmune phase,* which is accomplished by the cells of the reticuloendothelial system (RES). The duration of the nonimmune phase is shortened as the dose of antigen is lowered and may be as short as 20 hr. Thereafter, the appearance of antibody in the serum leads to the formation of antigen-antibody complexes which are more rapidly phagocytized. This accelerated disappearance of the antigen is known as the *immune elimination phase.*

The available data suggest that soluble protein antigens disappear from the blood in three separate phases, designated as equilibration, metabolism, and immune elimination (Fig. 7-2). Recent findings concerning the equilibration and metabolism phases provide a perfect illustration of antibody formation as a dynamic rather than a static process. It is generally agreed that half of the protein disappears from the blood within 24 hr. and that this represents an equilibration with extravascular plasma proteins. As noted earlier, however, 50 percent of the radiolabel of soluble proteins of low or high molecular weight is excreted in 1 hr. and 70 percent in 24 hr. The finding that the material in the urine is heterogeneous with respect to physical properties and that much of it is associated with RNA indicates that the antigen is rapidly metabolized as well as equilibrated during the first 24 hr.

After the first day the metabolism phase usually continues for 6 or 7 days but may persist for 12 days or longer if the dose of antigen is high. During this interval a constant amount of antigen remaining in the circulation is eliminated in unit time. Thus, there is a steady decline which follows an exponential curve. When plotted semilogarithmically, the elimination of antigen follows a straight line.

In the equilibration and metabolism phases the disappearance of antigen apparently follows the normal catabolic processes by which the host handles its own proteins. With the synthesis of antibody by about the seventh day, the

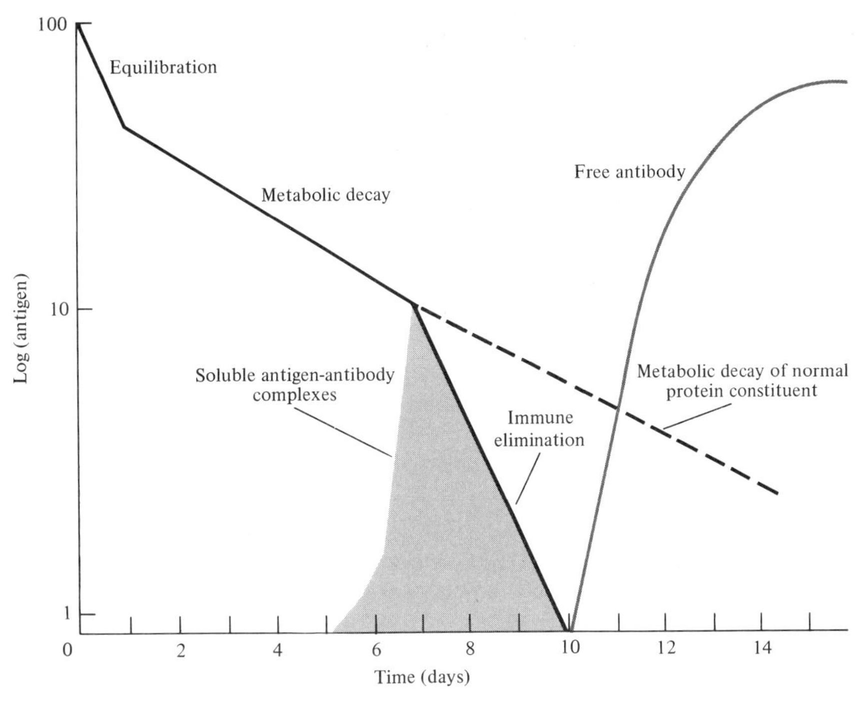

Figure 7-2 Disappearance of a soluble protein antigen from the blood: equilibration, metabolism, and immune elimination. *(F. J. Dixon, Harvey Lect., 58:21-52, 1963.)*

immune elimination phase is ushered in, soluble antigen-antibody complexes are formed, and the remaining antigen is rapidly removed from the circulation by the RES. As will be emphasized later, soluble antigen-antibody complexes, especially those present in slight antigen excess, can be biologically active in inducing anaphylaxis experimentally and are intimately involved in the pathogenesis of serum sickness.

Equilibration of pneumococcal and other bacterial polysaccharide antigens between the vascular and extravascular compartments occurs quickly, and localization within the RES generally resembles that seen with protein antigens. The subsequent fate of polysaccharide antigens, however, is quite different from that observed with proteins. Metabolism of bacterial polysaccharides proceeds at an unusually slow rate. Persistence of polysaccharide antigens within macrophages can be demonstrated for several months. The immune elimination phase is greatly delayed, and most important, the kinetics of antibody formation is strikingly different from that associated with protein antigens. For example, in man antibody production may continue for as long as 8 years following a single injection of 50 μg pneumococcal polysaccharide.

Secondary Contact If, after an interval of 10 days or more, a particulate or soluble antigen is injected intravenously into a sensitized animal (one that already had primary contact with the antigen), the rate of disappearance of the antigen from the circulation is greatly accelerated. The rate at which antigen is removed is proportional to the concentration of circulating antibody at the time of injection. Immune elimination occurs immediately if the antibody level is high. Even in the absence of detectable antibody, the immune elimination phase appears much earlier than on primary contact. For example, immune elimination of a soluble protein antigen may begin on the second day and may be completed by the fourth day.

Reactions to Injected Antigens

At the Tissue Level Antibody formation and tissue reactions to injected antigens are a function of the RES. The tissues primarily involved include the bone marrow, spleen, lymph nodes, lungs, and local granulomas. Other components of the RES play a limited role in antibody formation. The liver and the kidneys, for example, may take up and metabolize the antigen but may contribute little to the total synthesis of antibody.

Localization within the RES is dependent upon the physical state of the antigen and the route of inoculation. After intravenous injection of soluble protein antigens, the bulk of antibody formation occurs in the bone marrow, with lesser amounts synthesized in the spleen and the lungs. Following inoculation of particulate antigens by the intravenous route, the spleen and the lungs make a greater contribution and the bone marrow a lesser contribution to antibody production. The role of the lymph nodes in the production of antibody is most evident following intradermal or subcutaneous inoculation of the antigen. Both particulate and soluble antigens are rapidly fixed in the regional draining nodes, and antibody formation occurs first in the nodes on the side where the antigen was injected. When antigens are injected intramuscularly in the presence of complete Freund's adjuvant, a granuloma forms, and the bulk of the antibodies are synthesized locally within the granuloma. If, however, antigen and adjuvant are inoculated into the footpad, antibody formation is found in association with the bone marrow, spleen, homolateral lymph nodes, and the lumbar and cervical nodes.

Although the bone marrow makes an important contribution to antibody protection regardless of the physical state of the antigen and the route of injection, antibody activity per unit mass is never high because the total bulk is so great. Furthermore, the diffuse distribution of the bone marrow does not permit convenient quantitation. Consequently, most studies of antibody formation have been concerned with the roles of the spleen, lymph nodes, and local granulomas. The basic tissue reaction within the spleen and the lymph nodes is associated with the formation of germinal or lymphocytopoietic centers. These appear 3 to 4 days after primary antigenic stimulation and increase in size for 10 to 20 days.

The Cellular Basis of Antibody Formation As indicated previously, antibody formation is intimately associated with the RES and the lymphoid tissue and cells of the body. Further examination of lymphoid ontogenesis, the development of immunocompetence, and cellular synergism will provide additional details on this intimate association.

Ontogenesis of Lymphoid Cells and Tissues Lymphocytopoietic activities are a ramification of the general hematopoietic development of the individual. Initially, multipotential stem cells arise in the primitive streak area and migrate to the yolk sac and area vasculosa of the developing embryo. With continued proliferation of the cells, there is a migration from these primary areas, leading to the colonization of primitive hematopoietic centers in the fetal liver and bone marrow. Subsequently, the migrating cells colonize the rudimentary myeloid and lymphoid centers in the bone marrow, spleen, thymus, and gut-associated areas (in birds, the bursa of Fabricius). In the lymphoid and myeloid centers, the multipotential stem cells fall under the inductive influence of organ rudiments. When inductive elements arise from mesenchymal tissue, the multipotential stem cell differentiates to a unipotential myeloid stem cell. Inductive factors arising from epithelial elements, however, result in differentiation of the multipotential stem cell into a *unipotential lymphoid stem cell*, or *progenitor cell* (Fig. 7-3).

The Thymus The primary lymphoid centers of concern to this discussion are the thymus in all vertebrates and the bursa of Fabricius in birds, or its analogue in mammals. The epithelial elements of the thymus are derived by budding and specialization of the third and fourth pharyngeal pouches in humans and become evident by about the sixth week of gestation. Between the sixth and eighth weeks of gestation lymphoid development of the thymus occurs, and by about the tenth week the thymic cortex and medulla are delineated. The cortex is composed primarily of lymphocytes, and the medulla is composed of epithelial cells, lymphocytes, and Hassall's corpuscles. Cellular

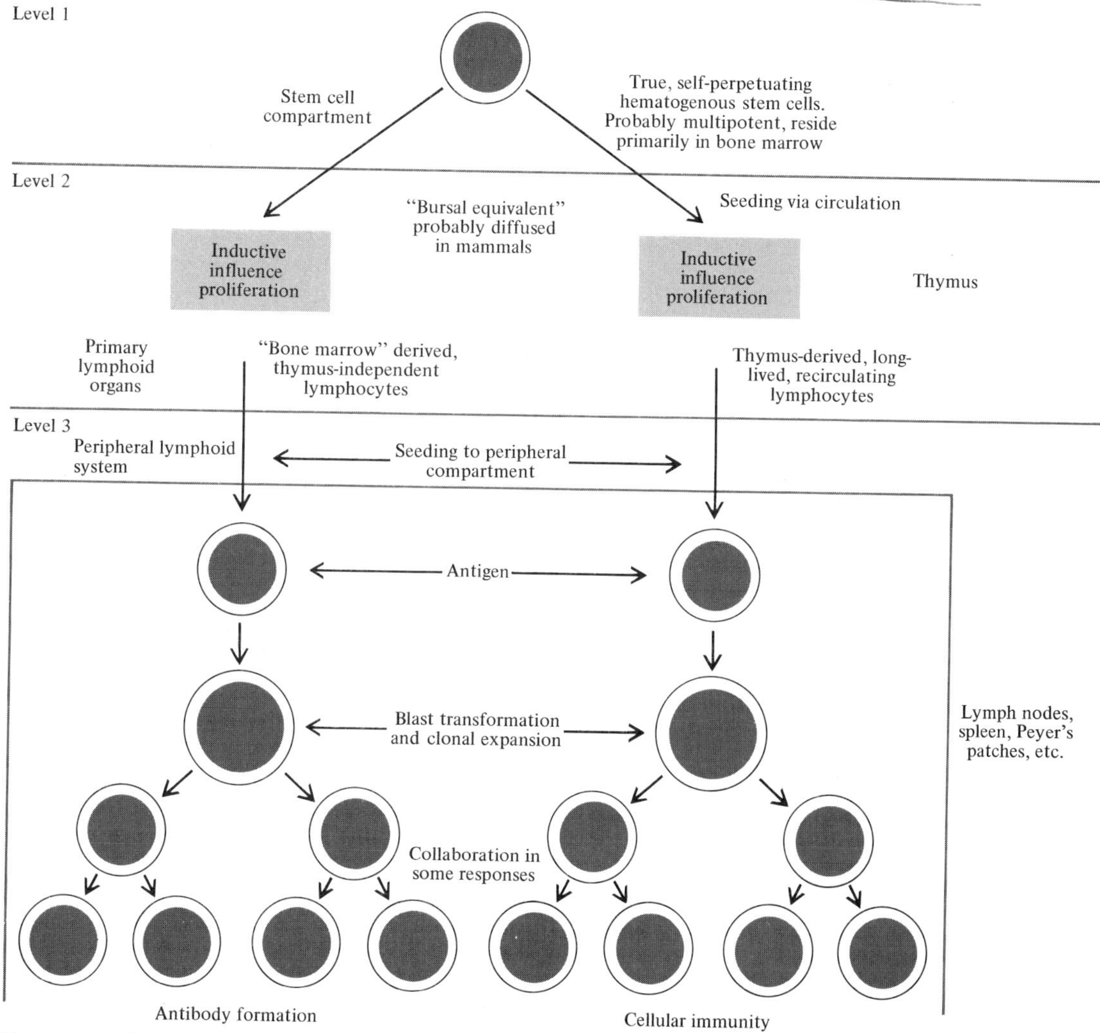

Figure 7-3 A schematic overview of the three main functional compartments of the lymphoid system. (*G. J. V. Nossal and G. L. Ada, Antigens, Lymphoid Cells and the Immune Response, New York, Academic Press, Inc., 1971.*)

proliferation proceeds at a high rate in the cortical lymphocytes and at a much lower rate in the medullary lymphocytes. The proliferation is *antigen-independent* and is probably motivated by humoral factors (hormones?) released by thymic epithelial elements.

In the fetal thymus the proliferative activity reaches a level higher than that in any of the other lymphoid centers. After birth, lymphocytopoietic activity in the thymus decreases with age but remains at a higher level in the adult thymus than in other lymphoid tissues. Approximately 95 percent of the cells resulting from thymic lymphocytopoiesis never leave the thymus but die in situ after a life span of 3 to 4 days. The surviving 5 percent of thymocytes acquire a new surface antigen—the theta antigen—and migrate from the thymus to seed the diffuse cortical tissue and paracortical nodules of secondary or peripheral lymphoid tissue (lymph nodes and the splenic white pulp, Figs. 7-3 and 7-4).

Cells bearing the theta antigen and seeding the peripheral lymphoid centers are referred to as thymus-derived, thymus-dependent, or T cells, and the areas of lymphoid tissues that they populate are referred to as thymus-dependent areas. T cells provide the bulk of the circulating

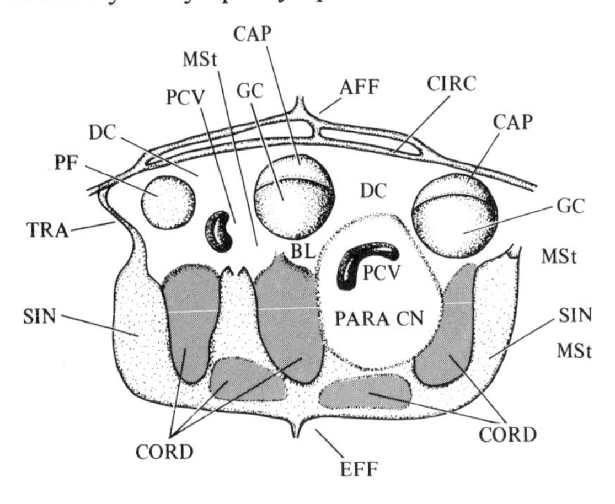

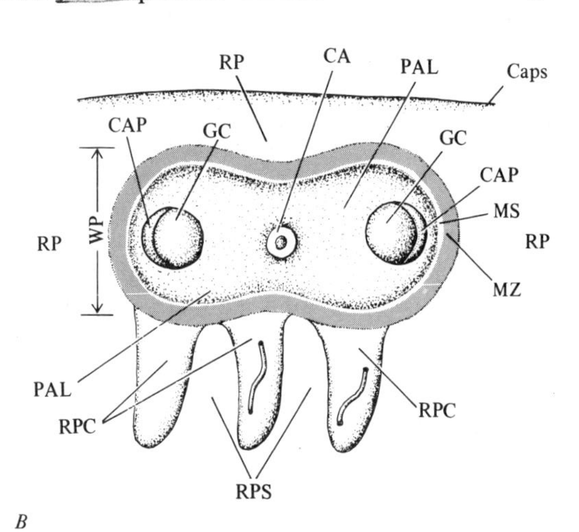

Figure 7-4 Schematic views of an antigenically stimulated lymph node and the spleen of an immunized animal. *(A)*. Schematic view of a section through an antigenically stimulated lymph node. AFF, afferent lymphatic vessel; CIRC, circular sinus; TRA, trabecular sinus; PF, primary lymphoid follicle; DC, diffuse cortex of lymph node; GC, germinal center; CAP, antigen-trapping area of "cap" of germinal center, rich in dendritic follicle cells; PCV, postcapillary venule; MSt, "muddy stream" area where lymphocytes leave cortex and enter medullary sinus through valvelike area; BL, areas where blast cells can be seen, possibly moving from germinal center into medullary cord; PARA CN, paracortical nodule which hypertrophies during cellular immune responses; CORD, medullary cord of lymph node rich in antibody-forming cells; SIN, medullary sinus, rich in macrophages and prime site of antigen capture; EFF, efferent lymphatic. *(B)*. Schematic view of the organization of the spleen as seen through a section from an immunized animal. Caps, capsule; RP, red pulp; WP, white pulp; MZ, marginal zone; MS, marginal sinus; PAL, periarteriolar lymphocyte sheath; CA, central arteriole; GC, germinal center; CAP, caplike area of germinal center rich in dendritic follicle cells; RPC, red pulp cords rich in antibody-forming cells; RPS, red pulp sinuses engaged in erythrocyte destruction and some erythropoiesis and myelopoiesis. *(G. J. V. Nossal and G. L. Ada, Antigens, Lymphoid Cells and the Immune Response, New York, Academic Press, Inc., 1971.)*

lymphocytes found in the bloodstream. Actually, T cells exhibit a kinetic, migratory behavior.

Blood bearing T cells enters the lymph node by vessels penetrating the hilum of the node and is transported farther into the node by arterioles and capillaries. The blood is carried into the thymus-dependent areas of the node by postcapillary venules, characterized by tall cuboidal endothelial cells. Although the concept has been recently challenged, it is generally held that T cells have the propensity for passing through the endothelial cells. Certain characteristics of T cells associated with the presence of particular surface carbohydrates facilitate their penetration of the plasma membranes of the endothelial cells, passage through the cytoplasm, and exit on the far side. Enzymatic removal of surface carbohydrates from the T cells can prevent emigration of the lymphocytes.

On a similar basis, T cells can enter the diffuse cortex of the node and "home" in on their anatomical niche. From the cortex, the T cells can migrate from the lymph node by way of efferent lymphatic channels; they then pass through the thoracic duct, from which they enter the circulatory system. If T cells leave the circulation to enter tissues other than the lymphoid centers, they can percolate through the tissue spaces via the lymphatic channels and return to the lymph nodes by way of afferent lymph ducts. Such recirculation patterns are a constant feature of T cells and will recur for the life of the cells.

T cells are prime components of the immune system of the immunocompetent individual and are vitally and intimately involved in antibody production, delayed hypersensitivity, graft rejection, graft versus host reactions, autoimmunity, immunological memory, immunological surveillance, and immunological tolerance, all of which will be dealt with in subsequent sections and chapters.

Gut-associated Lymphoid Centers In all mammals, including man, tissue analogues to the bursa of Fabricius are not known with certainty. Some investigators suggest that gut-associated centers such as the tonsils, adenoidal tissue, appendix, and Peyer's patches may be bursal analogues, while others prefer the concept of a diffuse bursal analogue spread throughout the tissues of the body. Stem cells colonize the gut-associated lymphoid centers during the first half of the embryonic period and begin to differentiate and proliferate into lymphoid progenitor cells. Differentiation and proliferation is antigen-independent, but evidence indicates that humoral factors or inducers generated by the reticulo-epithelial elements of the primary lymphoid organs are important in directing both differentiation and proliferation of the stem cells.

Stem cells proliferate and differentiate in a manner analogous to that of the T cell, acquire specific surface antigens (B antigens, hence B cells), and migrate to and populate secondary lymphoid tissue. In the secondary lymphoid centers, B cells form aggregates of lymphoid cells mixed with reticular cells (primary lymphoid follicles) and are the thymus-independent areas of peripheral or secondary lymphoid centers (lymph nodes, splenic red pulp, Figs. 7-3 and 7-4). The B cells are the source of all antibody-producing cells in the body.

Development of Immunocompetence From conception to birth, the human fetus develops in a highly protective environment, shielded from chemical and physical trauma by the homeostatic mechanisms afforded by the embryonic membranes, the uterus, and the physiological and immunological apparatus of the mother. In such a benign environment, embryonic development is usually completed uneventfully, and individuals are born with many of their own defense mechanisms in a relatively naïve state.

For a long period of time it was held that the human neonate arrived with an immature rather than a naïve immune system and that the system achieved maturity and full development only in the postnatal period. Investigations using animal models, premature human births, aborted human fetuses, and infants born with congenital infections or born of mothers with agammaglobulinemia have indicated that the normal human neonate is born with an immune system marked more by naïveté than by immaturity.

A normal human neonate, born after an uneventful gestation period, is equipped with a number of immune defense and allied mechanisms in a state of some readiness to meet the challenge of a new and often hostile world. The peripheral lymphoid tissues at birth are only moderately developed, as is reflected by minimal follicular activity and poor demarcation between the cortex and medulla. Germinal centers and plasma cells are virtually absent. As antigenic challenge begins to impinge on the individual, there is a rapid response in the form of increased follicular activity, proliferation of lymphocytes, production of germinal centers (masses of plasma cells), and the production of antibody.

The development of the naïve but ready immunological defense system can be traced in prenatal life in the perspective of the ontogenesis of tissues and cells discussed above. Organ cultures derived from uninfected fetuses have the capacity to produce IgM and IgG as early as the twentieth week of gestation. More recent evidence has indicated that synthesis of IgM may begin as early as the eleventh week, and IgG production may begin by the twelfth week of gestation. In the normal uninfected fetus, synthesis of IgM, IgG, and IgE is usually extremely low, and IgA and IgD synthesis is not detectable. Nonetheless, the data indicate that immunocompetence is present at an early gestational age (11 weeks, Fig. 7-5).

About the middle of the second month of gestation, maternal IgG traverses the placenta and appears in the fetal circulation; this can be detected by allotypic differences, specificity to a variety of antigens the fetus was never exposed to, and the use of isotopically labeled maternal IgG. The contribution of maternal IgG increases rapidly during the last half of the gestation period and is almost fully equilibrated with the fetal circulation a month before birth. On the other hand, concentrations of IgM and IgE found in fetal cord blood are unrelated to maternal concentrations, an indication of the capacity of the fetus to synthesize these immunoglobulins. The presence of maternal antibody in the fetal circulation affords specific protection with a battery of antibodies built up during 20 to 30 years or more of maternal immunological experience (Fig. 7-5).

Thus, the neonate has an immune system capable of synthesizing immunoglobulins and a maternal endowment of IgG at adult concentrations (Fig. 7-5). For the first 3 months of postnatal life, the infant is well protected from antigenic challenge by maternal IgG (with at least one exception: respiratory syncytial virus infection). From the moment of birth, however, maternal IgG is being catabolized by the infant's metabolic machinery, and the level continually declines until about 6 months of age when maternal IgG has virtually disappeared. As the concentration of maternal IgG falls, the opportunities for antigenic challenge of the infant's immune system steadily increase. The synthesis of immunoglobulins picks up during the first 9 months after birth, with the production of IgM, IgG, IgE, and IgA rising during the first 3 months and IgD appearing in about 8 months (Fig. 7-5). Since the infant's IgG concentration normally begins to rise immediately after birth while maternal IgG is declining, the total amount of IgG in the infant's blood never drops much below 40 percent of adult concentrations, and by the sixth month the concentration of IgG begins to rise. By puberty, adult immunoglobulin concentrations are attained.

Confirmatory evidence of the responsive po-

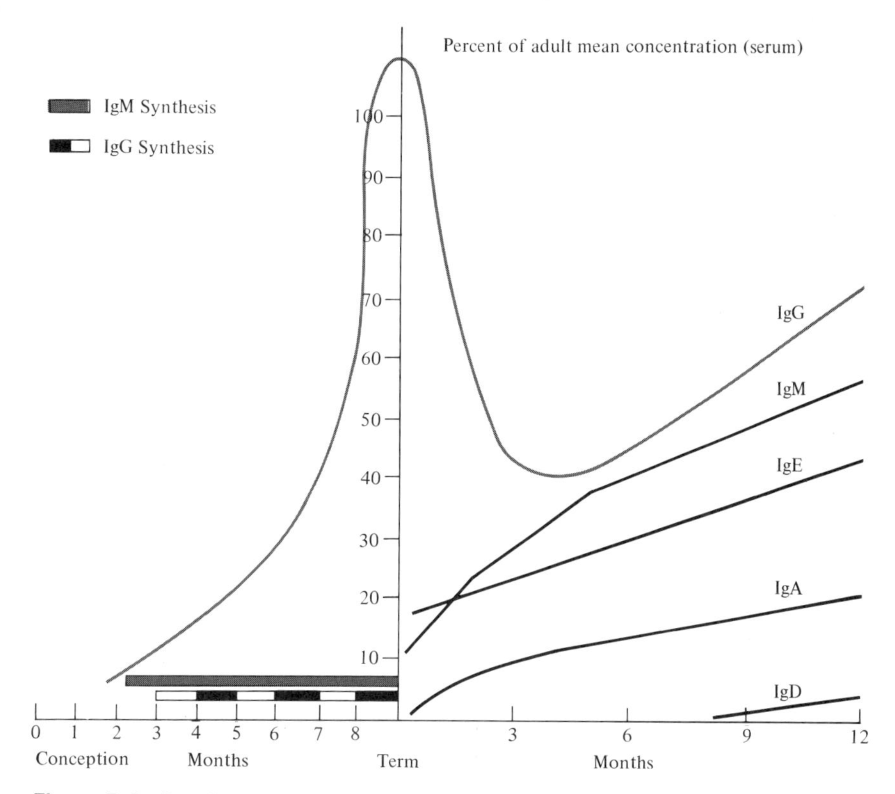

Figure 7-5 Development of immunoglobulins: serum concentrations during early human development. *(C. B. S. Wood, J. R. Coll. Physicians Lond., 6:246–258, 1972.)*

tential of the fetal immune system comes from studies of fetuses congenitally infected with rubella, herpes simplex, toxoplasma, cytomegalovirus, and syphilis. In many of these cases, cord bloods have elevated amounts of immunoglobulins, particularly of IgM. A concentration of 30 mg/100 ml of IgM is considered evidence of in utero infection. IgM concentrations in cord blood of congenitally infected fetuses may be as high as 270 mg/100 ml in rubella, 130 mg/100 ml in toxoplasmosis, and 36 mg/100 ml in cytomegalovirus disease. In severe cases of intrauterine infections, IgA concentrations may be as high as 11 mg/100 ml versus normal concentrations of approximately 2 mg/100 ml. Since neither IgM nor IgA can pass the placenta, the elevated immunoglobulin concentrations are taken as a priori evidence of fetal synthesis.

The development of allied mechanisms of defense parallels the ontogeny of the immune system. After 4 months of gestation, sporadic mast cells can be identified in the tissues of the fetus, and by 5 months, large numbers of mast cells are present. At 5 months, the fetus is capable of mounting an adult-type inflammatory response, albeit not as pronounced because of a paucity of infiltrating cells. Phagocytic cells are present at the time of development of the vasculature, are quite capable of efficient phagocytosis (provided that opsonic antibodies are present), possess intracellular bactericidal activity, and can synthesize interferon at or near adult concentrations. There is also evidence that the fetus can mount cell-mediated immune responses at the fourth to fifth months of gestation, as has been shown by graft rejection and the development of skin reactions to chemicals such as dinitrochlorobenzene.

These data strongly suggest that the fetus and the neonate are equipped with a functional defense system which normally develops unchallenged. After birth, antigenic challenges repeatedly impinge on the system, and adult sophistication develops through experience.

Cellular Synergism in Antibody Formation Prior considerations have dealt with the development of two separate lines of lymphoid cells, T cells and B cells, which occupy different areas in the same lymphoid tissues. Intimately associated with these two cell types is the macrophage. T cells, B cells, and macrophages constitute the important responsive elements of the immune system.

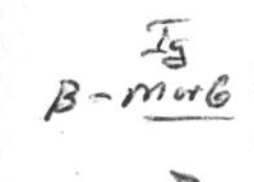

B Cells B cells are the source of antibody-forming cells (AFC) and are endowed with specific surface receptors located in the plasma membrane which appear to be IgM and IgG. The receptors are specific for individual determinant groups on antigenic molecules. All receptors on a particular B cell are directed toward and are specific for a single determinant group, and antibody molecules eventually produced by an AFC in response to antigenic stimulation have all the characteristics associated with the receptors (specificity, light and heavy chain markers, and allotypy).

T Cells T cells are capable of reacting with antigen, forming blast cells, and proliferating, but they do not form plasma cells and do not produce antibody. Because of their properties, T cells are referred to as *antigen-reactive cells* (ARC). The ability of T cells to interact with antigen also resides in surface receptors located in the plasma membrane. Available data indicate that T cell receptors are present in low concentration and cannot be definitely characterized as any of the known immunoglobulins, although some evidence is suggestive of IgM characteristics.

Receptors of B and T Cells Prelabeling the surfaces of B and T cells by radioiodination or by the use of tagged antiglobulin sera reveals an extremely rapid metabolic turnover of receptors. The half-life of B cell surface immunoglobulin is about 2 hr., while that of the T cell is 4 to 6 hr. If this indicates a slow shedding of receptors, then both B and T cells can be regarded as slowly secreting immunoglobulin molecules. In a number of instances, it has been demonstrated that following interaction with antigen or antiglobulin sera or plant lectins, receptors of AFC tend to cluster or aggregate to one pole of the cell, usually in the area over the Golgi apparatus, an epiphenomenon termed *capping*, which may represent an important step in determining what subsequent response the cell makes.

Antigen Capture and Distribution Most of the antigen introduced into the body is fairly rapidly disseminated, broken down, and excreted. The process is so efficient that within 48 hr. less than 1 percent of the original antigen is found in the lymphoid tissues, but this concentration is adequate to induce antibody formation. The response is dependent on several factors, including the physical state of the antigen and ingestion and digestion by macrophages.

Depending on the route by which it gains entrance, antigen becomes trapped or localized in one or another lymph node or tissue for extended periods of time and is responsible for eliciting antibody information. The antigen may be retained or trapped in two distinct manners and sites in the lymph node: by the macrophages or by the dendritic cells in the follicles.

Antigen taken up by macrophages can be handled in several ways, depending on the antigen. For most antigens, the bulk is pinocytosed, subjected to digestion by lysosomal enzymes, degraded, and eliminated without eliciting an immune response. For antigens which are nonmetabolizable, or at best slowly metabolized, the fate can be one of continuing residence in the phagolysosomes of the cell without noticeable degradation, release upon death of the cell, phagocytosis by a new macrophage, and repetition of the process. Polyvinylpyrrolidone and numerous bacterial polysaccharides exhibit such cycles and are eliminated at an extremely slow pace. In the case of metabolizable antigens, a small portion escapes degradation and survives on or near the surface of the macrophage and in this form proves to be immunogenic.

The second mode of antigen retention, capture by the dendritic cells of the lymph node follicles, represents a more specialized form of retention in that it requires the presence of antibody. Evidence indicates that antibody, especially IgG, attaches to the dendritic cell surfaces by means of the Fc fragment and is thus free to bind the antigen by means of its $F(ab)_2$ fragment. Antigen trapping of this type occurs more readily in individuals previously immunized with the antigen. In any event, both forms of antigen retention present undegraded, native antigen at the surface of cells in areas of the body through which the traffic of lymphocytes is heavy, allowing ample opportunity for contact between antigen and lymphocyte.

Interaction of Antigen and Cells Leading to Antibody Formation Depending on the antigen, the interaction of cells with antigen leading to antibody formation can take several pathways. In appropriate concentrations, some antigens can interact directly with AFC. Such antigens typically possess large numbers of a repeating *epitope* on the surface, can stimulate B cells directly, and are poor inducers of delayed hypersensitivity, i.e., fail to stimulate T cells to any extent. Polymerized flagellin, ferritin, polyvinylpyrrolidone, and polysaccharides are examples of thymus-independent antigens, since they can stimulate B cells without the participation of T cells (Fig. 7-6*A*).

Basically, the interaction of B cells with thymus-independent antigens in appropriate concentrations can cause cross-linking of receptor sites on the individual B cell. Presumably, cross-linking of receptor sites through interaction with repeating epitopes of the antigen (or by antiglobulin antibodies) can cause conformational changes in the Fc fragment and can lead to biochemical reactions in the membranes. The reactions in the membrane are transmitted to the interior of the cell (via changes in cAMP?), which then undergoes transformation to blast and plasma cells which produce antibody (Fig. 7-6).

Antigens which present a pattern of repeating epitopes are quite efficient in initiating antibody production following direct contact with B cells. In addition, antigens which tend to aggregate and are thus likely to have repeating epitopes may also function in this way. Concentration is a significant factor, since several antigens which normally aggregate but have—through mechanical manipulation (ultracentrifugation)—been rendered highly disperse, soluble, nonphagocytizable, and relatively insusceptible to capture, not only fail to stimulate the cells under these conditions, but actually deactivate the cells, rendering them tolerant, or unresponsive.

The roles of the macrophage and the dendritic cells become more understandable in view of the concept that the antigen must make contact with a B cell in order to initiate antibody production. The retention of undegraded antigen on the surface of macrophages of the RES (1) places the antigen in the heaviest lymphoid traffic and (2) provides for retention of several molecules of the antigen in close proximity, thus presenting an antigenic matrix with a number of repeating epitopes and facilitating cross-linking of B cell receptors. In like manner, the concentration of antigen molecules on the surfaces of dendritic cells by antibody can present a similar antigenic matrix to the reactive B cell (Fig. 7-7).

A second possible mechanism involving the macrophage was proposed when it was discovered that RNA-rich phenol extracts of macro-

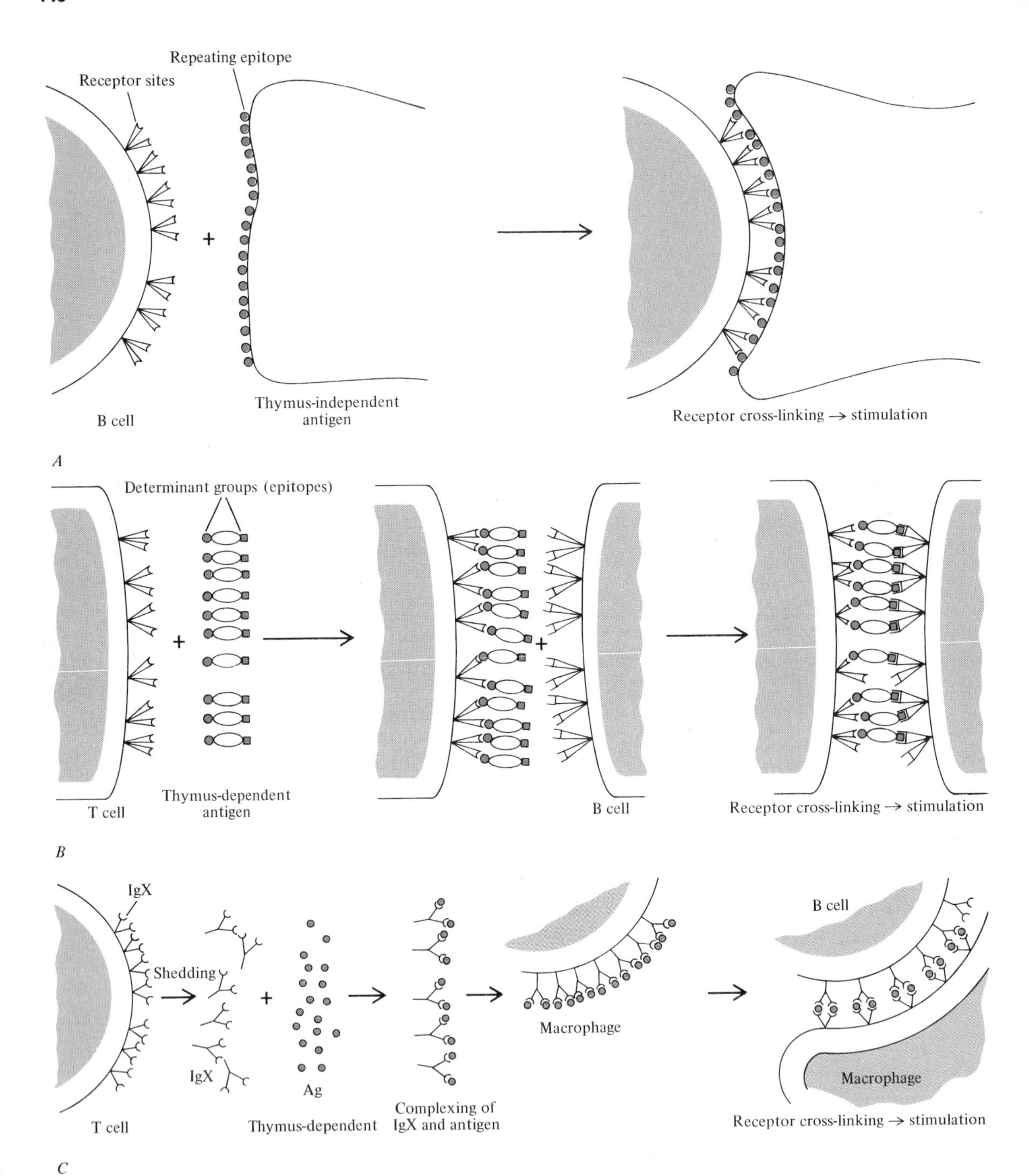

Figure 7-6 Schematic presentation of antigenic stimulation of B lymphocytes. *(A)* Interaction of B cells and thymus-independent antigen. *(B)* Synergistic interaction of T and B cells with thymus-dependent antigen. *(C)* Synergistic interaction of T cells, B cells, and macrophages with a thymus-dependent antigen.

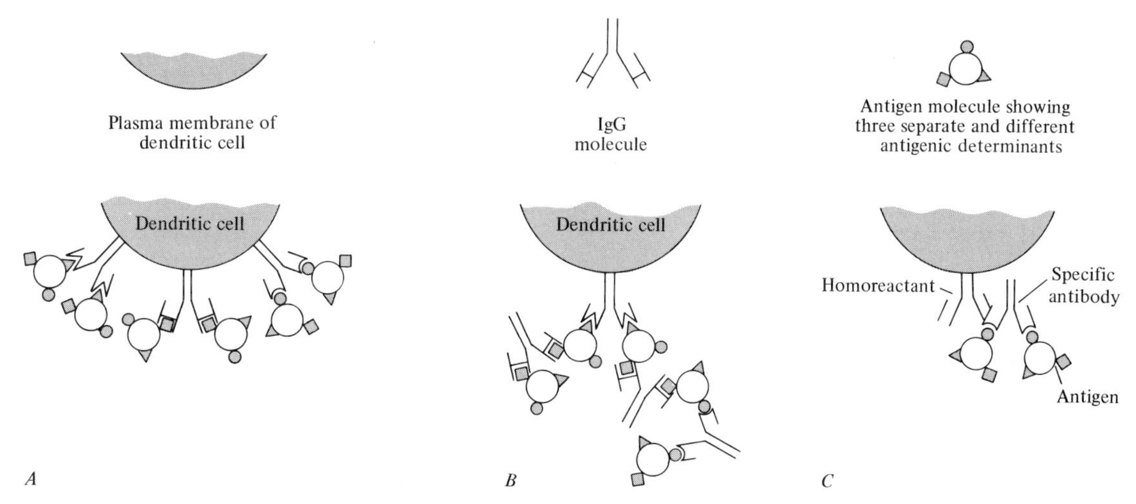

Figure 7-7 Localization of antigen at the surface of dendritic cells. The diagrams demonstrate three ways in which molecules of antigen may be localized at the surface of the follicle dendritic cell. *(A)* A simple mechanism in which the antigen is coupled via one antigenic determinant to the antibody molecule (IgG) which in turn is linked to the cell membrane via the Fc portion of the molecule. If the antigen in question contained n antigenic determinants, $n - 1$ would remain exposed. Different patterns of antigenic determinants would be exposed according to the specificity of each antibody molecule. It also follows that free hapten molecules, if bound in this way, would be "immunologically silent." *(B)* The "build-up" mechanism which would occur if large amounts of antigen and antibody were present. Electron micrographs of germinal centers frequently show a homogeneous, electron-dense material between dendritic cell processes which may represent layers of antigen-antibody complexes. *(C)* An additional mechanism of antigen fixation which invokes the presence of "homoreactant" and allows the trapping of Ig or an Ig-antigen complex via the Fab portion of the molecule in syngeneic situations. These mechanisms may constitute a "fail-safe" approach by the body to ensure follicular localization of antigen. Similar but rather more complex diagrams could be drawn for antibodies of other classes than IgG. *(G. J. V. Nossal and G. L. Ada, Antigens, Lymphoid Cells and the Immune Response, New York, Academic Press, Inc., 1971.)*

phages that had phagocytized antigen were capable of stimulating B cells to initiate production of specific antibody. Further evidence indicated that antigen or antigenic fragments can become firmly complexed with macrophage RNA and that in this form the antigen is much more immunogenic than in the uncomplexed state; i.e., it becomes a *superantigen.* The superantigen complex has been demonstrated to be capable of passing from the macrophage to the lymphocyte and stimulating the lymphocyte to initiate antibody production. Passage of superantigen requires contact between lymphocyte and macrophage, an observation that can be verified microscopically. An intriguing bit of recently reported evidence revealed the presence of a reverse transcriptase in small lymphocytes. In view of the finding of RNA in the superantigen, the transfer of information to the lymphocyte by the RNA can be envisaged with the antigenic fragment acting as a key to the lymphocyte door.

T cells can also interact with antigens in a specific manner by means of their receptors. In a number of instances, it has been demonstrated both in vivo and in vitro that collaboration between T and B cells is essential to produce antibody against the antigen. Antigens requiring collaborative effort on the part of T and B cells are referred to as thymus-dependent antigens and include heterologous erythrocytes, heterologous serum proteins, and a variety of protein-hapten conjugates. Data obtained from experiments with protein-hapten conjugates give some insight into the mechanisms involved. Basically, T cells interact with determinant groups on the carrier protein and tend to concentrate the conjugate on their surfaces. In this way, an antigen matrix is formed, with the hapten portion of the conjugate facing outward. Thus, the T cell presents the B cell with a repeating epitope (hapten) dominating. B cells capable of reacting with the hapten are stimulated to initiate the production of hapten-specific antibody (Fig. 7-6*B*). Evidence has also been obtained that the T cell function can be replaced by something released from the T cell. In this instance, it is believed that the T cell is shedding its surface receptors. As stated earlier, T cell receptors appear to be immunoglobulins but are of an undefined class; hence they are designated IgX. The released IgX molecules complex with carrier molecules of the conjugates and form an aggregate of IgX-conjugates with the hapten portion outward and dominant. The aggregate presents the B cell with a repeating epitope and stimulates the B cell to initiate the synthesis of hapten-specific antibody (Fig. 7-6*B*).

Cellular collaboration involving a three-cell system has been established for several antigens, including sheep erythrocytes. The picture derived from the data suggests that IgX is released by T cells and interacts with the antigen, forming an IgX-antigen matrix which binds to the surface of macrophages. Macrophage-bound matrices then stimulate B cells to initiate the formation of antibody (Fig. 7-6*C*).

After the B cell has been triggered either directly or through collaborative efforts with other cells and antigen, it undergoes a series of changes which culminate in the production of antibody. The B cell first transforms into a blast cell within 24 hr. after stimulation by the antigen. In contrast with the unstimulated blast cell, which has a division time of 38 hr., blast cells that are forming antibody divide every 10 to 12 hr. Shortly thereafter, the blast cells are transformed into immature plasma cells which are the most numerous cell type at the height of the primary antibody response and are responsible for the greatest production of antibody. In contrast with their normal doubling time of 16 hr., immature plasma cells divide every 7 hr. The immature plasma cells develop into mature plasma cells which synthesize antibody during their short half-life of 8 to 12 hr., but do not divide. (See the table on p. 151).

Thus, the active phase of antibody formation may be equated with a rapidly replicating and differentiating population of cells of the blast-plasma cell series. Plasma cells are an invariable accompaniment of antibody formation, and their number is roughly proportional to the extent of the antibody response. Following primary antigenic stimulation the number of plasma cells usually increases for a period of 10 to 20 days and then quickly declines.

In addition to its key role in triggering the antibody-forming mechanism, the antigenically stimulated small lymphocyte develops *immunological memory*, the capacity to give a secondary response on subsequent contact with the same antigen. After an effective primary response immunological memory probably persists for the life of the individual. As will be evident later, immunological memory is a fundamental factor underlying prophylactic immunization and protection against infectious disease on secondary exposure.

Intracellular Events: Plasma Cells and Their Precursors When plasma cells and their precursors are actively synthesizing and secreting

Cellular Events Occurring after Primary Antigenic Stimulation

Stage	Cell type	Antibody content	Function
1	B cell	0	Direct stimulation of B cell by thymus-independent antigens
	B cell + macrophage	0	Antigen captured by macrophage; subsequent stimulation of B cell
	B cell + macrophage	0	Antigen processed by macrophage; B cell stimulated by superantigen
	B cell + T cell	0	Antigen matrix formed at T cell surface; B cell stimulated by antigen matrix
	B cell + T cell + macrophage	0	Antigen matrix formed by IgX and antigen; antigen matrix fixed to macrophage; B cell stimulated by antigen matrix
2	Stimulated small lymphocyte (B cell) ↓	0	Develops potential to form antibody
	Blast cell ↓	+	Divides more rapidly and forms antibody
	Immature plasma cell ↓	+ + +	Divides more rapidly, produces more antibody, and is present in greatest numbers
	Mature plasma cell	+ + + +	Does not divide, has a short half-life, but synthesizes large amounts of antibody
3	Small lymphocytes (T cells and B cells) (memory cells)	0	Develop immunological memory, give secondary response on reexposure to antigen

antibody, they reveal a prominent basophilic cytoplasm, endoplasmic reticulum, and Golgi apparatus. The basophilic cytoplasm is pyroninophilic and thus contains a large amount of RNA. Ultrastructural studies of the developing plasma cell line show an extensive endoplasmic reticulum, the cytoplasmic machinery common to all cells whose primary function is the formation and secretion of protein. The Golgi apparatus, a bean-shaped area overlapping the edge of the nucleus, is also a feature of all glandular cells that secrete proteins. The fluorescent sandwich technique for the detection of antibody has demonstrated that antibody is concentrated in the basophilic areas of the cytoplasm that contain endoplasmic reticulum.

On Secondary Contact When a second injection of the same antigen is given to a sensitized host, the sequence of cellular events is generally similar to that observed after primary immunization. The total production of antibody is much greater on secondary as opposed to primary contact. At the cellular level this finding is presumably based on the fact that there are a greater number of immunologically competent small lymphocytes (possessing immunological memory) as a result of the replication of these cells following primary antigenic stimulation. The second injection of antigen thus triggers a greater number of small lymphocytes to differentiate, replicate, and produce antibody.

The Kinetics of Antibody Formation

The forces set in motion by the injection of antigen into an immunologically competent host are determined by a large number of factors, including the nature and quantity of the antigen, the site at which it is introduced, the duration of the stimulus, the number of times it had been injected, and the interval between injections. In the preceding sections consideration has been given to the fate of the antigen and the kinetics of cellular events that are associated with antibody formation. In this section attention will be focused on the basic features of the primary and secondary responses, their regulation, and the parameters that affect the quality and magnitude of their expression. Special emphasis will be placed on the synthesis of 19S and 7S antibody.

Primary 19S Response: Particulate Antigens Following the immune elimination of antigen, free antibody appears in the serum. It is evident from the results included in Table 7-3 that a graded series of primary antibody responses can be recognized. In the first level of response, a threshold dose of antigen can elicit the formation of a small amount of 19S antibody which is synthesized at a low rate, but 7S antibody and immunological memory fail to develop. In the second level of response, a somewhat greater amount of 19S antibody is produced at a maximal rate, but 7S antibody and immunological memory are not induced. In the third level of response, after a maximal quantity of 19S is synthesized at a maximal rate, 7S antibody and immunological memory develop. The goal in primary prophylactic immunization is to use a quantity of antigen that will induce the formation of 7S antibody and immunological memory on initial injection. With potent antigens the amount required to achieve this result may be as little as 0.01 μg.

After immune elimination of an adequate dose of antigen, synthesis of circulating 19S antibody proceeds exponentially for 4 or 5 days.

Table 7-3 Types of Graded Primary Responses to Particulate Antigens*

Quantity of antigen†	Graded level of antibody response	Formation of 19S antibody	Amount of 19S antibody	Rate of 19S antibody formation	Formation of 7S antibody	Response to reinjection with 10,000 × antigen: Before 10 days, Prim.	Before 10 days, Sec.	After 10 days, Prim.	After 10 days, Sec.
1 ×	None	−	−	−	−	+	−	+	−
10 ×	First	+	+	Low	−	+	−	+	−
100 ×	Second	+	+ +	Maximal	−	+	−	+	−
1,000 ×	Second	+	+ + +	Maximal	−	+	−	+	−
	or								
	third				+	+	−	−	+
10,000 ×	Third	+	+ + + +	Maximal	+	+	−	−	+
100,000 ×	Third	+	+ + + +	Maximal	+	+	−	−	+

* Based largely on studies with phages, animal viruses, flagella, and sheep red blood cells.
† The figures used are intended to indicate relative values only.

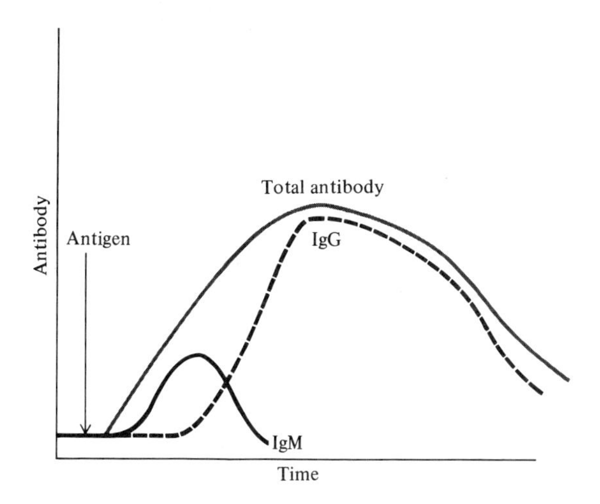

Figure 7-8 Schematic presentation of a primary antibody response to a particulate antigen.

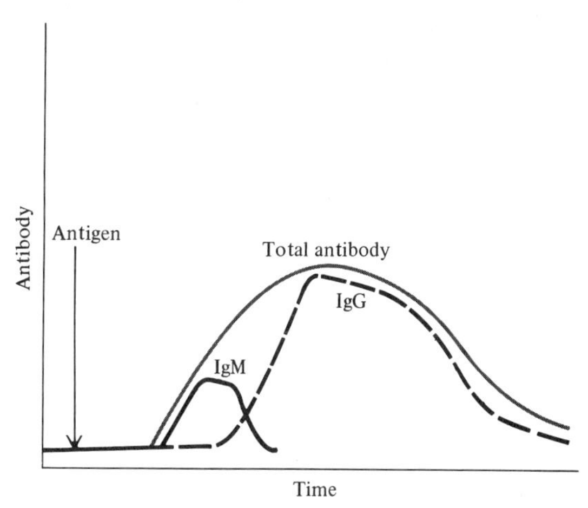

Figure 7-9 Schematic presentation of a primary antibody response to a soluble antigen.

During this interval when the log of the antibody concentration is plotted against time, a straight line is obtained. The length of time needed to double the concentration of antibody may be as little as 6 hr. Thereafter, the rate of 19S antibody synthesis slows, continues for another 5 days, and then ceases. At this time (10 days after appearance of antibody), 19S antibody has a half-life comparable to that of passively administered 19S antibody (Fig. 7-8).

Primary 19S Response: Soluble Antigens The early 19S antibody response to soluble protein antigens is generally similar to that found with particulate antigens. There is, however, usually a delay of 7 days or more after injection of antigen before serum antibody can be measured, and the relative amount of 19S antibody detected is much less than that induced by particulate antigens (Fig. 7-9). For example, the 19S response elicited by a soluble protein antigen is only about 5 percent of the magnitude of that obtained when the same amount of the antigen is absorbed onto acrylic particles prior to injection.

The Latent Period in the Primary 19S Response The time between the injection of antigen and the presence of free antibody in the serum is known as the latent period. The physical state of the antigen, its chemical nature, and the quantity injected can influence the duration of the latent period. With some particulate antigens, including ϕX phage and poliovirus, 19S antibody has been detected in 16 hr. With sheep red blood cells, on the other hand, the latent period is usually longer than 5 days. The quantity of antigen injected alters the length of the latent period but in a different manner, depending upon the antigen. For example, with ϕX phage the latent period is shortened as the quantity of antigen is lowered, whereas with sheep red blood cells the latent period is decreased as the dose of antigen is increased. With soluble protein antigens the latent period is usually 1 to 2 weeks.

The observed differences in the duration of the latent period with the same or with different antigens should be interpreted cautiously because they may be artifacts. The delay noted with some antigens may be caused by the relative insensitivity of antibody assays. A concentration of 10^{10} molecules per milliliter is required to detect circulating antibody in the most sensitive assays, and precipitation of soluble protein antigens by antibody is known to be the least sensitive assay method. Thus, it is possible that antibody formation may commence at similar times even though a detectable level of antibody occurs at different times after injection of antigen. Accordingly, the latent period in the primary 19S antibody response represents the time required for the antigen to be processed by the macrophage and to come into effective contact with a potentially responsive small lymphocyte. As soon as this is accomplished, antibody synthesis is initiated. With many antigens this time may be measured in minutes and hours rather than days or weeks.

Primary 7S Antibody Response: Particulate Antigens As noted in Table 7-3, if the quantity of antigen injected is adequate, 7S antibody will be found in the serum. There is general agreement concerning the sequential appearance of 19S and 7S antibody, although the longer latent period for 7S may be partly associated with the lesser sensitivity of assay methods for 7S as opposed to 19S.

With various particulate antigens, 7S antibody has been detected as early as the first day or as late as 2 weeks after injection. Whenever it appears, initial synthesis of 7S antibody is exponential for about 4 days with a doubling time as short as 8.5 hr. Thereafter, 7S antibody synthesis continues at a slow rate, presumably for the life of the individual, provided that the initial antigenic stimulus was adequate. This is in striking contrast to the synthesis of 19S antibody, which is usually limited to about 10 days (Fig. 7-8). As with 19S, 7S antibody synthesis may begin within hours but may not be detected for several days.

Primary 7S Antibody Response: Soluble Antigens The sequential appearance and synthesis of 7S antibody after injection with soluble protein antigens is generally similar to that observed with particulate antigens except for the greater delay in detection of 7S antibody (Fig. 7-9). In contrast to the formation of 19S antibody to soluble protein antigens, the time of onset and the magnitude of the 7S antibody response appear to be independent of the physical state of the antigen.

Secondary (Anamnestic) Antibody Response In comparison with a primary antibody response, a secondary antibody response usually can be induced by a smaller dose of antigen in a shorter period of time, producing peak titers that are higher and that persist longer. The increased production of antibody is a 7S response. The amount of 19S antibody that is synthesized in the secondary response is usually equivalent to that in a primary response. It is often difficult to demonstrate 19S antibody because of the presence of preexisting antibody, because of the inhibiting effect of antibody on the secondary response, and because of the large excess of newly synthesized 7S antibody, usually ten times the level produced in the primary response, and sometimes higher. However, under appropriate conditions it can be shown that synthesis of 19S precedes the synthesis of 7S in the secondary response.

Although its detection may be delayed for a few days, depending on the concentration of preexisting antibody, the kinetics of the secondary response indicate that exponential synthesis of 7S antibody is initiated almost immediately after challenge and continues for 5 days with a doubling time as short as 6.5 hr. The rate of synthesis falls and continues at the depressed level for 10 days or longer. During this interval the decline in synthesis of 7S antibody is more rapid than in the primary response. Thereafter, production of 7S antibody continues for the life of the individual at a lower rate (Fig. 7-10).

While the features of the secondary response apply to most particulate antigens and most soluble protein antigens, sheep red blood cells are an exception to the rule that the peak titers

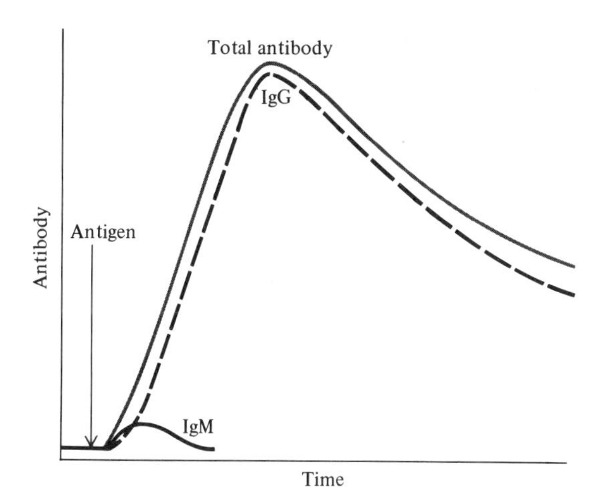

Figure 7-10 Schematic presentation of a secondary (anamnestic) response to soluble antigen.

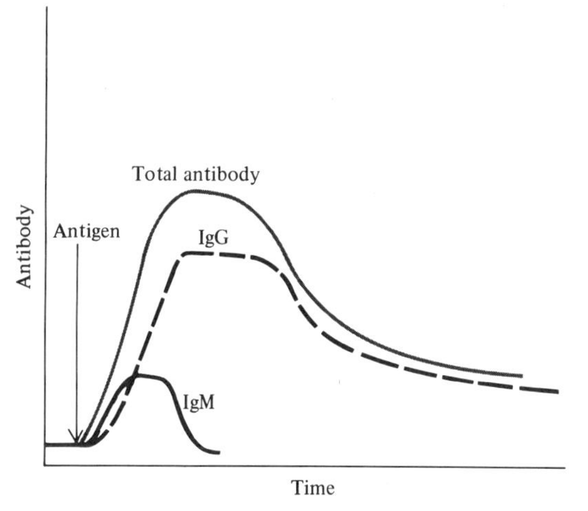

Figure 7-11 Schematic presentation of a secondary (anamnestic) response to a particulate antigen.

are ten times (or more) higher in the secondary as compared with the primary response. Little difference in peak titers is found in the primary and secondary responses to sheep red blood cells. In other respects, however, the reinjection of sheep erythrocytes induces a typical secondary response (Fig. 7-11).

The Response to Polysaccharide Antigens The kinetics of the antibody response to polysaccharide antigens is quite different from that observed with particulate and soluble protein antigens. Generally, there is an exaggerated primary response and a failure to demonstrate a typical secondary response on reinjection of the polysaccharide. The O somatic lipopolysaccharide antigens of *Salmonella* induce a predominantly 19S antibody response which persists for a year or more with only trace amounts of 7S, and a secondary response is difficult to produce. A single injection of 50 μg of pneumococcal polysaccharide in man stimulates the production of a high concentration of antibody that is maintained at relatively high levels for 3 to 6 years. Reinjection after 8 years fails to elicit a typical secondary response. Following immunization of man with dextran similar results are generally found. In the case of dextran, 7S is the predominant antibody that is formed.

The explanation of the unusual features of the immune responses stimulated by polysaccharide antigens is not known. As will be documented later, however, in the case of particulate and soluble protein antigens, synthesis of 19S antibody continues as long as the antigen persists. Thus, it is reasonable to assume that the long duration of the primary 19S response with polysaccharides is related to their slow metabolism. As pointed out earlier, bacterial polysaccharides may persist for several months inside macrophages.

Immunological Memory The capacity to give a secondary response following specific antigenic challenge is known as immunological memory. Characteristically, memory is associated with the synthesis of 7S antibody. It is evident from the results included in Table 7-3 that antibody formation is not invariably accompanied by the development of immunological memory. If the primary response is limited to the synthesis of 19S antibody, memory cannot be demonstrated. On the other hand, if 7S antibody is formed on primary antigenic stimulation, immunological memory develops.

The duration of immunological memory is a function of the dose of antigen employed for primary stimulation and the interval between the primary and the secondary injections of the antigen. At low doses of antigen, immunological memory increases for about 3 months, begins to decline after about 6 months, and is dependent on the dose used for secondary challenge. At higher doses of antigen, memory usually persists for the life of the individual and is mostly independent of the amount of antigen reinjected.

The precise time when immunological memory develops is known to vary with the quantity and the physical state of the antigen. Perhaps the ability to demonstrate memory can be equated with the complete cessation of 19S antibody synthesis which can occur as early as 10 days after injection of the antigen. Thereafter, the ability to give a more effective secondary response (increased immunological memory) increases with the interval between injections. The simplest explanation for this observation is the continued replication of immunologically competent small lymphocytes. The fact that memory is carried by small lymphocytes has been amply documented. For example, if small lymphocytes are obtained from an animal 15 months after a primary injection with antigen and are transferred to an irradiated recipient, the recipient will give a secondary antibody response when challenged with antigen.

Qualitative Changes in Antibody: Avidity Antibody obtained from different individuals or from the same individual at different times after primary, secondary, or repeated injection of antigen may differ as much as 10,000-fold in its capacity to bind antigen. The *avidity* of an antibody is defined as the dilutional stability of an antigen-antibody complex and can be measured by diluting the complex and observing the extent of dissociation of the antigen from the complex. A large number of investigations have established that qualitative changes in antibody avidity are associated with various phases of the immune response and the physical state of the antigen. Some of the findings on these changes are itemized below.

1 19S antibody is more efficient than 7S antibody in binding to particulate antigens.
2 Early 19S antibody has a low avidity, but this increases as the antibody titer rises between the fourth and tenth days and then declines.
3 Primary 7S antibody increases in avidity between the second and the fourth weeks.
4 Secondary 7S antibody avidity rises more rapidly, subsequently shows only a slight decrease, and is much greater than the avidity of primary 19S or 7S antibody.

One possible explanation for the increased avidity of antibody during the course of immunization is that antigen acts as a selective agent for the preferential stimulation of cells that form antibody of high avidity. This possibility is consistent with the fact that antigen can stimulate the mitosis of immunologically competent small lymphocytes.

From another point of view it is important to recall that most antigens have a variety of determinant groups unequally distributed on their surfaces. The early antibodies are probably directed against the predominant determinant group. As immunization continues, an increasing number of the different determinant groups elicit the formation of antibody specific for the particular determinant group. With time and additional injections of antigen there exists a population of antibody molecules containing specific antibodies for each of the determinant groups. According to this line of reasoning, avidity is a property of a population of antibody molecules. If specific antibodies are complexed with a number of different determinant groups on the surface of the antigen molecules, the chances are that a more avid complex of antigen-antibody molecules will be formed.

In reality, then, avidity can be thought of as

the closeness of the "fit" of an individual antibody molecule with a specific determinant group and as a property of a population of antibody molecules reacting with different determinant groups to form a more stable complex.

Regulation of Antibody Formation

Effect of Antigen Earlier considerations have indicated that the quantity of antigen can regulate the relative rate of 19S antibody formation, can determine whether or not a primary 7S response and immunological memory will occur, and can affect the duration of immunological memory. In addition, several lines of evidence, including those listed below, reveal that 19S antibody synthesis is dependent on the persistence of antigen.

1 The slower the metabolism of antigen, the longer the synthesis of 19S antibody continues.
2 The depletion of antigen could account for the short duration and abrupt cessation of 19S antibody formation.
3 Formation of 19S antibody can be prolonged if another injection of antigen is given prior to the expected cessation of 19S antibody synthesis.
4 The administration of specific antibody can prevent or reduce 19S antibody synthesis.

Thus, it appears that antigen must persist for the continued synthesis of 19S antibody and that removal of antigen can terminate 19S formation.

With respect to the role of antigen in the long-term production of 7S antibody the data are much less convincing. Consequently, a number of explanations have been proposed to account for the prolonged synthesis of 7S antibody. These include the following possibilities:

1 Continued synthesis of 7S antibody is dependent upon the persistence of an amount of antigen (one molecule per antibody-forming cell) that cannot be detected by the most sensitive methods available.
2 Initial contact with antigen may lead to a permanent derepression of the cell that is manifested by the formation of 7S antibody.
3 Messenger RNA from macrophages which have come in contact with the antigen may be transferred to small lymphocytes and can stimulate them to synthesize 7S antibody.

Although the latter two explanations are attractive theories, experimental confirmation of their validity is lacking. On balance, the data support the conclusion that antigen is of major importance in maintaining and stabilizing the formation of 7S antibody for a period of at least 40 days after injection. Since the findings are based on the role of antibody as a feedback inhibitor of its own synthesis, it will be helpful to enlarge the discussion to consider the broader aspects of the regulatory role of antibody.

Effect of Antibody Under appropriate conditions passively administered antibody inhibits the formation of 19S and 7S antibody as well as the development of 7S immunological memory. There are, however, marked differences in inhibiting capacity of various populations of antibody molecules. For example, primary 7S antibody is more efficient than 19S antibody in suppressing antibody synthesis, secondary 7S is more efficient than primary 7S, and antibody becomes increasingly efficient with increasing number of injections of the antigen.

Only when specific 19S antibody is passively transferred at the same time as the antigen can the primary 19S response be blocked. If secondary 7S antibody is given 3 days after the antigen, at a time when 19S antibody is being synthesized at a maximal rate, there is partial suppression of the primary 19S response, and the primary 7S response and 7S immunological memory fail to develop. The experimental data demonstrate that the events that determine 7S antibody formation and 7S immunological memory are not completed within 3 days and that these events are dependent on antigen.

More recently, precise studies at the cellular

level using the direct and indirect hemolytic plaque tests have clarified the role of antibody in suppressing 7S antibody synthesis and the role of antigen in maintaining 7S antibody synthesis. The inhibiting effect of passively transferred antibody is not apparent for 48 to 72 hr. This indicates that antibody does not suppress synthesis in already committed cells, but that it operates by removing from the system the stimulus (antigen) for the maintenance of antibody synthesis. The sensitivity of the 7S antibody-forming system to feedback inhibition by antibody decreases with time after injection of the antigen. However, the fact that inhibition can still be found when the transfer of antibody is delayed for 40 days after injection of the antigen suggests that during this period antigen is a major factor in the continuing synthesis of 7S antibody.

Thus, feedback inhibition by antibody operates at various stages in the synthesis of 19S and 7S antibody, represents an important mechanism for the regulation of antibody formation, and is mediated through interaction with antigen. This latter conclusion is warranted because of the specificity of the inhibition and because passively transferred antibody and a reduced quantity of antigen influence the kinetics of antibody formation in a comparable way. Feedback inhibition as discussed above and the induction of tolerance (Chap. 11) are two regulatory mechanisms in suppression of antibody production that have been closely studied. Several other regulatory mechanisms inherent in the immune system and its components have been proposed, and some evidence has been obtained for them.

Effect of T Cells T cells may have a regulatory effect on antibody production by B cells. Results of studies in which depletion or elimination of T cell populations was accomplished by neonatal thymectomy, x-irradiation, or the application of antilymphocyte antiserum specifically directed toward theta antigen-bearing cells showed enhanced primary antibody responses to such antigens as protein-hapten conjugates, pneumococcal polysaccharides, keyhole limpet hemocyanin, and polyvinylpyrrolidone. The enhanced antibody response to these antigens by T cell deprivation was related predominantly to the increased production of IgM antibodies. Restoration of T cell populations in the deprived animals resulted in decreased ability to produce antibody against the antigens.

Another aspect of the suppressive activities of T cells is associated with antigenic competition. When animals are immunized with two antigens simultaneously or in close sequence, antibody formation to one or both antigens is depressed (*antigenic competition*). In studies employing protein-hapten conjugates or two different heterologous red blood cells, it was found that antigenic competition was a T cell-dependent phenomenon, that it did not occur in thymus-deprived animals, and that restoration of T cell populations restored the competition phenomenon. The magnitude of the competition observed was directly related to the size of the T cell population present and occurred irrespective of specific circulating antibodies. The interpretations of these competition studies plus those involving enhanced antibody response to certain antigens in the absence of T cells suggest strongly that the T cells release soluble factors which have an inhibitory or suppressive effect on the B cells.

A characteristic feature of thymus-dependent antigens is that the response is predominantly, if not solely, a production of IgM. Under appropriate conditions in thymus-deprived animals, even thymus-dependent antigens can elicit IgM responses, indicating that IgM production is less thymus-dependent than IgG production. This has been demonstrated using hapten-protein conjugates and heterologous erythrocytes as antigens. The data strongly suggest that one of the regulatory influences of the T cell may be the shift of antibody production from IgM to IgG.

The phenomenon can be extrapolated to mean that, in the absence of T cells, the physicochemical properties of the antigen may determine whether a particular subset of B cells can be stimulated or not. The phenomenon can also be related to a regulation of the selective pressure placed on the B cell population and consequently the increase in specific affinity of antibodies produced in the response. As the production shifts to IgG, the avidity of the antibody population shifts to a higher level. This in turn leads to a more efficient removal of antigen from the system. As the level of antigen present is reduced, the competition for antigen between circulating antibody and the receptors on the surfaces of the lymphocytes increases. This type of competition statistically favors the cells with receptors of higher affinity, which in turn produce antibody of higher affinity. As this competition increases, therefore, the avidity of the antibody population increases rapidly.

It has also been suggested that the T cell is involved not only as an antigen-focusing cell (antigen matrix). For example, antigen-coated particles, carrier-tolerant T cells, or antigen-coated B cells used as focusing surfaces failed to cooperate with B cells in thymus-deprived animals. This is interpreted to mean that antigen focusing alone is insufficient and that specifically activated T cells are essential for antibody responses to thymus-dependent antigens. In conjunction with the power to switch antibody production from IgM to IgG, this concept suggests a more profound function for the T cell population.

A number of experiments indicate that the T cell population can release soluble factors which enhance antibody response. These factors are considered to be distinct from the proposed IgX. The studies involved T cells not specifically directed toward the antigen under investigation. T cells are stimulated in vivo by introducing them into a test animal of a different strain and causing them to mount a graft versus host reaction (Chap. 10) or in vitro by exposing the cells to small amounts of antilymphocyte serum or to plant-derived mutagens (phytohemagglutinin, concanavalin A, pokeweed mitogen). The presence of the stimulated T cells or the supernatants of in vitro incubations of the stimulated cells enhanced several aspects of antibody formation against an antigen to which the T cells had not been sensitized and was presumably mediated by soluble products released by the T cells.

In primed animals the T cells or their released products caused a spontaneous rise in specific antibody titers in the absence of further antigenic challenge. If the antigen was a protein-hapten conjugate, an enhanced secondary response to the hapten could be elicited in the presence of these T cells by a cross-reacting protein-hapten conjugate (same hapten, different carrier), indicating that the proposed soluble factors can abrogate the requirement for carrier specific T cells and can enhance B cell memory directed toward the hapten. The soluble factors presumably are nonspecific, have a short half-life, and act rapidly. While the studies cited above are at best artificial situations, specific antigenic stimulation of both the T and B cells in the normal immune response allows release of those factors in close proximity to the B cells, thereby enhancing their reaction to the antigen in both primary and secondary responses.

Thus, the T cell can and may play a central role in the regulation of some, if not all, antibody production. The picture is paradoxical in that the T cells apparently have both suppressive and enhancing influences. The exact situation in which either of these influences is brought to bear is unknown. Factors such as the physicochemical state of the antigen, the amount of antigen, the amount of specific antibody present, and the number of cells involved may all be directive in these instances. Additionally, one must consider the possibility that there are subsets of the T cell population with either enhancing or suppressing powers but not both, and the dominant influence would then depend on which subset of cells was stimulated by the existing conditions.

Route of Inoculation

The influence of the route of inoculation of the antigen on antibody production depends on a delicate balance between the speed and efficiency with which the antigen is taken up by macrophages and the rate at which it is excreted. The uptake and excretion in turn are primarily functions of the physical state of the antigen. The situation can be best illustrated when a protein antigen is inoculated by various routes in the soluble and in the particulate (alum-precipitated) form.

When a soluble antigen is injected intravenously or intraperitoneally, it is relatively inefficient because most of the antigen is excreted in the urine in a few hours. An equivalent concentration of the antigen is more effective when given by the intramuscular, subcutaneous, or intradermal routes because the antigen is released slowly from the site of inoculation, thus providing a greater opportunity for contact with the macrophages. However, when the antigen is converted to the particulate form by precipitation with alum, it is more effective by the intravenous and intraperitoneal routes than by the intramuscular, subcutaneous, or intradermal routes. The explanation is related to the fact that a particulate antigen is more rapidly and efficiently taken up by macrophages than is a soluble antigen and that with particulate antigens uptake is more rapid after intravenous and intraperitoneal injection than following introduction by other routes.

Characteristically, then, the intravenous route of inoculation is best adapted to particulate antigens. The antibody response develops rapidly and the peak titer attained is high, but the rate of decline is fast. Soluble antigens, on the other hand, are best suited to inoculation by the intramuscular, subcutaneous, or intradermal route. The antibody response is delayed and the peak titer attained is low, but the rate of decline is more gradual.

Adjuvants and the Enhancement of Antibody Production

In human immunization many antigens are inoculated by the subcutaneous or intramuscular rather than by the intravenous route primarily because the risk of fatal anaphylactic reactions is reduced. The low efficiency associated with subcutaneous or intramuscular injection of antigen has led to a search for methods that will enhance the production of antibody. The result has been the discovery of a variety of materials which function as *adjuvants,* substances which when mixed with antigens greatly enhance the intensity and duration of the antibody response (Fig. 7-12).

Not only can adjuvants enhance antibody production, but they can convert an apparently nonantigenic substance to an effective antigen. Unfortunately, however, adjuvants may lead to the production of certain autoimmune diseases (Chap. 11), to increased hypersensitivity of the delayed type (Chap. 8), and to severe local reactions.

Enhancement of antibody production by an adjuvant apparently stems primarily from the slow release of the antigen from the site of inoculation. The following events are associated, in turn, with the slow release of antigen.

1. Delay in absorption of the antigen by macrophages
2. Delay in metabolism and processing of the antigen by macrophages
3. Delay in stimulation of small lymphocytes and in the initiation of antibody production
4. Delay in immune elimination of the antigen

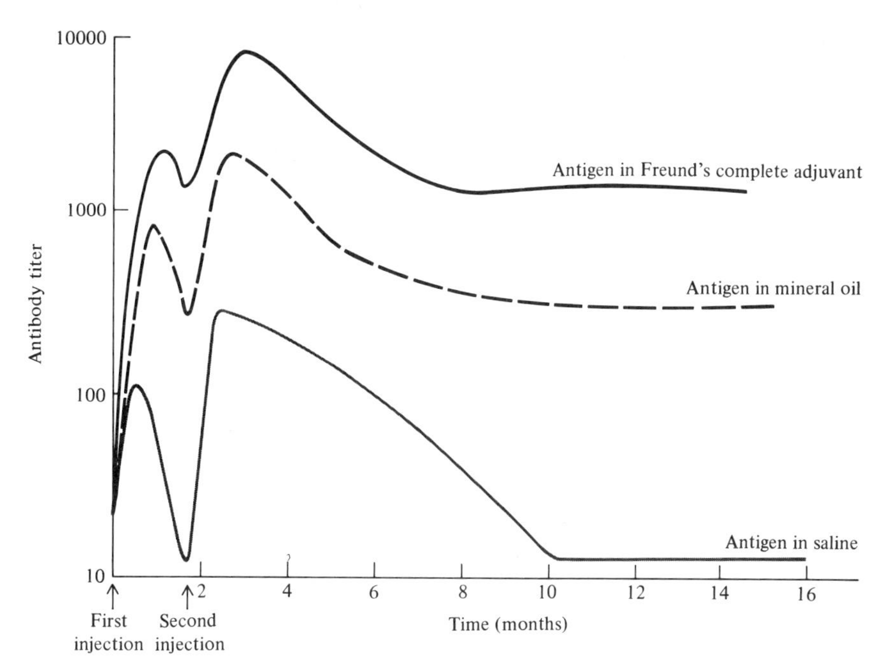

Figure 7-12 The effect of adjuvants on antibody responses to an antigen (killed *Salmonella typhi*).

5 Prolonged antigenic stimulation of small lymphocytes within the regional lymph nodes
6 A progressive influx of inflammatory cells into the site of inoculation, leading to the production of a local granuloma which contains plasma cells and their precursors from the second to the seventh weeks, local formation of antibody, and further delay in the release of antigen from the area
7 The appearance of impressive medullary collections of plasma cells in the regional nodes and occasionally in remote nodes and in the spleen

The net result of the adjuvant is to greatly increase the intensity and duration of the antibody response, to induce immunological memory which is essentially maximal in extent, and perhaps to permit the development of a secondary response. Antibody production within the granuloma is a minor factor in the action of the adjuvant, since excision of the granuloma 2 weeks after injection of the antigen has no demonstrable effect. Earlier excision of the inoculation site (1 week after injection) causes only a slight diminution in the enhancing effect of the adjuvant.

Although a large number of materials are known to function as adjuvants, those employed in human immunization are limited for the most part to aluminum salts, bacterial endotoxins, and water-in-oil emulsions (incomplete Freund's adjuvant). Prevention of diphtheria and tetanus is based on universal immunization of infants and young children with either alum-precipitated toxoids or with toxoids absorbed on aluminum phosphate gel. Usually the toxoids are combined with *Bordetella pertussis* vaccine which also exerts an adjuvant effect. The active ingredient in the pertussis vaccine is the lipopolysaccharide endotoxin. Similar enhancement of antibody production can be achieved with purified lipopolysaccharides obtained from several other gram-negative bacteria including species of *Salmonella* and *Brucella.* The mechanism of the adjuvant effect of bacterial endotoxin is not known, but it has been suggested that cells damaged by endotoxin release DNA precursors which may accelerate the replication of cells that are producing antibody.

Two types of water-in-oil emulsions exert a comparable adjuvant effect in man. In the Freund type of adjuvant, mineral oil is converted to a water-in-oil emulsion by an emulsifying agent such as Arlacel A (mannide monooleate). More recently, preparations containing peanut oil emulsified by Arlacel A and stabilized by aluminum monostearate have been utilized. The chief advantage of the latter emulsion is that all components of the adjuvant are metabolized over a period of a few months, whereas mineral oil is more slowly metabolized and may even contain some components that are nonmetabolizable. Antigen dissolves in the watery phase of the emulsion and is released slowly from the site of inoculation. The oil apparently facilitates the dispersal of antigen to antibody-forming tissues beyond the regional lymph node.

Despite the fact that far greater efficacy in the extent and duration of the immune response can be achieved with aqueous vaccine-in-oil adjuvants than with alum, none of the emulsion adjuvants have been licensed by regulatory agencies in the United States. Experimentally, however, the water-in-oil adjuvants have been used extensively, especially in connection with influenza virus vaccine and with repository or emulsion therapy for allergies. By contrast, influenza vaccine contained in water-in-oil emulsion has been licensed for use in man in Great Britain.

Water-in-oil emulsions with added mycobacteria (complete Freund's adjuvant) provide a greater enhancement of the antibody response than can be obtained without the mycobacteria. The tissue reaction is much more extensive and resembles a tuberculous granuloma. The regional lymph nodes may be occupied by granuloma tissue, and there are extensive medullary collections of plasma cells in the remote lymph nodes and in the spleen. The extent of the tissue necrosis has precluded the use of this type of adjuvant. The adjuvant effect can be reproduced when peptido-glycolipids associated with the wax D fraction of human strains of *Mycobacterium tuberculosis* are added to a water-in-oil emulsion.

In addition to the classical depot-type adjuvants, recent studies have revealed immunoenhancing activities associated with a variety of substances which provide further insight into the possible mechanisms of the classical adjuvants.

Polyanionic substances such as polyacrylic acids and dextran sulfate have demonstrated the ability to restore IgM and IgG responses to thymus-dependent antigens, such as sheep red blood cells, in adult, thymectomized, irradiated, bone-marrow reconstituted animals. Since T cell activity is absent in these animals, the results indicate that these *charged* compounds can replace T cell activity in these antibody responses.

In experiments using aged animals or thymectomized animals in which T cell activity is low or absent and animals which were low responders to various antigens, synthetic double-stranded polynucleotides were able to restore normal antibody responses. In normal animals, the compounds are able to enhance antibody responses. The mechanism by which the polynucleotides may operate is through the adenyl cyclase–cAMP (cyclic adenosine monophosphate) system. The compounds stimulate the formation of cAMP in lymphocytes, and elevated levels of cAMP have demonstrated the ability to enhance immune responses to a number of antigens.

More recently, classical adjuvants have been shown to require the presence of T cells in order to exhibit an immunoenhancing effect. Thus, thymus-deficient animals fail to respond to the effects of LPS endotoxin from *E. coli* or from *B. pertussis* unless the T cell populations are restored. Adjuvants like LPS may work by stimulating the production of immunoenhancing, soluble substances produced by T cells as discussed previously, which in turn stimulate the B cells to a more vigorous response.

Host Factors in Antibody Production

In the preceding discussion of factors influencing antibody production it was assumed that antigen was injected into an immunologically competent host. An extensive, expansive, controversial, and contradictory literature provides ample testimony to the fact that the response to antigenic stimulation varies with the species, age, genetic constitution, and environmental background of the host and to the fact that the response can be modified by numerous physical, chemical, and operative procedures.

Obviously, a comprehensive analysis of the problem is beyond the scope of this text. Fundamentally, however, host-induced influences on antibody production operate directly or indirectly through an effect on macrophages, small lymphocytes, or derivatives of the latter cells.

In the ensuing section an effort will be made, through the use of selected examples, to illustrate the basic principles involved. Whenever possible, emphasis will be placed on variations in man's response to antigenic stimulation.

Species Antibody production is limited to vertebrate animals. As the phylogenetic scale goes up among the most primitive vertebrates, the cyclostomes, there is a rising level of immunologic reactivity and an increasingly differentiated and complex immunologic mechanism. Hagfish, which have no macrophages or plasma cells, are devoid of immunoglobulins, cannot remove or metabolize antigens, and cannot form antibody. Sea lampreys clear circulating antigen slowly, show a single, faint immunoglobulin band on immunoelectrophoresis, and produce an equivocal antibody response. Elasmobranchs require 30 days to clear antigen from the circulation on primary injection, but only 7 days on reinjection of antigen. The primary antibody response is feeble, but the secondary response is vigorous. However, precipitating antibody cannot be demonstrated even in the secondary response. On the other hand, multiple immunoglobulin bands appear on immunoelectrophoresis. In teleosts, precipitin formation provides evidence for the gradual evolutionary emergence of an immunologic response characteristic of higher vertebrates.

In higher vertebrates there are numerous examples in which a given antigen stimulates the formation of antibody in one species but not in another, or in some members of the species but not in others. In most carefully studied cases the ability to form antibody to a particular antigen is controlled by a simple dominant Mendelian factor. Precisely how the genetic control operates is uncertain, but inability to produce antibody may be due to failure of macrophages to metabolize the antigen or failure of small lymphocytes to recognize the antigen. The balance of evidence favors the latter possibility.

It is probable in certain instances, however, that failure of a species to respond may be due to the close chemical relationship of the antigen with the antigens in the tissues of the host. Every animal is tolerant to the multitude of antigens and determinant groups contained in its own tissues. Consequently, it is not surprising that some naturally or artificially synthesized antigens may cross-react on the basis of chemical similarity with the host's own antigens. Since the host is tolerant to its own antigens, it should not produce an antibody response when challenged with an identical antigen present in other materials.

Cross-reacting, or heterophil, antigens often occur in widely separated phylogenetic groups. When the cross-reacting antigen is responsible for the development of sheep hemolysins (antibodies that hemolyze sheep red blood cells in the presence of complement), it is known as a *heterophil Forssman* antigen. Among the antigens capable of inducing sheep hemolysins after immunization of rabbits are such apparently diverse antigens as gram-negative and gram-positive bacteria, yeast, and the tissues of fish, bird, and mammals. Other heterophil systems include antigens shared by human group O red blood cells and gram-negative bacteria; by human group A red blood cells, the paratyphoid bacillus, and type XIV pneumococcus; by group A streptococcal antigens and human and rabbit cardiac and skeletal muscle; by group A type 12 streptococci and human glomerular membrane; and by enveloped viruses and host cell membranes.

Age Most human neonates are born with a plasma concentration of IgG equivalent to that in the mother but are devoid of IgM, IgA, IgD, and IgE. This situation arises because IgG readily traverses the placenta while IgM, IgA, IgD, and IgE do not and because the neonate synthesizes little immunoglobulin. In accord with these observations, neonatal lymph nodes have poorly developed lymphoid nodules, and germinal centers and medullary foci of plasma cells are absent. A similar picture is obtained with animals maintained under germ-free conditions on an antigen-free diet. Such animals are devoid of antibody, plasma cells, and germinal centers.

Synthesis of IgG usually begins when the infant is 1 to 3 months of age and then rapidly increases until the plasma levels reach adult values between 1 and 2 years of age. Meanwhile, the placentally transferred IgG falls off with a half-life of about 15 days and is gradually replaced by active synthesis of IgG by the infant. Between the fifth and twelfth weeks, net synthesis by the infant equals the amount of maternal IgG being metabolized, and the plasma level of IgG reaches its lowest level (300 to 600 mg/100 ml). Thereafter, the infant synthesizes increasing amounts of IgG, and the plasma concentration rises steadily until adult levels are attained (Fig. 7-13).

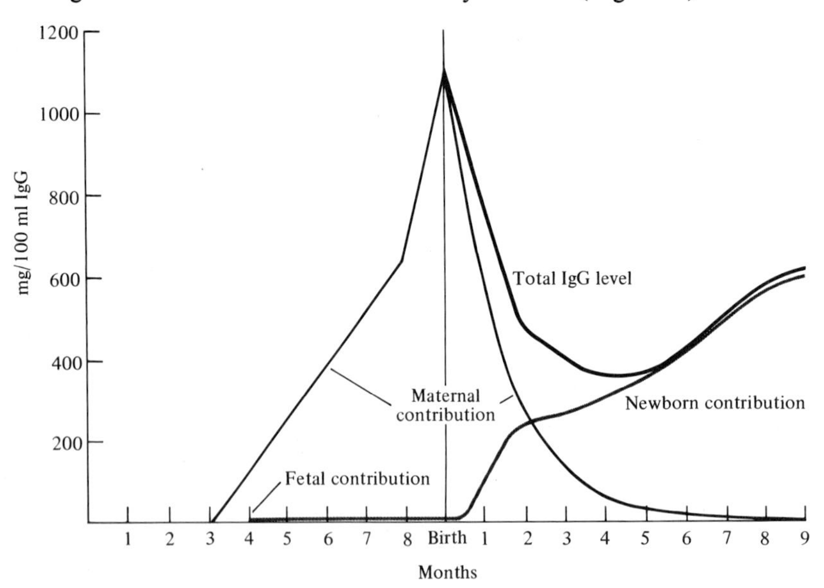

Figure 7-13 Schematic presentation of probable development of IgG levels in the fetus and newborn. (*M. R. Allansmith, B. H. McClellan, and M. Butterworth, J. Pediatr., 75:1231–1244, 1969.*)

More clear-cut but wholly compatible results are obtained from studies of infants born to mothers with agammaglobulinemia (hypogammaglobulinemia). These neonates are virtually devoid of antibody. Synthesis of immunoglobulin is evident at about the fourth week and increases steadily until adult levels are attained around the end of the first or second year (Fig. 7-14). In these infants, it is apparent that the formation of IgM, and probably also IgA, precedes the appearance of IgG.

The ontogenesis of human immunological response, however, develops much earlier than might be surmised from the preceding considerations. Small lymphocytes appear after about 8 or 10 weeks of gestation. Their function may involve the acquisition of tolerance to the antigens in the fetus. Apparently these small lymphocytes are potentially immunologically competent; at least, the transfer of fetal lymphocytes to irradiated adult recipients can restore antibody-forming capacity.

As with primitive species, with the human neonate, and with the response of an immunologically competent host, IgM is the first antibody produced. In the presence of infection synthesis of IgM can begin about the third month of gestation and can continue throughout embryonic life. Why tolerance of the fetus and the infant to rubella virus fails to develop, even when the mother is infected prior to conception, is especially puzzling. The continued synthesis of IgM, however, can be accounted for by the persistence of the antigen.

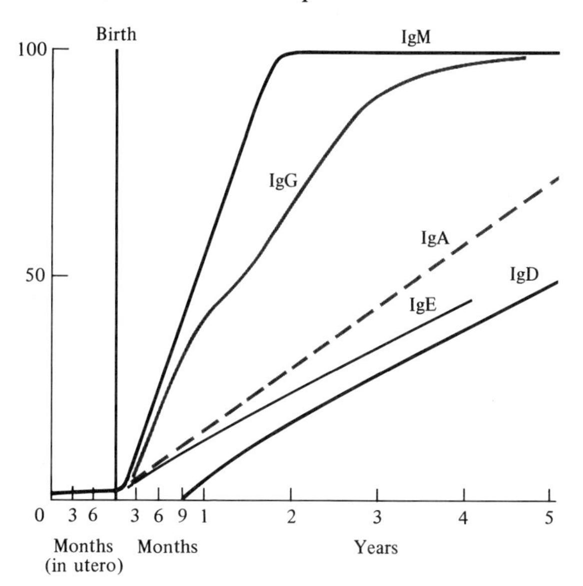

Figure 7-14 Synthesis of immunoglobulins in infants born of agammaglobulinemic mothers.

In the absence of in utero infection, synthesis of IgM begins immediately after birth when the infant is exposed to the antigens in the environment. The level of IgM in the plasma increases and at 1 year of age is about 75 to 90 percent of the adult level.

There is suggestive evidence that a small amount of IgG may be synthesized beginning about the seventh month of gestation, but rarely will this exceed 0.1 percent of the adult level. Synthesis of IgA commences about 2 weeks after birth. The plasma level of IgA rises slowly so that only 40 to 50 percent of the peak value is present at 1 year of age, the maximal concentration being attained between 4 and 12 years of age.

In view of the foregoing consideration it is not surprising that infants under 3 months of age require a greater dose of antigen if they are to produce an antibody response that is equivalent to that of the older infant. Both immunological naïveté and feedback inhibition by placentally transferred IgG operate to reduce the effectiveness of a given dose of antigen. The initial and subsequent synthesis of immunoglobulins in infants born of mothers with hypogammaglobulinemia is comparable to infants born with maternal IgG. Consequently, immunological naïveté is probably a more important factor than feedback inhibition in the requirement for a greater dose of antigen in the young infant.

Genetic Constitution In man, definitive evidence for genetic control of antibody production is provided by the inheritance of agammaglobulinemia (hypogammaglobulinemia). Most cases of inherited agammaglobulinemia occur in males and are transmitted by the female as a sex-linked recessive trait. The total level of plasma immunoglobulins is usually 25 mg/100 ml or less, involves IgM, IgA, and IgG and probably IgD and IgE as well, and is not associated with accelerated metabolism of immunoglobulins. Consequently, the defect is due to a lack of antibody-producing cells.

In addition to the deficit in immunoglobulins, the tissues of children with inherited agammaglobulinemia are virtually devoid of plasma cells, and the lymph nodes fail to develop germinal centers. There are, however, adequate numbers of small lymphocytes in the circulation and in the various lymphoid tissues. Accordingly, these patients can develop delayed hypersensitivity (Chap. 8) in response to antigenic stimulation.

Patients with inherited agammaglobulinemia experience repeated infections with pyogenic cocci, *Candida*, and with a protozoan parasite, *Pneumocystis carinii*. Most of the children have repeated episodes of pneumonia, but recurrent meningitis, septicemia, otitis media, sinusitis, and conjunctivitis are also frequently encountered. By contrast, the response to viral infection is similar to that of normal children. Control of the disease is based on prophylactic intramuscular injection of commercially available human immunoglobulin in a dose of 100 to 150 mg/kg of body weight at monthly intervals, an amount calculated to maintain the plasma concentration of IgG above 100 to 150 mg/100 ml. In addition, appropriate antibiotics are used to control any infections that may develop.

Two other inherited diseases are known to be associated with immunological abnormalities. Ataxia telangiectasia is a progressive neurological and vascular disease frequently characterized by a poorly developed thymus, a deficiency in IgA, severe sinopulmonary infection, failure to develop delayed hypersensitivity (Chap. 8), and prolonged survival of skin allografts (Chap. 10). The Swiss, or lymphopenic, form of agammaglobulinemia, or thymic alymphoplasia, the most extreme immunological deficiency, is inherited as an autosomal recessive characteristic in males and females and involves an arrest in the development of the thymus and the thymus-dependent lymphoid tissues. There is a great paucity of small lymphocytes, plasma cells, and immunoglobulins. The problem of infections is greatly increased, extending to all types of microorganisms, and the children rarely survive the first year despite heroic efforts to preserve their lives with thymic grafts and with infusions of bone marrow, fetal liver, and fetal thymus cells.

In addition to the foregoing examples, it is probable that many cases of acquired agammaglobulinemia and dysgammaglobulinemia are inherited, but the evidence is less satisfactory.

Physical, Chemical, and Operative Procedures Paradoxically, many of the most potent immunosuppressive agents are also capable of enhancing antibody synthesis. Any given agent may produce a wide spectrum of effects, extending from increased antibody formation to complete inhibition of the immune response. Suppression or enhancement of antibody production is largely dependent upon when the agent is given in relation to antigenic challenge and is influenced to a lesser extent by the dose of the agent and the intensity of the antigenic stimulus.

Most of the powerful immunosuppressive agents are potent lymphocytotoxic agents but may also be responsible for causing marked lymphoid hyperplasia. X-rays, nitrogen mustards, 6-mercaptopurine, thioguanine, azathioprine, methotrexate, 5-fluoro-2-deoxyuridine, cortisone, prednisone, cyclophosphamide, penicillamine, colchicine, and endotoxin are examples of such agents. Suppression of antibody formation by these agents can be ascribed primarily to the destruction or inhibition of small lymphocytes. On the other hand, it is probable that the release of nucleic acids from cells injured by one of these agents is responsible for both the hyperplastic lymphoid tissue and the enhanced production of antibodies.

Nucleic acids and nucleic acid digests are known to increase antibody formation in the absence of cytotoxic agents and to restore antibody synthesis in treated animals. When nucleic acids are released from the killed or injured cells and taken up by small lymphocytes, protein synthesis, cell growth, and cell division are stimulated. Introduction of antigen when there is pronounced hyperplasia of lymphatic tissue leads to the enhanced production of antibody. The precise time enhancement can be demonstrated varies with the agent. For example, with x-rays enhancement is evident when the antigen is given a few hours prior to irradiation, whereas maximal suppression of antibody production occurs when the antigen is given 24 hr. after irradiation. On the other hand, maximal enhancement of antibody formation can be shown when a small dose of antigen is injected 5 days after a 1-week course of 6-mercaptopurine, whereas complete suppression is achieved if the antigen is administered while the animal is under treatment with the drug (Fig.7-15). If 6-mercaptopurine is given a few days after the antigen, 19S synthesis may be prolonged, but 7S antibody synthesis and memory may fail to develop.

Since antibody formation is a special problem in protein synthesis, it is not surprising that a broad range of protein and nucleic acid inhibitors, in doses below the toxic level, suppress the production of antibody. Demonstration of their inhibiting effect on antibody synthesis, however, requires the use of sensitive techniques. The data included in Table 7-4 indicate the dose of the inhibitor which produces a 90 percent or greater suppression of the secondary antibody response to bovine serum albumin by in vitro cultures of rabbit lymph node fragments. The use of this sensitive technique has also provided an experimental model for the evaluation of the inhibitory effect of acetylsalicylic acid (aspirin), salicylic acid (2-hydroxybenzoic acid), gentisic acid (2,5-dihydroxybenzoic acid), and gentisate (5-hydroxysalicylate), which have long been used therapeutically in rheumatic conditions and may function by blocking pyridoxal activity in the synthesis of amino acids and proteins. For maximal inhibition of the secondary antibody response, each of the drugs must be present at the time the antigen is placed in contact with the lymph node fragment and must be kept in contact with the fragment, especially for a period of 9 days, which represents the induction period in this system. Little inhibition is produced if the drug is added after the ninth day, although 90 percent of the antibody is formed after the ninth day.

Table 7-4 Inhibitors of the Secondary Response in Vitro

Agent	Concentration producing 90% or greater suppression
Puromycin	3 μM (1.6 μg/ml)
Chloramphenicol	20–50 μg/ml
Actinomycin D	0.003–0.01 μg/ml
Sodium salicylate	1.5 mM (240 μg/ml)
Aspirin	2.0 mM
Gentisate	0.5 mM

Source: From C. T. Ambrose, *J. Exp. Med.*, 124:461–482, 1966.

Various operative procedures are known to exert a marked effect on antibody formation. Ablation of the thymus, the circulating small lymphocytes, and to a lesser extent, the spleen leads to suppression of the immune response. When small amounts of particulate antigens are injected intravenously into splenectomized animals or humans, antibody production is greatly depressed. If, however, the particulate antigens are injected intraperitoneally or intradermally, antibody synthesis is unaffected.

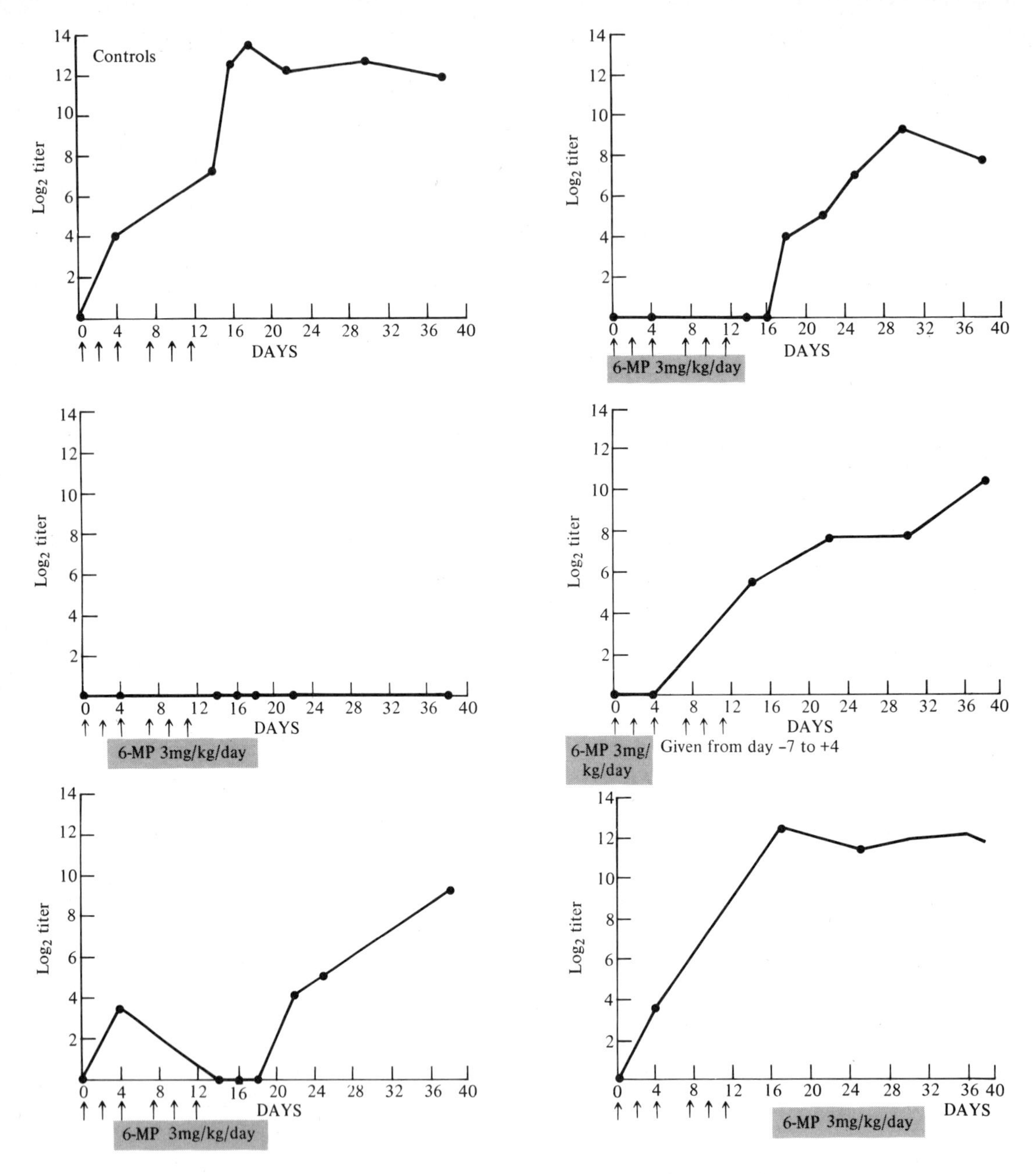

Figure 7-15 The effect of 6-mercaptopurine on antibody production. Course of immune response in control and 6-MP treated rabbits. Each vertical arrow represents antigenic injection. Time and duration of administration of 6-MP is also indicated. Each value depicted in the graph represents the average titer for the group. (*R. Schwartz, J. Stack, and W. Dameshek, Proc. Soc. Exp. Biol. Med., 99:164-167, 1958.*)

The profound effects on the immune response produced by neonatal thymectomy or by depletion of small lymphocytes by chronic drainage from a thoracic duct fistula in rats and mice are interrelated observations. The thymus does not contain immunologically competent cells, but it seeds the peripheral lymphoid tissues with small lymphocytes. The absence or removal of small lymphocytes is associated, in turn, with suppression of 7S antibody formation, prolonged survival of allografts (Chap. 10), and failure to develop delayed hypersensitivity (Chap. 8). Complete restoration of immunological reactivity in neonatally thymectomized animals can be achieved through the administration of viable thymus, small lymphocytes, or peripheral lymphoid tissue (bone marrow, spleen, lymph node) containing small lymphocytes.

These findings are paralleled in man in patients with ataxia telangiectasia or thymic alymphoplasia, inherited diseases accompanied by a poorly developed thymus.

Summary

Antibody production in an immunologically competent host is influenced by the chemical nature, physical state, quantity, and persistence of the immunogen (antigen); the rate at which it diffuses from the site of inoculation; the number of times it is injected and the interval between injections; and the concentration and avidity of the specific antibody present in the host.

On primary stimulation with an adequate dose of a particulate or soluble protein antigen in a host lacking placentally transferred or cross-reacting antibody, the antigen is metabolized by the macrophages of the reticuloendothelial system and antigenic fragments are transported to small lymphocytes. On contact with the antigenic fragment the small lymphocytes transform into a rapidly replicating and differentiating population of cells of the blast-plasma cell series which synthesize 19S (IgM) antibody exponentially for a period of 4 or 5 days. After another 5 days the formation of 19S antibody is shut off by the exponential formation of 7S (IgG) antibody which continues for about 4 or 5 days. Feedback inhibition by increasingly avid 7S gradually turns off 7S synthesis, but small lymphocytes develop immunological memory, which usually persists for the life of the host.

Immunological memory, the capacity to give a secondary response on subsequent contact with the same antigen, usually can be induced by a smaller dose of antigen in a shorter period of time, producing peak titers that are higher and that persist longer. The increased formation of antibody on second contact with the antigen is a 7S response. Synthesis of 19S precedes 7S and is equivalent to that produced in the primary response. The simplest explanation of the secondary response is that antigen stimulates a greater number of small lymphocytes possessing immunological memory to differentiate, replicate, and synthesize antibody.

ANTIGEN-ANTIBODY INTERACTION

Specificity

Specificity, the outstanding feature of antigen-antibody interaction, is based on complementarity in chemical structure between determinant groups on the surface of the antigen and combining sites on the surface of the antibody. The complementary chemical structures are associated with about 1 percent of the surface of the antigen and antibody molecules but are nonetheless responsible for the formation of antigen-antibody complexes. Ordinarily, the size of the critical reactive sites approximates five to seven amino acid or sugar residues on the antigen and an equivalent number of complementary amino acid residues on the antibody.

The binding forces between antigen and antibody are apparently associated with weak attractive forces that operate over a short range and do not involve strong ionic or covalent bonds. These forces include the mutual attraction between all atoms (van der Waals forces), coulombic or electrostatic attraction between oppositely charged ionic groups, and attraction between polar nonionic groups such as hydrogen bonds. Because of the weakness and short range of these forces, the firmness of the union is a function of the closeness of the fit or the complementary spatial configuration between the determinant group on the antigen and the combining site on the antibody.

Combination in Multiple Proportions

The second most important characteristic of antigen-antibody interaction is the fact that antigens and antibodies combine in multiple proportions. Most antibody molecules are divalent, having two identical combining sites located on opposite ends of the cylindrical molecule (as indicated previously, IgM and IgA may have a greater valence). Antibody can form a bridge between antigen molecules when the combining sites on the antibody molecule react with the same determinant group on two antigen molecules. Antigens, however, are multivalent, usually containing 5 to 10 determinant groups per molecule, although they may have 200 or more. There are usually several different groups on one antigen molecule, and these are present in varying concentrations. Thus, an antigen molecule has the potential for combining with numerous antibody molecules, while an antibody molecule is usually limited to combining with two antigen molecules. The expression used to describe this relationship is that antigens and antibodies combine in multiple proportions.

Other Features of Antigen-Antibody Interaction

The rate of association of antigen and antibody is extremely rapid, probably occurring within a few milliseconds, and does not require an electrolyte. The formation of insoluble antigen-antibody complexes, however, requires the presence of electrolyte and is dependent on the relative concentrations of antigen and antibody. Under optimal conditions the insoluble complex is formed within a few seconds, but may develop much more slowly under other circumstances and varies widely with the particular test procedure employed.

The union of antigen with antibody is reversible. The rate of dissociation of antigen-antibody complexes, however, is generally slow. The half time of dissociation is directly related to the avidity of the antibody and has been estimated to vary between 2 hr. and more than 8 days. Thus, despite its reversibility, the combination of antigen with antibody is relatively firm.

Analysis of the concentration of free antigen, free antibody, and antigen-antibody complexes in equilibrium mixtures has led to the conclusion that interaction between antigen and antibody is due to a series of bimolecular reactions which follow the law of mass action. Difficulty has been encountered, however, in the interpretation of equilibrium constants because of the heterogeneity of antibody molecules reacting with a particular determinant group on the antigen and because most antigens contain different determinant groups.

Detection and Measurement of Antigen and Antibody

The fundamental importance of antigen-antibody reactions is associated with their role in the prevention of, modification of, or recovery from infection; with their use in directly or indirectly establishing the identity of the causative agent; and with their activity in altering tissue responses to the detriment of the host (Chap. 8). A variety of in vitro and in vivo techniques are available for detection and measurement of antigen when the antibody is known or of antibody when the antigen is known. With the exception of the ferritin and fluorescent antibody methods, antigen-antibody reactions are a two-stage process involving the initial (invisible) combination of antigen and antibody and the secondary (visible) manifestation of their interaction.

The observed reaction is dependent upon the physical, chemical, and biological properties of the antigen, the antibody, and the antigen-antibody complex and occasionally may require additional components such as complement. The major systems employed to demonstrate antigen-antibody reactions are precipitation, agglutination, complement-fixation, neutralization, and the induction of specific tissue reactions or variants of these procedures. Quantitative procedures have been developed for each of these test systems and have provided highly specific and sensitive analytical tools for the assay of proteins, polysaccharides, hormones, enzymes, and other antigenically active materials.

Limitations of the Unitarian Theory of Antibodies

As antigen-antibody methods were developed, antibodies were designated according to the manifestations observed in the test. Thus, the terms precipitins, agglutinins, lysins, opsonins, and antitoxins were used for the antibodies that participated in precipitation, agglutination, lysis, phagocytosis, and neutralization of toxins. Proposed 50 years ago, the unitarian theory holds that a single antigen induces the formation of only one kind of antibody which under appropriate experimental conditions can be responsible for any of the observed reactions.

Although the unitarian theory focused attention on the similarities between various antigen-antibody reactions, it is no longer tenable. It is now recognized that antibodies that react with the same antigen molecule may have different functions and that the functional activity of an antibody cannot be measured in terms of weight of protein. As noted earlier, most antigens contain a number of chemically distinct determinant groups, each of which is responsible for the production of different classes of antibody immunoglobulins. Within each class there is marked heterogeneity in the antibody population, and there are striking qualitative changes in the antibodies at various stages in the immunization process. These properties are reflected in antigen-antibody reactions in a variety of ways. For example, antibodies can combine with an antigen but fail to precipitate, IgM antibodies may be as much as 1,000 times as active as IgG in causing agglutination and hemolysis, and IgG is much more efficient in producing precipitation than IgM.

THE PRECIPITIN REACTION

Optimal Proportions

When a soluble antigen is mixed with antibody in the presence of electrolyte (0.15 *M* sodium chloride) at an appropriate temperature, an insoluble complex of antigen and antibody, or precipitate, may result. *Precipitin tests* ordinarily require high concentrations of antibody and consequently are less sensitive in detecting antigen or antibody than most other immunological reactions (Table 7-5). The explanation is related to the size and surface area of the antigen, which increase inversely with the cube of the diameter. Thus, a soluble antigen requires a

Table 7-5 Sensitivity of Common Serological Procedures for Detecting Antibody

Method	μg of antibody N/ml*
Precipitation	
Ring test	4
Gel diffusion	7.5
Quantitative	10
Bacterial agglutination	0.01
Passive hemagglutination	0.004
Complement fixation	0.1

* Approximate values.

much greater amount of antibody in proportion to its size than does a particulate antigen such as a microorganism in order to achieve a visible insoluble complex. In addition, it is known that 7S antibody is more efficient than 19S in combining with soluble antigens, whereas 19S antibody, which is much larger, is much more efficient than 7S in combining with particulate antigens.

The formation and composition of a precipitate are dependent on the relative concentrations of antigen and antibody in the reaction mixture. If, for example, a series of increasing amounts of antigen is added to a series of tubes containing constant amounts of antibody, floccules form in one of the mixtures sooner than in the others. The ratio of antigen to antibody in this mixture is approximately the *equivalence ratio,* or the *optimal proportion ratio*. The amounts of precipitate progressively decrease on each side of the optimal proportions ratio (Fig. 7-16).

Quantitative Precipitin Curve

If the precipitates formed in the series of tubes used to determine the optimal proportions ratio are washed and assayed for nitrogen (N), the concentration of antibody N in the precipitates can be obtained by subtracting the amount of antigen N from the total N. In this way the quantitative course of the precipitin reaction can be followed in a series of reaction mixtures containing a constant amount of antibody and increasing concentrations of antigen. When the micrograms of the total and antibody N are plotted against the micrograms of antigen N, a *quantitative precipitin curve* is obtained. Because the quantitative precipitin curve is fundamental to an understanding of antigen-antibody reactions and because it led to the development of immunochemistry, it merits careful attention. To assist the reader the pertinent data are not only illustrated graphically in Figure 7-16 but are also supplemented by a list of the essential findings and by hypothetical molecular arrangements of the antigen-antibody complexes in various portions of the curve according to the lattice hypothesis.

The following findings are based on the quantitative precipitin curve (Fig. 7-16):

1. The amount of antibody precipitated increases to a maximum with increasing addition of antigen and then falls off rapidly.
2. In the zone of antibody excess, antibody can be detected in the supernatant after removal of the precipitate.
3. In the equivalence zone, where the optimal proportion ratio is found, neither antigen nor antibody can be detected in the supernatant after removal of the precipitate.
4. In the zone of antigen excess, antigen can be detected in the supernatant after removal of the precipitate.
5. The maximum amount of antibody N in the precipitate is found when there is a trace of antigen in the supernatant.
6. The ratio of antibody N to antigen N in the precipitate decreases with increasing concentration of antigen.
7. In the zone of antigen excess, as well as in the equivalence zone and the zone of antibody excess, the ratio of antibody N to antigen N in the precipitate is appreciably greater than one.
8. Most of the N in the precipitate represents antibody N even in the zone of antigen excess.
9. When the molecular weights of the antigen and antibody are known or assumed, the molecular ratio of antibody to antigen can be calculated in the various regions of the curve and expressed diagrammatically in the form of a lattice.
10. The quantitative data permit the determination of the valence of the antigen and the antibody.
11. The curve provides incontrovertible proof that antigens and antibodies combine in multiple proportions; i.e., an antigen molecule can bind a variable number of antibody molecules depending upon the valence of the antigen and the concentration of each reagent, and that an antibody molecule usually binds two molecules of antigen.
12. In addition to free antibody in the zone of antibody excess and free antigen in the zone of antigen excess, soluble antigen-antibody complexes of variable composition are formed.

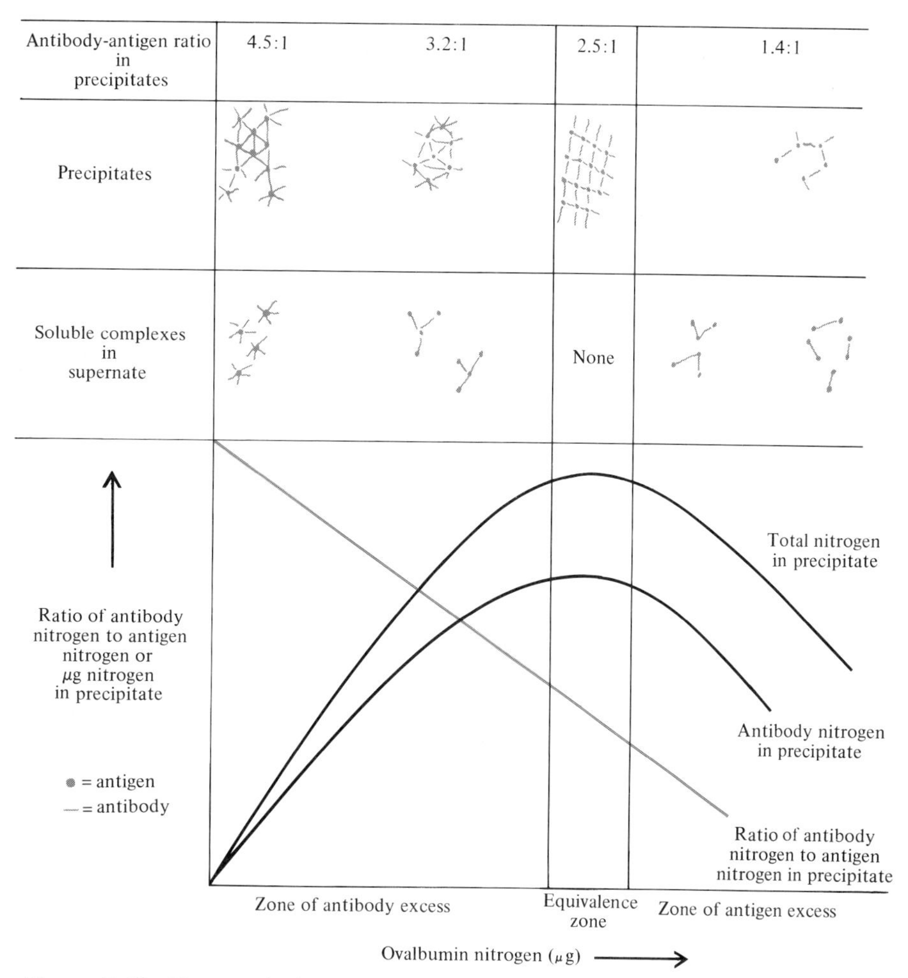

Figure 7-16 The quantitative precipitin reaction of ovalbumin (valence = 5) with rabbit anti-ovalbumin antibody. (*Modified from J. H. Humphrey and R. G. White, Immunology for Students of Medicine, 3d ed., Oxford: Blackwell Scientific Publications, Ltd., 1970.*)

The molecular ratios of antibody to antigen illustrated in Figure 7-16 represent those obtained with egg albumin, an antigen which has a valence of 5. Quantitative precipitin curves obtained with other antigens generally indicate that the molecular composition of the precipitate is a function of the valence of the antigen. For example, the molecular antibody-to-antigen ratio in the equivalence zone is about 2.5 to 1 for egg albumin which has a molecular weight of 42,000 and 83 to 1 for hemocyanin which has a valence of 231 and a molecular weight of more than 6 million. However, the basic features of the quantitative precipitin curve are similar for all soluble antigens.

Lattice Hypothesis

The lattice hypothesis is a generally accepted concept designed to account for the formation of antigen-antibody precipitates (Fig. 7-16). It is based on the combination of multivalent antigen with divalent antibody in multiple proportions to form an aggregate, lattice, or complex of large size. In the lattice hypothesis, an antibody molecule forms a bridge between two molecules of antigen, and an antigen molecule binds a variable number of antibody molecules, depending on its valence and the concentration and avidity of antibody. The precipitate may be visualized as a three-dimensional arrangement of alternating antigen and antibody molecules. The data revealed by the quantitative precipitin curve are in accord with the lattice hypothesis but do not specify the mechanism of precipitation in precise physicochemical terms.

Coprecipitating (Nonprecipitating) Antibody

In carrying out the quantitative precipitin curve, the antigen is added in one portion to the antibody. In the equivalence zone, neither antigen nor antibody can be detected in the supernatant after the removal of the precipitate. If, however, small amounts of egg albumin (equal in total concentration to the quantity used in the equivalence zone) are added serially to the antibody until no more precipitate is formed, the amount of antibody N in the precipitate is 22 percent less than that precipitated by adding the antigen in one portion. Antibody which is not included in the precipitate on serial addition of small amounts of antigen can coprecipitate with antigen-antibody complexes at optimal proportions.

Detection of coprecipitating antibody is dependent upon the ability of antigen and antibody to combine in multiple proportions in molecular ratios that vary with the concentration of the reactants. The finding of coprecipitating antibody represents another reflection of heterogeneity in the avidity of antibody. The more avid antibody molecules combine with the early additions of antigen to form a precipitate, leaving the less avid coprecipitating antibodies free in the supernatant. Coprecipitating antibodies are probably found in all antibody preparations, forming a large proportion of early 19S antibody, decreasing with appearance of primary 7S antibody, and being present in minimal quantity in secondary 7S antibody. Thus, the concentration of coprecipitating antibody varies inversely with the avidity of the antibody, the duration and intensity of immunization, and the number of injections of the antigen.

Qualitative Precipitin Tests

The Ring Test When a small test tube or capillary tube containing undiluted or slightly diluted antiserum is carefully layered with antigen, the antigen and antibody diffuse into one another over a wide range of concentrations. A positive reaction is indicated within a few minutes by the formation of a visible ring, or precipitate, at the interface where the antigen and antibody are present in an optimal proportions ratio. The ring test is widely used in forensic medicine to identify proteins, especially stains of blood and seminal fluid. As little as 1 μg of antigen may be detected by the ring test.

Agar (Gel) Diffusion Tests Several modifications of the ring test have been developed by allowing antigen, antibody, or both reactants to diffuse through a gel or semisolid medium such as *agar*. These methods provide greater precision and, within limits, permit recognition of the number of components present in the solutions of antigen and antibody. In the Oudin procedure of *single diffusion in one dimension,* antigen solution is layered over a column of agar containing antibody in a test tube. As the antigen diffuses through the agar, a moving boundary line or band of precipitate develops, behind which the excessive antigen concentration causes the precipitate to dissolve. The time required to form the band of precipitate may vary from a few hours to a few days, depending on the concentration of the reactants. A single band may be taken as one criterion of the purity of the antigen-antibody system. If mixtures of antigens and antibodies are present, multiple bands of precipitate develop because of differences in molecular size, electrical charge, rate of diffusion, and relative concentration of the reactants in the different antigen-antibody systems.

In the procedure involving *double diffusion in one dimension* antibody is incorporated into agar, a column of agar is superimposed, and the antigen solution is placed above. A band of precipitate appears in the agar where each antigen and antibody meet in optimal proportions.

The Ouchterlony procedure of *double diffusion in two dimensions* permits direct comparison of various antigens and antibodies. Agar is poured on a flat surface, such as a petri plate or a slide, and is allowed to harden. The reactants are placed in wells cut out of the agar. Each band of precipitate that forms in the agar between the wells containing antigen and antibody reflects the combination of an antigen-antibody system in optimal proportions as in the procedures involving diffusion in one dimension. Several antigens can be tested with a single antiserum located in the central well on one petri plate or slide. The patterns of the precipitating bands formed between the wells permit the detection of identical antigens in different mixtures or the recognition of nonindentical material (Fig. 7-17). When identical antigens located in adjacent wells react with antibodies diffusing from the central well, the bands of precipitate fuse *(reaction of identity)*. If the antigenic samples contain no common determinant group, the bands of precipitate intersect *(reaction of nonidentity)*. If the antigens share determinant groups but also have distinct determinant groups, the bands of precipitate fuse but the antigen used to produce the antiserum shows a

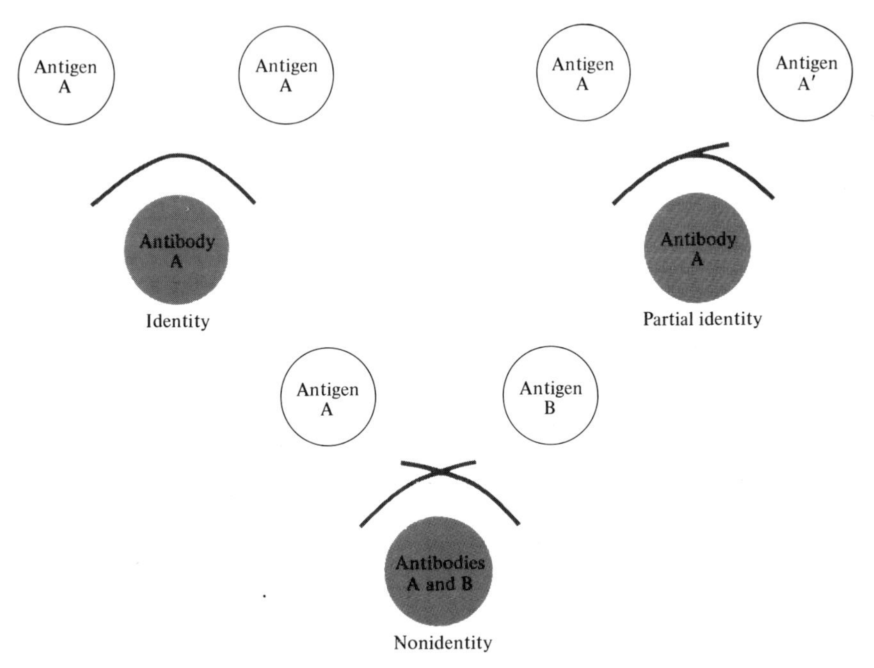

Figure 7-17 Precipitin reactions in a double diffusion system in agar. A precipitin band forms where antigen and antibody combine in optimal proportions.

spur projecting out beyond the point of fusion *(reaction of partial identity).* The antibody molecules which do not cross-react diffuse past the bands of fusion where they combine with the distinct determinant groups on the antigen.

Immunoelectrophoresis Immunoelectrophoresis combines electrophoresis with double diffusion in two dimensions. The components of a complex protein mixture such as serum are placed in a central well and are separated by electrophoresis in agar. Troughs are cut in the agar parallel to the direction of migration and on each side of the electrophoretically separated components. Antiserum is then added to the two troughs. After a few days the antibody diffusing from the troughs forms a band of precipitate with each of the electrophoretically separated proteins. Immunoelectrophoresis is a powerful method for resolving and identifying antigens and antibodies in a mixture. For example, with this procedure human serum can be resolved into 30 or more antigens. This technique is especially useful in screening the serum of patients suspected of having agammaglobulinemia or one of the dysgammaglobulinemias.

Hapten Inhibition of Precipitation

No reaction has played a more important role in leading to an understanding of the chemical basis of antigenic specificity than *hapten inhibition of precipitation.* When a hapten is incorporated into the structure of proteins by diazo or peptide linkage, it confers a new antigenic specificity on the protein and frequently masks the antigenicity of carrier protein. In addition to directing the antigenic specificity of hapten-protein conjugates, the hapten can combine with antibody against the conjugate. Since a hapten has a valence of one (i.e., represents a single determinant group), lattice formation cannot occur. Hapten attached to the combining sites on antibody to the hapten-protein conjugate which are complementary to the hapten results in the formation of a soluble complex in the absence of precipitation. Proof that this occurs is indicated by the failure of the conjugate to precipitate with specific antibody whose combining sites have bound the hapten. This is the reaction known as hapten inhibition. Different haptens can be compared by determining the minimal concentrations required to prevent precipitation in a standard quantitative system. Thus, it is possible to obtain a quantitative measure of the antigenic reactivity of hapten groups modified in different ways.

BACTERIAL AGGLUTINATION

In bacterial agglutination, antibodies specifically directed toward antigenic components of the bacterial cell surface can cross-link organisms, causing them to clump in large masses. While both IgM and IgG can agglutinate bacteria, IgM is the more efficient. The many antigens toward which the antibodies may be directed include various components of slime layers or capsules, cell walls, and flagella. Bacterial agglutination tests can be performed by several different methods including tube tests, hanging-drop preparations, and slide tests. The tube agglutination tests which are run in a series of test tubes with a standard suspension of organisms and serial dilutions of antiserum are the most accurate for determining antibody titers. The slide agglutination test is made by adding a drop of bacterial suspension to a drop of a dilution of antiserum and observing the agglutination under the microscope. The advantage of the slide test is speed, economy of reagents, and the ability to run many tests in a short time.

Because of the extreme sensitivity of the agglutination tests, they have proved to be extremely useful in the research laboratory and in the diagnostic laboratory. Serological identification of suspected infectious agents is of importance in the epidemiology of disease as well as in providing the basis for a reliable decision on which antimicrobial agent to use in therapy. Many organisms have been identified and classified to an exquisite degree by agglutination methods. Such infectious agents include the pneumococci, pasteurella, brucella, salmonella, and shigella. Additionally, diagnosis of specific infection may be made in part by the demonstration of agglutinating antibodies in the patient's serum. In many cases, the actual rise in serum antibodies does not exceed a titer of 1:500 but may go as high as 1:5,120 as in the case of brucellosis. In experimental immunization, titers as high as 1:50,000 are not uncommon for agglutinating antibodies.

The principal limitations of bacterial agglutination tests are that they cannot be (1) used with many bacteria that agglutinate spontaneously, i.e., in the absence of specific antibody, or (2) developed for quantitative analysis of antigen-antibody interactions. In the latter case, the bulk of the N in the antigen (bacteria) is unrelated to the surface antigens that participate in the agglutination reaction. Since only a few molecules of antibody are required to cause the bacteria to agglutinate, the difference between the total N in the agglutinated material and that found in the antigen (bacteria) alone is insufficient for accurate quantitation.

COMPLEMENT AND COMPLEMENT FIXATION

Complement (C′) is a multifactorial system found in the blood which can mediate and amplify a number of immune reactions. The system consists of nine protein components (Table 7-6) which act in a sequential cascade (Fig. 7-18). Normally the components exist as inactive proteins in the blood, but when participating in the cascade many of the proteins exhibit enzymatic activity.

The triggering of the cascade occurs during immune reactions involving IgG or IgM. Conformational changes in the antibody molecules occur which unmask sites on the Fc portions of the molecules. Complement component one, C1, composed of three subunits (q, r, and s, held together by calcium ions) interacts with the unmasked sites on the Fc portion by means of binding sites on subunit q. This interaction in turn sequentially activates r and s, producing an

Table 7-6 Physicochemical Characteristics of the Components of Complement

Terminology	Molecular weight	Electrophoretic mobility	Normal serum concentration (μg/ml)
C1	—	—	—
C1q	400,000	$\gamma 2$	190
C1r	168,000	β	?
C1s	79,000	$\alpha 2$	120
C4	240,000	$\beta 1$	430
C2	117,000	$\beta 2$	30
C3	185,000	$\beta 1$	1,300
C5	185,000	$\beta 1$	75
C6	125,000	$\beta 2$	60
C7	—	$\beta 2$	—
C8	150,000	$\gamma 1$	+
C9	79,000	α	+

Source: From S. Ruddy, I. Gigli, and K. F. Austen, *N. Engl. J. Med.*, 287:489–495, 1972.

esterolytic activity in subunit s. Esterase then acts on C4, splitting it into two fragments, the larger of which enters the cascade.

Basically, the *complement cascade* is a series of reactions resulting in the cleavage or fragmentation of components by enzymatic activity associated with preceding components. The larger fragments usually participate in the complement cascade, while the smaller fragments do not. However, the smaller fragments often possess biological activity. It is through the biological activity of these smaller fragments that complement becomes involved in inflammatory reactions (Fig. 7-18).

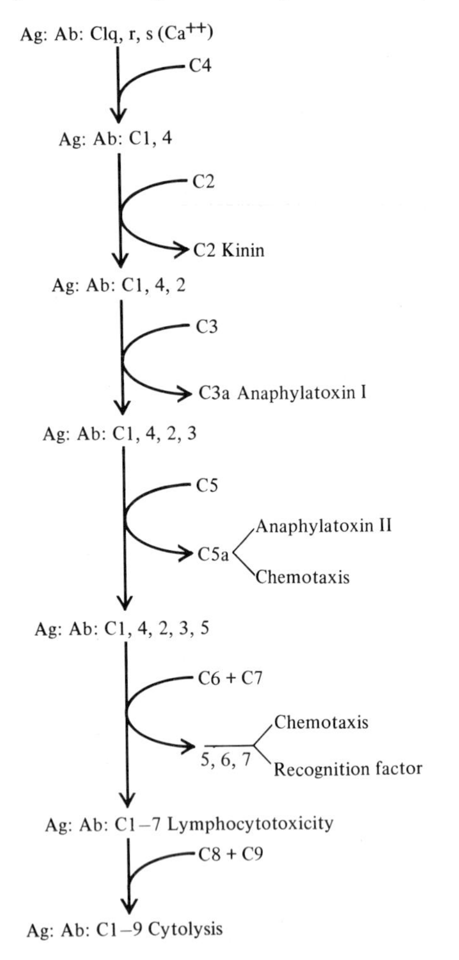

Figure 7-18 Sequential interactions of the components of complement with antigen-antibody complexes.

Certain control mechanisms govern the complement cascade and its active fragments, including enzymatic instability and the presence of inhibitors in the serum proteins. For example, C2 is a highly unstable component and its enzymatic activity, in the form of $\overline{C4, 2}$, is subject to rapid decay, as is the activity associated with C5. Protein inhibitors exist for C1, the C3b fragment, and/or C6, while an enzyme cleaves arginine from the fragments C3a and C5a, inactivating their anaphylatoxic activity.

There are a number of biological activities associated with various complexes and fragments that occur as the complement cascade progresses (Table 7-7). If the antigen involved in the reaction is a cell (mammalian cell or red blood cell) or if the antigen-antibody reaction takes place on the surface of such a cell, the addition of the full cascade of complement to the surface of the cell results in cell lysis. Many, if not all, of these fragments and complexes can occur free in the fluid phase with the consequent activities listed in Table 7-7. Thus, a number of reactions can occur locally when complement is activated by antigen-antibody reactions. In addition, complement endows antibacterial immune reactions with bactericidal powers in which many gram-negative bacteria can be killed or lysed by the action of complement and specific antibody. The bactericidal activity is enhanced by lysozyme. Gram-positive organisms seem to be much more resistant to the cidal action of complement.

A second pathway of activation for complement exists which bypasses the usual sequence of reactions and allows complement from C3 to C9 to be activated without the participation of C1, 4, and 2. Several protein factors substitute for these early components and serve the purpose of activating C3. These protein factors include properdin (a β-globulin present in trace

Table 7-7 Biological Activities of the Complement Cascade

Complex or fragment	Activity	Effect
C1,4	Virus neutralization	Must be present for effective neutralization of herpesvirus
C1,4,2	Virus neutralization	Enhances neutralizing effect of antibodies
C2-kinin	Vasoactive peptide	Bradykinin-like increase in vascular permeability
C3a	Anaphylatoxin I	Histamine release from mast cells; effective at 10^{-13} to 10^{-14} *M*
	Leukoattractant	Chemotaxis for neutrophils
C1,4,2,3	Phagocytosis	Makes cells and antigen-antibody complexes more susceptible to phagocytosis
	Virus neutralization	Enhances viral neutralization
	Immunocytoadherence	Causes antigen-antibody complexes to adhere to RBC, platelets, neutrophils
C5a	Anaphylatoxin II	Histamine release from mast cells
	Leukoattractant	Attracts polymorphonuclear leukocytes and monocytes
C5,6	LPS inactivation	"Detoxifies" LPS
$C\overline{5,6,7}$	Prepares for lysis	Can adsorb to unsensitized bystander cells and make them susceptible to lysis by C8,9
	Leukoattractant	Attracts neutrophils
C1-7	Prepares for lysis	Makes cells susceptible to lysis
	Lymphocytotoxicity	Makes cells more susceptible to sensitized "killer" lymphocytes
C1-9	Lysis	Integrity of target cell membrane destroyed, cells are nonselectively permeable
	Bactericidal	Gram-negative bacteria are lysed in presence of lysozyme; gram-positive bacteria are killed without lysis

amounts, with a molecular weight of 223,000), factor A (a euglobulin, with a molecular weight of 180,000), factor B (a glycine-rich glycoprotein, C3 proactivator), factor D (a euglobulin, C3 proactivator convertase, with a molecular weight of 40,000), and factor E (a protein, with a molecular weight of 160,000), required in the activation of complement by the cobra venom factor. These factors permit activation of C3 through C9 by such diverse substances as zymosan (carbohydrate from yeast cell walls), endotoxin, antigen-antibody aggregates, and insoluble polysaccharides. The alternate mechanism is at present an area of intense research, and some of the biological activities associated with the classical pathways of complement cascade can be generated by the alternate pathway without the immunological specificity associated with the classical pathway. However, a specific site on the hinge region of IgG4, IgA1, and IgA2 which can activate complement by the alternate pathway does allow expression of immunological specificity. A proposed pathway for alternate mechanisms is presented in Figure 7-19.

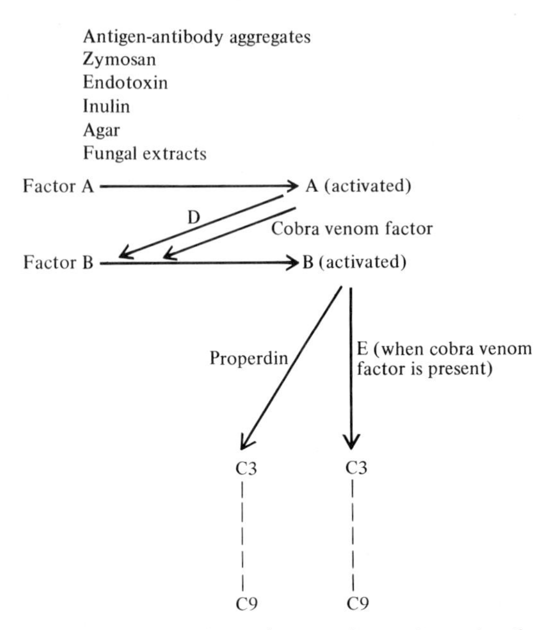

Figure 7-19 Alternate pathways of complement activation.

The lytic action of complement on red blood cells has provided the investigator and the diagnostician with a potent and extremely sensitive tool to detect the presence of antibodies against a wide variety of antigens, particularly those of microbial origin. While tests employing the principle of complement fixation in the presence of antigen-antibody reactions appear in several modifications, the underlying concept is identical. The test for complement fixation employs two systems: (1) the test system in which antibodies against a suspected antigen (or vice versa) are to be detected and (2) an indicator system in which sheep red blood cells and lytic antibodies against sheep red blood cells (hemolysins) are used.

Serum from an individual who is suspected of having been infected with the microorganism (antigen) in question is sampled and heated to 56°C for 30 min. to destroy any complement activity in the serum. To the inactivated test serum is added some of the suspected antigen and a known amount of complement, and the mixture is incubated. The red blood cells are incubated with the hemolysin to produce sensitized red blood cells (red blood cells with anti-RBC antibody attached). When aliquots of the test system are added to aliquots of the indicator system, one of two things can happen. If antibodies specific for the suspected antigen are present in the test serum, then they would have combined with the antigen, and the known amount of complement added would be fixed (consumed in the cascade). In such instances no complement would be free in the test system, and when an aliquot is added to the indicator system nothing will happen. If, however, no specific antibodies are present in the test serum, no complement will be fixed, and all of it will remain free. When an aliquot of this test system is added to the indicator system, the free complement will be activated by the sensitized red blood cells, the cascade will ensue, and lysis of the red blood cells will occur. Thus, the end points of the test indicate the presence or absence of specific antibody in the test serum. No lysis in the indicator system is a positive test, indicating the presence of specific antibody in the serum; lysis in the indicator system is a negative test, indicating the absence of specific antibody in the test serum.

THE COOMBS' TEST

The direct *Coombs' test* (antiglobulin test) is a method for the detection of antibodies or complement fixed to the surface of particulate carriers (cells, red blood cells). The antibodies detected by this test are unique in that they themselves are incapable of causing agglutination (or hemolysis) of the particulate carriers in vitro. If, however, antibodies directed against immunoglobulins or against the third or fourth components of complement are added to these coated carrier particles, agglutination will occur, indicating the presence of these immunoglobulins on the surface of the cells. The indirect Coombs' test is performed to detect circulating antibody which is incapable of agglutinating cells. Washed red blood cells are added to a sample of the suspect serum. Circulating antibody binds to these cells and then may be detected by adding anti-immunoglobulin antibodies which will agglutinate the coated cells.

BIBLIOGRAPHY

Abdou, N. I., and Abdou, N. L.: "Immunoglobulin Receptors on Human Leucocytes: III. Comparative Study of Human Bone Marrow and Blood B Cells: Role of IgM Receptors," *Clin. Exp. Immunol.,* 13:45-54, 1973.

Abrahams, S., Phillips, R. A., and Miller, R. G.: "Inhibition of the Immune Response by 7S Antibody," *J. Exp. Med.,* 137:870-892, 1973.

Azar, H. A., and Potter, M. : *Multiple Myeloma and Related Disorders,* New York: Harper & Row, Publishers, Incorporated, 1973.

Bernier, G. M.: "Structure of Human Immunoglobulins: Myeloma Proteins as Analogues of Ab," *Progr. Allergy,* 14:1-36, 1970.

Borek, F.: "Immunogenicity," in A. Neuberger and E. L. Tatum (eds.), *Frontiers of Biology,* Amsterdam: North-Holland Publishing Company, 1972.

Davie, J. M., and Paul, W. E.: "Immunological Maturation. Preferential Proliferation of High-Affinity Precursor Cells," *J. Exp. Med.,* 137:200-204, 1973.

Day, E. D.: *Advanced Immunochemistry,* Baltimore: The Williams & Wilkins Company, 1972.

dePetris, S., and Raff, M. C.: "Normal Distribution, Patching and Capping of Lymphocyte Surface Immunoglobulin Studied by Electron Microscopy," *Nature [New Biol.],* 241:257-259, 1973.

Dresser, D. W.: "The Role of T-Cells and Adjuvant in the Immune Response of Mice to Foreign Erythrocytes," *Eur. J. Immunol.,* 2:50-57, 1972.

Dwyer, J. M., and Mackay, I. R.: "The Development of Antigen-binding Lymphocytes in Foetal Tissues," *Immunology,* 23:871-879, 1972.

Feldmann, M., and Nossal, G. J. V.: "Cellular Basis of Antibody Production," *Q. Rev. Biol.,* 47:269-302, 1972.

Gery, I., Kruger, J., and Spiesel, S. Z.: "Stimulation of B-Lymphocytes by Endotoxin: Reactions of Thymus-deprived Mice and Karyotypic Analysis of Dividing Cells in Mice Bearing T_6T_6 Thymus Grafts," *J. Immunol.,* 108:1088-1091, 1972.

Gottlieb, A. A., and Schwartz, R. H.: "Antigen-RNA Interactions," *Cell. Immunol.,* 5:341-362, 1972.

Gutman, G. A., and Weissman, I. L.: "Lymphoid Tissue Architecture. Experimental Analysis of the Origin and Distribution of T-Cells and B-Cells," *Immunology,* 23:465-479, 1972.

Jones, W. R., Kaye, M. D., and Ing, R. M. Y.: "The Lymphoid Development of the Fetal and Neonatal Appendix," *Biol. Neonate,* 20:334-345, 1972.

Katz, D. H., and Benacerraf, B.: "The Regulatory Influence of Activated T-Cells on B-Cell Responses to Antigen," *Adv. Immunol.,* 15:94, 1972.

———, and Unanue, E. R.: "Critical Role of Determinant Presentation in the Induction of Specific

Responses in Immunocompetent Lymphocytes," *J. Exp. Med.,* 137:967-990, 1973.

Milton, J. D., and Mowbray, F. F.: "Reversible Loss of Surface Receptors on Lymphocytes," *Immunology,* 23:599-606, 1972.

Möller, G. (ed.): "Antigen-binding Lymphocyte Receptors," *Transplant. Rev.,* 5:3-166, 1970.

Raff, M. C.: "T and B Lymphocytes and Immune Responses," *Nature,* 242:19-23, 1973.

Ross, G. D., Rabellino, E. M., Polley, M. J., and Grey, H. M.: "Combined Studies of Complement Receptor and Surface Immunoglobulin-bearing Cells and Sheep Erythrocyte Rosette-forming Cells in Normal and Leukemic Human Lymphocytes," *J. Clin. Invest.,* 52:377-385, 1973.

Rowe, D. S., Hug, K., Faulk, W. P., McCormick, J. N., and Gerber, H.: "IgD on the Surface of Peripheral Blood Lymphocytes of the Human Newborn," *Nature [New Biol.],* 242:155-157, 1973.

Ruddy, S., Gigli, I., and Austen, K. F.: "The Complement System of Man," *N. Engl. J. Med.,* 287: 489-495, 545-549, 592-596, and 642-646, 1972.

Sawyer, M. K., Forman, M. L., Kuplic, L. S., and Stiehm, E. R.: "Developmental Aspects of the Human Complement System," *Biol. Neonate,* 19:148-162, 1971.

Schmidtke, J. R., and Johnson, A. G.: "Regulation of the Immune System by Synthetic Polynucleotides: I. Characteristics of Adjuvant Action on Antibody Synthesis," *J. Immunol.,* 106:1191-1200, 1971.

Schwartz, R. S.: "Immunoregulation by Antibody," *Progr. Immunol.,* 1:1081-1092, 1971.

Tomasi, T. B.: "Structure and Function of Immunoglobulin A," *Progr. Allergy,* 16:81-213, 1972.

Uhr, J. W., and Möller, G.: "Regulatory Effect of Antibody on the Immune Response," *Adv. Immunol.,* 8:81-127, 1968.

Unanue, E. R.: "The Regulatory Role of Macrophages in Antigenic Stimulation," *Adv. Immunol.,* 15:95-165, 1972.

———, Karnovsky, M. J., and Engers, H. D.: "Ligand-induced Movement of Lymphocyte Membrane Macromolecules: III. Relationship between the Formation and Fate of Anti-Ig-Surface Ig Complexes and Cell Metabolism," *J. Exp. Med.,* 137:675-689, 1973.

Chapter 8

The Allergic State: Hypersensitivity

Arthur E. Krikszens and Bernard A. Briody

PERSPECTIVE

Allergy refers to an altered state of reactivity to an antigen usually acquired as a consequence of prior exposure to the same or a closely related antigen. This altered state of reactivity broadly encompasses three reactions: (1) increased reactivity to the antigen (hypersensitivity, allergy, or hyperergy), (2) decreased reactivity to the antigen (hyposensitivity, hypoergy), or (3) lack of reactivity to the antigen (anergy). Allergic reactivity resides in the tissues and cells of the individual and exhibits immunological specificity.

Material covered in this chapter is concerned with hypersensitivity, is concentrated almost exclusively on human hypersensitive reactions, and emphasizes the mechanisms associated with atopy, immune complex diseases, delayed hypersensitivity, and cell-mediated immunity. An understanding of these reactions is essential in order to achieve a fundamental appreciation of immunological surveillance, immunosuppression, autoimmune disease, tolerance, transplantation, and enhancement, all of which will be considered in succeeding sections of the text.

Allergens

Allergens are substances capable of eliciting an allergic response. Included in the category of allergens are frankly antigenic materials (foreign proteins of plant or animal origin and microbial agents, components, and metabolic products) and haptens (cosmetics, drugs, detergents, solvents, and numerous other low molecular weight compounds used in industrial and commercial processes).

Sensitization

Initial exposure to an allergen "primes," or sensitizes, the individual to subsequent contact with the same allergen *(sensitization)*. There is, however, a latent period of variable duration during which reintroduction of the antigen produces little or no clinical response. After the latent period, reexposure of the individual to the same allergen can elicit an allergic, or hypersensitive, reaction with clinical manifestations.

The pathophysiology underlying clinical expression of hypersensitive reactions is virtually independent of the properties of the allergen but is strongly influenced by the genetic background of the individual, the cellular and tissue response to the allergen, and its portal of entry (i.e., peripheral injection, inhalation, ingestion, dermal contact). An extremely minute amount of allergen may be sufficient to elicit a response in a sensitized person, causing a reaction which is frequently violent and disproportionate to the concentration of the allergenic stimulus.

Classification

Historically, the classification of hypersensitive reactions was based on the time required for a sensitized individual to develop overt clinical manifestations upon reexposure to the antigen. Immediate hypersensitivity reactions became apparent in several minutes to hours after reintroduction of the allergen, whereas delayed hypersensitivity reactions appeared only after several hours or days. As knowledge grew, it became evident that hypersensitivity reactions represent a spectrum or continuum of overlapping responses which have been arbitrarily divided into four types (Table 8-1). The balance of the chapter is designed to examine each category and to gain insight into the mechanisms responsible for each particular reaction.

TYPE I: ANAPHYLACTIC RESPONSES

Systemic Reactions

Experimental anaphylaxis in the guinea pig is the prototype for illustrating the mechanisms and clinical expression of type I responses. If a guinea pig is injected intraperitoneally with a small amount of ovalbumin and, after a latent period of 2 to 3 weeks, is reinjected intravascularly with a higher concentration of ovalbumin, a dramatic sequence of events rapidly ensues. Within minutes the animal becomes irritable, sneezes, coughs, experiences respiratory distress, exhibits convulsions, and dies; this syndrome is known as *anaphylactic shock,* or *systemic anaphylaxis.* The initial antigenic stimulation is termed the *sensitizing dose,* and subsequent stimulation is termed the *shocking dose.*

Autopsies of guinea pigs that succumb to anaphylactic shock reveal that the major organs and tissues affected are the lungs, gastrointestinal tract, and the vasculature. Pulmonary involvement is especially prominent, as is evidenced by enlarged lungs of lower specific gravity inflated with trapped air. Death is caused by suffocation or inability to exhale the CO_2 released in the lungs because of bronchiolar constriction (smooth muscle contraction) and edema (increased vascular permeability). Tissues or organs prominently involved in anaphylactic reactions are referred to as *target tissues,* or *shock organs.* Species variation in target

Table 8-1 Classification of Hypersensitivity Reactions

Type of reaction	Reaction time for clinical manifestation	Mediators	Clinical examples
Type I: classical immediate hypersensitivity	15–20 min.	IgE, IgG, complement, pharmacological agents: Histamine SRS-A Prostaglandins ECF-A Kinins	Anaphylaxis, asthma, hay fever, allergic rhinitis, and insect, food, and drug allergies
Type II: cytolytic and cytotoxic reactions	Variable: hours to days	IgG, IgM, complement	Drug-induced diseases: Thrombocytopenia Agranulocytosis Hemolytic anemia Hemolytic disease of the newborn, Goodpasture's syndrome, autoimmune diseases
Type III: immune complex diseases	Variable: minutes to days	IgG, IgM, IgE, complement, neutrophils, eosinophils, lysosomal hydrolases	Arthus reaction, serum sickness, extrinsic allergic alveolitis
Type IV: delayed hypersensitivity, cell-mediated immunity	Hours to days	T lymphocyte, macrophage, soluble mediators TF, LTF, MIF, etc.	Contact dermatitis, graft rejection, autoimmune disease, cell-mediated immunity to infectious diseases

tissues is apparent, for in man, skin, mucous membranes, lungs, and vasculature are involved; in dogs, the liver is singled out; and in rabbits, the heart is the shock organ. Fatal anaphylactic shock in man is associated with laryngeal edema, pulmonary emphysema, and vascular collapse.

Cutaneous Reactions

When a small shocking dose of antigen is administered intradermally to a sensitized guinea pig, the anaphylactic reaction will generally be confined to the injected area. The localized response is characterized by the formation of a wheal and flare. The *wheal* is a pale, central area of puffiness due to edema and is surrounded by a *flare* associated with hyperemia and subsequent erythema. Cutaneous anaphylactic reactions can be elicited in many different species and represent important tools used to identify the causative allergen in human anaphylactic reactions.

Mechanisms Involved

Investigation into the mechanism of type I responses has indicated that several components are involved and that more than one mechanism can be involved, depending on the circum-

Table 8-2 Some Properties of Human IgE and IgG

Property	Human IgE (reagin)	Human IgG
Tissue fixation:		
Homocytotropic	++++	− + (rare)
Heterocytotropic	−	++++
Complement fixation	−	+
Loss of ability to fix to tissue after heating at 56°C for 30 min.	+	−
Persistence at fixation site	Weeks to months	2 to 4 days

stances. Specific sensitivity to an allergen can be transferred from a sensitized person to a normal person with serum. This form of adaptive immunity is known as *passive sensitization* and represents a straightforward demonstration that sensitivity is associated with soluble substances in the serum. Further observations have revealed that the active factors present in serum are antibodies.

Depending on the species of animal being investigated and upon the circumstances of the experiment, two classes of antibody have been implicated in anaphylactic responses. Both IgE and IgG have been demonstrated to be involved in the type I responses in various animal species (Table 8-2). In man the overwhelming majority of anaphylactic reactions are associated with IgE.

In anaphylaxis two distinct mechanisms can operate to produce the same end result. One mechanism involves IgE (*reagin* or *homocytotropic antibody*) and can occur when (1) a shocking dose of allergen makes contact with specific IgE fixed to mast cells or (2) a shocking dose of allergen forms soluble complexes with specific circulating IgE and the complexes fix to mast cells by means of the Fc fragment of IgE (Fig. 8-1). As a consequence of the reaction of allergen-IgE complexes on the surface of mast cells, the pharmacological mediators of anaphylaxis are released.

The second mechanism involves IgG (*heterocytotropic antibody*) and occurs when the shocking dose of allergen makes contact with specific circulating IgG. Soluble antigen-antibody complexes are formed, and complement is activated when fixed to the Fc fragment of IgG. In fact, in the absence of prior sensitization, anaphylaxis can be induced by a single injection of large numbers of soluble antigen-antibody complexes formed in antigen excess. By either procedure, peptide fragments of complement termed *anaphylatoxins I* and *II* are produced which in turn cause the release of the pharmacological mediators of anaphylaxis (Fig. 8-2). Anaphylaxis involving IgG and complement is known as *aggregate anaphylaxis.*

Skin Tests

Detection of IgE Skin tests, such as the Prausnitz-Küstner passive transfer reaction (P-K test), can be used to detect the presence of IgE (homocytotropic) or IgG (heterocytotropic) antibody in the serum of a sensitized person. If a small volume of serum (0.1 ml) from a sensitized person is injected intradermally into a normal person, and after a latent period of 24 to 48 hr. the sensitizing allergen is injected into the

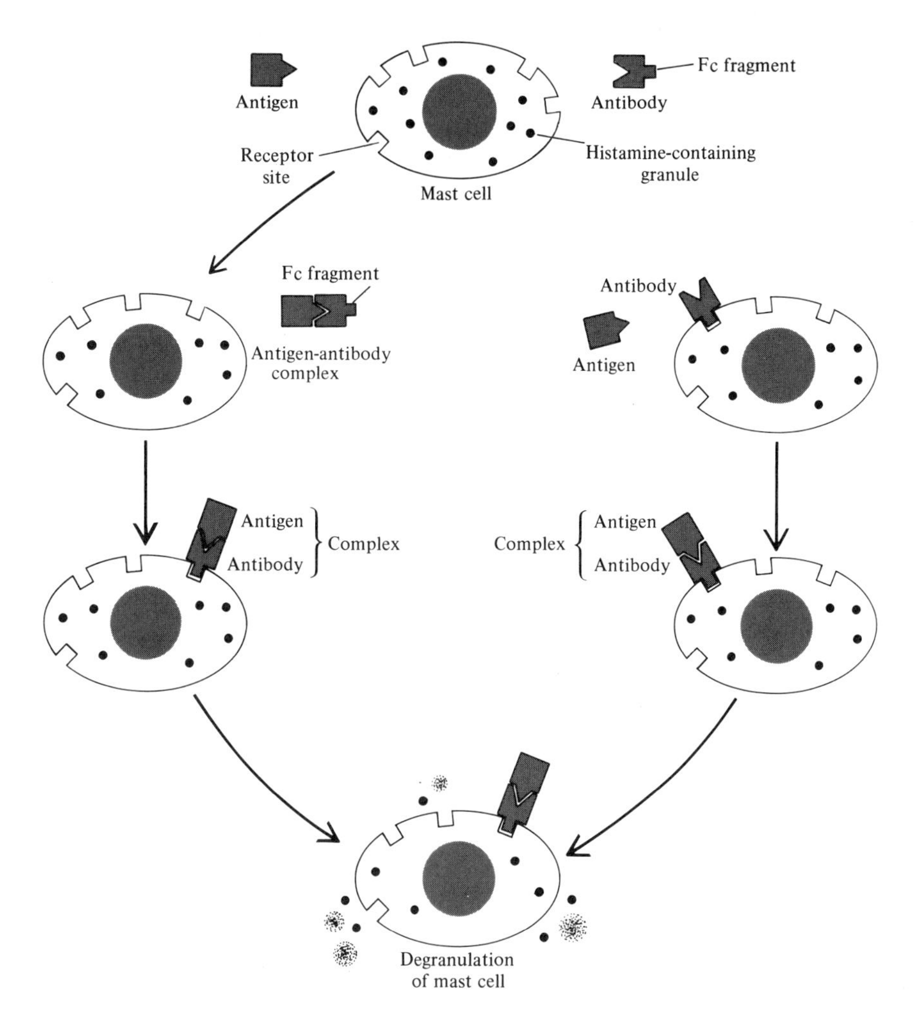

Figure 8-1 Schematic presentation of the degranulation of mast cells as a result of the interaction of antigen, IgE antibody, and cell surface receptor sites.

same site, a wheal-and-flare reaction occurs within a few minutes and forms the basis of the Prausnitz-Küstner (P-K) skin test in man. The active factor present in the sensitizing serum can persist at the site for 4 weeks or more, and the test is exquisitely sensitive, since 1×10^{-5} μg of antibody N will suffice to prepare the target cells for a wheal-and-flare reaction.

That the active factor in the donor's serum is IgE-specific for the allergen in question is based on several lines of evidence, including the following:

1 Sensitizing (reaginic) activity of the serum can be removed by precipitation with antibody (IgG) specific for the Fc fragment of human IgE.
2 On purification the distributions of sensitizing activity and IgE are parallel.
3 Purified IgE has high sensitizing activity which can be removed by antibody (IgG) specific for the Fc fragment of human IgE.

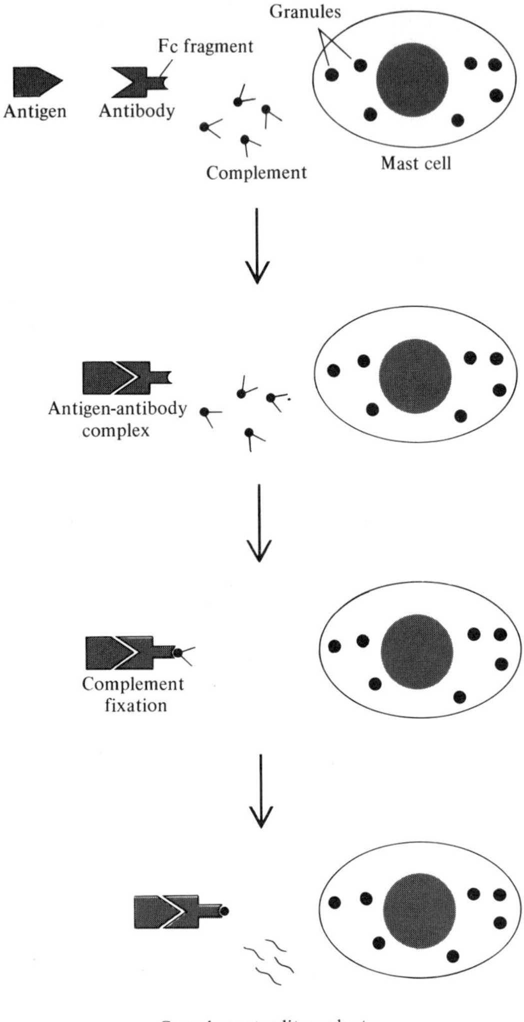

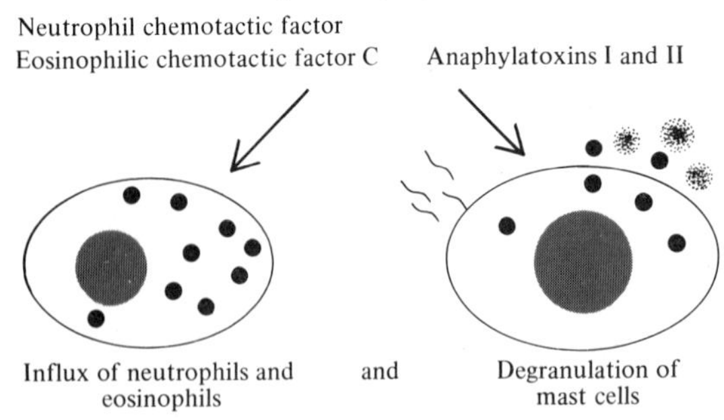

Figure 8-2 Schematic presentation of the degranulation of mast cells and the chemotaxis of neutrophils and eosinophils by split products released as a result of the interaction of antigen, IgG antibody, and complement.

4 The wheal-and-flare reaction can be induced not only by the sensitizing allergen but by antibody (IgG) specific for the Fc fragment of human IgE.
5 The wheal-and-flare reaction can be blocked if isolated Fc fragments of human IgE or human IgE myeloma proteins are injected prior to the sensitizing serum.
6 The wheal-and-flare reaction can be induced by soluble IgE-allergen complexes without prior sensitization of the site.
7 The wheal-and-flare reaction can be induced by aggregates of IgE without prior sensitization of the site.
8 Purified IgE can be used to passively sensitize human lung fragments, leukocytes, and mast cells so that the pharmacological mediators of anaphylaxis will be released on exposure to specific allergen.
9 The reaction in item 8 can be induced by antibody (IgG) specific for the Fc fragment of human IgE as well as by the allergen.
10 The reaction in item 8 can be blocked by isolated Fc fragments or by human IgE myeloma proteins when brought into contact with target cells prior to the sensitizing serum.

In summary, the Fc fragment of IgE is a key to the anaphylactic wheal-and-flare reaction, since its inactivation in purified IgE results in the loss of sensitizing activity, but not of allergen-binding activity. The data cited above demonstrate that IgE, whether alone or in combination with the allergen, adsorbs onto receptor sites on target cells by means of the Fc fragment; these sites can be blocked either by isolated Fc fragments or by the Fc fragment of intact IgE myeloma proteins. While attached to target cells, IgE retains two combining sites for the specific allergen as well as antigenic determinant groups on the Fc fragment that can react with specific (IgG) antibody. Presumably, when the specific allergen combines with IgE on the surface of target cells, conformational changes are induced within the Fc fragment, thus activating enzymes that lead to the release of the pharmacological mediators of anaphylaxis. Similar alterations probably occur when antigenic determinant groups on the Fc fragment of IgE combine with specific (IgG) antibody.

Detection of IgG In contrast with human IgE, which fixes to the surface of human target cells for several weeks, human IgG rapidly diffuses from the injection site and quickly becomes unavailable to react with the antigen. On the other hand, human IgG exhibits heterocytotropism and will fix to the target cells of other species. For example, when a small volume (0.1 ml) of serum from a sensitized person is injected intradermally into a normal guinea pig after a latent period of less than 48 hr., intravascular injection of the antigen along with Evans blue dye leads to an immediate wheal-and-flare reaction in the previously prepared site, as indicated by leakage of the blue dye (passive cutaneous anaphylaxis, or PCA, reaction). Because of its molecular weight and size, the dye is normally confined to the intravascular compartment. However, as a consequence of IgG-antigen reaction on the surface of target cells, pharmacological mediators of anaphylaxis are released that produce increased vascular permeability, thus permitting the dye to escape into the prepared site. The PCA reaction can be demonstrated with 5×10^{-3} μg antibody N.

Preformed soluble antigen-IgG complexes formed in antigen excess can elicit a wheal-and-flare reaction after intradermal injection into a normal guinea pig (aggregate anaphylaxis). Thus, although the visible manifestations of the reaction are the same, aggregate anaphylaxis requires complement and operates through a different mechanism than does the P-K reaction.

Atopic Reactions (Atopy)

As noted earlier, the overwhelming majority of anaphylactic reactions in man are associated with IgE. Approximately 10 percent of the population inherit a tendency to overproduce IgE, are subject to anaphylactic reactions involving the skin and mucous membranes as a consequence of natural exposure to a wide variety of environmental allergens, and are prime candidates to develop fatal anaphylactic shock after natural or artificial exposure to allergenic materials. Such persons are referred to as *atopics*, the phenomenon is known as *atopy*, and the response to the allergen is designated an *atopic reaction;* the clinical syndrome is appropriately referred to in such terms as atopic dermatitis, atopic rhinitis, and atopic conjunctivitis.

Thus, an estimated 20 million atopics in the United States suffer anaphylactic reactions upon exposure to environmental pollutants, animal or plant products (foods, pollens, dander, feathers, fur, infectious agents, insect secretions), and drugs. In addition, acute episodes of hay fever (atopic or allergic rhinitis) may progress to a chronic and debilitating disease (asthma) characterized by bouts of respiratory distress, overinflation of the lungs, coughing, and rattling or whistling respiratory sounds (rhonchi).

Characteristically, the allergenic material comes into contact with the skin directly or by the airborne route and with the mucous membranes directly or by the airborne route (conjunctiva), following inhalation (respiratory tract), or following ingestion (gastrointestinal tract). Clinical expression of atopic reactions is commonly referable to the portal of entry of the allergen (dermatitis, conjunctivitis, rhinitis, gastrointestinal distress), but there are many exceptions. For example, urticaria (wheal-and-flare reactions, vesicular eruptions of the skin, hives, blisters) may occur from ingestion, inhalation, injection, or direct contact with the antigen. Such considerations and the ensuing discussion emphasize that the atopic state is a generalized rather than a localized condition.

Overproduction of IgE in Atopics Atopics have the genetic capacity to produce plasma concentrations of IgE (1 to 7 μg per milliliter) that are ten times higher than those of normal persons. As indicated by the data included in Table 8-3, a partial explanation for the overproduction of IgE in atopics is based on immuno-

Table 8-3 Association of IgA Deficiency with Atopic Reactions

Population	Immunoglobulin deficiencies	IgA deficiencies	Atopic reactions	Maximal IgA concentration	Age incidence of atopic reaction
Normal subjects	0.16%	0.05%	—	Adult	—
Atopics	7.00%	6.70%	10%	Adult	Increases to adulthood

Source: Adapted from H. S. Kaufman and J. R. Hobbs, *Lancet,* 2:1061–1063, 1970.

logical deficiency in synthesis of IgA. In a normal population 0.16 percent are immunologically deficient, and 0.05 percent have a specific IgA deficiency. When a subpopulation of atopics is examined, 7 percent are immunodeficient, and 6.7 percent have a specific IgA deficiency. Thus, the overall incidence of immunological deficiency among atopics is 44 times that in normal persons, specific IgA deficiency is 134 times that in normal persons, and other immunoglobulin deficiencies (IgG, IgM, IgD, IgE) are less than three times that in normal persons (0.3 percent compared to 0.11 percent).

A theory can be formulated to account for the overproduction of specific IgE in atopics. As noted in Chapter 7, the distribution of gut-dependent lymphocytes having the potential to synthesize IgA and IgE following antigenic stimulation is closely parallel, especially in submucosal areas. IgE-producing cells in normal persons are generally shielded from intensive antigenic stimulation by the far greater number of IgA cells and by secretory IgA, which is uniquely resistant to acid and proteolytic enzymes. However, in atopics the IgA shielding mechanism is not operative, and exposure to antigen results in massive stimulation of IgE cells, elevated plasma concentrations of specific IgE, and fixation of IgE on the surface of target cells throughout the body. In normal persons antigen can escape the secretory IgA surveillance mechanism and make contact with potential IgE-producing cells, but the intensity of the antigenic stimulus is such that synthesis of specific IgE always remains below the threshold level required for an anaphylactic response. In summary, IgA deficiency in atopics is significantly reflected in a paucity of secretory IgA which permits the allergen to reach potential IgE-producing cells unimpeded, thereby causing an exaggerated specific IgE response. When allergenic reexposure occurs, an atopic reaction quickly ensues.

Obviously, the IgA deficiency theory of atopy is an oversimplification of a highly complex phenomenon. However, other possible mechanisms, such as the presence of an excess number of potential IgE-producing cells, greater synthesis of IgE per cell, or more permeable mucosal membranes in atopics, have no experimental basis of support.

The Cells Involved

Several types of cells may become involved in atopic reactions as a consequence of the fixation of IgE to receptor sites on the plasma membrane. Attachment of IgE to the plasma membrane occurs by means of the Fc portion of the molecule. Union of IgE and receptor site thus leaves the IgE allergen-binding sites unobstructed. Experimental observations indicate that the allergen must be at least divalent and must bridge two adjacent IgE molecules to initiate the reaction. Cells prominently involved in anaphylactic responses in man include mast cells, basophils, platelets, neutrophils, and eosinophils. IgE-allergen complexes formed at the surface of the target cell or attaching to the cell after formation elsewhere cause profound effects. Conformational changes induced within the Fc fragment activate the cyclic AMP-adenyl cyclase-phosphodiesterase system and lead to the release of pharmacological mediators from the target cells which amplify the response through action on other surrounding cells and tissues. In man, the target tissues and shock organs most often involved (skin, lungs, gut) contain an abundant supply of mast cells and provide ready access to extrinsic antigenic stimulation.

Pharmacological Mediators

Histamine In man, histamine accounts for the major manifestations of anaphylactic responses. Histamine is found primarily in the granules of the ubiquitous mast cell, in the granules of the circulatory basophil, and in platelets. When released in the skin, histamine is capable of exciting sensory nerves, resulting in burning and itching sensations. In addition, histamine elicits an axon reflex, resulting in dilation of the surrounding arterioles and subsequent hyperemia, producing the flare effect. Histamine also causes contraction of the vascular endothelial cells, resulting in rupture of intercellular joints, increased permeability, and edema, which produces the wheal effect.

Another important pharmacological response induced by histamine is *smooth muscle contraction.* Consequently, histamine can involve diverse tissues, including the vasculature, intestines, uterus, and especially the bronchioles. In addition, histamine is a secretagogue, stimulating secretion by a number of tissues.

Clinical manifestations induced by histamine in man include pain, itching, and wheal-and-flare reactions (urticaria) in the skin; swelling of mucous membranes (turbinates in hay fever, bronchial mucosa in asthma); bronchiolar contraction; pylorospasm; and stimulation of lacrimal, nasal, pulmonary, and digestive secretions. Systemic anaphylactic reactions are associated with pulmonary emphysema, obstructing laryngeal edema, circulatory collapse with a profound drop in blood pressure, and shock. Histamine can be released in lethal quantities, but its half-life is short, and it is susceptible to inactivation and removal by enzymatic oxidation or methylation. Therefore, although it is important during the initial stages of anaphylactic reactions, including fatal shock, histamine cannot be held responsible for the more chronic or prolonged effects of such reactions.

Slow-reacting Substance of Anaphylaxis The importance of a second mediator, slow-reacting substance of anaphylaxis (SRS-A), which causes slow, prolonged contraction of smooth muscle, is becoming increasingly evident. SRS-A probably is composed of at least two substances: (1) One is released from cells by lecithinase A and has the properties of an unsaturated fatty acid similar to prostaglandins; (2) the other is released from sensitized human lung cells after interaction with antigen and is an *acidic lipid* distinct in its characteristics from prostaglandins. The precise structures of these components are not yet known. The pulmonary smooth muscles of man are particularly sensitive to the action of SRS-A.

Experimental animal observations indicate that immunological release of SRS-A can involve either mast cells or neutrophils. IgE-mediated anaphylactic reactions, especially those involving a limited number of soluble IgE-allergen complexes, induce the release of SRS-A from mast cells. Complement-dependent release of SRS-A from neutrophils and mast cells is mediated by soluble antigen-IgG complexes.

In contrast with histamine, smooth muscle contraction induced by SRS-A requires more time to develop, can persist for several hours, and is not relieved or prevented by antihistaminic drugs.

Kinins Kinins are polypeptides which can contract smooth muscle, increase vascular permeability, cause vasodilatation, and produce pain. The kinins are generated from a polypeptide precursor, *kininogen* (serum α-globulin), by enzymes known as *kallikreins*. Plasma kallikrein cleaves off a nonapeptide known as *kallidin I (bradykinin)* from the precursor polypeptide, while tissue kallikrein cleaves off a decapeptide known as *kallidin II (lysyl-bradykinin)*. Kinins have long been implicated in inflammation, and the cascade of kinin formation requires activation of kallikreins which occur as inactive forms, or proenzymes. As with histamine, the kinins are subject to rapid enzymatic inactivation.

Serotonin Serotonin (5-hydroxytryptamine) is found primarily in the mucosal layer of the gastrointestinal tract, in brain tissue, and in platelets. Although serotonin is a potent mediator in systemic anaphylactic responses in rats and mice, in which it causes smooth muscle contraction and increased vascular permeability, its importance in man in this respect is not compelling.

Prostaglandins Fourteen different prostaglandins have been identified in tissues and have been classified into four separate groups: prostaglandins A, B, E, and F (PGA, PGB, PGE, PGF). Antigen-induced release of prostaglandins E and F has been demonstrated in several instances, but their precise role in anaphylactic reactions remains vague. Group E compounds, in particular PGE_1 and PGE_2, are potent smooth muscle relaxants, whereas some group F compounds induce prolonged smooth muscle contraction. On the other hand, prostaglandins E and F can produce vasodilatation. In this connection, PGE_1 and PGE_2 can inhibit the release of histamine and SRS-A, and the effect of PGF_2 has not yet been elucidated.

Eosinophilic Chemotactic Factors The eosinophilic chemotactic factor of anaphylaxis (ECF-A) is probably responsible for the marked eosinophilia observed in many hypersensitive reactions. ECF-A is a small molecule (molecular weight, 500 to 1,000) that is inactivated at 100°C in alkaline solution and is not associated with complement. Another chemotactic factor—the *eosinophilic chemotactic factor of complement* (ECF-C)—represents a split product of C5 (C5a) released during the complement cascade associated with soluble antigen-IgG complexes.

Mechanism of Releasing Pharmacological Mediators

The mechanism by which the pharmacological mediators of anaphylaxis are released is beginning to be unraveled. Apparently, IgE-mediated release of histamine and SRS-A is intimately involved with the adenyl cyclase-phosphodiesterase system of the cells. A number of β-adrenergic agents (epinephrine, isoproterenol) increase the activity of membrane-bound adenyl cyclase which in turn raises intracellular levels of cyclic AMP (cAMP) and inhibits IgE-mediated release of histamine and SRS-A. Cytoplasmic phosphodiesterase normally exerts a controlling effect by breaking down cAMP into 5′-AMP, thus regulating the levels of cAMP. Inhibitors of phosphodiesterase, such as the methylxanthines (theophylline and caffeine), permit a rise in intracellular levels of cAMP and also inhibit IgE-mediated release of histamine and SRS-A. IgE-mediated release of histamine and SRS-A occurs without disruption or destruction of the target cells. Current evidence indicates that IgE-mediated release of histamine from mast cells is an active secretory process triggered by low levels of cAMP (Fig. 8-3).

The role of the eosinophil in the release of mediators remains obscure. However, clinical and experimental studies have demonstrated that eosinophils are intimately involved in reactions associated with the release of histamine. Originally, eosinophils were believed to function

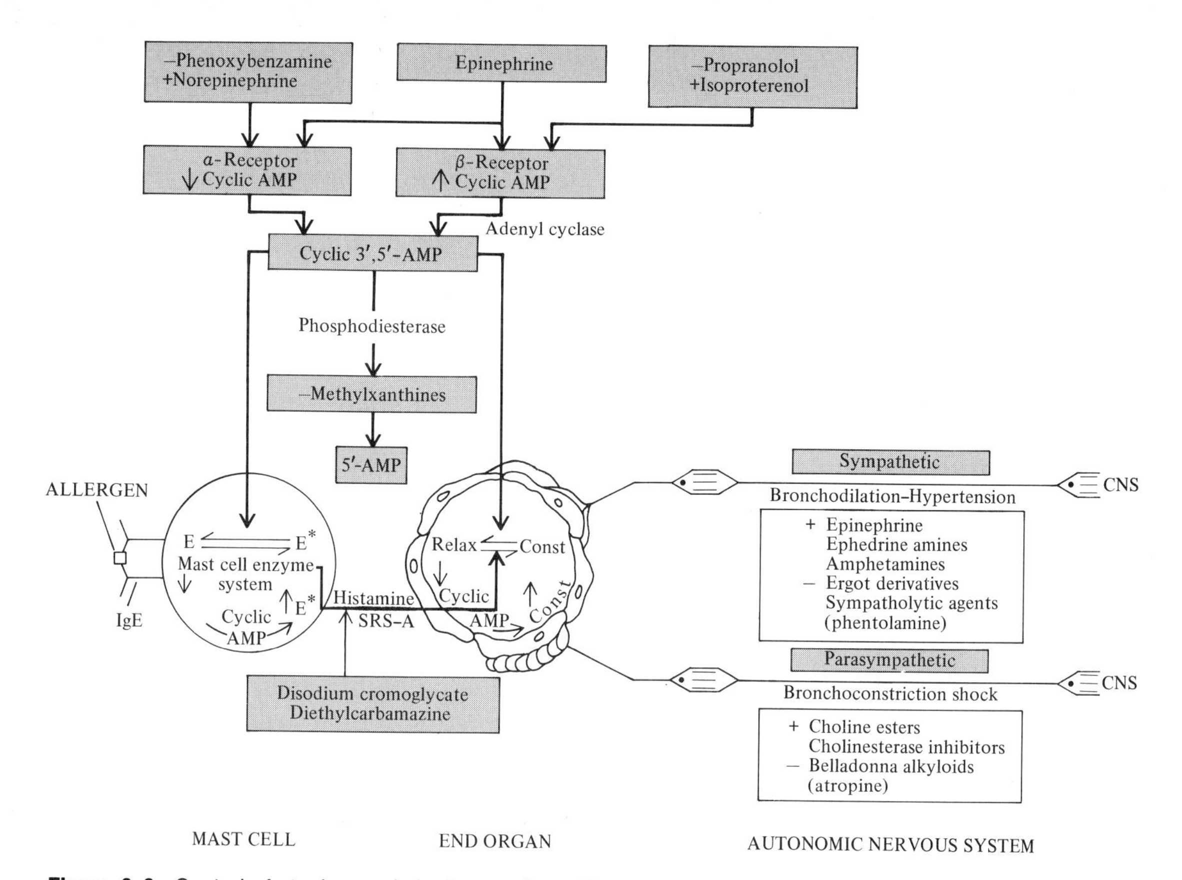

Figure 8-3 Control of atopic-anaphylactic reactions. The end result of unleasing an anaphylactic reaction depends upon the sensitivity of the mast cell to stimulation and the state of excitability of the end organ. Mast cell sensitivity depends upon the amount of IgE receptor available and the level of cyclic AMP; cyclic AMP levels are decreased by stimulation of α-adrenergic receptors and increased by stimulation of β-adrenergic receptors. Decreased cyclic AMP causes formation of active enzyme which increases the sensitivity of the mast cell for release of mediators, while increased cyclic AMP lowers mast cell sensitivity. Similar receptors control cyclic AMP and the level of excitability of the end organ smooth muscle. The magnitude of an anaphylactic reaction may be controlled by drugs which affect α- and β-adrenergic receptors. The excitability of the end organ is also controlled by the autonomic nervous system which provides an additional point at which drugs may be used to influence anaphylactic reactions and a mechanism whereby emotions, via central nervous system (CNS) connections with the autonomic nerves, may modulate anaphylactic reaction. *(From S. Sell, Immunology, Immunopathology and Immunity, Hagerstown, Md., Harper & Row, Publishers, Inc., 1972.)*

as scavengers with a predilection for antigen-antibody complexes and were thought to neutralize histamine, since a substance is present in eosinophilic granules that inhibits histamine. Recently, however, it has been shown that substances released from eosinophils in the area of the anaphylactic reaction can cause the release of histamine from mast cells.

Even less is known concerning the mechanism by which anaphylatoxins I and II effect the release of mediators from mast cells. As noted earlier, the anaphylatoxins are produced as split products of C3 and C5 in the complement cascade set in motion by soluble antigen-IgG complexes.

Therapy

Immunotherapy: Desensitization or Hyposensitization Specific desensitization *(hyposensitization)* is often used in the treatment of atopics, especially those in whom the clinical manifestations of hay fever and asthma due to pollens cannot be controlled effectively by drugs. There are two basic procedures, or mechanisms, involved in specific desensitization, both requiring the injection of allergen in concentrations that fail to induce anaphylactic responses.

Occasionally, in life-threatening emergency situations it is necessary for a physician to administer an antiserum or drug to which the patient is allergic. In the absence of effective alternative therapy, the physician must attempt to desensitize the patient immediately. Under such conditions, specific desensitization consists of a series of carefully graded injections of the allergen every 20 to 60 min., beginning with extremely small doses and continuing over a period of 6 to 8 hr. or until the patient fails to respond to an amount of the allergen equivalent to about one-tenth of the required therapeutic dose. At this point, the full therapeutic dose can be administered. Although this method of densitization removes the threat of anaphylactic shock, it does not obviate the subsequent appearance of a hypersensitive reaction known as *serum sickness.* Caution must prevail at each step in the desensitization procedure, and a syringe containing a solution of epinephrine or Adrenalin must be available in the event that an anaphylactic response develops. Presumably, this emergency desensitization depends upon the slow, gradual, and temporary exhaustion of the intracellular stores of histamine in mast cells.

More commonly, elective desensitization is initiated 3 months before the hay fever season. The offending allergen is given in a series of subcutaneous weekly or biweekly injections, commencing with minute doses of the allergen; dosage is gradually increased, and in many cases, the interval between doses is also increased. As many as 50 injections may be required in order to relieve or eliminate the seasonal clinical manifestations of hay fever, a goal that is realized for 80 to 90 percent of the patients.

An alternative method of elective desensitization employs depot therapy, which involves a single injection of the allergen emulsified in an adjuvant. Slow release of the allergen from the adjuvant leads to continuous antigenic stimulation, thereby achieving the same objective accomplished by serial injections. Unfortunately, the most efficient adjuvants are not metabolizable and result in the formation of sterile abscesses, granulomas, and persistent nodules at the site of injection. Naturally, there is a continuing search for equally potent adjuvants without the harmful side effects of currently available products.

In any event, the efficacy of elective desensitization procedures depends on the anamnestic formation of high plasma concentrations of IgG which function by preventing or reducing interaction of allergen with IgE. Presumably, the allergen combines with IgG in the zone of antibody excess, and the complex fixes complement and is swept away by phagocytic cells, thus precluding contact of the allergen with IgE.

Drug Therapy While prophylaxis is the more desirable goal, alleviation of the manifestations of atopic reactions remains the bulwark of clinical medicine. The most common drugs used for treatment of atopic reactions are antihistaminic drugs which specifically antagonize the effects of histamine. Corticosteroids are efficient in controlling many manifestations of hypersensitivity, but in view of serious side effects, prolonged therapy should be reserved for conditions which are refractory to other therapeutic regimens such as asthma. Diethylcarbamazine, a compound that interferes with the formation and release of SRS-A from sensitized cells, is promising as a prototype anti-SRS-A agent, if not as a therapeutic tool. Disodium cromoglycate is effective in reducing asthmatic responses in sensitized persons and appears to function by preventing release of the pharmacological mediators of anaphylaxis even after the allergen has adsorbed onto target cells. β-adrenergic catecholamines (epinephrine, isoproterenol, ephedrine) are active bronchodilators and provide rapid and dramatic relief of asthma and are the most potent available drugs for the treatment of anaphylactic shock.

Avoidance Therapy The most obvious and rational approach to prevention and control of atopic reactions is for the patient to avoid contact with the offending allergen(s). Avoidance therapy is highly effective in the case of food and drug allergens and in allergens associated with clothing, household furnishings, and bedding manufactured from plant or animal products. Avoiding contact with the allergen is less effective where arthropod bites and stings are concerned and is rarely practical where infectious agents, pollens, and other airborne particles (dust containing allergens) are concerned. Nonetheless, it is often surprising how much progress can be achieved in reducing the intensity of atopic reactions induced by atmospheric pollutants by modifying the process of household cleaning, by substituting hot water or radiant heating for forced air heating, by sleeping in a filtered, air-conditioned room, and by living in an appropriately humidified environment.

TYPE II: CYTOLYTIC AND CYTOTOXIC RESPONSES

Cytolytic and cytotoxic reactions induced by allergens can lead to the lysis of cells *(cytolysis)* or to the death of cells without lysis *(cytotoxicity)*. The formed elements of the blood—erythrocytes, leukocytes, and platelets—are especially prone to cytolytic and cytotoxic reactions. The antigens involved are membrane components (blood group antigens, for example) or haptens that conjugate directly with the cellular membrane or complex first with plasma proteins and then attach to the membrane.

Haptens involved in cytolytic and cytotoxic reactions frequently include drugs such as quinidine, amidopyrine, chlorpromazine, penicillin, chloramphenicol, and sulfonamides. Occasionally, haptenic sensitization affects more than one cell type, but more commonly a single cell type becomes the target. Cell destruction requires the continued presence of the drug, and when administration of the drug is halted, recovery ensues but may be somewhat delayed.

In terms of mechanism, antibodies may already have been formed against the antigen, as occurs in blood transfusion reactions, or antibodies may be formed against extraneously introduced cross-reacting membrane antigens or against membranes modified by interaction with drugs (hapten-carrier complexes). The antibodies involved are primarily IgG and IgM, which can fix complement. Since the union of antigen and antibody takes place at cell surfaces, the activation of the complement cascade leads to damage of those cells which accommodate the reaction. The complement-damaged cells can undergo intravascular and extravascular destruction. Usually, intravascular destruction is the direct result of complement-mediated lysis. Extravascular destruction of the opsonized cells occurs primarily in the spleen, liver, and lungs.

The cells are sequestered within the scavenger reticuloendothelial cells of these organs, immunologically mediated lysis presumably ensues, and metabolic disposition of the destroyed cells takes place.

Type II responses in man include blood transfusion reactions in which blood group antigens in erythrocyte membranes are the inciting factors, hemolytic disease of the newborn in which Rh antigen on fetal and neonatal erythrocytes is the target of maternally formed antibodies, and drug-induced hemolytic anemias, leukopenias, and thrombocytopenias.

TYPE III: IMMUNE COMPLEX RESPONSES OR IMMUNE COMPLEX DISEASES

The Arthus Reaction

One of the type III prototype reactions can be provoked when a sensitized person with a high titer of circulating antibody is reinjected with the antigen (Arthus reaction). The antibodies involved are of the IgG class that can precipitate with antigen and fix and activate complement. The requirement for a high titer of precipitating antibody indicates that the person has experienced one or more anamnestic responses to the antigen before becoming actively sensitized.

Arthus reactions in sensitized persons vary, depending on the route of administration and the dose of the antigen. For example, following intradermal injection of the antigen, a focal area of inflammation and necrosis can develop in 6 to 12 hr. (cutaneous Arthus reaction). Following intravascular injection of the antigen, focal inflammatory and necrotic areas can appear in several tissues and organs in 6 to 12 hr. (systemic Arthus reaction). When the antigen is injected by other routes (subcutaneous, intramuscular, intraperitoneal), both the extent and the distribution of the lesions closely correspond to the dose.

The focal inflammatory reactions vary in severity and may progress from hyperemia to erythema to edema to hemorrhage and necrosis. The histopathology and chronology of the sequence are characteristic of Arthus reactions. Although all the mechanisms involved in the Arthus phenomenon are not yet fully established, a closer examination of the process does provide insight into the genesis of the reaction.

Formation of Microprecipitates Introduction of the antigen into a sensitized person with a high titer of antibody results in the formation of antigen-antibody complexes of varying size, some of which deposit in the tissues. Experimental evidence indicates that only the larger complexes are capable of depositing in the manner characteristic of the Arthus reaction, i.e., in the form of *microprecipitates* (Fig. 8-4). As indicated earlier, IgG subclasses capable of fixing complement play an important role. Fixation and activation of complement trigger off the sequence, leading to the development of typical lesions.

Initially, deposits of acidophilic material are found in the lumina and walls of blood vessels and are accompanied by local disturbances of the microcirculation, including hyperemia, edema, erythema, and hemostasis. The early changes are transient in appearance and are probably caused by complement-mediated, anaphylatoxin-induced release of histamine from mast cells, and/or by IgE-mediated action. In addition, activation of enzymes such as sulfhydryl (SH)-dependent proteases may lead to the release of vasoactive peptides from tissue and cellular substrates or the release of kinins from plasma substrates. The resulting increased permeability allows the immune complexes to pass between endothelial cells and lodge along the basement membrane of the blood vessels as well as in the lumen and on the endothelial surface.

The Role of Complement In addition to its role in the formation of anaphylatoxins and the release of histamine and other mediators, complement is associated with the generation of chemotactic substances (anaphylatoxin II or C5a and C$\overline{5, 6, 7}$) which cause a large influx of

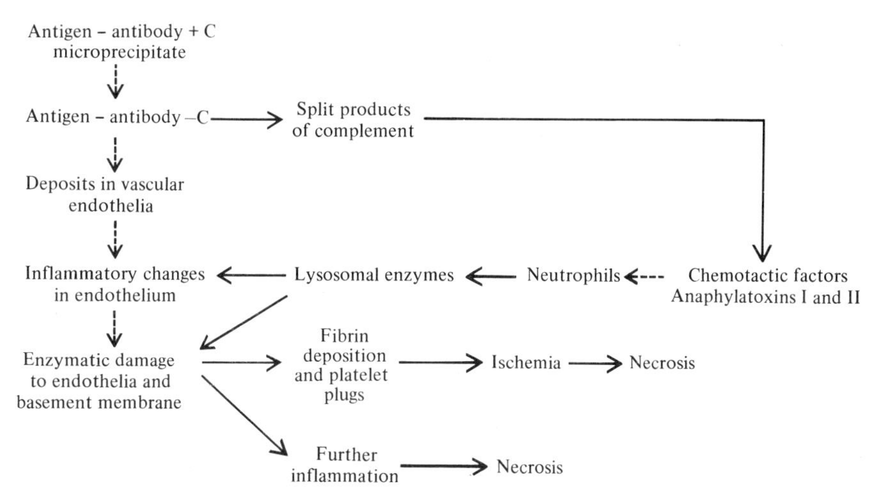

Figure 8-4 A flow diagram of the interactions between antigen-antibody reactions, inflammation, blood-clotting mechanisms, and necrosis.

neutrophils into the areas containing the microprecipitates. The neutrophils adhere to the precipitated complexes (immune adherence), to other neutrophils, and to the endothelial cells lining the lumen. Changes in the endothelial cell surfaces resulting from the action of enzymes tend to make the surface sticky. Thus, after passing through the interendothelial spaces, neutrophils lodge along the basement membrane.

The Role of Neutrophils in Releasing Lysosomal Enzymes The accumulating neutrophils begin to ingest the microprecipitates deposited on the endothelial cells and along the basement membrane. Some neutrophils die after ingesting relatively large numbers of antigen-antibody complexes and release lysosomal enzymes into the surrounding milieu. Other neutrophils, while not succumbing to the ingestion of antigen-antibody complexes, also release hydrolytic enzymes as a result of heightened phagocytic activity.

The release of lysosomal enzymes leads to amplification of the response. Acidic and neutral proteases released from lysosomes can act on serum and tissue substrates to release peptide mediators which, along with the mediators generated by the fixation of complement, increase the vigor and scope of the reaction. Many of the released enzymes (proteases, lipases, lecithinases) attack and destroy endothelial cells lining the blood vessels, exposing connective tissue in the walls of the blood vessels. The exposed connective tissue can activate platelets which can subsequently clump and form platelet plugs in the smaller blood vessels. Concomitantly, activation of the blood-clotting cascade through the action of lysosomal enzymes and through surface activation by exposed connective tissue elements results in the formation of fibrin. The combined effect of the fibrin and platelet plugs leads to occlusion of the smaller blood vessels, resulting in ischemia and necrosis (Fig. 8-5).

Serum Sickness

The Classical Syndrome About 70 years ago von Pirquet and Schick described another immune complex prototype reaction that appeared

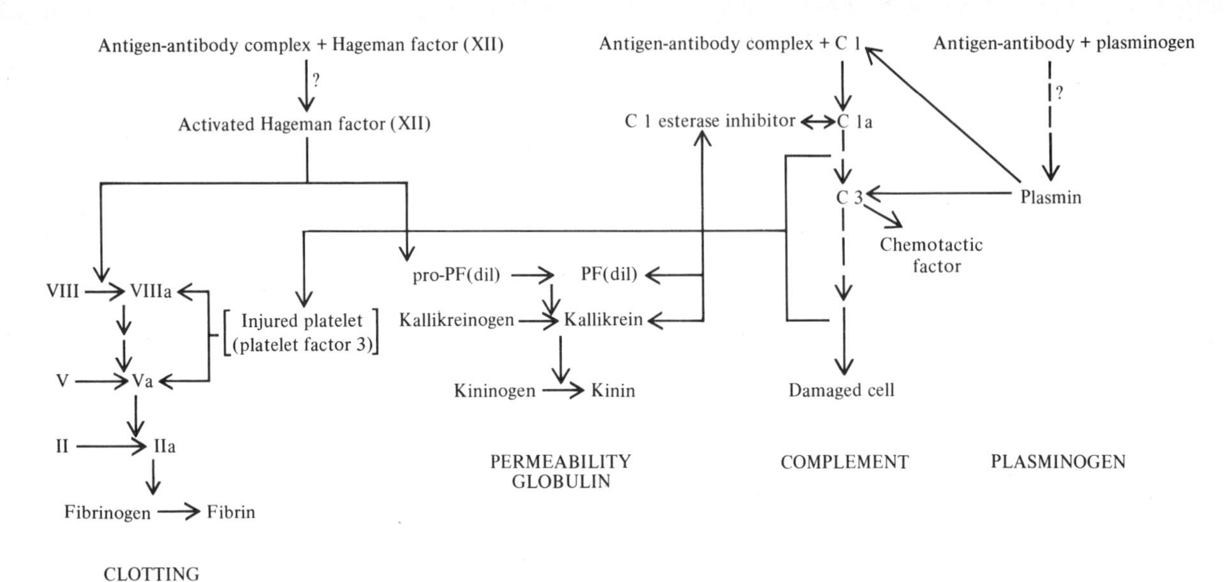

Figure 8-5 Interrelations of antigen-antibody activated enzyme systems. (*From E. L. Becker, Proc. R. Soc. Med., 173:383-392, 1969.*)

7 to 12 days following a single injection of a high concentration of foreign serum protein. Serum sickness can be induced by a variety of antigens and haptens, especially by drugs, and the syndrome includes arthritis, glomerulonephritis, vasculitis, neuritis, myocarditis, endocarditis, skin eruptions, fever, lymphadenopathy, abdominal pain, nausea, and vomiting.

Since the turn of the century the incidence of serum sickness has largely paralleled the therapeutic and prophylactic use of tetanus, diphtheria, and other antitoxins and pneumococcal, meningococcal, *Hemophilus influenzae,* and other antisera. Effective use of these reagents necessitated the injection of large amounts of antiserum or serum fractions, which were frequently prepared in horses. Serious untoward reactions often developed, sometimes in the majority of patients. With the development of active immunization and chemotherapy, the demand for antiserum therapy abated, and the incidence of serum sickness declined. However, antiserum prepared in horses is still utilized in counteracting intoxication with botulinum toxin and snake venoms, in rabies prophylaxis, and in therapy of gas gangrene. More recently, the increasing use of horse antihuman lymphocyte serum as an immunosuppressive adjunct in organ and tissue transplantation has again made serum sickness a cause for concern. In addition, the widespread use of penicillin, sulfonamides, tetracyclines, aspirin, barbiturates, phenylethylhydantoin, iodides, thiouracil, and other drugs is responsible for many current cases of serum sickness.

The Immune Elimination Curve If a normal previously unexposed person is injected intravenously with a high concentration of the antigen (e.g., 10 ml of horse serum) and is monitored periodically for antigen, antibody, and complement levels in the blood from the time of injection, through the development of clinical manifestations, to the complete subsidence of the disease, it is possible to correlate the dynamics of the humoral immune response to the antigen with the development and subsidence of the disease (Fig. 8-6). Typically, the onset of serum sickness occurs 7 to 12 days after injection of the antigen and is characterized by fever, urticaria, lymphadenopathy, myalgia, and arthritic manifestations. Concomitantly, or shortly thereafter, glomerulonephritis and vasculitis appear.

Immune elimination of the antigen and the formation of antibody are positively correlated with the development of the syndrome (Fig. 8-6). The antigen equilibrates between the vascular and intravascular compartments, and metabolism of the antigen proceeds. Shortly thereafter, antigenic stimulation of immunocompetent cells is initiated, and antibody production commences. In spite of steady metabolic elimination of the antigen, antibody production begins when there is a large excess of antigen in the blood. As the antibody concentration in the circulation rises, more and larger soluble antigen-antibody (IgG) complexes are formed, still in antigen excess. As antibody production and immune complex formation continue, increasing quantities of complement are activated and fixed, leading to a fall in the plasma concentration of complement.

Even though the immune complexes are soluble, the fixation of complement causes them to adhere to cellular elements of the blood and probably to the endothelial lining of the smaller vessels. In addition, the filtering action of the kidneys leads to accumulation of the complexes in the glomeruli. The antigen-antibody-complement complexes thus become inflammatory foci scattered throughout the tissues and infiltrated with neutrophils.

With the continued rise in antibody production the complexes increase in size and become more amenable to phagocytosis by infiltrating

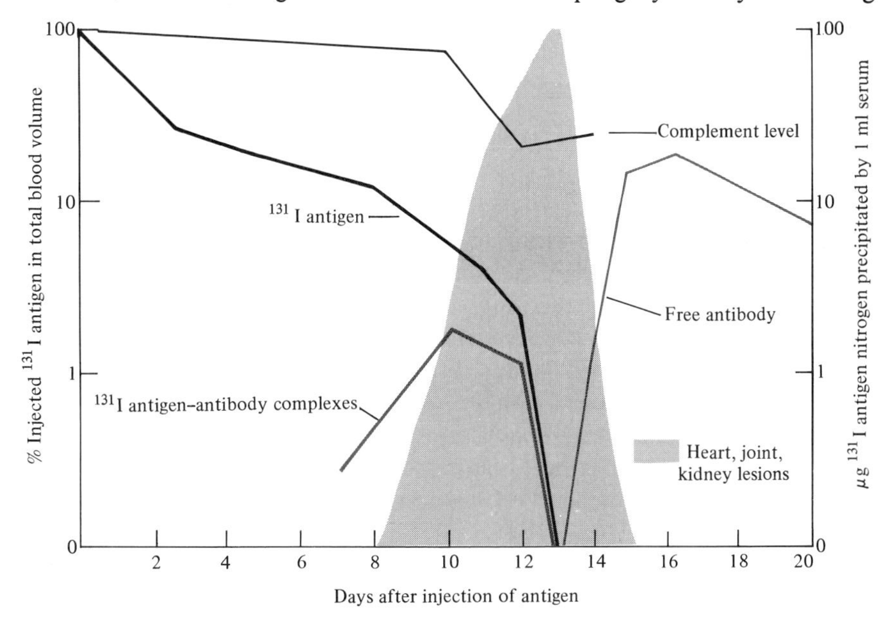

Figure 8-6 The immune elimination curve. The sequence of events in classic "one-shot" serum sickness parallels the record of an experiment involving injection of ^{131}I-labeled bovine serum albumin into a rabbit. As detectable antigen-antibody complexes appear in the circulation, complement drops to less than half normal values, morphological lesions appear in heart, blood vessels, joints, and kidneys. Shortly after all antigen-antibody complexes are eliminated, free antibody appears in circulation, and inflammatory lesions rapidly disappear. (*From F. J. Dixon, Harvey Lect., 58:21–52, 1963.*)

neutrophils and eosinophils. This leads to a more rapid and efficient removal of the immune complexes from the system. Thereafter, the inflammatory lesions gradually disappear, the complexes are eliminated, and free antibody appears in the serum. As the titer of free antibody rises in the serum, the manifestations of serum sickness rapidly subside, usually without serious sequelae. Precisely, the elimination of the immune complexes as foci of inflammation causes subsidence of the disease.

The Role of IgE Both IgG and IgE have been implicated in serum sickness. Urticaria (wheal-and-flare skin reactions) is a frequent component of the syndrome, and it is believed to be a manifestation of IgE-antigen interaction. Presumably, mediators released by the interaction of antigen with IgE fixed on the surface of mast cells initiate edema, thus enhancing the inflammatory response. On the other hand, the vasculitis and arthritis resemble the Arthus reaction and are due to antigen-IgG mediation which activates the complement cascade and leads to an influx of neutrophils.

Accelerated and Immediate Serum Sickness If a person has had prior contact with the antigen or hapten and has produced IgG which has subsequently disappeared from the circulation, reinjection of the antigen or hapten may initiate an anamnestic response and a more rapid development of the syndrome in 3 to 6 days (accelerated serum sickness). In accord with the nature of the anamnestic response, a lower concentration of antigen or hapten will suffice to induce the accelerated response.

If by virtue of prior contact with the antigen or hapten a person has a high concentration of circulating IgG at the time the antigen or hapten is reinjected, anaphylactic shock (immediate serum sickness) may develop within a few minutes. Obviously, the clinical manifestations of immediate serum sickness are distinct from and more severe than those encountered in serum sickness or accelerated serum sickness. In terms of mechanism, immediate serum sickness is a form of aggregate anaphylaxis mediated by IgG and complement and is appropriately considered a type I response.

TYPE IV: DELAYED HYPERSENSITIVITY RESPONSES

In man, delayed hypersensitivity represents a category of immune responses that is an integral accompaniment of most, if not all, microbial infections, is critically involved in contact dermatitis, is the principal mechanism of graft rejection (Chap. 10), is the underlying basis for the pathogenesis of the majority of autoimmune diseases (Chap. 11), and is an important factor in recovery from intracellular infections (cell-mediated immunity). Less certain and remaining controversial is the role which delayed hypersensitivity may play in the pathogenesis of disease processes initiated by microorganisms.

When an antigen or hapten is injected intradermally into an appropriately sensitized person, the reaction becomes apparent in 5 to 24 hr. and may show progressive changes for 2 to 3 days or more. The hallmark of delayed hypersensitivity is the appearance of *induration,* a raised, firm, hard area at the site of injection involving T lymphocytes and macrophages and usually surrounded by erythema. Increasing tissue damage may result in a definite area of necrosis which is followed by healing and repair and in severe reactions, scarring.

Systemic reactions may ensue if a sufficiently large amount of antigen enters the circulation of a sensitized person. In man, the clinical signs include leukopenia and fever developing in 8 hr. and subsiding 24 hr. after moderate doses of antigen. At high antigen concentration, leukopenia and fever may occur in 2 to 3 hr. and may be followed by general malaise, hypothermia, increasing prostration, and death.

Induction

The Antigen Induction of delayed hypersensitivity is strongly influenced by the concentration and physical state of the antigen, the route by which the antigen enters the body, and whether or not the antigen is present within an inflammatory focus. For example, a vigorous antibody response will develop when a soluble protein antigen is injected intravenously, but little or no delayed hypersensitivity will be induced. On the other hand, both delayed hypersensitivity and antibody formation will result if the same quantities of antigen are injected by any route into an active inflammatory focus produced by an irritant such as turpentine. When the physical state of the antigen is altered by adsorption on aluminum hydroxide precipitates, delayed hypersensitivity and antibody formation are induced more efficiently by a variety of routes including intramuscular injection.

The most efficient way to induce delayed hypersensitivity is to incorporate the antigen into an adjuvant complex containing water-in-oil emulsions with or without killed microorganisms or endotoxins (Chap. 7). In addition to enhancing antibody production, adjuvants will stimulate the development of delayed hypersensitivity to soluble protein antigens by any route. In terms of promoting the induction of delayed hypersensitivity, adjuvants presumably function by localizing the antigen within an inflammatory focus and by limiting the rate of release of the antigen. In these respects, an adjuvant creates an environment similar to that encountered in most microbial infections which are accompanied by delayed hypersensitivity.

Pure Delayed Hypersensitivity Responses Analysis of the mechanisms involved in the induction of delayed hypersensitivity is complicated by the concurrent formation of antibody. However, the difficulty can be circumvented by several procedures which permit the induction of delayed hypersensitivity in the absence of antibody production *(pure delayed hypersensitivity responses)*. For example, if a highly purified soluble protein antigen is injected in minute concentration (fraction of a microgram) by the intradermal route, pure delayed hypersensitivity will result. Other appropriate methods include the intradermal or subcutaneous injection of antigen-antibody precipitates formed in antibody excess or the inclusion of soluble or insoluble antigen-antibody complexes in an adjuvant. Another procedure involves the injection of proteins heavily conjugated with hapten; this leads to the induction of delayed hypersensitivity to the protein and the formation of antibody specific for the hapten. In addition, some proteins such as gelatin present a limited number of determinant groups to the immune system and are virtually nonimmunogenic in terms of producing antibody. However, gelatin can elicit delayed hypersensitivity uncomplicated by the presence of antibody.

Antigenic Determinants: Number and Size Although the procedures for eliciting pure delayed responses appear to be diverse, there is a common operating denominator which serves to reduce the number of antigenic determinants available at any given point in time for stimulation of the immune system. In general, delayed hypersensitivity requires a smaller immunogenic stimulus than does antibody formation. Fractions of a microgram of the antigen can induce a delayed response, whereas hundreds of micrograms or even milligram quantities of the antigen are needed for antibody production.

The size of the antigenic determinant responsible for inducing delayed hypersensitivity is larger than that required to produce antibody. For example, in experiments involving a series of related peptides of increasing size as haptens, it was found that a peptide of hexamer size had 96 percent of the antibody-binding capacity of the heptameric peptide, but only the heptamer could induce a delayed response. Thus, the size of the determinant group required for induction of delayed hypersensitivity is exquisitely and critically dependent on the addition of a single amino acid.

Carrier Specificity In addition to providing evidence of the need for a larger antigenic determinant, studies of hapten-protein conjugates have revealed that the specificity of delayed hypersensitivity is a function of both hapten and carrier. For example, when a hapten used for sensitization is coupled to a different carrier, the new hapten-carrier complex will fail to elicit a delayed response; whereas the original hapten-carrier conjugate will induce a typical delayed reaction, thus demonstrating the role of carrier specificity in delayed hypersensitivity. The accumulated data indicate that the larger antigenic determinant essential for inducing delayed hypersensitivity is composed of both hapten and carrier (Fig. 8-7).

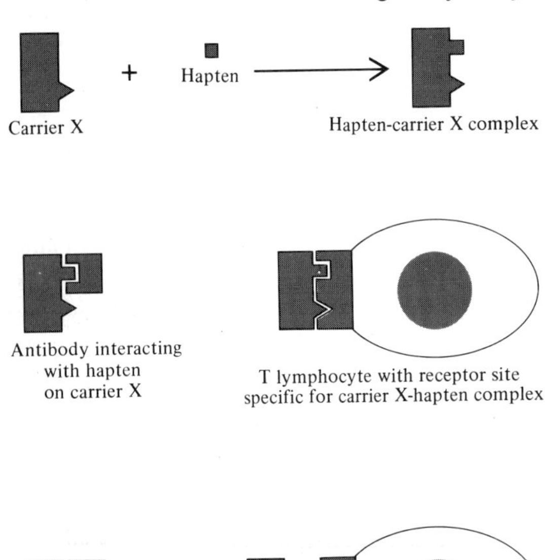

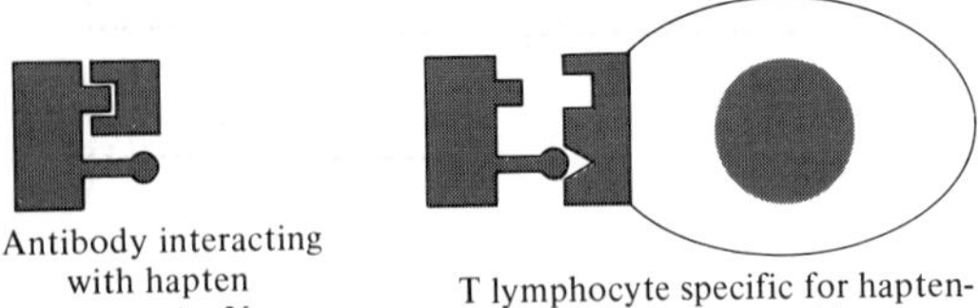

Figure 8-7 Schematic presentation of the specificity of T lymphocytes for hapten-carrier complexes.

Adjuvant-induced Delayed Hypersensitivity As noted earlier, adjuvants facilitate the induction of delayed reactions. When an antigen is incorporated in a water-in-oil emulsion containing killed tubercle bacilli (Freund's complete adjuvant), delayed hypersensitivity can be induced toward both the antigen and the tubercle bacilli. A more detailed examination of tubercle bacilli has shown that wax D is the active component involved in the adjuvant-induced response.

In terms of presumed mechanism, the adjuvant stimulates an inflammatory response at the site of injection which involves an influx of cells, including circulating immunocompetent T lymphocytes, which represent the key to the reaction. With time the inflammatory reaction provides a greater opportunity for more and more T cells to come in contact with and respond specifically to the antigen. Concomitantly, the slow release of antigen from the adjuvant complex limits the number of determinant groups available at any given point in time for stimulation of T cells. Consequently, delayed hypersensitivity develops before antibody production can be detected. On the basis of these and other observations, several investigators suggest that delayed hypersensitivity is one step in the production of antibody and that adjuvants, by increasing the inflammatory reaction, enhance or exaggerate the delayed response at the expense of antibody formation.

Histopathology

A closer examination of the sequential development of induration, the hallmark of a delayed response following intradermal injection of antigen into a sensitized person, provides greater insight into the mechanisms involved. Within a few hours increased vascular permeability leads to the leakage of fluid from dermal and subdermal vessels. Although the increased permeability closely resembles that induced by mediators of anaphylactic responses such as histamine, it cannot be inhibited by antihistamines.

In the first 3 to 4 hr. and particularly in the more severe reactions, the influx of neutrophils is similar to that encountered in Arthus reactions. Thereafter, the proportion of lymphocytes and macrophages in the infiltrate escalates rapidly. At 24 hr. macrophages predominate (80 percent) and continue to increase in proportion to other cells for another 24 to 72 hr. Thus induration is caused by a massive infiltration of cells, especially of macrophages.

Contact Dermatitis

A specialized and clinically significant form of delayed hypersensitivity can be induced and elicited by exposure of the skin to a large number and wide variety of low molecular weight compounds (contact dermatitis). Many of the active materials are organic chemicals and solvents used in industrial processes or present in cosmetics, drugs, or plant products (poison ivy, poison sumac). In addition, contact dermatitis can be caused by divalent metallic ions such as nickel and beryllium. None of the active components are antigenic unless combined with carrier proteins, in which case they act as haptens.

Recent experimental studies are instructive in illustrating the mechanism whereby contact dermatitis is produced. If guinea pig skin is painted with dinitrochlorobenzene (DNCB), and the animal is reexposed to the same compound a few weeks later, a typical delayed hypersensitivity reaction will develop at the challenge site. When the experiment is repeated with ^{14}C-labeled DNCB, the fate of the compound can be followed sequentially. The results indicate that DNCB penetrates into cutaneous structures probably via the pores and/or its solubility in lipids and into other tissues. Twenty percent of the radioactive label is excreted in the urine, 75 percent is disseminated into noncutaneous tissues, and 5 percent remains in the skin where it is present largely as residues of 2,4-dinitrophenyllysine and S-dinitrophenylcysteine in epidermal proteins. The delayed hypersensitivity response is specifically directed toward the hapten-carrier complex composed of the altered epidermal protein with the attached dinitrophenyl groups.

Extensions of such experiments have disclosed the following:

1 The active chemicals must conjugate with epidermal proteins, forming covalent bonds.
2 Contact dermatitis shows carrier specificity, since the response can be elicited only with identical hapten-carrier protein complexes.
3 Intact lymphatic pathways between the skin and regional lymph nodes are essential, indicating that hapten-epidermal protein conjugates are transported to the nodes and/or that sensitized cells travel to and from the site and the nodes.
4 Similar delayed reactions can be induced in mucous membranes as well as in skin.

The Cells Involved

From the preceding discussions it is evident that the cellular component is the major factor involved in delayed hypersensitivity. The critical role of cells was demonstrated in 1940 by Landsteiner and Chase who found that delayed hypersensitivity could be transferred with viable cells but not with serum from a sensitized person. Since then it has been shown that the cells actually involved in transferring delayed sensitivity are the circulating small lymphocytes (T lymphocytes).

Upon receipt of sensitized T lymphocytes, a normal person will respond to the antigen with a typical delayed hypersensitivity reaction. Furthermore, mixtures of sensitized T cells and antigen injected locally in normal persons elicit a delayed response. Transfer of delayed sensitivity by T cells is called *adoptive immunity* and clearly illustrates that delayed hypersensitivity is dependent upon the interaction of T cells with antigen. Thus T cells are the key to the immunological specificity of the delayed response and the initiator of subsequent events associated with the response.

The work of numerous investigators indicates that T cells combine with antigen by means of specific receptor sites on the surface. The receptors probably are integral components of the T cell membrane and resemble immunoglobulins but have not actually been identified as immunoglobulins of any of the known classes. Receptors are present in T cells that have never been exposed to antigen. According to *clonal selection theory,* receptor sites on previously unsensitized T cells are precommitted to combine specifically with one or, at most, a few antigenic determinants. Whenever the receptors react with the proper determinants, that T cell will become sensitized. Thereafter, when a sensitized T cell reacts with the specific determinant, a delayed response will be initiated which involves blastogenesis and at least limited cellular division of the T cell in the regional node.

The small lymphocytes involved in delayed hypersensitivity are of thymic origin and are long-lived cells that comprise 90 percent or more of the circulating lymphocyte pool. In the course of circulation through the body, the T cells cycle several times daily by leaving their position in the paracortical areas of lymphoid tissue, entering the blood by way of efferent vessels, passing through the endothelial cells lining the walls of postcapillary vessels into the tissue spaces, traversing the lymphatic channels into the lymphatic ducts, and returning to the lymphoid centers.

Antigen may interact with appropriate T cells in a number of ways. For example, circulating T cells with specific receptor sites may combine with the antigen at a peripheral site; T cells in the regional node may react with antigen coming there through the draining lymphatics; or T cells in lymphatic tissue throughout the body may filter out antigen that has escaped into the circulation. Wherever the interaction occurs, the T cells undergo blastogenesis and cellular division which results in the production of specifically sensitized cells and expansion of the number of reactive T cells. From the blastogenetic centers the sensitized T cells can enter the circulation, seed other lymphatic tissues, or accumulate at sites where the antigen is deposited or injected.

Although T cells hold the key to the development of delayed hypersensitivity which cannot develop in their absence, they represent but a small fraction of the total cellular response to the antigen. The predominant cell is the macrophage which accumulates primarily in perivascular areas at the site of antigenic deposits. The macrophages are derived from blood monocytes which pass between vascular endothelial cells in response to antigenic challenge. In passing from the blood to the tissue spaces, the macrophages increase in size, number of mitochondria, number of granules that appear dense in phase contrast microscopy, capacity to take up neutral red dye, phagocytic activity, number of lysosomes, and concentration of acid hydrolases and are referred to as activated macrophages.

Lymphokines and the Mechanisms of Cell Recruitment and Tissue Damage

Statement of the Problem Numerous studies utilizing histopathological, autoradiographic, and electron microscopic techniques have established that during the course of a delayed hypersensitivity response the accumulation of specifically sensitized small lymphocytes is by no means striking. On the other hand, the reaction site is massively infiltrated with cells, preponderantly composed of macrophages. How can a minute amount of antigen trigger such a massive cellular response? Why are so many cells attracted to the site when so few cells are specifically sensitized to the antigen? What signals are released that can account for a sequence of events that leads to necrosis in response to a minute concentration of antigen? In essence the problem is one of recruitment and activation of large numbers of cells capable of reacting specifically with the antigen. The answer is associated with the specific release of lymphokines from sensitized T cells in response to antigenic stimulation. Thus, lymphokines are the mediators of delayed hypersensitivity and are the factors responsible for recruitment of cells and eventually for the subsequent tissue damage.

Lymphokines Responsible for Immunological Specificity

Dialyzable Transfer Factor An important breakthrough occurred in 1954 when Lawrence and his associates found that killed cells or cell extracts of sensitized human lymphocytes could transfer specific sensitivity to a normal person and labeled this active component the transfer factor. Sensitivity transferred in this manner persisted for months or years. Subsequent studies have partially characterized this transfer factor (Table 8-4) and have demonstrated that it can be released from sensitized T cells by freezing and thawing and by mechanical pressure.

The effect of this transfer factor is not restricted to the site of injection but leads to a generalized state of sensitivity in the recipient in a matter of hours with maximal sensitivity being achieved in a few days. The action of transfer factor is not evident until the recipient is challenged with specific antigen and responds with a typical delayed reaction.

In vitro studies of the effect of transfer factor on normal lymphocytes are particularly instructive. Addition of transfer factor to the lymphocytes produces no discernible response. However, if specific antigen is added to the mixture of transfer factor and normal lymphocytes, approximately 5 percent of the cells undergo blastogenesis. The transformation of normal lymphocytes to blast cells in the presence of transfer factor and antigen can be elicited only by the antigen that sensitized the lymphocytes from

Table 8-4 Some Properties of Dialyzable Transfer Factor

Biological	Biochemical	Immunological
Properties of whole extract: Prompt onset (hours); Long duration (> 1 year); Equal intensity	Soluble, dialyzable, lyophilizable	Not an immunoglobulin
Dissociable from transplantation antigens	Molecular weight < 10,000	Not immunogenic
Small quantities yield magnified effects	No protein, albumin, α- or γ-globulin	Immunologically specific
	Orcinol positive	Converts normal lymphocytes in vitro and in vivo to antigen-responsive state
	Polypeptide/polynucleotide composition	Transformation and clonal proliferation of converted lymphocytes exposed to antigen
	Inactivated at 56°C for 30 min.	Informational molecule/derepressor/receptor site
	Resists pancreatic RNase	
	Retains potency (5 years)	

Source: H. S. Lawrence, *Adv. Immunol.*, 11:195, 1969.

which the transfer factor was extracted, thus indicating that transfer factor is extremely specific in the information it transfers to normal lymphocytes. Consequently, the key function of transfer factor is to confer immunological specificity to recipient lymphocytes, thereby magnifying the pool of sensitized lymphocytes.

In vivo experiments correlate well with the in vitro data. When transfer factor is injected into a normal person, he will respond with a delayed hypersensitivity reaction when challenged intradermally with the specific antigen. In addition, when lymphocytes are removed at a later date from the recipient of the transfer factor and are exposed to the antigen in vitro, they will undergo blastogenesis, an indication that the recipient lymphocytes had been sensitized in vivo by transfer factor.

As indicated by the properties included in Table 8-4, dialyzable transfer factor is a nonimmunogenic molecule of small size which can convey immunologically specific information; this is demonstrated when it converts normal lymphocytes in vitro and in vivo to an antigen-responsive state. The fact that dialyzable transfer factor can be released in 30 to 60 min. from sensitized lymphocytes exposed to specific antigen suggests that it is a preformed molecule. Although the precise chemical composition of transfer factor has not yet been determined, likely candidates are a short chain, protease-resistant polypeptide or a short, double-stranded, RNase-resistant RNA fragment or a combination of polypeptide and RNA. Some investigators have speculated that transfer factor may act as a *derepressor*.

Nondialyzable Transfer Factor With the discovery and partial characterization of the dialyzable transfer factor interest in the small lymphocyte gathered momentum. Within the past several years more than a dozen lymphokines have been detected following antigenic stimulation of sensitized T cells. In addition, it has been found that lymphokines can be released from sensitized small lymphocytes by mitogenic agents such as plant lectins.

As noted earlier, dialyzable transfer factor is released in 30 to 60 min. when sensitized lymphocytes are challenged with the antigen. If incubation of cells and antigen is continued for 24 hr., a nondialyzable transfer factor is released which is synthesized by the cell after exposure to the antigen. When tested in vitro, nondialyzable transfer factor is potent in converting normal lymphocytes to an antigen-responsive state. Whereas dialyzable transfer factor can convert 5 percent of normal lymphocytes to an antigen-responsive state, nondialyzable transfer factor (lymphocyte transforming factor) can convert 20 percent of a normal lymphocyte population to the antigen-responsive state. Little is known concerning the physical and chemical properties of nondialyzable transfer factor and its activity in vivo. A diagrammatic comparison of some of the properties of dialyzable and nondialyzable transfer factors is included in Figure 8-8.

RNA Transfer Factor Evidence indicates that RNA extracts prepared from the lymph nodes of sensitized persons are capable of converting normal lymphocytes to an antigen-responsive state. The biological activity is associated with RNA fractions in the 8S to 18S range and is sensitive to RNase and phosphodiesterase. Active preparations are free of dialyzable transfer factor, but their in vivo function has not yet been determined.

Evaluation of Transfer Factors in Delayed Hypersensitivity Responses

Each of the three transfer factors discussed above has the unique capacity to transfer immunologically specific information to normal lymphocytes in the absence of antigen. Detection of the information transfer depends upon

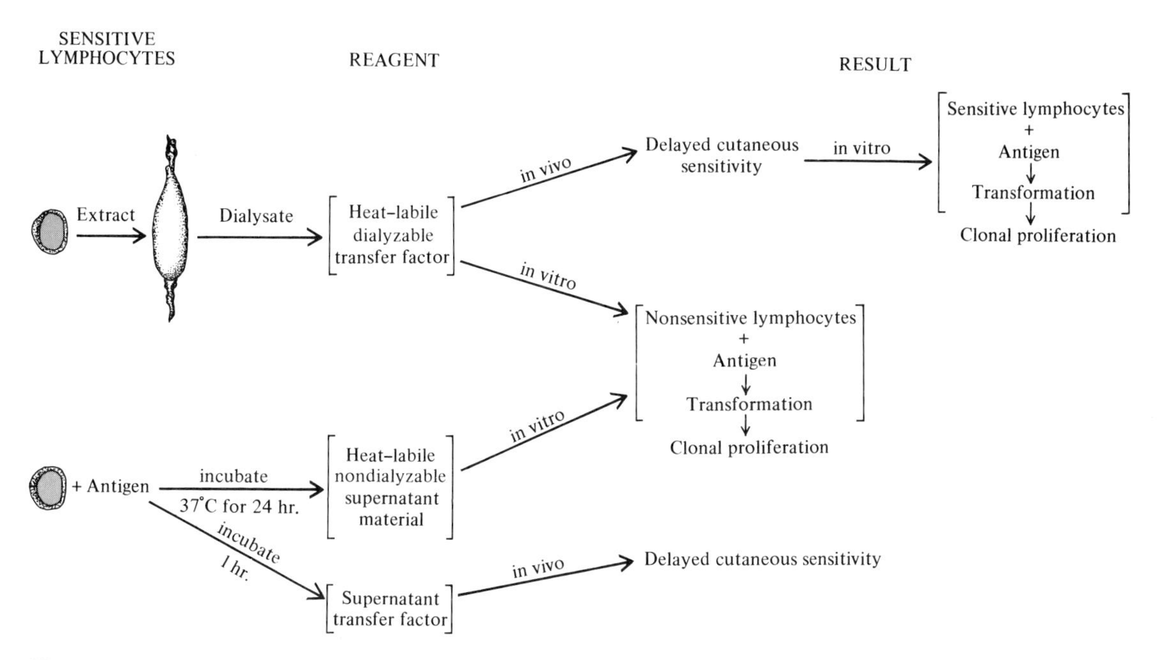

Figure 8-8 Diagrammatic comparison of in vivo and in vitro activities of dialyzable transfer factor, antigen-liberated transfer factor, and lymphocyte transforming factor. (*From H. S. Lawrence, Adv. Immunol., 11:195–266, 1969.*)

the knowledge that the converted lymphocytes will undergo blastogenesis and clonal proliferation when exposed for the first time to the specific antigen, a response identical to that occurring when antigen-sensitized lymphocytes are reexposed to the antigen.

It is difficult to escape the conclusion that in the process of inducing delayed hypersensitivity an antigen stimulates appropriate lymphocytes either to synthesize or to code for the synthesis of a set of transfer factors. When the sensitized lymphocytes are reexposed to the antigen, several events occur which amplify the reaction.

1 Dialyzable transfer factor is rapidly released and converts normal lymphocytes to an antigen-responsive state.
2 Synthesis of the more potent nondialyzable transfer factor is induced, and the transfer factor is released over a longer period of time.
3 Blastogenesis and clonal proliferation of sensitized and converted lymphocytes ensue and continue for a period of 4 to 5 days, especially in the regional lymph nodes (Fig. 8-9).
4 The circulating lymphocyte pool and lymphatic tissue are populated with antigen-responsive cells.

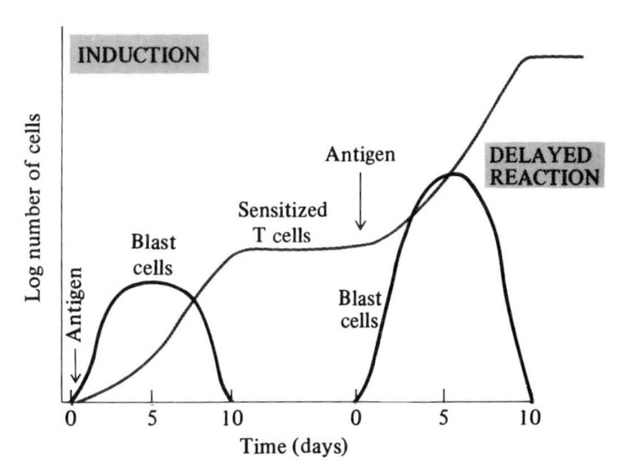

Figure 8-9 Blast cells and sensitized T cells in the paracortical areas of lymph nodes.

Thus, a minute amount of antigen acting on a few sensitized lymphocytes can lead rapidly to the conversion, recruitment, and distribution of a large population of antigen-responsive cells. Nonetheless, the response is probably limited to a maximum conversion of 20 percent of lymphocytes exposed to the antigen and therefore cannot account for the massive increase in the total number of cells observed in sites undergoing delayed response.

Other Lymphokines

Migration Inhibitory Factor Search for an explanation of the predominance of activated macrophages in delayed responses led to the discovery of a number of other lymphokines which are released from sensitized lymphocytes by antigen and are responsible for the recruitment of macrophages. One of the best-studied lymphokines involved in enlisting macrophages is the migration inhibitory factor (MIF).

A convenient method for demonstrating the action of MIF is the capillary tube migration inhibition technique. In principle, a mixed population of macrophages and sensitized lymphocytes in a ratio of 99 to 1 is placed in a series of capillary tubes. When incubated in the absence of antigen, the macrophages migrate from the tube in a fan-shaped pattern. However, when incubated in the presence of antigen, migration of the macrophages is inhibited. Appropriate control tubes indicate that inhibition of macrophage migration requires both sensitized lymphocytes and antigen (Fig. 8-10).

Subsequent studies have confirmed that antigen stimulates sensitized lymphocytes to release a soluble mediator (MIF) commencing at 6 hr. and continuing for 4 days. Inhibitors that block RNA and protein synthesis prevent the formation and release of MIF, thus indicating that the message for MIF synthesis is transcribed and translated after sensitized lymphocytes come in contact with the antigen. Additional properties

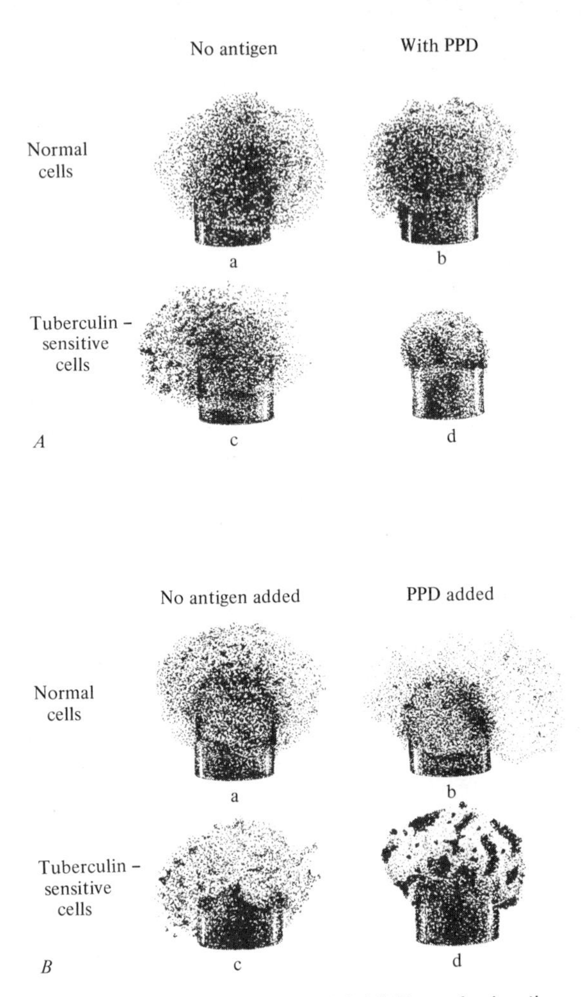

Figure 8-10 Antigen-induced inhibition of migration of peritoneal cells from sensitized animals. *A.* Migration of peritoneal cells from normal and tuberculin-sensitive guinea pigs with purified protein derivative (PPD). Photographs were taken after 24 hr. of incubation. *(a)* Normal cells without antigen; *(b)* normal cells in PPD 15 μg/ml; *(c)* tuberculin-sensitive cells without antigen; *(d)* tuberculin-sensitive cells in PPD 15 μg/ml. Migration is inhibited. *B.* Effect of PPD on normal and tuberculin-sensitive cells when added after the cells have migrated for 20 hr. in normal media. Photographs were taken after 40 hr. total incubation. *(a)* Normal cells, no PPD added; *(b)* normal cells, PPD added at 20 hr.; *(c)* tuberculin-sensitive cells, no PPD added; *(d)* tuberculin-sensitive cells, PPD added at 20 hr. *(From J. R. David, S. Al-Askari, H. S. Lawrence, and L. Thomas, J. Immunol., 93:264–273, 1964.)*

Table 8-5 Migration Inhibitory Factors

Species	Inducer	Cell source	Culture time	Target cell	Production inhibited by	Molecular weight (Sephadex)	Inacti-vated at	Electrophoretic mobility (R_f)	Destroyed by	pH stability	Laboratory
Guinea pig	PPD, Tumor antigens	LNC, PXL	6–96 hr.	GP-PX cells	Mitomycin, puromycin	25,000 and 55,000	80°C		*	2–10	Bloom, Bennett
	OCB-BGG, Con A	LNC	24 hr.	GP-PX cells	Actinomycin, puromycin	35,000 to 55,000	80°C	Pre-albumin	4 mg. insol. trypsin, 4 mg. insol. chymotryp-sin, and 100 mg. neur-aminidase		Remold, David
Human	PPD, SKSD, PHA, PKM, vaccinia vi-rus	PBL	72 hr.	GP-PX cells		50,000	80°C				Thor
	PPD, SKSD	PBL	72 hr.	GP-PX cells		55,000					Remold, David
	None	Lym-pho-blast lines	4–6 hr.	Lym-pho-blast lines							Glade, Broder

* Resistant to 1 mg. insoluble trypsin and to 1 mg. insoluble chymotrypsin

Note: Con A = concanavalin A; GP-PX = guinea pig–peritoneal exudate cells; LNC = lymph node cells; OCB-BGG = o-chlorobenzoyl–bovine gamma globulin; PBL = peripheral blood lymphocytes; PHA = phytohemagglutinin; PKM = pokeweed mitogen; PPD = purified protein derivative of tuberculin; PXL = peritoneal exudate lymphocytes; SKSD = streptokinase–streptodornase.

Source: After B. R. Bloom and P. R. Glade (eds.), *In Vitro Methods in Cell-mediated Immunity,* New York: Academic Press, Inc., 1971, p. 571.

of purified and partially characterized MIF are included in Table 8-5.

MIF differs fundamentally from transfer factors in that it lacks immunological specificity and species specificity. However, macrophages recruited to the site of delayed reactions do appear to have specific surface protein receptors for interaction with MIF that can be removed by treatment with trypsin. As with transfer factors, MIF can be released from sensitized lymphocytes by plant lectins.

When infiltrating macrophages interact with MIF, their mobility is sharply curtailed and they remain in the area as long as MIF is secreted by the antigen-responsive sensitized lymphocytes. The action of MIF on macrophages is reflected in such morphological changes as depressed ruffling of pseudopodial membranes and increased microtubular and lysosomal contents.

Additional Lymphokines Acting on Macrophages Three other apparently distinct lymphokines affect macrophages. Chemotactic factor is responsible for chemotaxis of macrophages, and its activity depends on the establishment of a gradient of decreasing concentration from the point of secretion by the antigen-stimulated sensitized lymphocytes. A macrophage-aggregating factor is a lymphokine that may provide a mechanism for clumping macrophages, thereby restricting their movement and inducing the formation of giant cells. Along with MIF, macrophage-activating factor is thought to be partly responsible for the increased lysosomal activity of macrophages that is a significant feature of delayed reactions.

Mitogenic Factors Supernatants obtained from sensitized lymphocytes stimulated by antigen contain several incompletely characterized *mitogenic factors;* the interactions of these factors with each other and with other lymphokines remain obscure. Presumably, mitogenic factors are involved in stimulating blastogenesis, growth, and clonal proliferation of antigen-responsive lymphocytes. Some of the mitogenic factors are apparently antigen-specific, some are species-specific, and others can stimulate across species lines.

Lymphotoxin: A Cytotoxic Lymphokine Cellular and tissue damage involves lymphocytes, macrophages, and their products and varies directly with the scope and magnitude of the delayed reaction. Lymphotoxin (LT), the best-characterized cytotoxic molecule, is produced rapidly by sensitized lymphocytes in response to antigen, is dependent on active protein synthesis, and can damage or lyse cells. Target cells vary in susceptibility to LT. Lymphocytes and macrophages are relatively resistant to LT and are damaged only by high concentrations.

The exact mechanism of cytotoxicity is obscure, but it is known that LT is especially potent, since less than 1 μg per milliliter can damage susceptible target cells. The rate and extent of cell destruction varies with the sensitivity of the target cell and the LT concentration. Apparently, LT does not penetrate target cells but interacts with the cell membrane, producing damage in selected sites. Since various polyanions (polyvinylpyrrolidone, DNA, soluble RNA) can compete with LT for membrane sites, LT may be a polyanion. The susceptibility of target cells may be partly determined by their metabolic state. Actively metabolizing cells are resistant to LT but become eight to ten times more susceptible when their energy metabolism and biosynthetic capabilities are inhibited.

Other Cytotoxic and Regulatory Lymphokines Other factors that may be involved in cytotoxicity or in regulation of delayed responses include proliferation inhibition factor (PIF), cloning inhibitory factor (CLIF), interferon, and inhibitor of DNA synthesis (IDS). PIF and CLIF can block in vitro proliferation of a number of cell types, but their precise functions remain to be elucidated. Interferon lacks cytotoxicity, and nothing is known of its role in regulating delayed hypersensitivity, but it does prevent replication of intracellular parasites and conceivably could limit the magnitude of delayed reactions caused by such parasites. IDS does not inhibit blastogenesis but can reversibly prevent mitosis of lymphocytes. Although the role of IDS in delayed hypersensitivity is unknown, it is possible that IDS exerts a negative control on antigen-responsive lymphocytes by holding the population in check and preventing a "snowballing" effect.

Skin Reactive Factor Factors with phlogistic (inflammatory) potential are associated with sensitized lymphocytes. One of these, *skin reactive factor* (SRF), can elicit a typical indurated lesion similar to that seen in delayed hypersensitivity when injected intradermally in guinea pigs. The inflammatory activity of SRF is not blocked by drugs that antagonize histamine, serotonin, or SRS-A, but there is some suggestion that kinins and the Hageman factor may be involved in production of induration.

Lymph Node Permeability Factor Extracts of lymph nodes from sensitized persons contain another phlogistic lymphokine, a *lymph node permeability factor* (LNPF). When injected intradermally, LNPF increases the permeability of the local blood vessels and causes an extensive influx of leukocytes which quickly become monocytic in character, i.e., a sequence of events typically observed in delayed hypersensitivity.

LNPF is present in sites undergoing tuberculin reactions and is known to accumulate in contact dermatitis caused by dinitrochlorobenzene. Apparently, LNPF is not released from sensitized lymphocytes upon contact with antigen but only after the sensitized lymphocytes have been damaged. Obviously, once released, LNPF can accelerate the inflammatory reaction and lead to the accumulation of cells.

Little is known concerning the chemical properties of LNPF. Activity is associated with a component that is antigenic, has a molecular weight greater than 100,000, is resistant to proteolytic enzymes, and is heat-stable at 100°C for 20 min. Current preparations of LNPF contain significant quantities of RNA ($>$ 7 percent), and some LNPF activity may be due to RNA. Purified RNA is known to possess similar permeability-inducing capacity. However, LNPF activity is resistant to RNase.

Lymphocytic Chalone In addition to lymphokines, other soluble substances may be involved in regulating delayed hypersensitivity reactions. A chalone is a molecule synthesized by a tissue which exerts an antimitotic effect specific for that tissue. Lymphocytic chalone is a protein synthesized by lymphocytes that can inhibit transformation and proliferation of lymphocytes, DNA and antibody synthesis (Chap. 7), and graft-versus-host reactions (Chap. 10) in which lymphocytes are critically involved. Presumably, lymphocytic chalone functions partly by way of the adenyl cyclase-cAMP system. Antigenic stimulation may block the action of lymphocytic chalone, thus permitting sensitized lymphocytes to undergo blastogenesis and clonal proliferation. When antigen is eliminated, the antagonism is relieved, and the chalone once again exerts its antimitotic effect. Therefore, a regulatory feedback control mechanism can be proposed for lymphocytic chalone in immune responses, including delayed hypersensitivity.

Postulated Mechanism of Delayed Hypersensitivity Reactions

On the basis of the foregoing considerations, a sequence of events can be postulated to account for delayed responses (Fig. 8-11). Although the mechanisms involved can be most clearly ob-

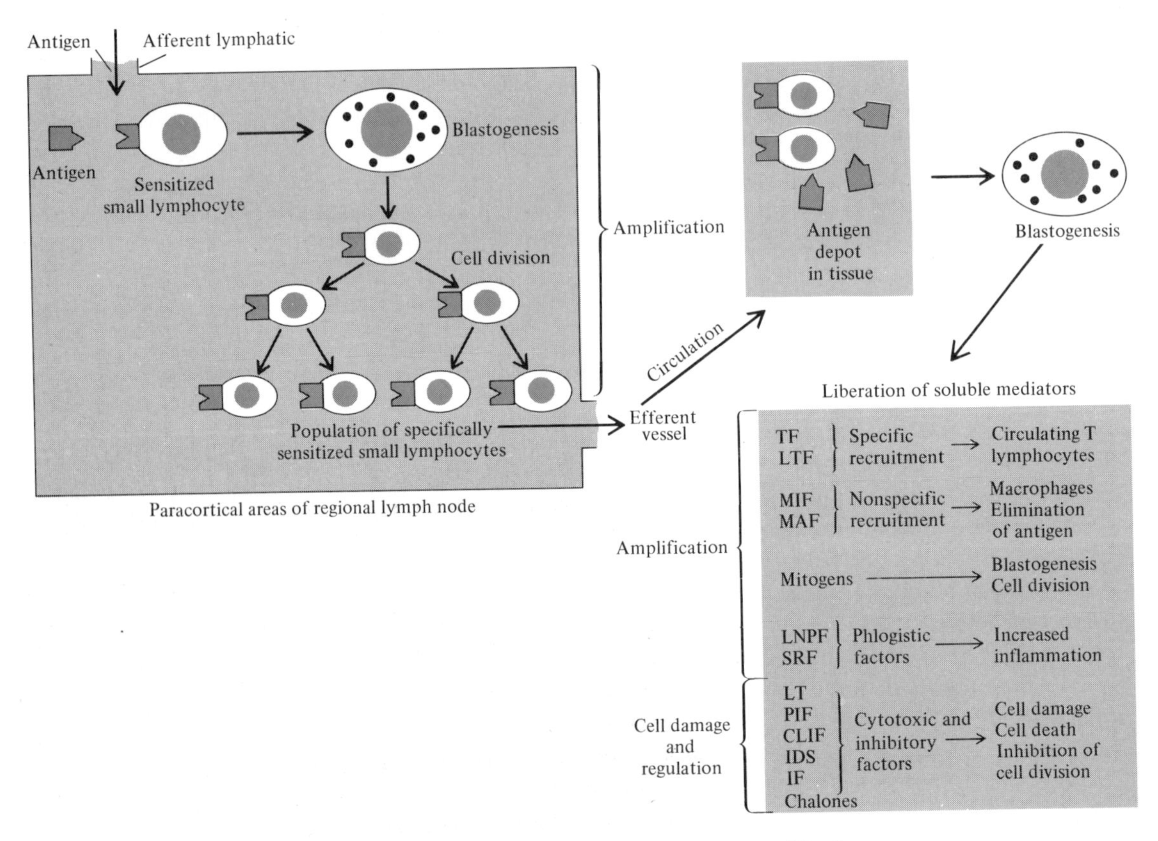

Figure 8-11 Schematic presentation of the mechanisms leading to the amplification and pathogenesis of delayed hypersensitivity reactions.

served following peripheral exposure (contact dermatitis) or injection, it is essential to emphasize that similar reactions can and do occur in any tissue or organ in the body, provided that an infectious agent or other antigen and appropriate T lymphocytes can interact.

Basically, the process of sensitization involves:

1 Combination of an antigenic determinant with a specific receptor site on the surface membrane of a small lymphocyte (T cell)
2 Transformation of the T cell into a large blast, lymphoblast, or immunoblast cell (blastogenesis)
3 Clonal proliferation of the blast cells, usually in the paracortical areas of the regional lymph node
4 Reversion of the blast cells to antigen-responsive T cells (sensitized lymphocytes)

The sensitized T cells contain preformed dialyzable transfer factor and the genetic information to synthesize lymphokines upon reexposure to the antigenic determinant. In addition, the sensitized lymphocytes retain the inherent capacity of all T cells to cycle several times daily between the vascular and extravascular compartments and to populate the paracortical areas of lymphatic tissue throughout the body. Thus, a general state of delayed hypersensitivity to the antigenic determinant exists throughout the body that is totally dependent upon sensitized T cells.

Consequently, a sensitized person has an increased number of T cells committed to specific interaction with the antigenic determinant, thereby enhancing the prospect of more rapid and extensive contact upon reexposure. Keeping in perspective the fact that much is uncertain and remains to be elucidated, the following postulated mechanism of delayed hypersensitivity reactions focuses on a sequence of events that is in accord with current observations (Fig. 8-11).

1 The cause of the increased vascular permeability which initiates the inflammatory reaction and leads to an influx of leukocytes is not known.
2 Sensitized T cells in the circulation and in the lymph nodes interact with the antigenic determinant, undergo blastogenesis and clonal proliferation, release preformed dialyzable transfer factor, and begin to synthesize other lymphokines.
3 Dialyzable transfer factor converts normal lymphocytes to an antigen-responsive state, causing an immediate amplification of the response.
4 An expanded number of sensitized T cells migrates into the sites containing the antigen and responds by releasing dialyzable transfer factor and by synthesizing and gradually releasing increasing concentrations of other lymphokines.
5 The release of lymphokines in the area of the antigen restricts the movement of macrophages, causes a chemotactic influx of macrophages, and results in their adherence to each other and to sensitized T cells, thus leading to a massive accumulation of activated macrophages.
6 The synthesis and release of other lymphokines builds up, and the reaction increases more rapidly in intensity. Mitogenic factors stimulate lymphocyte growth; nondialyzable transfer factor and RNA transfer factor accumulate in concentration, causing a sharp rise in antigen-responsive lymphocytes; lymphotoxin release commences; and skin reactive factor and lymph node permeability factor enhance the inflammatory response.
7 Increased production and release of lymphotoxin from sensitized T cells and of lysosomal enzymes from activated macrophages lead to a further progression of the inflammatory response, cellular and tissue destruction, and hemostatic disturbances including microthrombus formation and coagulation.

Postulated Regulation of Delayed Hypersensitivity Reactions

In the absence of regulatory mechanisms, the enhancement, amplification, and vigor of delayed hypersensitivity reactions would probably continue for a prolonged interval. However, the antigen is gradually eliminated by the lysosomal enzymes of macrophages, and less antigen is available to stimulate sensitized T cells. Concomitantly, regulatory lymphokines (proliferation inhibition factor, cloning inhibitory factor, and inhibitor of DNA synthesis) and lymphocytic chalone reduce the capacity of sensitized T cells to respond to the antigen, thereby shutting off the synthesis of the reaction-enhancing lymphokines. The latter may also be inactivated by lysosomal enzymes released from activated macrophages and cells destroyed by lymphotoxin. In addition, a certain amount of dilution results from the leakage of fluid from the vasculature and from lysed cells. Thus, despite a dramatic cellular response, a delayed hypersensitivity reaction can subside quickly, and healing and repair can ensue.

Cytophilic Antibody: An Alternate Mechanism Involved in Delayed Reactions?

An alternate explanation for the immunological specificity and sequence of delayed hypersensitivity responses involves the concept of *cytophilic antibody* which by definition has a predilection for receptor sites on the surface of certain cells. Factors with cytophilic antibody activity can be detected in IgM and IgG and in serum alpha globulins. Presumably, cytophilic antibody is elicited by antigenic stimulation of T lymphocytes (Fig. 8-12). Titers of cytophilic antibody are usually low but may be raised somewhat when antigen is combined with complete adjuvant and injected intraperitoneally.

One of the intriguing properties of cytophilic antibody in connection with delayed hypersensitivity is its ability to attach to trypsin-sensitive receptors on the surface of macrophages. Consequently, suggestions have been made that attachment of an antigenic determinant to cytophilic antibody on the surface of macrophages

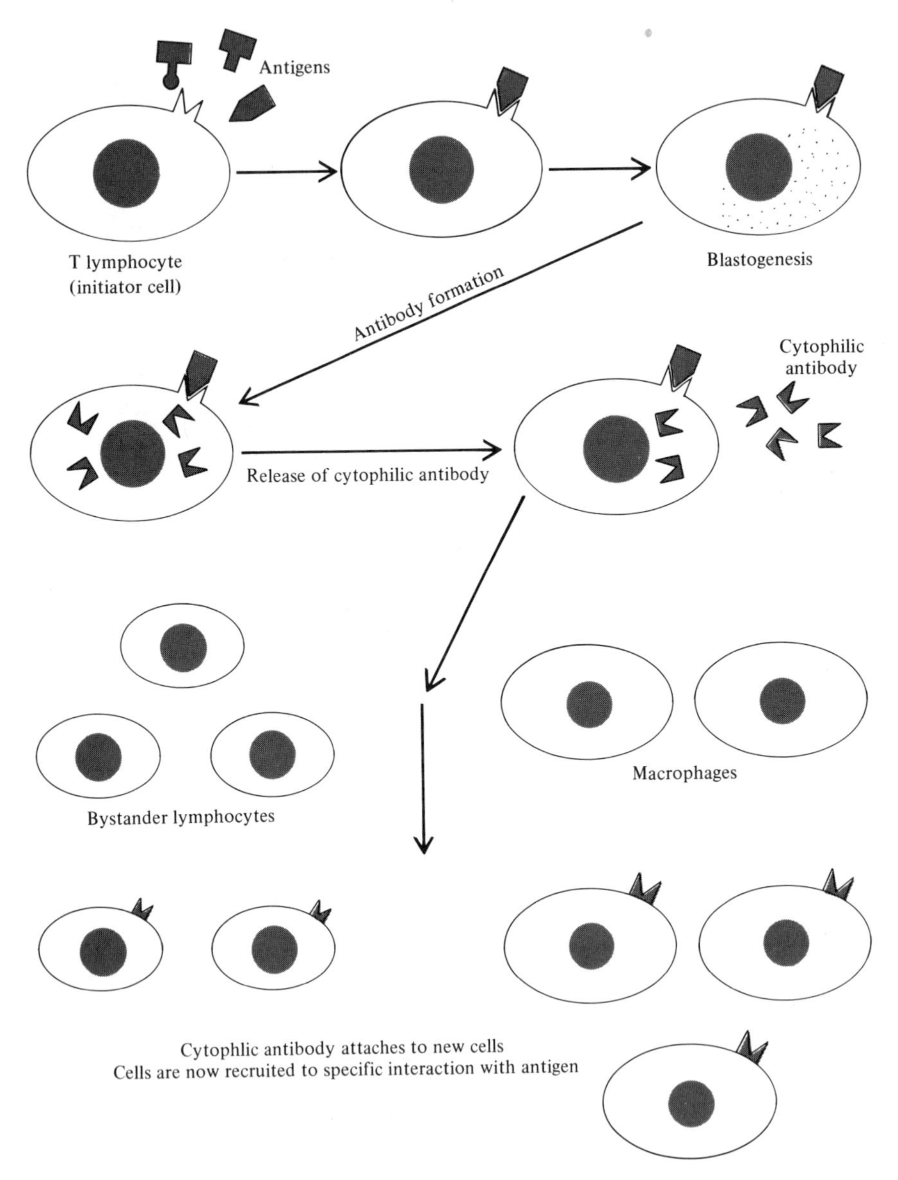

Figure 8-12 Schematic presentation of the possible role of cytophilic antibody in the recruitment of cells for delayed hypersensitivity reactions.

can account for inhibition of macrophage migration, clumping and adherence of macrophages, and sensitization of cells. Passive transfer of delayed hypersensitivity by serum is unsuccessful, but proponents of the cytophilic antibody theory argue that the failure is due to the low concentration of cytophilic antibody in serum. Furthermore, it is postulated that sensitized T cells can transfer delayed hypersensitivity to a normal person only because a small proportion of the transferred T cells can produce cytophilic antibody when stimulated by antigen. At present there is no conclusive evidence to show whether or not cytophilic antibody plays a vital role in delayed hypersensitivity reactions. However, on the basis of available data, most immunologists hold that sensitized T cells mediate delayed hypersensitivity through the production and release of lymphokines following contact with the antigenic determinant.

CELL-MEDIATED IMMUNITY

Another name for a delayed hypersensitivity response is a cell-mediated response. Originally, the term cell-mediated was used to designate hypersensitivity reactions that could be transmitted from a sensitized to a normal person by transferring cells (subsequently shown to be sensitized T lymphocytes), but not serum. Hypersensitivity responses that could be passively transferred by serum were called humoral, or antibody-mediated, reactions.

As knowledge developed, it has become increasingly apparent that cell-mediated (delayed hypersensitivity) responses are vitally involved in recovery from many infections, and conversely, recovery is delayed or fails to occur if there is a paucity or absence of T cells, even though antibody production is unimpaired. The concept of cell-mediated immunity is considered separately in order to emphasize its role in recovery from infection and not because it differs in any way from delayed hypersensitivity responses. In addition to delayed hypersensitivity and cell-mediated immunity, specific interaction of sensitized T cells with antigen forms the basis of most autoimmune diseases, the rejection of transplanted tissues and organs, immunological surveillance, and protection against cancer (Chaps. 10 and 11).

Intracellular infections

Infections that are most effectively controlled and eliminated by cell-mediated immunity are those caused by facultative or by obligate intracellular parasites. Facultative intracellular parasites include bacteria *(Mycobacterium, Salmonella, Brucella, Pasteurella, Listeria),* fungi *(Histoplasma),* and protozoa *(Leishmania, Trypanosoma).* Obligate intracellular parasites include viruses, rickettsiae, chlamydiae, and some protozoa (*Plasmodium, Toxoplasma,* and perhaps *Pneumocystis*).

In a number of infections, the sequence of cutaneous reactivity and histopathology is characteristic of delayed hypersensitivity responses, and upon reinfection with the same microorganism an accelerated response occurs. In addition immunity to a number of microbial infections, not necessarily limited to those caused by facultative or obligate intracellular parasites, can be transferred by sensitized T cells or transfer factor but not by serum. These observations, together with the demonstration that a microorganism can induce the synthesis and release of lymphokines from sensitized T cells, indicate that cell-mediated immunity is an immunologically specific reaction of the delayed hypersensitivity type.

Under the influence of antigen-induced release of lymphokines from sensitized T cells, activated macrophages (occasionally called angry or immune macrophages) exhibit increased phagocytic, biosynthetic, and cidal power. The cidal force is associated with a rise in the number of lysosomes, an augmented concentration of hydrolytic enzymes and cidal basic proteins, and an enhanced ability to discharge the lysosomal contents into phagosomes containing the microorganisms. Thus, activated macrophages are much more effective than normal macrophages in ingesting and killing microorganisms and in eliminating them by lysis or digestion. One macrophage factor operating to kill ingested microorganisms is a basic, cationic protein termed *monocytin*.

Specific and Nonspecific Components of Cell-mediated Immunity

Once it is activated under the influence of lymphokines released from sensitized T cells by antigen, the increased cidal power of macrophages is nonspecific. For example, macrophages activated as a consequence of a delayed hypersensitivity reaction involving *Salmonella typhosa* have an enhanced capacity to destroy unrelated bacteria, including *Mycobacterium, Listeria,* and *Brucella,* and animals possessing such activated macrophages are resistant to lethal doses of these microorganisms. The persistence of activated macrophages is dependent upon the continued release of lymphokines from sensitized T cells stimulated by specific antigen. After removal of the antigenic stimulus, release of lymphokines diminishes, activated macrophages disappear, and nonspecific resistance fades. However, the specific component of cell-mediated immunity persists indefinitely, since it is associated with long-lived sensitized T lymphocytes.

Several investigators have succeeded in clearly dissecting the specific and nonspecific components of cell-mediated immunity. For example, mice infected with *Mycobacterium tuberculosis* generally develop both skin reactivity and resistance to infection. However, if infected with extremely high doses of mycobacteria, the mice acquire nonspecific resistance, but become anergic and fail to show skin reactivity to the bacteria. On the other hand, lymphocytes from anergic mice are quite capable of transferring cutaneous delayed hypersensitivity to normal recipients. Thus, peripheral manifestations of delayed hypersensitivity are not necessarily an accurate reflection of cell-mediated immunity.

Viral Infections

Viruses represent a special category of obligate intracellular infections for a variety of reasons. In virus infections, the extracellular stage is often short. Many viruses are passed from cell to cell by membranous extensions and invaginations. Other viruses, viral genomes, or viral genes are transmitted vertically from generation to generation during cellular division (Chaps. 2, 3, and 11). Some viruses have an outer coat (membrane or envelope) derived from host cell membranes (Chap. 2). Other viruses can induce or expose new antigens on the surface membrane of infected cells (Chap. 2). These factors often complicate the picture of cell-mediated immunity, but basically the mechanism is essentially the same as that involved in delayed hypersensitivity reactions. In fact, lymphokines and lysosomal enzymes appear to be of overriding importance in recovery from most, if not all, viral infections by digesting viruses and the cells in which they replicate.

An additional factor, formerly thought to play a more significant role in recovery from viral infections, is interferon, a species-specific but not virus-specific lymphokine. The importance of interferon should not be overemphasized. For example, in the presence of normal or elevated concentrations of antibody and interferon, but under conditions in which T cells are suppressed, depressed, or absent, recovery from viral infections is seriously impaired, and a fatal outcome often results. Thus, the paramount importance of cell-mediated immunity in recovery from viral infections is amply documented.

Deficiencies in Cell-mediated Immunity

Deficiencies in cell-mediated immunity are based on genetic defects or can be acquired during the course of other diseases (Hodgkin's disease, lymphocytic leukemia, cancer, measles, hepatitis, leprosy), following immunization (measles), following immunosuppressive therapy (Chaps. 10 and 11), or following severe burns. A common feature in each of these situations is the vulnerability of the affected person to progressive intracellular infections caused by temporary or permanent suppression of T lymphocytes. Consideration of acquired T cell deficiencies and the therapeutic utility of specific transfer factors and nonspecific induction of delayed hypersensitivity in their managemant will be discussed in Chapters 10 and 11. In the ensuing sections, a few genetic defects will be briefly mentioned to illustrate their roles in immune deficiency disease.

DiGeorge Syndrome

In patients with congenital absence of thymus and parathyroids *(DiGeorge syndrome),* the major deficiency is in cell-mediated immunity; characteristics of this syndrome include failure to induce delayed hypersensitivity, failure to respond to plant lectins, and failure to release lymphokines. Antibodies can be produced, especially against thymus-independent antigens, and plasma cells and germinal centers are present in lymph nodes. Patients with DiGeorge syndrome often have severe infections and usually die in the course of infections caused by viruses, fungi, or *Pneumocystis carinii.* Efforts to achieve immunological reconstitution by thymic transplantation have met with some success (see also Chap. 10).

Combined Deficiency Syndromes (Swiss Agammaglobulinemia)

In the combined deficiency syndromes, both cellular and antibody responses are depressed. Generally, affected infants quickly acquire a succession of pyogenic and viral infections, including those caused by *Pseudomonas,* varicella virus, *Candida,* and *Pneumocystis carinii. Swiss agammaglobulinemia* is inherited as an autosomal recessive trait and represents a severe form of immunodeficiency with a short-term survival. However, a few successful reports of immunological reconstitution with bone marrow transplants have been recorded (see also Chap. 10). Patients with these syndromes regularly respond to immunization with vaccinia virus or BCG vaccine for tuberculosis with progressive disease.

Ataxia telangiectasia is an autosomal recessive disease characterized by impaired delayed hypersensitivity and commonly associated with depressed IgA activity. Clinically, affected children have neurologic abnormalities, cutaneous and ocular arterial and capillary dilatations (telangiectasia), and recurrent and severe pulmonary infections.

Wiskott-Aldrich syndrome is a sex-linked inherited disease in males who show defective delayed hypersensitivity reactions and often have depressed concentrations of IgM. Clinically, the disease is associated with thrombocytopenia, eczema, and recurrent infections.

BIBLIOGRAPHY

Bach, F. H., and Good, R. A. (eds.): *Clinical Immunobiology,* vol. I, New York: Academic Press, Inc., 1972.

Bloom, B. R., Ceppellini, R., Cerottini, J.-C., David, J. R., Kunkel, H., Landy, M., Lawrence, H. S., Maini, R., Nussenzweig, V., Perlmann, P., Spitler, L., Rosen, F., and Zabriskie, J.: "In Vitro Methods in Cell-mediated Immunity:" A Progress Report, *Cell. Immunol.,* 6:331-347, 1973.

Engers, H. D., and Unanue, E. R.: "The Fate of Anti-Ig-Surface Ig Complexes on B Lymphocytes," *J. Immunol.,* 110:465-475, 1973.

"FASEB Conference. Membranes in Growth, Differentiation and Neoplasia," *Fed. Proc.,* 32:19-108, 1973.

Garcia-Giralt, E., La Salvia, E., Florentin, S., and Mathé, G.: "Evidence for a Lymphocytic Chalone," *Rev. Eur. Etud. Clin. Biol.,* 15:1012-1015, 1970.

Granger, G. A., Laserna, E. C., Kolb, W. P., and Chapman, F.: "Human Lymphotoxin: Purification and Some Properties." *Proc. Natl. Acad. Sci. USA,* 70:27-30, 1973.

Houck, J. C., and Chang, C. M.: "A New Sensitive Assay for Macrophage Inhibitory Factor," *Proc. Soc. Exp. Biol. Med.,* 142:800-803, 1973.

Kaliner, M., Orange, R. P., and Austen, K. F.: "Immunological Release of Histamine and Slow Reacting Substance of Anaphylaxis from Human Lung IV. Enhancement by Cholinergic and α-Adrenergic Stimulation," *J. Exp. Med.,* 136:556-567, 1972.

Kaufman, H. S., and Hobbs, J. R.: "Immunoglobulin Deficiencies in an Atopic Population," *Lancet,* 2:1061-1063, 1970.

Krueger, G. R. F.: "Morphology of Chemical Immunosuppression," *Adv. Pharmacol. Chemother.,* 10:1-90, 1972.

Lance, E. M., Gillette, S. C., Goldstein, A. L., White, A., and Zatz, M. M.: "On the Mode of Action of Thymosin," *Cell. Immunol.,* 6:126-131, 1973.

Lopes, J., Nachbar, M., Zucker-Franklin, D., and Silber, R.: "Lymphocyte Plasma Membranes: Analysis of Proteins and Glycoproteins by SDS-Gel Electrophoresis," *Blood,* 41:131-140, 1973.

McCombs, R. P.: "Diseases Due to Immunologic Reactions in the Lungs," *N. Engl. J. Med.,* 286:1186-1194, 1245-1252, 1972.

McLean, R. H., and Michael, A. F.: "Properdin and C3 Proactivator: Alternate Pathway Components in Human Glomerulonephritis," *J. Clin. Invest.,* 52:634-644, 1973.

Möller, G. (ed.): "Antigen Recognition in Cell-mediated Immunity," *Transplant. Rev.,* 10:3-176, 1972.

———(ed.): "Interaction between Humoral Antibodies and Cell-mediated Immunity," *Transplant. Rev.,* 13:3-141, 1972.

Müller-Eberhard, H. J., and Götze, O.: "C3 Proactivator Convertase and Its Mode of Action," *J. Exp. Med.,* 135:1003-1008, 1972.

North, R. M.: "Importance of Thymus-derived Lymphocytes in Cell-mediated Immunity to Infection," *Cell. Immunol.,* 7:166-176, 1973.

Orange, R. P., Murphy, R. C., Karnovsky, M. L., and Austen, K. F.: "The Physicochemical Characteristics and Purification of Slow-reacting Substance of Anaphylaxis," *J. Immunol.,* 110:760-770, 1973.

Parker, C. W., and Smith, J. W.: "Alterations in Cyclic Adenosine Monophosphate Metabolism in Human Bronchial Asthma: I. Leukocyte Responsiveness to β-Adrenergic Agents," *J. Clin. Invest.,* 52:48-59, 1973.

Pfueller, S. L., and Lüscher, E. F.: "The Effects of Immune Complexes on Blood Platelets and Their Relationship to Complement Activation," *Immunochemistry,* 9:1151-1166, 1972.

Pick, E., and Turk, J. L.: "The Biological Activities of Soluble Lymphocyte Products," *Clin. Exp. Immunol.,* 10:1-23, 1972.

Pirofsky, B., Davies, G. H., Ramirez-Mateos, J. C., and Newton, B. W.: "Cellular Immune Competence in the Human Fetus," *Cell. Immunol.,* 6:324-328, 1973.

Savilahti, E.: "IgA Deficiency in Children: Immunoglobulin-containing Cells in the Intestinal Mucosa, Immunoglobulins in Secretions and Serum IgA Levels," *Clin. Exp. Immunol.,* 13:395-406, 1973.

Shands, J. W., Jr., Peavy, D. L., and Smith, R. T.: "Differential Morphology of Mouse Spleen Cells Stimulated in Vitro by Endotoxin, Phytohemagglutinin, Pokeweed Mitogen and Staphylococcal Enterotoxin B," *Am. J. Pathol.,* 70:1-24, 1973.

Simon, H. B., and Sheagren, J. N.: "Migration Inhibitory Factor and Macrophage Bactericidal Function," *Infect. Immun.,* 6:101-111, 1972.

Smith, R. W., Terry, W. D., Buell, D. N., and Sell, K. W.: "An Antigenic Marker for Human Thymic Lymphocytes," *J. Immunol.,* 110:884-887, 1973.

Spreafico, F.: "Biological Activities of Antilymphocyte Serum," *Adv. Pharmacol. Chemother.,* 10:257-338, 1972.

Taichman, N. S., Movat, H. Z., Glynn, M. F., and Broder, I.: "Further Studies on the Role of Neutrophils in Passive Cutaneous Anaphylaxis of the Guinea Pig," *Immunology,* 21:623-635, 1971.

Valentine, F. T., and Lawrence, H. S.: "Cell-mediated Immunity," *Adv. Intern. Med.,* 17:51-93, 1971.

Williams, T. W., and Granger, G. A.: "Lymphocyte in Vitro Cytotoxicity: Mechanism of Human Lymphotoxin-induced Target Cell Destruction," *Cell. Immunol.,* 6:171-185, 1973.

Chapter 9

Immunohematology

Arthur E. Krikszens and Bernard A. Briody

PERSPECTIVE

Man's desire to transfer blood from one individual to another dates back to antiquity, but the attempt to make this transfer successfully was usually characterized by failure. The discovery of the major blood groups by Landsteiner in 1900 put whole blood transfusion on a more practical, scientific basis. Since then, *immunohematology* has expanded tremendously and has made valuable contributions to clinical and forensic medicine, genetics, and anthropology. In clinical medicine, the beneficial results achieved by whole blood transfusion have made it one of modern medicine's most powerful and routine lifesaving procedures. On the other hand, the risk of inadvertently transmitting hepatitis virus to the recipient must always be weighed by the physician before whole blood is administered.

The differences between and within the blood groups are based on the chemical and conformational structure of antigenic determinants on the surface membrane of erythrocytes. The antigens involved belong to one of two groups of genetically determined isoantigens *(alloantigens)* of medical importance to man. The other group involves the HL-A transplantation antigens discussed in Chapter 10. The blood group antigens represent systems of antigenic determinants found on the surfaces of erythrocytes and other body cells. The antigens appear to be the products of *alleles* or of closely linked genes and are inherited according to simple Mendelian laws. The major blood group systems (ABO and Rh) exhibit independent segregation.

While the ABO and Rh systems are the most significant clinically, a number of other blood group systems are recognized. Many of these have clinical, genetic, and anthropological importance because of their prevalence in selected populations, whereas the distribution of others is restricted to certain families and ethnic groups.

THE ABO BLOOD GROUP SYSTEM

Isoantigens and Isoantibodies

Basically, the ABO classification depends on the presence or absence of two *isoantigens,* A and B, present on the surface of erythrocytes. A peculiarity of the system is that each individual develops isoantibody to the absent isoantigen(s). Thus, if isoantigen A is absent, isoantibody α is present in the plasma. Isoantibodies presumably arise early in postnatal life as a result of exposure to bacterial and plant polysaccharide antigens that cross-react with the blood group antigens. The ability to produce isoantibodies to the inherited isoantigen is turned off by self-recognition or natural tolerance, whereas isoantibodies against the noninherited isoantigens are formed following stimulation by exogenous cross-reacting antigens.

Genetics

The presence of a specific isoantigen on the erythrocyte surface is dependent on the presence of the corresponding gene. Three allelic genes are involved—A, B, and O. Genes A and B are codominant, while the O gene is recessive to the other two. The resulting genotypic and phenotypic combinations are included in Table 9-1.

After the discovery of the ABO antigens, attempts to obtain active blood group substances from erythrocytes met with limited success. Active substances could be extracted with ethanol but not with aqueous solutions. It was found, however, that ABO antigenic specificities along with several other blood group antigens could be detected as water-soluble molecules in human secretions, particularly in saliva and gastric juice. Besides the ABO specificities, the Lewis specificities Le^a and Le^b and the H specificity were found. Detailed genetic and chemical analyses of the various water-soluble blood group specificities led to an understanding of their interrelationships.

The chemical structures involved in the antigenic specificities presumably arise from closely related but independent gene systems—ABO, Hh, Lele, and Sese. The alleles Se and se control the secretion of A or B substances, but have no effect on the expression of the A and B antigens on the erythrocyte surface. The Se gene in either the SeSe or Sese state results in secretion, whereas the se gene in the sese state only shuts off the secretion of A and B antigens. About 20 percent of individuals with A or B antigens on their erythrocytes fail to secrete A or B substances and are probably sese genotypes.

O erythrocytes react preferentially with agglutinins in certain cattle sera. The agglutination can be inhibited by secretions not only from O individuals but also from A, B, and AB individuals as well. Since AB individuals cannot have O genes, the active substance in these se-

Table 9-1 The ABO Blood Group System

Genotype	Phenotype	Isoantigens on erythrocytes	Isoantibody in serum
AA AO	A	A	β (anti-B)
BB BO	B	B	α (anti-A)
AB	AB	AB	None
OO	O	None	α and β

cretions as well as on the O erythrocytes cannot be a product of the O gene. The factor involved has been termed the H substance and is a product under control of the H and h genes. H gene is dominant and codes for the production of H substance, whereas the h gene is recessive. An hh individual lacks not only H substance but A and B antigens as well.

The presence of large amounts of H substance on O erythrocytes is the result of the absence of A and B antigens, since H substance is the direct structural precursor of A and B antigens. Thus, the H and ABO genes are closely related in terms of phenotypic effects but are genetically independent.

The other system in which genes are inherited independently of the ABO, Hh, and Sese genes is the Lewis system, controlled by two alleles—Le and le. The Le gene is dominant and gives rise to Le^a phenotypes, whereas the le gene in the lele state results in the absence of the Le phenotype. Another specificity, Le^b, is believed to be the consequence of the interaction of H and Le genes.

Chemical Basis of Immunospecificity

In reality, the gene products are enzymatic proteins termed glycosyltransferases, and the blood group substances reflect the structural relationships between the products of these enzymes. Water-soluble blood group substances are abundantly secreted in saliva, gastric juice, meconium, and especially in ovarian cyst fluid. Active substances, purified from these sources, are glycoproteins and have a molecular weight ranging from 3×10^5 to 1×10^6. Purified preparations of A, B, H, and Le^a antigens contain 85 percent carbohydrate and 15 percent amino acids, are qualitatively identical in carbohydrate and peptide composition, and are antigenically specific on the basis of their carbohydrate moieties. The same five sugar residues are present in each blood group antigen: D-galactose, L-fucose, N-acetyl-D-galactosamine, N-acetyl-D-glucosamine, and N-acetylneuraminic acid (sialic acid), but one of these sugars appears to be immunodominant in each of the antigens analyzed. The antigens are constructed as a firm backbone of peptides with large numbers of short oligosaccharide chains attached at intervals. Extensive analyses of the enzymes and the antigenically active glycoproteins using immunochemical, chemical, and enzymatic methodology have revealed that the genes specify glycosyltransferases which act sequentially on common precursor molecules, the resulting antigenic specificity depending upon which genes are present and how far the sequence progresses.

A diagrammatic representation of the complex interrelationships is shown in Figure 9-1. Precursor I differs from precursor II in the linkage of the terminal galactose, I having β-1,3 and II having β-1,4. Precursor II can cross-react with type XIV pneumococcal polysaccharide. In several of the steps in the sequence the particular specificity is determined by the position and number of the fucosyl groups substituted on the precursor molecules.

In the case of A and B substances, the preceding specificities of H and Le^a moieties are masked by the addition of terminal nonreducing sugars. Sialic acid residues are the most variable components found in active substances, their point of attachment is in doubt, and their complete removal has no apparent effect on the immunospecificity of the blood group substances. Subgroups are recognized in A and B, but the immunochemical basis of the subgroups has not yet been elucidated.

Most of the data concerning the various blood group antigens have been derived from analyses of water-soluble secretory substances. The fact remains, however, that blood group specificities on the surface of erythrocytes are glycolipids. Nevertheless, while the glycolipids have not been studied extensively, their immunospecificity resides in carbohydrate (oligosaccharide) moieties that are closely similar, if not identical, to those in the secretory glycoproteins.

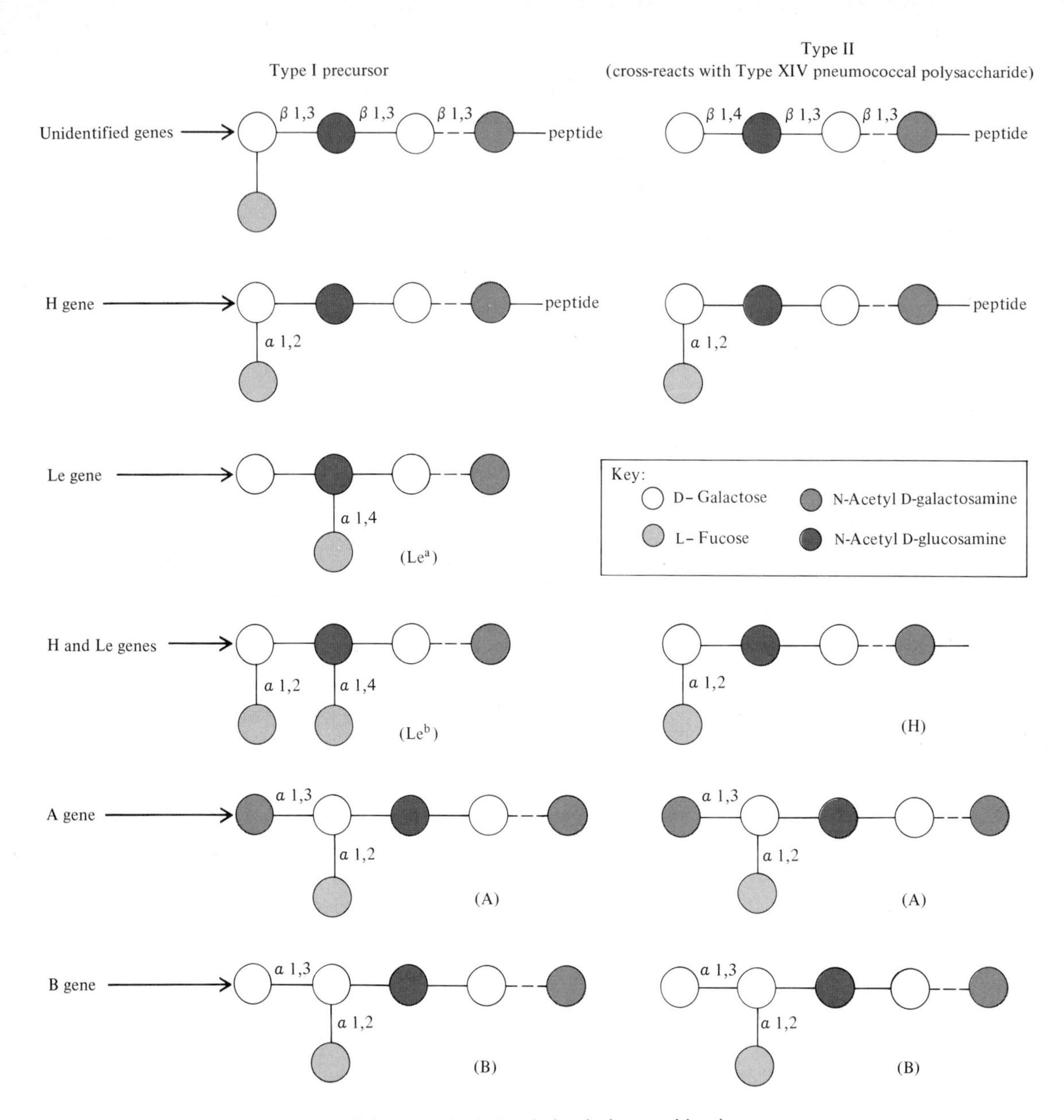

Figure 9-1 Proposed structures of the carbohydrate chains in human blood groups controlled by H, Le, A, and B genes. (*Based on data from W. M. Watkins, Science, 152:172-181, 1966. Copyright 1966, by the American Association for the Advancement of Science.*)

THE Rh BLOOD GROUP SYSTEM

In 1940, Landsteiner and Wiener found that sera from rabbits and guinea pigs immunized with *rh*esus monkey erythrocytes cross-reacted with 85 percent of the human erythrocytes tested; the remaining 15 percent were nonreactive. Reactive erythrocytes were termed *Rh positive,* while those that failed to react were labeled *Rh negative.* Since then, a system involving 30 or more immunospecificities and a vast number of complex allelic interactions has evolved. The original Rh factor of Landsteiner and Wiener is not included but is known to be an antigen shared by man and rhesus monkeys—the LW antigen—which may be a precursor of the Rh antigens. Knowledge of the serology and genetics of the Rh group has far outstripped chemical and immunochemical analyses. In fact, little is known concerning the chemical nature of the Rh antigens, although there have been claims of inhibition of specifically reactive antibodies by gangliosides derived from brain tissue and by compounds containing neuraminic acid. Interpretation of the results has been difficult and not as fruitful as anticipated.

Two theories are extant in the field of Rh blood groups. The Wiener theory postulates a single genetic locus accommodating a large number of alleles. In addition, according to Wiener anti-Rh antibodies against a particular Rh antigen can be heterogeneous because they are directed toward portions of the molecule. The Fisher-Race theory maintains that Rh antigens are determined by three basic pairs of closely linked genes, each of which can be represented by a dominant or recessive allele. Thus, each parent contributes a set of three genes: C or c, D or d, and E or e. The symbol D designates the most important Rh antigen. Each dominant gene and each recessive gene is apparently representative of a series of alleles the number of which seems to be increasing steadily. The exception to the foregoing is the d allele, which has not yet been detected and, therefore, denotes only the absence of D. In addition, there is evidence that the genes can act in combination to produce compound antigens with characteristics of both gene products, thus increasing the complexity. The most common genotype-phenotype combinations of Rh antigens among Caucasians are CDe (41 percent), cde (38 percent), and cDE (15 percent).

HEMOLYSIS CAUSED BY BLOOD GROUP ISOANTIBODIES

Transfusion Reactions

Transfusion across blood group incompatibility barriers may result in intravascular hemolytic reactions or rapid removal of the erythrocytes from the vasculature by the reticuloendothelial system. In the case of ABO blood group antigens, the reaction may be due to isoantibodies present in the serum of the recipient or antibodies produced by accidental immunization through previous transfusions.

In the case of Rh antigens, isoantibodies do not develop; therefore, hemolytic reactions involving the Rh system proceed only if the recipient had been previously immunized with the Rh antigen in question. The D antigen is the most important of the Rh antigens, and hemolysis due to Rh incompatibility occurs most frequently in the D negative (Rh negative) individual who has been given Rh positive whole blood or blood derivatives contaminated with Rh positive erythrocytes. In addition, pregnant women who are exposed to Rh positive erythrocytes during parturition will produce isoantibodies and transfer them across the placenta during a subsequent pregnancy, leading to erythroblastosis fetalis. Other isoantigens in other blood group systems can sensitize man, especially when donor blood is used for repeated transfusions in the same patient.

Hemolytic Disease of the Newborn (Erythroblastosis Fetalis)

In many cases, following parturition, an Rh negative mother becomes sensitized to fetal erythrocytes containing Rh antigens inherited from the father. Subsequent pregnancies result in anamnestic responses in the mother, the production of IgG capable of passing the placenta, and hemolytic reactions in the fetal circulation.

The majority of cases of hemolytic disease of the newborn, however, are due to ABO incompatibility. Of the remaining cases (about one-third), most are induced by Rh incompatibility, and only a minute fraction are associated with other blood group incompatibilities. In ABO incompatibilities, about half the cases occur in first pregnancies, whereas Rh incompatibilities develop during subsequent pregnancies.

Prophylaxis of Rh antibody-induced hemolytic reactions is readily achieved by preventing maternal sensitization to Rh antigen on fetal erythrocytes. The procedure involves the intramuscular administration of 1,000 to 5,000 μg of anti-D IgG to the mother within 36 hr. of delivery or abortion. The anti-Rh IgG causes rapid removal of the Rh positive fetal erythrocytes from the maternal circulation before sensitization can occur.

BIBLIOGRAPHY

Dimitrov, N. V., and Nodine, J. H. (eds.): *Drugs and Hematologic Reactions,* New York: Grune & Stratton, Inc., 1973.

"Editorial: Fetal/Maternal Incompatibility," *Lancet,* 2:958-959, 1972.

Kabat, E. A.: *Blood Group Substances,* New York: Academic Press, Inc., 1956.

Neely, C. L., and Draus, A. P.: "Mechanisms of Drug-induced Hemolytic Anemia," *Adv. Intern. Med.,* 18:59-76, 1972.

Prankerd, T. A. J.: "Idiopathic Thrombocytopenia Purpura," *Clin. Hematol.,* 1:327-337, 1972.

"Prevention of Rh Sensitization: Report of a WHO Scientific Group," *WHO Tech. Rep. Ser.,* no. 468, 1971.

Race, R. R., and Sanger, R.: *Blood Groups in Man,* Oxford: Blackwell Scientific Publications, Ltd., 1962.

Watkins, W. M.: "Blood Group Substances," *Science,* 152:172-181, 1966.

Zmijewski, C. M., and Fletcher, J.: *Immunohematology,* New York: Appleton-Century-Crofts, 1972.

Chapter 10

Transplantation Immunology

Arthur E. Krikszens and Bernard A. Briody

PERSPECTIVE

Interest in the transplantation of tissues and organs is probably as old as man and is conceptually, graphically, and sculpturally entrenched in Greek mythology. Although blood transfusions (allografts) and skin autografts have been performed successfully in man for about 150 years, it is only in the past 30 years that the immunogenetic principles of transplantation biology have been elucidated. Concomitantly, for the past 3 decades the transplantation of human tissues and organs has become a more practical, albeit imperfect, therapeutic procedure. There are many problems associated with the field of transplantation, including the ethical, moral, social, economic, and legal aspects of tissue and organ procurement; methods of tissue and organ preservation; the selection of recipients and donors; and the refinement of surgical techniques. The central problem, however, is that of graft rejection, a phenomenon that is immunological in nature. Consequently, the material in this chapter is concerned with an understanding of the immunological and genetic basis of graft rejection, with how immunosuppression can be utilized to mediate graft survival, with an awareness of the hazards of immunosuppression, and with the conditions under which graft-versus-host reactions develop.

TERMINOLOGY

Before proceeding to a discussion of rejection phenomena, it will be helpful to tabulate the

Table 10-1 Terminology of Transplantation Immunology

Noun	Adjective	Definition
Autograft	Autologous	A graft from one site to another in the same individual
Isograft	Isogeneic, syngeneic	A graft between individuals of the same genetic constitution (identical twins or members of a highly inbred group of animals after 20 or more generations of brother $\times$ sister matings)
Allograft (homograft)	Allogeneic	A graft between genetically dissimilar individuals of the same species
Xenograft	Xenogeneic	A graft between individuals of different species
—	Orthotopic	Pertaining to a graft placed in its normal anatomic position
—	Heterotopic	Pertaining to a graft placed in an unnatural anatomic position
—	Allovital	Pertaining to a graft that is expected to perform its normal function
—	Allostatic	Pertaining to a graft that is expected to serve as a nonviable mechanical support
Isoantigens (alloantigens)	—	The genetically determined antigenic differences between individuals of a species
Isoantibodies (alloantibodies)	—	Immunoglobulins that react specifically with isoantigens
Transplantation antigens (histocompatibility antigens)	—	The genetically determined antigens on the surface membrane of grafted cells that decide whether a graft is accepted or rejected
Histocompatibility genes	—	Genes responsible for the formation of transplantation antigens
Histocompatibility (H) loci	—	The chromosomal locations of histocompatibility genes
Histocompatibility alleles	—	The series or family of alternative genes present at each of the histocompatibility loci which are codominant (end products being demonstrable in heterozygotic progeny)

descriptive terms used in transplantation immunology which have immunological, genetic, anatomic, and functional significance (Table 10-1). Clinically, the major activity at present is concerned with the use of allografts.

GRAFT REJECTION (HOST-VERSUS-GRAFT REACTIONS)

Although the pioneering investigations of Little, Snell, Gorer, and others had established that transplanted tumors in mice were rejected because they contained genetically determined isoantigens not present in the recipient, it was Medawar who first critically analyzed the fate of skin allografts and demonstrated the basic pathophysiology and immunological nature of graft rejection. The classic observations of Medawar were extended and amplified by numerous investigators and are summarized in the ensuing sections.

First-set Rejection (Primary Rejection)

Under conditions in which both donor and recipient are healthy normal individuals, an allograft attempted for the first time will invariably be rejected. The process of graft rejection has a characteristic, sequential, and reproducible pathophysiology; each stage of the process is outlined below, along with the essential immunological components of the reaction.

The Afferent Arm of the Response (Days 1 and 2) Following surgical implantation of an orthotopic allograft of skin, healing ensues, vascularization develops, and the graft appears morphologically and functionally healthy and vigorous. Concomitant with the establishment of the microcirculation, the T lymphocytes of the recipient become sensitized to the transplantation antigens in the graft in a variety of ways. T cells migrate into the graft, recognize the foreign transplantation antigens, and are sensitized. Some of the sensitized T lymphocytes under the continuing stimulation of the transplantation antigens undergo blastogenesis and mitotic division within the graft, producing an increasing population of antigen-responsive cells. Other sensitized T cells leave the graft via the afferent lymphatic channels and undergo blastogenesis and mitotic division in the regional lymph nodes. As a consequence of surgical trauma, transplantation antigens are solubilized and drained into the local lymph nodes where T lymphocytes are sensitized. In addition, a few donor or passenger leukocytes, rich in transplantation antigens, migrate from the graft and sensitize recipient T cells in the draining lymph nodes.

Central Lymphoid Response (Days 2 and 3) The growing population of T cells specifically sensitized to the transplantation antigens migrates out of the paracortical areas of the regional lymph nodes and seeds other lymphoid tissue throughout the body, causing a generalized delayed hypersensitivity. Since the sensitivity is associated with the long-lived T lymphocytes responsible for delayed hypersensitivity memory, the recipient can remain sensitized for life.

The Efferent Arm of the Response (Days 4 to 9) Inflammation becomes evident by about the fourth day, and there is a progressive and extensive invasion of the graft by sensitized T lymphocytes and macrophages, but plasma cells are conspicuous by their absence. Stimulated by the transplantation antigens in the graft, the antigen-responsive sensitized T cells synthesize and release a battery of lymphokines that lead to cellular destruction and tissue damage. Since the transplantation antigens are present on the surface membranes of the donor cells, T cells are frequently seen attached to the grafted cells prior to evidence of their cytotoxic activity. Eventually, as the endothelial linings of the blood vessels within the graft are damaged, thrombosis occurs, vascular occlusion results, and the graft becomes ischemic.

Sloughing of the Graft (Day 10) With extensive necrosis developing throughout the grafted tissue, the graft assumes a scab-like appearance and sloughs off from the recipient. *First-set rejection* is completed before antibody production against the transplantation antigens reaches a peak and pursues an identical chronological course in agammaglobulinemics, thus proving that it is independent of antibody formation.

Second-set Rejection (Accelerated Rejection)

When a second skin allograft from the same donor is implanted in a recipient after rejection of the first allograft, more rapid destruction of the graft occurs because the recipient has an expanded population of antigen-responsive sensitized T cells as a result of prior exposure to the transplantation antigens. Vascularization commences but does not progress extensively before the sensitized T lymphocytes initiate a violent reaction in the depth of the graft. Necrosis develops early, and sloughing is usually complete in 6 days.

White-Graft Rejection

If allografts are attempted in recipients who have high concentrations of circulating antibodies against transplantation antigens, explosive rejection occurs. As soon as vascularization of the graft is attempted, the antibodies attach to the transplantation antigens on the surface membrane of the grafted cells and initiate a cytotoxic, complement-mediated reaction that destroys the cells and prevents further vascularization. In effect, the graft is choked to death with ischemia, and total rejection can occur so rapidly that sensitized T cells rarely participate in the reaction.

Clinical Experiences in Rejection

Experiences with renal transplantation in man indicate that graft rejection rarely follows the classic features outlined above, primarily because of the therapeutic use of immunosuppressive agents or techniques that prolong the survival of the graft. The rejection phenomena frequently represent a mixture of responses which is reflected in clinical nomenclature. For example, hyperacute or acute humoral rejection is essentially equivalent to white-graft rejection and results when a graft is performed in the presence of antibodies against transplantation antigens. Theoretically, the antibodies may be present because of previous cross-reacting grafts, blood transfusions, blood group antigens, cross-reacting antigens present in pathogenic bacteria, or antigenic stimulation by fetal cells consequent to parturition.

Acute or intermediate rejection is essentially equivalent to first- or second-set rejection in that it is mediated primarily by sensitized T cells. Acute or intermediate rejection crises develop after the first week and up to 2 years following transplantation. Local radiation can attenuate, reduce, or abolish this type of rejection crisis, suggesting that the reaction is caused by the invasion of cells which are susceptible to radiation.

Late or chronic rejection is the major pattern of rejection seen in persons who have had prolonged immunosuppressive therapy. In these cases, damage to the graft is a slow, chronic process associated with the production of antibody which occurs in spite of the immunosuppression. The main point of antibody action is on the vascular walls. Years may be required before the graft is finally destroyed, but when fully developed the process is essentially irreversible.

FACTORS MEDIATING GRAFT REJECTION

Transplantation Antigens (Histocompatibility Antigens)

As noted in Table 10-1, transplantation antigens are genetically determined antigens located on the surface membrane of tissue cells; their presence or absence decides whether a graft is accepted or rejected. For example, isografts between individuals of the same genetic constitution have identical transplantation antigens and are always accepted. On the other hand, allografts have genetically determined transplantation antigens that are foreign to the recipient. Consequently, recipient T lymphocytes will mount an immunological response (delayed hypersensitivity) to the donor transplantation antigens and in the process will destroy the allograft.

Although transplantation antigens fall into several groups or systems, each of which is capable of eliciting an immune response under allogeneic conditions, one or two groups or systems exert a predominant influence on the magnitude and intensity of the rejection process. Such groups of transplantation antigens are usually termed the major histocompatibility systems. In a number of animal species the major histocompatibility systems are comparable, and many concepts applicable to the human systems represent an extrapolation from experimental studies of the animal systems.

The Human Leukocyte-Locus A System in Man

The human leukocyte-locus A (HL-A) system, as the name implies, was first detected in leukocytes, but the histocompatibility antigens are found in all nucleated cells in the body. As the major histocompatibility locus in man, HL-A antigens are comparable to the H-2 system in mice, AgB system in rats, B system in chickens, H-I system in rabbits, DL-A system in dogs, RhL-A system in monkeys, and CL-A system in chimpanzees.

In dealing with major histocompatibility systems, a general rule can be formulated which states that the greater the disparity (histoincompatibility) between the donor and recipient, the more rapid and violent will be the rejection. Minor histocompatibility systems can contribute to the rejection response in cumulative fashion. For example, even if donor and recipient are identical in their major histocompatibility loci, differences in minor transplantation antigens can eventually lead to rejection. Thus, the greater the number of differences in both major and minor loci between donor and recipient, the more vigorous will be the rejection.

Characteristics of HL-A Antigens

Numerous attempts have been made to separate transplantation antigens from the plasma membrane of leukocytes and to purify and characterize them physically, chemically, and immunologically. Solubilization of the antigenic components has been tried using four different approaches: (1) detergents and detergent-like compounds, (2) proteolytic enzymes, (3) chaotropic agents, and (4) sonic energy. Much diversity exists in the character of the antigens released by these methods which is partly dependent on the technique used.

Water-soluble substances with antigenic activity have been obtained with molecular weights ranging from 7,000 to more than 800,000. Chemically, some of the antigenic materials are composed of proteins with varying percentages of carbohydrate and lipid; others are glycoproteins, and some are proteins. Much evidence has accumulated which indicates that the protein or polypeptide moieties are responsible for alloantigenic activity, but enzymatic degradation, periodate digestion, and inhibition studies suggest a similar role for the carbohydrate moiety. In many of the antigens, the carbohydrate content represents 5 to 7 percent of the total molecule. Thus, the results of chemical analyses of HL-A antigens are inconclusive and must await further clarification.

HL-A Subloci and Polymorphism

Despite the uncertainty concerning the chemical nature of HL-A antigens, accumulated data indicate that there is a large number of transplantation antigens (extreme polymorphism) in the HL-A system. The marked polymorphism associated with transplantation antigens reflects the number of histocompatibility loci, the number of different alleles (alternative genes) at each locus, and their relative frequencies. There are two principal HL-A subloci (LA and Four), each of which is multiallelic. Every individual has maternally and paternally derived chromosomes, each bearing two alleles (LA and Four) which are inherited as a unit. The genes are codominant and code for a series of HL-A antigens. Thus, an individual heterozygous at each sublocus (LA and Four) expresses four major HL-A antigens, one LA and one Four antigen from each parent. Consequently, since there are several possible alleles at each sublocus, the probability of finding two randomly selected individuals in the general population with matching HL-A antigens is low (less than 1:8,000). Similar results obtain with parent-offspring analyses. With siblings, on the other hand, there is a 1:4 chance that they will have identical HL-A antigens.

When skin grafts are performed in an attempt to evaluate the significance of the HL-A system, the results are revealing. As expected, skin grafts in identical twins survive indefinitely. Even with single antigenic differences within the HL-A system, skin grafts are rejected within 10 days, an indication that the HL-A antigens are part of a major histocompatibility system in man. Skin grafts between siblings with identical HL-A antigens survive for 20 to 40 days before being rejected. The data indicate that matching of HL-A antigens cannot be equated with complete histocompatibility and that graft survival also reflects differences in minor histocompatibility antigens. Unfortunately, clinical experience in regard to HL-A identity and persistence of renal transplants is similarly disappointing because of the cumulative effect of minor incompatibilities. Nonetheless, grafts from sibling donors with identical HL-A antigens are always preferable because they function better, provoke fewer rejection episodes, and survive longer under comparable or less vigorous immunosuppressive therapy than do grafts from nonidentical HL-A donors.

The ABO Blood Group Histocompatibility System

The unique success of blood transfusions, the most widely employed therapeutic allografts, derives from two essential aspects: (1) the simplicity and efficacy of donor-recipient matching procedures and (2) the deficiency of HL-A antigens in human erythrocytes. For example, erythrocytes from ABO-compatible donors fail to sensitize man against skin allografts.

On the other hand, the ABO blood group antigens comprise the other major histocompatibility system in man. As noted in Chapter 9, if donor erythrocytes are transfused into an incompatible recipient, a severe or fatal reaction can ensue as a consequence of the agglutination of the cells, complement-mediated lysis, and destruction of the antibody-coated cells in the spleen. Skin grafts implanted into ABO-incompatible recipients show accelerated rejection, and AB erythrocytes or A and B antigens derived from the gastric mucosa of hogs and horses can sensitize group O human volunteers so that subsequent skin grafts from AB, A, or B donors are rejected prematurely (second-set rejection). In addition, renal allografts from an A or B donor to an O recipient show an acute second-set or white-graft rejection characterized by a failure to establish circulation in the graft accompanied by distention and thrombosis of afferent arterioles and glomerular capillaries with sludged erythrocytes, presumably mediated by preformed circulating isoantibodies. The accumulated data indicate that ABO antigens are part of a major histocompatibility system and are also present on the surface of fixed tissue cells.

The Y Histocompatibility System

In mice and rats, one of the minor histocompatibility systems is associated with the heterogametic male sex. The sex-linked Y antigen represents an exception to the rule which states that isografts survive indefinitely. In isogeneic mice and rats, isografts from males to females are rejected slowly or with moderate speed, whereas other isografts are always accepted. Accumulated evidence confirms that the rejection of male isografts by female recipient mice is due to the presence of a transplantation antigen determined by a locus on the Y chromosome. In mice, the Y antigen seems to be a species-determined factor rather than an isogeneically inherited characteristic. The extent and significance of the Y system in man is still under investigation. Meanwhile, however, whenever possible in human transplants, male allografts to female recipients should be avoided.

Cell-mediated Immunity

The involvement of cells as effectors of allograft rejection is amply documented. The pathophysiology and chronology of first- and second-set rejection indicate that the basic reaction is one of delayed hypersensitivity, or cell-mediated immunity. The findings that allograft sensitivity can be transferred by cells and by transfer factor, but not by serum, and that rejection occurs at the expected time in agammaglobulinemics substantiate the fundamental significance of delayed hypersensitivity in graft rejection. It follows, therefore, that the active cells involved in graft rejection are T lymphocytes and macrophages.

Alloantigenic stimulation leads to blastogenic and mitotic activity in the antigen-responsive T lymphocytes. The derived immunoblasts or blast cells are much larger than the T lymphocytes, have little or no endoplasmic reticulum, and actively synthesize nucleic acid and protein; the protein is synthesized on small clusters of ribosomes scattered randomly in the cytoplasm instead of on membrane-associated ribosomes. Through mitotic activity the immunoblasts build up a population of sensitized cells that revert to their lymphocyte form and seed lymphatic tissue throughout the body.

The efferent arm of the response then accumulates numerous sensitized T cells within the graft as the inflammatory response begins. The sensitized T cells localize in the small blood vessels of the graft and pass through the endothelial cells into the grafted tissue. Contact with the transplantation antigens in the graft causes the synthesis and release of lymphokines by the sensitized T cells and the recruitment and activation of other lymphocytes and macrophages.

As the inflammatory response progresses, tissue damage and destruction within the graft become more evident. The mechanism of cell destruction is primarily associated with direct contact of the sensitized T cells with the graft cells and, to a lesser extent, through the action of released lymphotoxin on the graft cells. After combining with the transplantation antigens on the plasma membrane of the graft cells, the sensitized T cells remain adherent to the target cells until the latter are killed, often by lysis (the so-called kiss of death). The precise factors involved in the death of the target cells are unknown but may well be associated with lymphotoxin. The absolute number of lymphocytes observed in the rapid and massive destruction of the graft are presumably supplemented by an influx of macrophages which amplify the response and enhance the tissue damage by releasing lysosomal enzymes.

Perhaps the most critical target cells in the graft are the endothelial cells of the vascular bed. The incoming sensitized T cells adhere to the endothelial cells early in the rejection process, causing their destruction and exposing the underlying connective tissue, thereby leading to thrombus formation, platelet activation, and the clotting cascade. Thereafter, ischemic necrosis of massive areas of the grafted tissue ensues, and rejection is complete.

Humoral Immunity

While antibody is not essential for graft rejection, it may become involved at any stage in the process, especially in human renal transplantation. As noted earlier, antibody is a practical consideration because blood group isoantibodies in the recipient or HL-A antibodies present at the time of the transplant can lead to an acute or hyperacute rejection of the allograft. In addition, the late development of antibody in immunosuppressed patients appears to be particularly important in chronic rejection of renal transplants several years after their implantation.

Both IgM and IgG classes can participate in allograft rejection, their destructive effects being mediated by complement. After antibody combines with HL-A or other transplantation antigens on the plasma membranes of the grafted cells, complement can be bound. The net result is not only the cytotoxic effect on the grafted cell but also the release of anaphylatoxins, the infiltration of neutrophils, thrombus formation, and ischemic necrosis quite analogous to the Arthus reaction.

FACTORS MEDIATING GRAFT SURVIVAL

Currently, one of the most active areas of immunological investigation involves concerted efforts to prolong the survival of allografts both experimentally and in clinical practice. Apart from accurate histocompatibility testing, which will be considered in a subsequent section, graft survival can be prolonged by several mechanisms, including appropriate anatomical and physiological conditions, variations in the immune response, and a battery of intervention procedures including biological, chemical, and physical agents and surgery. However, the plethora of methods employed is ample testimony to the difficulty of the problem and the lack of a safe and effective remedy. Nonetheless, much progress has been achieved, and hopefully, additional gains can be realized without seriously compromising the overall immunological integrity of the allograft recipient.

Immunologically Privileged Sites

Uterine allografts of naturally implanted embryos represent the outstanding example of effective resolution of allogeneic transplantation and constitute an essential prerequisite for the evolution of mammals. The human fetus, for example, develops into an allograft of impressive proportion without either sensitizing the mother or being responsive to existing or induced maternal sensitivity. In addition, many heterotopic allografts (those placed in an unnatural anatomic position) are accepted, occasionally indefinitely in the recipient. Thus, the concept of immunologically privileged sites connotes that there are certain favored sites in which heterotopic allografts can survive for prolonged periods in the recipient, apparently exempt from immunological rejection.

There appear to be three mechanisms whereby tissues can achieve an immunologically privileged status:

1 Protection or quarantine of the allograft within a matrix impenetrable to immunocompetent cells (uterus and cartilage)
2 Absence of a lymphatic drainage system (brain and hamster cheek pouch) or an ineffective lymphatic drainage system (testis)
3 Lack of vascularity or relative avascularity (meninges, cornea, and anterior chamber of the eye)

Thus, it is apparent that survival of allografts in immunologically privileged sites is dependent upon blockage of afferent, efferent, or both afferent and efferent arms of the rejection response. In pregnancy, for example, the trophoblast functions as a protective barrier for both the fetus and the mother. In cartilage allografts, for which survival for years is the rule, the chondrocytes are surrounded by a matrix of sulphated mucopolysaccharides which excludes them from antigenically stimulating the recipient. In corneal allografts, survival is permanent as long as the grafts remain unvascularized. The corollary to these observations also pertains. If the trophoblastic or cartilagenous matrices are removed or if vascularization or lymphatic drainage is established in the privileged sites, typical first-set rejection of the allografts results.

Immunological Enhancement

One of the apparent paradoxes in immunology concerns the phenomenon of immunological enhancement, which may be defined as the prolongation of allograft survival by means of actively or passively produced antibodies specific for the transplantation antigens in the graft. Since enhancement requires the presence of specific antibody, it is probably distinct from tolerance, which occurs under conditions which prevent or suppress antibody production. On the other hand, the function of the antibody may be to favor the development of low zone tolerance by reducing the concentration of transplantation antigens available for stimulation of T or B cells.

Enhancing antibodies may be elicited by active immunization or introduced by passive immunization, or both. Experimentally, for example, functional renal transplants (allografts) can persist for more than 200 days in rats receiving an intravenous injection of donor spleen cells 1 day before the graft and passive immunization with antiserum prepared in animals of the recipient strain against donor spleen and lymph node cells. The prime mediators of enhancement appear to be IgG antibodies, but there is confusion concerning the particular subclass involved, since both complement-fixing (IgG1) and noncomplement-binding (IgG2) antibodies have been incriminated. In some systems, the action of antibody appears to be dose-dependent. Small, passively administered doses of antibody tend to prolong graft survival, whereas large doses shorten the time required for rejection.

Naturally, in the absence of definitive data and because of widely disparate experimental conditions, theoretical explanations for enhancement are numerous and conflicting. Afferent blockade is stated to occur because antibodies combine with the transplantation antigens and prevent them from stimulating the immune system of the recipient. Efferent blockade is assumed to function because antibodies combine with the transplantation antigens, thereby preventing their interaction either with sensitized T cells or with cytotoxic antibodies or both. This scheme necessarily requires that enhancement occur after antibodies are produced, since the interference is with the activities of T and B cells. Central blockade may result when antibodies suppress the proliferation of T cells or the formation of cytotoxic antibody by feedback inhibition. Although available evidence can be cited in support of each theory and may represent, in fact, a composite at the afferent, central, and efferent levels of the immune response, the authors favor a more fundamental biological explanation based on the selective survival of grafted cells with IgG2 adherent to their surface, the selective destruction of grafted cells with adsorbed IgG1 mediated by complement, and the development of low zone tolerance associated with the limited but continuous release of transplantation antigens. Admittedly, the only evidence in favor of the latter theory is that experimentally IgG2 is highly efficient in promoting enhancement, that it does suppress the formation of sensitized T cells, that the Fc fragment of IgG2 depresses T cells (central depression of allograft immunity), that the $F(ab)_2$ fragment of IgG2 blocks the lytic action of IgG1 in the presence of complement, and that human IgG2 and $F(ab)_2$ against HL-A donor antigens are clinically useful in renal transplantation.

Immunosuppression

Utilizing a variety of techniques, often in combination, the experimental biologist and the clinician can intervene in ways that will, in some cases, effectively prolong the survival of allografts. The procedures are designed to suppress the cell-mediated response. Ideally, prolongation of allograft survival should specifically and selectively suppress the development of delayed hypersensitivity to the transplantation antigens in the graft without seriously compromising the ability of the immune system to respond to other antigens. Indeed, partial success has been achieved, and prospective progress can be anticipated. For example, on the basis of available experimental and clinical data, it is not unreasonable to assume that most immunosuppressive agents are clinically effective primarily because they facilitate the development of immunological tolerance to the transplantation antigens in the allograft. Unfortunately, at the same time, the immunosuppressive agents seriously hamper the cell-mediated immunological surveillance mechanism of the recipient, as is indicated by an unusually high incidence of intracellular infections and cancer in patients receiving prolonged immunosuppressive therapy.

Apart from immunological enhancement and tolerance, numerous immunosuppressive agents may interfere with humoral as well as cell-mediated immunity or may inhibit different phases in the immune response (afferent, central, efferent). The various immunosuppressive agents frequently exhibit differential susceptibility for selected cells and tissues, are dose- and time-dependent, and exert synergistic effects when used in combination.

Radiation Whole-body x-irradiation is one of the oldest methods of destroying lymphatic tissue but is rarely used today. A dose of 200 to 600 rads causes a temporary but severe pancytopenia and is frequently accompanied by a sharp increase in life-threatening infections. Permanent impairment of the immune system results when 1,500 rads are employed and often necessitates bone marrow or lymphocyte transplantation, which is associated in turn with graft-versus-host rejection. X-irradiation produces intracellular lesions in the mitotic apparatus and in DNA replicating mechanisms and induces maximal immunosuppression when administered a few hours to a few days prior to transplantation.

Local irradiation of the allograft after implantation or during rejection crises (acute episodes in which functional activity of the transplant is impaired) is of some value, especially when combined with other immunosuppressive agents. The beneficial effects of local irradiation are probably due to the destruction of immunocompetent cells within the graft. Extracorporeal irradiation of blood passing through an arteriovenous shunt is aimed directly at the destruction of the T lymphocytes of the recipient and appears to be of value when used in conjunction with other agents.

Surgical Ablation Thymectomy, splenectomy, and lymphadenectomy performed in an effort to remove lymphatic tissue have generally failed to prolong graft survival. Experimentally, neonatal thymectomy will significantly promote allograft acceptance but is impractical in man. Adult thymectomy is intended to deplete the T cell population but requires other immunosuppressive agents to reduce the circulating and stationary pools of T cells. Splenectomy can remove one-third of the lymphoid tissue in the body and can depress antibody formation, but the remaining lymphatic tissue compensates for ablated tissue, and allografts are rejected without delay. Similar conditions pertain to lymphadenectomy.

Thoracic Duct Drainage Originally exploited with great success in animal experiments, physical removal of T lymphocytes by chronic thoracic duct drainage is used in man as an initial immunosuppressive procedure as well as an adjunct to other agents. The method involves cannulation of the thoracic duct and the removal of several liters of lymph daily from the recipient, followed by plasmaphoresis of the lymphocytes and recirculation of the lymph. The result is suppression of delayed hypersensitivity and prolongation of allograft survival, but the procedure is cumbersome, requires careful monitoring of the circulating lymphocyte pool over an extended period of time, and is associated with an increased risk of serious microbial infection.

Biological Agents Apart from the potential use of antigen or antibody in producing immunological enhancement and antigen in inducing immunological tolerance, there are a number of biological agents that can delay allograft rejection when administered singly or in combination with other agents. Clinically useful biological agents include the corticosteroids and antilymphocyte globulin (antibody). Antibiotics (chloramphenicol, tetracyclines, puromycin, actinomycin D, mitomycin C), enzymes (asparaginase), and plant alkaloids (colchicine, vinblastine, vincristine) are also available, but their therapeutic use is limited because of their toxicity and diverse side effects.

Corticosteroids Although corticosteroids cannot be used alone in primary immunosuppression, a number of natural and synthetic congeners are integral components of current therapeutic regimens. The steroids vary in potency and in their toxicity for different species. Fortunately, man is resistant to the toxic effects of corticosteroids, and the drugs can be administered for prolonged periods without encountering toxic reactions. Prednisone, the most widely used immunosuppressive steroid, intervenes at many points in the immune response but is especially potent as an anti-inflammatory agent in inhibiting the effector phase of graft rejection. For this reason, prednisone is particularly valuable in reversing rejection crises. The corticosteroids can produce other diverse effects including stabilization of lysosomal membranes, lymphocytolysis, depression of cellular metabolism, and inhibition of primary and secondary humoral and cellular immune responses, but their value in prolonging allograft survival is considered to derive principally from their anti-inflammatory action and not from a direct attack on the immune system.

Antilymphocyte Antibodies Even though Metchnikoff raised the issue at the turn of the twentieth century, only in the past 10 years has the therapeutic use of antilymphocyte serum (ALS) and its purified derivatives, antilymphocyte globulin (ALG) and antilymphocyte immunoglobulin (ALIgG), become an exciting reality in transplantation immunology. ALS is generally prepared in horses following immunization with human lymphocytes derived from the thymus, lymph nodes, recirculating pool, stillborn infants, or cadavers and is subsequently fractionated into the gamma globulin fraction (ALG) or is further separated into ALIgG.

Antilymphocyte antibodies are selectively active against T cells and cause a dramatic fall in the circulating lymphocyte pool within a few hours. Concomitantly, there is a depletion of the paracortical, thymus-dependent areas of the central lymphoid tissue. The mode of action of antilymphocyte antibodies appears to depend on combination with the predominant T cells in the recirculating pool, complement-mediated lysis, and sequestration and destruction within the liver and spleen. B lymphocytes remain virtually unaffected, and humoral responses are generally intact.

Preparations of antilymphocyte antibodies constitute the most potent immunosuppressive agents therapeutically available. For example, when used experimentally, antibodies against T cells can greatly extend the survival of xenografts as well as allografts and can even abolish a preexisting state of graft sensitivity. Clinical impressions concerning the value of antibodies against T cells are generally favorable, but an accurate assessment is difficult because the antilymphocyte preparations are invariably combined with other immunosuppressive agents and vary widely in potency, dosage, route, and duration of treatment. Probably the antibodies against T cells will be especially valuable in the management of rejection crises. Although antilymphocyte antibodies are generally nontoxic in the dosages required to suppress rejection and are selectively active against T cells, there are potential drawbacks and hazards associated with their therapeutic use, including rejection when their administration is discontinued, anaphylaxis, serum sickness, and immune complex renal disease. In addition, since antibodies against T cells leave the humoral response intact, eventual rejection can be induced by cytotoxic and cytolytic antibodies against the transplantation antigens in the allograft, or antibodies against the T cells can be inactivated by the humoral response of the recipient.

Antilymphotoxin Antibody Another approach to the problem of suppressing graft rejection is based on the production and use of antibody against species-specific lymphotoxin, an antigenic lymphokine intimately involved in the destruction of target cells in cell-mediated immunity. The limited data available indicate that antilymphotoxin antibody is highly effective in suppressing graft rejection and may prove to be clinically useful. In cell culture experiments, antilymphotoxin antibody prevents the release of lymphotoxin even when cell contact is made between sensitized T lymphocytes and their target cells. After contact with the target cells and antilymphotoxin antibody, the sensitized T lymphocytes enlarge and disappear from the culture. In view of these findings, antilymphotoxin antibody may be especially valuable in reversing rejection crises.

Immunosuppressive Drugs Many of the drugs listed in Table 10-2 were first used in cancer chemotherapy, but several alkylating agents and antimetabolites can also prolong the sur-

Table 10-2 Properties of Selected Immunosuppressive Drugs

Type and agent	Action	Immunosuppressive result
Alkylating Agents Nitrogen mustards (cyclophosphamide) Sulfur mustards Busulfan Triethylenemelamine	Alkylate and cross-link DNA, RNA, and proteins; interfere with nucleic acid synthesis; active against rapidly dividing cells	Can suppress primary and secondary antibody responses; suppress delayed hypersensitivity responses
Antimetabolites Folic acid antagonists Aminopterin Amethopterin	Prevent conversion of folic acid to folinic acid; inhibit synthesis of purines and DNA	Can suppress primary and secondary antibody responses; suppress delayed hypersensitivity responses
Purine analogues 6-Mercaptopurine Azathioprine	Interfere with the interconversion of nucleosides; inhibit DNA synthesis	Suppress primary IgG production; suppress delayed hypersensitivity responses
Pyrimidine analogues Cytosine arabinoside Adamantyl cytarabine	Inhibit DNA polymerase and formation of deoxycytidine; can be converted to a nucleotide and incorporated into nucleic acid	Can suppress primary and secondary antibody responses; suppress delayed hypersensitivity responses

vival of allografts. The most valuable and widely used drug in clinical immunosuppression is *azathioprine,* a purine analogue that interferes with DNA synthesis, suppresses delayed hypersensitivity, and inhibits IgG production. Azathioprine can be administered orally, is broken down to 6-mercaptopurine, and then is converted to the active ribotide which competes with inosinic acid for enzymes involved in guanylic and adenylic acid synthesis and inhibits the synthesis of a precursor of inosinic acid (5-phosphoribosylamine) by a feedback mechanism. When administered following the antigen, agents such as azathioprine, cyclophosphamide, and amethopterin are probably immunosuppressive for two major reasons: (1) They inhibit the active proliferation of antigen-responsive T cells, and (2) they facilitate the development of immunological tolerance.

Combined Immunosuppressive Agents Since no single agent has yet been clinically applied to prolong allograft survival and to reverse rejection crises that arise, synergistic combinations of agents and procedures have evolved into more or less successful immunosuppressive regimens. A report from the Kidney Transplant Registry indicates that the most successful scheme for prolonging the survival of renal allografts includes the use of prednisone, azathioprine, actinomycin D, and localized irradiation of the graft after implantation. Rejection crises developing after transplantation are controlled primarily by massive doses of prednisone. Evaluation of antilymphocyte antibodies and antilymphotoxin antibodies is proceeding cautiously and may ultimately prove to be so beneficial as to largely replace the current regimen.

Under the stimulus of effective combined immunosuppressive therapy and with the passage of time, there is a strong clinical impression that the recipient makes a natural accommodation to the allograft. In other words, if a graft functions for a year, there is a high probability that it will survive for many more years. Two major reasons are cited for these observations: (1) Immunological tolerance has been developed, and (2) the endothelium of the recipient replaces the graft endothelium and acts as a shield against rejection.

Immunological Surveillance

The greatest hazard associated with therapeutic prolongation of allograft survival is the creation of immunological cripples who are at the mercy of intracellular infections and cancer. As noted in Chapter 8, cell-mediated immunity is primarily responsible for the elimination of and recovery from intracellular infections. At therapeutic dosage, most immunosuppressive agents destroy T lymphocytes without seriously impairing B lymphocytes. With more widespread and prolonged use of immunosuppressive drugs in transplantation and particularly in the treatment of autoimmune diseases and with long-term study of patients with immunological deficiency diseases and autoimmune diseases, it is becoming increasingly apparent that there is a sharply increased incidence of malignancy in patients whose T lymphocytes are absent, depressed, suppressed, perverted, or exhausted. These findings have led to the suggestion that the major evolutionary function of cell-mediated immunity is to provide surveillance against immunologically altered cells, including those with neoplastic potential. Thus, immunological surveillance is a protective mechanism that eliminates neoplastic cells that continuously arise as a consequence of somatic mutation because they contain new antigens in their plasma membranes which are recognized as foreign and are destroyed by antigen-responsive T lymphocytes. Obviously, if T cells are missing, reduced, or cannot function, immunological surveillance is ineffective, and malignancy will result.

The validity of the concept of immunological surveillance is supported by a number of experimental observations. For example, carcinogenesis in animals is greatly enhanced by immunosuppressive drugs and antilymphocyte antibodies. Practically every potent experimental carcinogen is also a powerful immunosuppressive agent. Neoplastic cells occasionally carried over with renal allografts survive, replicate, and metastasize in the immunosuppressed recipient, whereas they are known to be promptly rejected by individuals whose T lymphocytes are not immunosuppressed.

HISTOCOMPATIBILITY MATCHING

Because histocompatibility matching of donor and recipient combined with less vigorous immunosuppression is currently the most logical approach to transplantation, strenuous efforts are being directed toward effective and practical testing procedures. While exact matching in man is possible only in the case of identical twins, the less the disparity between donor and recipient, the greater the chance of graft survival. Two major groups of transplantation antigens (ABO blood groups and HL-A) must be considered, and minor antigens should be evaluated whenever possible.

Assuming ABO compatibility, which can be achieved without difficulty, the chief complexities are introduced by HL-A matching, and a battery of in vitro and in vivo tests have been devised in an attempt to evaluate histocompatibility in this system. As a base line, and in the absence of immunosuppression, it is apparent that even one or two allelic differences in HL-A antigens are critical. In one series of experiments, for example, human skin allografts persisted for 24.9, 14.4, and 11.6 days respectively in volunteers with 0, 1, and 2 HL-A allelic differences.

Serological Tests

A number of serological tests have proved valuable as initial screening procedures to assay the similarity of HL-A antigens among hundreds of potential donors and recipients; these tests are reproducible, speedy, economical, and readily adaptable to computer analysis. In essence, the tests utilize antisera usually specific for a limited number of HL-A antigens and obtained from patients receiving multiple transfusions of whole blood, multiparous women sensitized to fetal antigens defined by paternally derived genes absent in the mother, and individuals deliberately immunized with skin grafts or leukocyte injections.

Since HL-A antigens are present in relatively high concentration on the plasma membrane of circulating leukocytes, these cells are widely employed in serotyping. Lymphocytes, granulocytes, and platelets have been assayed for HL-A antigens by a variety of methods, including leukoagglutination, complement-mediated lymphocytotoxicity, complement fixation, immune adherence, mixed hemagglutination, and immunofluorescence procedures. The cells of prospective donors are compared with those of the recipient in their reactions with a panel of antisera specific for selected HL-A antigens. The most compatible donors have cells that combine with the same antisera as the cells of the recipient, as determined quantitatively by one or more of the indicated tests.

One-way Mixed Leukocyte Culture (MLC) Test

Together with preliminary screening by serotyping, the selective use of the MLC test forms the basis for most current schemes for matching histocompatibilities of donors and recipients. The one-way MLC test depends upon the fact that some immunocompetent T lymphocytes, when exposed to HL-A incompatible antigens, will transform into large blast cells, take up tritiated thymidine, and divide. The degree of stimulation is a measure of the histocompatibility difference between donor and recipient lymphocytes.

In practice, the MLC test is made unidirectional by killing donor lymphocytes by x-irradiation or preventing their response by treatment with mitomycin C. Thus, only recipient lymphocytes undergo blastogenesis and mitosis when exposed to incompatible HL-A antigens on donor lymphocytes in mixed cell cultures. The MLC test can be quantitated by determining the incorporation of tritiated thymidine. When recipient lymphocytes fail to take up and incorporate the radiolabel, it can be concluded that donor and recipient lymphocytes have the same HL-A antigens. Not only does the one-way MLC test correlate well with serotyping of HL-A antigens, but it is also capable of detecting some, but by no means all, of the minor transplantation antigens. Consequently, even when totally compatible by the MLC test, donor allografts can be eventually rejected by the recipient.

An interesting but as yet unexplained factor in performance of the MLC test is that even though it is the response of T lymphocytes that is measured, the presence of macrophages is apparently essential for the reaction, since highly purified populations of lymphocytes respond poorly.

Normal Lymphocyte Transfer (NLT) Test

The NLT test depends upon the intensity of the delayed hypersensitivity reaction (2 days) occurring at the intradermal site where viable lymphocytes from a prospective recipient are injected into a prospective donor. The NLT test presumably represents a graft-versus-host reaction in which the injected T lymphocytes respond to the HL-A antigens of the prospective donor, the severity of the reaction being a measure of the disparity in HL-A antigens. Consequently, a minimal or negative reaction is considered evidence of HL-A compatibility. Apart from the hazards of injecting viruses (especially hepatitis virus) or malignant cells, the NLT procedure has the major drawback of sensitizing the T lymphocytes of the prospective donor to the transplantation antigens of the recipient.

The Third-man Test

In this test a neutral individual (third man) is first sensitized with a skin graft or lymphocytes from the prospective recipient. After he has rejected the recipient graft, the third man is challenged with skin grafts or lymphocytes from prospective donors. If the prospective recipient and donor share at least one major antigen, the third man rejects the donor graft in a second-set rejection. The chief drawback which makes the procedure unsuitable for clinical use is that the third man selects only donors who share transplantation antigens, not donors who differ with respect to major antigens.

Current Clinical Practice

While the complexities and difficulties of histocompatibility matching are not completely resolved, much progress has been achieved. The development of serotyping procedures, the availability of antisera specific for different HL-A antigens, and the evaluation of data derived from panels of antisera have facilitated the use of computerized data retrieval systems in organizing large pools of potential donors in matching programs on a national or continental basis (Eurotransplant, Scandiatransplant, and the program at the University of California at Los Angeles). Thus, a few potential HL-A compatible donors can be selected and subsequently examined by the one-way MLC test with recipient lymphocytes. Schemes such as these should make the use of cadavers more practical as a source of organ transplants. Among other factors, the pursuit of more effective matching procedures is critically dependent upon the isolation and characterization of HL-A and other transplantation antigens.

GRAFT-VERSUS-HOST REACTIONS

The three requirements for graft-versus-host reactions (GVHR) are:

1 The allograft must contain T lymphocytes.
2 The recipient must have transplantation antigens absent in the allograft donor.
3 The recipient must be incapable of rejecting the immunocompetent T cells in the donor allograft.

Inability to reject allogeneic T lymphocytes might be due to the fact that the recipient is immature (fetus), has immunological deficiency disease, has been accidentally irradiated or otherwise immunosuppressed, or fails to recognize the donor T cells as foreign, whereas the donor lymphocytes can become sensitized to the transplantation antigens in the host. The latter case is an experimental situation in which T lymphocytes derived from either inbred parent AA or BB and injected into F_1 hybrid progeny mice (AB) will (1) be accepted by the hybrid progeny, (2) react immunologically to the transplantation antigens inherited from the other parent and produce a fatal GVHR. Death of the hybrid mice is preceded by a *runting syndrome* characterized by inhibition of growth, splenomegaly, and hemolytic anemia.

In man, GVHR are encountered following allogeneic transplants of bone marrow, leukocytes, or thymus in efforts to reconstitute immunodeficient children, to repopulate lymphatic tissue irreversibly damaged in radiation accidents, to treat leukemic patients who have been therapeutically immunosuppressed, and to provide replacement of blood by intrauterine transfusion in the prevention of erythroblastosis fetalis or Rh disease. The syndrome observed in man includes fever, loss of weight, anemia, splenomegaly, diarrhea, and rash. As with host-versus-graft reactions, the greater the disparity in transplantation antigens between donor and recipient, the more severe will be the GVHR. Differences in HL-A antigens, for example, can be fatal.

Following the transfer of allogeneic T lymphocytes to the immunologically incompetent recipient, the donor cells colonize the spleen and lymphoid centers of the recipient. In these locations the donor T cells react to the incompatible transplantation antigens in the recipient and undergo blastogenesis and mitosis, leading to the formation of a large population of sensitized lymphocytes. Thereafter, the destruction of recipient tissue mediated by lymphokines accelerates, splenomegaly becomes more prominent, and the sensitized T cells function as the lymphatic tissue of the recipient even to the extent that donor skin grafts are readily accepted. Although the GVHR may proceed to a fatal outcome, fortunately in many situations GVHR have a finite duration. The explanation for this finding is not apparent, and consequently, numerous suggestions have been offered, including immunological enhancement, immunological tolerance, mutual chimerism or immunological tolerance between donor and recipient, eventual senesence and death of the donor lymphocytes, and in some cases, regeneration of the suppressed or incompletely destroyed lymphatic tissue of the recipient.

BIBLIOGRAPHY

Biggar, W. D., Park, B. H., and Good, R. A.: "Immunological Reconstruction," *Annu. Rev. Med.,* 24:135-143, 1973.

Burnet, F. M.: *Immunological Surveillance,* New York: Pergamon Press, 1970.

Cinader, B.: "The Future of Tumor Immunology," *Med. Clin. North Am.,* 56:801-836, 1972.

Feldman, J. D.: "Immunological Enhancement: A Study of Blocking Antibodies," *Adv. Immunol.,* 15:167-214, 1972.

Fudenberg, H. H., Pink, J. R. L., Stites, D. C., and Wang, A. C.: *Basic Immunogenetics,* New York: Oxford University Press, 1972.

Leibovitz, S., and Schwartz, R. S.: "Malignancy as a Complication of Immunosuppressive Therapy," *Adv. Intern. Med.,* 17:95-124, 1971.

Loughridge, L. W. "Drugs and Other Agents in Renal Transplantation," *Progr. Biochem. Pharmacol.,* 7:498-520, 1972.

Möller, G. (ed.): "Lymphoid Cell Replacement Therapy," *Transplant. Rev.,* 9:3-72, 1972.

——— (ed.): "Stimulation of Lymphocytes by Allogeneic Cells, " *Transplant. Rev.,* 12:3-228, 1972.

Najarian, J. S., and Simmons, R. L.: *Transplantation,* Philadelphia: Lea & Febiger, 1973.

"Proceedings First International Symposium on

Clinical Organ Transplantation," *Transplant. Proc.,* 4:427-792, 1972.
Turnell, R. W., Clarke, L. H., and Burton, A. F.: "Studies on the Mechanism of Corticosteroid-induced Lymphocytolysis," *Cancer Res.,* 33:203-212, 1973.
Weston, W. L., Claman, H. N., and Krueger, G. G.: "Site of Action of Cortisol in Cellular Immunity," *J. Immunol.,* 110:880-883, 1973.
Winkelstein, A.: "Mechanisms of Immunosuppression: Effects of Cyclophosphamide on Cellular Immunity," *Blood,* 41:273-284, 1973.

Chapter 11

Autoimmunity

Arthur E. Krikszens and Bernard A. Briody

IMMUNOLOGICAL TOLERANCE (IMMUNOLOGICAL UNRESPONSIVENESS)

Two forms of immunological tolerance are recognized—natural and acquired. Immunological tolerance may be defined as a specific immunological reaction involving antigen (tolerogen), T and B lymphocytes, and complement occurring when an antigen is presented in a form or under conditions that induce the immune mechanisms of an immunocompetent individual to be unresponsive both on initial exposure and, for a variable period, upon subsequent challenge with the same antigen.

The ability of antigen to turn off immunoresponsive mechanisms (immunological tolerance) is essential for human survival, for otherwise immunological suicide would eliminate the human species. In addition, the establishment of immunological tolerance can enhance allogeneic transplantation, whereas a breakdown in tolerance can precipitate autoimmune disease. Paradoxically, the end result of acquiring or losing tolerance may be cancer. Obviously, then, an appreciation and understanding of tolerance are relevant to clinical medicine.

Natural Tolerance and the Clonal Selection Theory of Burnet

Burnet postulated that natural tolerance develops during fetal life as a mechanism to prevent individuals from mounting an immune response to their own antigens, and he formulated the *clonal selection theory* as a means to account for the immunospecificity of self-recognition (natural tolerance) and of responses to foreign antigens (humoral and cell-mediated immunity). Although it has been modified many times, the clonal selection theory stimulated an enormous amount of productive experimental research and successfully predicted two of the most fundamental concepts in immunology: (1) tolerance can be produced if foreign antigens are introduced during fetal development; (2) clonal proliferation of selected small lymphocytes occurs in response to antigenic stimulation.

Immunological recognition of ones' own antigens, known as autoantigens, is the result of an ontogenetic maturation process occurring during embryogenesis upon exposure to fetal antigens. Under normal conditions natural tolerance persists for the life of the individual but can be broken, leading in some cases to autoimmune disease and cancer. Although the phenomenon of natural tolerance is amply documented, the mechanism by which it occurs is obscure. Current evidence suggests that natural tolerance is not due to the elimination or loss of immunologically reactive small lymphocytes (forbidden clones) but to the inhibition or inactivation of genes required for a specific cell-mediated or humoral response.

According to clonal selection theory, clones of small lymphocytes committed to respond to one or a few antigenic determinants arise as a result of somatic mutation during embryogenesis when the mutation rate is extremely high. After immunological maturation, contact with the appropriate antigenic determinant causes the selected clones to transform into large blast cells, divide, and revert to sensitized small lymphocytes, thereby greatly expanding the population of antigen-responsive cells specifically capable of recognizing that determinant group (Chap. 7).

Acquired Tolerance

As predicted by Burnet and demonstrated by Medawar and others, exposure of the fetus to a foreign antigen can lead to a state of acquired tolerance specific for that antigen. Embryos treated in this manner developed into adults unable to produce sensitized lymphocytes or antibody upon challenge with the antigen. Subsequently, it was found that although acquired tolerance can be induced most readily before or during maturation of the immune system, it can also be produced under special circumstances in immunologically competent adults.

An analysis of the factors that influence the development of acquired tolerance is essential for a more adequate understanding of the phenomenon and as a prelude to a deeper appreciation of autoimmune disease and cancer. As noted in succeeding sections, in addition to the maturity of the immune system itself, the acquisition of tolerance is critically dependent upon the dose, physical state, complexity, and metabolizability of the antigen and the route by which it is administered. Furthermore, it is apparent that numerous procedures can facilitate, inhibit, or terminate tolerance and that T cells and B cells differ significantly in their susceptibility to induction and persistence of the tolerant state.

Dose of Antigen (Tolerogen)

As illustrated in Figure 11-1, when manipulated properly a variety of antigens can induce tolerance in immunocompetent individuals either in subimmunogenic concentration (low zone tolerance) or in amounts 10 to 100 times that required to elicit maximal antibody production (high zone tolerance). Depending on the antigen used, repeated small doses injected intravenously in picogram to fractions of a milligram quantities can cause low zone tolerance, as evidenced by the fact that the individual becomes unresponsive to subsequent challenge with an immunogenic concentration of the antigen. Experimental induction of low zone tolerance in mice may be accomplished with 10^{-1} μg of bovine or horse serum albumin, lysozyme, or ovalbumin, whereas as little as 10^{-7} μg of flagellin will suffice.

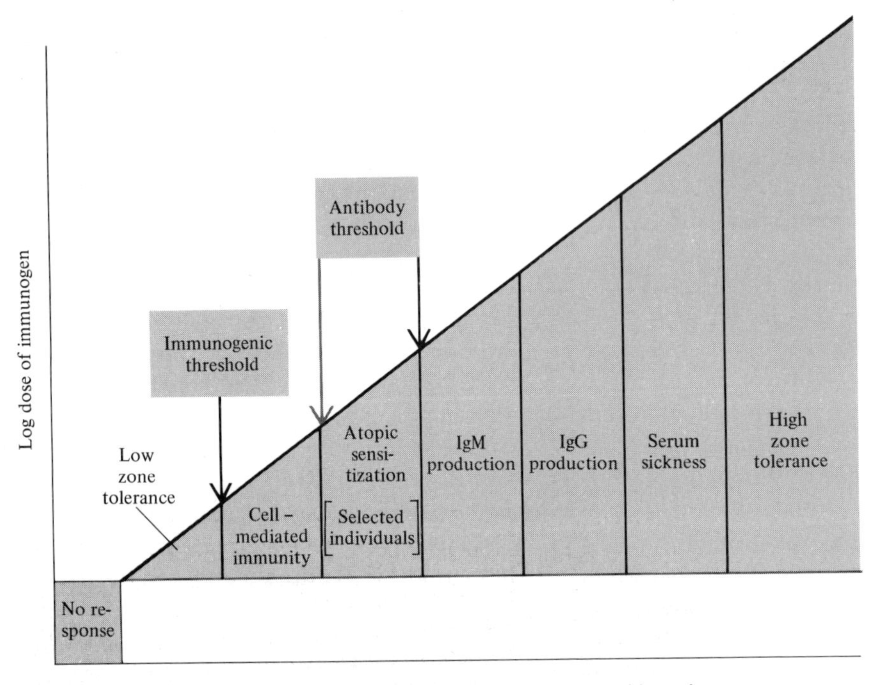

Figure 11-1 Immunospecific responses on primary contact with an immunogen.

Under comparable conditions 10,000 times greater concentrations of these antigens in a single intravenous injection are required to cause high zone tolerance. In man, it is estimated that production of high zone tolerance to bovine serum albumin and flagellin would require about 8 lb and 32 μg, respectively. Between low and high zone tolerance, the antigens exert immune responses that may result in sensitized T cells, antibody production, or both. Expressed on a logarithmic scale of increasing concentrations of the antigen, an orderly sequence of specific immunological reactions occurs involving low zone tolerance, delayed hypersensitivity, atopic sensitization, IgM production, IgG production, serum sickness, and high zone tolerance (Figure 11-1).

Physical State of the Antigen

Another factor, the physical state of the antigen, has a direct bearing on the specific immunological reaction that results. Soluble antigens of low molecular weight introduced orally or by intravenous injection—i.e., by routes that are unlikely to localize or concentrate the antigen—facilitate the induction of tolerance. On the contrary, aggregation of a soluble antigen, adsorption onto particulate matter, localization within an adjuvant, or the introduction of the antigen by the intradermal, subcutaneous, or intramuscular routes inhibits the development of tolerance.

Monomeric or deaggregated serum proteins (bovine and serum albumin, ovalbumin, bovine and human gamma globulin), as opposed to aggregated complexes or particulate antigens (bacteria, viruses, erythrocytes), are much more effective in causing tolerance. The general suitability of small, soluble antigens in inducing high zone tolerance is probably associated with their relatively simple molecular structure, diminished immunogenicity, rapid equilibration between vascular and extravascular compartments, persistence in the circulation, and perhaps most significantly, the known inability of macrophages to fix the antigens as a prelude to their reaction with T and/or B cells. Stated another way, an antigen that succeeds in making direct contact with a T cell, B cell, or both, without the intervention of other cells (T cells, B cells, macrophages) is more likely to induce tolerance and to inhibit the formation of sensitized cells and antibody.

The foregoing discussion is not meant to imply that tolerance cannot be induced by particulate antigens. As a matter of fact, lymphocytes from a closely related individual of the same species introduced in utero are accepted as autoantigens. When reexposed to the tolerogen (lymphocytes or skin graft) as adults, the grafts survive indefinitely. What apparently is required for particulate antigens to induce tolerance is the presence of a majority of surface antigenic determinants that are identical to those in the recipient plus a minimum that are different. In man, closely related particulate surface antigens may exist as cancer cells, as membranes surrounding group A streptococci (Chap. 14) or viruses (Chap. 2), or in a wide variety of tissue cells infected with viruses (Chap. 2).

Metabolizability of the Antigen

Inferred in the discussion of the physical state of the antigen is the question of the extent to which it is metabolized. Small, soluble, heterologous serum proteins that cannot be readily fixed by macrophages are metabolized slowly in contrast with their aggregated or particulate form. On a weight basis, pneumococcal polysaccharides which are metabolized at an extremely slow rate are especially potent inducers of tolerance. Note also that closely related particulate antigens would be metabolized slowly as would autoantigens.

Paradoxically, partial metabolism of the antigen may operate to facilitate the acquisition of tolerance. For example, bovine gamma globulin injected into the jugular vein of guinea pigs results in antibody production. However, when the antigen is injected into the mesenteric vein, the animals become tolerant. Presumably, bovine gamma globulin passes from the mesenteric vein to the liver where it is deaggregated into the monomeric form which facilitates tolerance. Similarly, intradermal injection of haptenic allergens leads to their complexing with epidermal proteins and the induction of delayed hypersensitivity, whereas the same haptens given orally cause tolerance.

Enhancement and Immunosuppression

Two of the most interesting procedures that facilitate the induction of tolerance are immunological enhancement (Chap. 10) with IgG2 or its Fc, Fab, and $F(ab)_2$ fragments and immunosuppression (Chap. 10). Available evidence suggests that both methods include specific and nonspecific components. Fab and $F(ab)_2$ are the specific factors and Fc the nonspecific element in enhancement. Although the dissection of the IgG2 molecule may seem unduly artificial, since it is normally secreted as a unit, the separate functions of the components are revealing and potentially useful therapeutically. Fab and $F(ab)_2$ probably operate at the level of surface receptors on T lymphocytes and may provide a selective mechanism accounting for the immunospecificity of enhancement. Fc, on the other hand, exerts a central depression on T cell function and may also be essential in the induction of tolerance. It must be emphasized, however, that precise information is conspicuous by its absence.

While specific when antigen is present and nonspecific in its absence, immunosuppression (Chap. 10) is only marginally specific in comparison with the general depression of T lymphocytes. Nonetheless, when the nonspecific effects abate, tolerance can persist for a prolonged period. In the case of immunosuppressed allografts (Chap. 10), tolerance conceivably can be permanent. Whether the result is due to the immunosuppressive regimen, to a combination of the initial immunosuppression plus the establishment of low zone tolerance or enhancement, or to another mechanism remains obscure.

Lymphocyte Stimulation and Complement

Two of the more instructive observations concerning the inhibition of tolerance involve nonspecific stimulation of lymphocytes and depression of complement. Whenever lymphocytes are stimulated by adjuvants, killed mycobacteria, endotoxin, or vitamin A, it is much more difficult to induce tolerance. Presumably, the proliferation of lymphocytes and the accompanying influx of cells provide an adequate opportunity for the antigen to interact with T cells, B cells, and macrophages, thus favoring cellular or humoral immunity rather than tolerance.

The fact that complement is essential for the development of tolerance, especially high zone tolerance, introduces another puzzling factor. Nonetheless, genetic defects in the complement system as well as agents known to depress or inactivate complement, such as cobra venom protein, vitamin A, and fumaropumaric acid, interfere with the production of tolerance. Theoretically, the requirement of complement for the induction of tolerance is logical if it is assumed that cytotoxic antibody is produced prior to the establishment of tolerance and that complement mediates the destruction of either antigen-responsive or memory cells.

In a number of experimental situations employing pneumococcal polysaccharide, bovine serum albumin, and human gamma globulin as antigens, it has been conclusively shown that sensitization including antibody production is a natural prelude to the induction of high zone tolerance. These findings have led to the formulation of the exhaustive differentiation theory of high zone tolerance. The theory assumes that all potential antibody-producing cells for the particular antigenic determinants are activated, the high concentration of antigen precludes the development of memory cells, eventually the antibody synthesizing plasma cells will die, the precursor cells (lymphocytes) capable of responding to the antigen will be exhausted, and the animals will become unresponsive. Perhaps complement is an essential element in the destruction of antigen-responsive cells or memory cells by cytotoxic antibody.

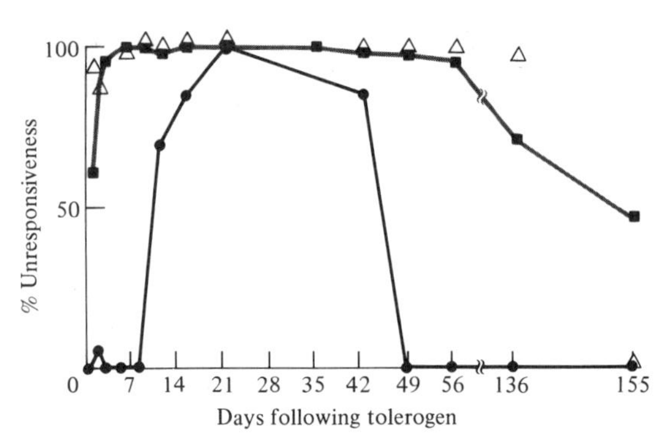

Figure 11-2 Kinetics of the induction of unresponsiveness in thymus and bone marrow cells. ■ thymus; ● bone marrow; △ deaggregated human gamma globulin injected donor. *(From W. O. Weigle, Clin. Exp. Immunol., 9:437–447, 1971.)*

The Cellular Basis of Tolerance

It is apparent that the immunospecificity of tolerance is a function of T lymphocytes or both T and B lymphocytes and that the ability to induce tolerance is inversely related to the immunogenicity of the tolerogen. Lymphocytes, but not serum, from a tolerant animal can transfer a specific state of tolerance to x-irradiated isogeneic animals (adoptive tolerance), thus clearly establishing the cellular basis of tolerance. Closer examination of the situation has revealed that T cells can become tolerant independently of B cells. Experimentally, as noted in Figure 11-2 and Table 11-1, induction of tolerance in T cells requires less tolerogen, develops more rapidly, and persists for a longer period of time

Table 11-1 Induction of Tolerance to Human Gamma Globulin in Adult Mice

	Percent unresponsiveness*	
Dose of tolerogen injected (mg)	In thymus	In bone marrow
0.1	96	9
0.5	99	56
2.5	99	70

* Eleven days after injection.
Source: W. O. Weigle, *Clin. Exp. Immunol.*, 9:437–447, 1971.

than in B cells. For example, T cells of mice injected intravenously with human gamma globulin became tolerant 2 days later and remained unresponsive for more than 100 days, whereas B cells became tolerant 21 days later and reverted to a responsive state in 49 days. The dose response curve of T cell and B cell populations also varies significantly (Table 11-1).

Further analysis of these and similar experiments has led to a number of significant findings and to the formulation of concepts that may have important implications in clinical medicine.

1 T cells can achieve tolerance rapidly in the absence of sensitization or antibody production and remain tolerant for a prolonged period.
2 The tolerant state in B cells is more difficult to induce, requires a greater concentration of the tolerogen, develops more slowly, and is finite in duration.
3 T cells are closely associated with low zone tolerance, whereas T cells and B cells are regularly involved in high zone tolerance.
4 Tolerance in T cells alone can prevent the initiation of a humoral response by B cells.
5 Induction of high zone tolerance is preceded by a potent antibody response which disappears and is succeeded by unresponsiveness (exhaustive differentiation).
6 Complement is required for the induction of high zone tolerance, but its role in low zone tolerance, if any, remains to be determined.
7 High zone tolerance, but not low zone tolerance, can be induced in the presence of memory cells.
8 While generally involving both T and B cells, natural tolerance may be limited to or maintained only by T cells; this may explain not only why it is partial or finite but also why it can be broken, resulting in autoimmune disease.

Termination or Breaking of Tolerance

Fundamental to an understanding of tolerance is the knowledge that it is partial (not complete) and temporary (not permanent). Even when induced in neonatal animals, tolerance is spontaneously terminated, and the animals become responsive to the tolerogen in about 6 months. The spontaneous recovery of immunocompetence clearly documents that induced tolerance is partial and temporary. Once tolerance is induced, it apparently can be maintained indefinitely by judiciously spaced intravenous injections of the antigen. Nonetheless, whether the continued presence of antigen is a prerequisite for the maintenance of tolerance is still questioned by some astute investigators, and the final answer awaits conclusive experimental support.

While natural tolerance can persist indefinitely in man, possibly as a result of the continuing circulation of minute quantities of sequestered or semisequestered antigens, abundant evidence is accumulating to show that the balance between tolerance and responsiveness to autoantigens is precarious. With advancing age the probability that natural tolerance will be lost steadily increases. In addition, a variety of stimuli can terminate natural tolerance either spontaneously or artificially. Basically, the conditions under which tolerance is broken can be categorized into those that are associated with the following:

1 The release of relatively high concentrations of sequestered or semisequestered antigens as a consequence of anomalies, obstruction, trauma, genetic defects in the lysosomal enzymes of phagocytic cells, inflammation, or malignancy.

2 The injection of autoantigens in combination with adjuvants.
3 Contact with reactive chemicals that can lead to antigenic alteration of the fluid or formed elements of the vascular system (Chap. 8).
4 Contact with or injection of a cross-reacting antigen that shares some antigenic determinants with an autoantigen but also has a number of antigenic determinants that are different from the autoantigen. Presumably, cross-reacting antigens interact with T cells of different specificity and can then make contact with responsive (nontolerant) B cells.

Mechanisms Responsible for Maintaining Tolerance

Accuracy demands the unequivocal statement that the mechanism of tolerance at either the cellular or the molecular level is unknown. Currently, the two most attractive theories, which are not mutually exclusive and may be wholly or partly valid, invoke an antibody feedback mechanism based on enhancement (Chap. 10) or an antigen-dependent depression or inactivation of T cell genes. The problem may not be quickly resolved, since picogram quantities of autoantigens might suffice to maintain tolerance by acting on T cells, while B cells may remain fully responsive but unactivated because an unknown T cell function is required for B cell activation. Similarly, if somatic mutations are associated with the loss of tolerance, it is not known if they are functional at the level of bone marrow stem cells, the thymocytes, the long-lived T cells, or combinations of these cells. However, despite these uncertainties and those involving complement and macrophages in natural tolerance, it is difficult to avoid the conclusion that, as experimental progress continues, we may unravel the problem to the extent that would provide a more hopeful prognosis for clinical intervention in transplantation, autoimmune disease, and cancer.

AUTOIMMUNITY

Autoimmune phenomena express the reality of cell-mediated and humoral responses to (1) native or endogenous antigens, (2) antigenically modified endogenous antigens, or (3) exogenous antigens that cross-react with endogenous antigens. Beyond this, however, there is little agreement as to what constitutes autoimmune disease and essentially no definitive information concerning the pathogenesis of recognized autoimmune diseases.

The criteria proposed by Witebsky, which are enumerated below, and those added by others have created some order out of the chaos, but few of these postulates can be validated, and human autoimmune disease remains an enigma.

Postulates for Classifying a Clinical Syndrome As an Autoimmune Disease

1 A cell-mediated or humoral response to the diseased tissue must be present.
2 The antigen causing the disease must be identified, isolated, and characterized.
3 The specific antigen must be capable of reproducing the disease in animals.
4 The experimentally induced disease must be capable of being transferred by immunocompetent cells or antibodies.

In the interest of illustrating some of the problems encountered as well as methods that might be employed to effect their resolution, the following sections are concerned with an indication of the types of antigens that are involved, an evaluation of the role of antibodies versus sensitized cells, an enumeration of findings consistent with an immunological basis for autoimmune disease, a description of the general features of some human autoimmune diseases, a review of pertinent animal experiments, and an appraisal of theories proposed to account for autoimmune disease.

Antigens Implicated in Autoimmunity

The antigens involved in autoimmunity generally fall into four categories: (1) late developing endogenous antigens which are anatomically segregated and to which the host is probably not tolerant, (2) sequestered or semisequestered endogenous antigens to which the host probably is ordinarily but partially tolerant at the T cell level, (3) antigenically modified endogenous antigens, or (4) cross-reacting exogenous antigens. Spermatozoa and a lens protein may be cited as examples of late-developing endogenous antigens to which the host is probably not tolerant by virtue of the fact that these antigens are synthesized within anatomically segregated tissues at a time when the host is immunocompetent. A much larger group of sequestered or semisequestered antigens is synthesized during embryonic life within tissues surrounded by a continuous basement membrane and largely, but not completely, shielded from contact with immunocompetent cells. Included within this category are antigens present within the thyroid, testis, adrenal cortex, lens, stomach, colon, brain, and skeletal and cardiac muscle. Collectively, such antigens are known as organ-specific antigens because they are restricted to a particular organ or tissue rather than the species. In addition, similar organ-specific antigens are found in the corresponding tissues of a wide range of different species.

Another group of antigens to which T cell tolerance probably is established are known as non-organ-specific antigens. These endogenous antigens are widely distributed in the tissues of individuals of the same and different species. Included in the category of non-organ-specific antigens are nuclei, DNA, histones, RNA, mitochondria, and microsomes.

Theoretically, endogenous antigens can be modified antigenically by a virtually unlimited number of agents, including enzymes excreted by invading microorganisms or those present in the normal flora and antigens coded for by viral genes but introduced temporarily or permanently into the surface structure of the plasma membranes of host cells (Chap. 2). Practically, the vast majority of clinically significant antigenic alterations occur following exposure of the skin to organic chemicals and solvents or plant products in the form of contact dermatitis (Chap. 8) or following exposure of the formed elements of the blood to drugs, leading to hemolytic anemias, leukopenias, and thrombocytopenias (cytolytic and cytotoxic complement-mediated responses, Chap. 9). Curiously, contact dermatitis is not usually classified an an autoimmune disease, whereas the drug-induced hemolytic anemias, leukopenias, and thrombocytopenias are included in this category. Clearly, however, both contact dermatitis and cytolytic and cytotoxic reactions represent immune responses to endogenous antigens modified by conjugation with haptens.

As is evident from the properties of organ-specific and non-organ-specific antigens, cross-reacting exogenous antigens are widely distributed in nature. Probably, in most cases exogenous cross-reacting antigens are brought into contact with human immunocompetent cells along with bacterial membranes and enveloped viruses. For example, gram-negative bacteria, pneumococci, and myxoviruses cross-react with human blood group substances. Among the group A streptococci, antigenic cross-reactions with human tissue antigens are relatively extensive, as indicated by the following examples: (1) group-specific carbohydrate and glycoprotein antigens cross-react with human sarcolemma and cardiac glycoprotein; (2) type 1, M protein cross-reacts with human HL-A antigens; (3) type 12 and type 5 membranes and cell walls stimulate T lymphocytes from patients with progressive glomerulonephritis.

Many viruses infecting man are enveloped with membranes which are partly derived from nuclear, intracytoplasmic, or plasma membranes of the host cell but which also include virus-specific antigens. It may be somewhat more than coincidental that only enveloped viruses are involved in postvaccinal and postinfectious encephalitis (Chap. 24) and in subacute sclerosing panencephalitis due to measles virus (Chap. 22). Perhaps, multiple sclerosis may represent the chronic form of such diseases. Included in the enveloped viruses are members of the pox-, herpes-, myxo-, and arbo- groups and rabies, rubella, and lymphocytic choriomeningitis viruses. In addition, infection with enveloped EB virus in infectious mononucleosis (Chap. 25) and with enveloped cytomegalovirus (Chap. 25) after blood transfusion or cardiopulmonary bypass perfusion results in a number of autoimmune reactions.

Autoantibodies

Autoimmune disease is blessed with a plethora of autoantibodies, often reactive with multiple antigens even when the disease is characterized by organ-specific pathology and for the most part representing the result rather than the cause of tissue damage. On the other hand, autoantibody can combine with the target antigen present on the surface membrane of erythrocytes, leukocytes, platelets, vascular endothelial cells, and glomeruli and in cooperation with complement can induce pathology in these sites (Chap. 8), and the tissue destruction can be passively transferred with antibody. In systemic lupus erythematosus (SLE), complexes of autoantibody, DNA, and complement adhere to the epithelial side of the glomerular basement membrane, give rise to lesions similar to those occurring in serum sickness, and are associated with a fall in serum complement during active phases of the disease (Chap. 8). Similar immune complexes are found in skin biopsies of patients with discoid lupus erythematosus.

Although most autoantibodies have no etiological role, reflect the release of altered antigens following tissue damage, presumably have the biological function of combining with and facilitating the disposal (immune elimination, Chap. 8) of modified tissue components, and are occasionally present in individuals without evident autoimmune disease, a battery of autoantibody tests is of diagnostic value. Included in this category are autoantibodies found in serum and checked for immunofluorescence on frozen sections of tissue, agglutination of circulating blood elements and antigen-coated particles, complement fixation, precipitation, or ability to damage cell cultures.

The available evidence suggests that the role of autoantibodies in the pathogenesis of autoimmune disease is restricted to those cells that are literally suspended or bathed in antibody. Autoantibody is unable to produce lesions in solid tissues either in vivo or in vitro.

Sensitized Cells

Although direct supporting data are lacking, many experts believe that autoimmune diseases largely represent delayed hypersensitivity responses. The strongest evidence that most autoimmune disease is the expression of cell-mediated immunity is based on experimental models of organ-specific disease which can be adoptively transferred with sensitized T cells but not with serum. Even though autoantibodies are frequently present, there is little or no correlation with the disease.

Experimental allergic encephalomyelitis (EAE) is the prototype model illustrating the role of delayed hypersensitivity in production of organ-specific disease. EAE can be regularly induced in animals when an encephalitogenic peptide composed of 11 amino acids, only 3 of which need be constant, is injected along with Freund's adjuvant and can be transferred with sensitized T cells. In addition to EAE, appropriate organ-specific antigens incorporated in Freund's adjuvant can experimentally produce peripheral neuritis, thyroiditis, gastritis, adrenal atrophy, uveitis, orchitis, and aspermatogenesis which resemble syndromes encountered in man. Both the human and experimental diseases present histopathological features consistent with delayed responses including infiltrates that are predominantly mononuclear and the ability to cause tissue damage in organized tissue (Chap. 10).

Human Autoimmune Diseases

A few selected examples will serve to illustrate the general principle that autoimmune diseases represent a confusing continuum or spectrum of overlapping clinical manifestations, pathological lesions, and immunological features whose pathogenesis is obscure (Table 11-2). Even in the organ-specific diseases such as thyroiditis, pernicious anemia, and myasthenia gravis the clinical picture, tissue damage, and immunological reactivity are rarely restricted to a single organ. On the other hand, there is a strong tendency for more than one autoimmune disease to be present in the same individual, as occurs in reciprocal thyroiditis and pernicious anemia, involvement of thymus and skeletal muscle in myasthenia gravis, and multiple tissue destruction in SLE and rheumatoid arthritis. For example, patients with SLE often develop hemolytic anemia, leukopenia, thrombocytopenic purpura, rheumatoid arthritis, dry keratoconjunctivitis and salivary gland disease (Sjögren's syndrome), and dermatomyositis (Table 11-2).

Apart from multiple autoimmune diseases and autoantibodies to multiple antigens occurring in the same individual, the incidence of autoantibodies and autoimmune disease increases with age, is highest among persons with generalized immunological deficiency or agammaglobulinemia, is higher in females than in males, is more prevalent in identical twin and first-degree relative cohorts of patients than in the random population, and on the basis of genetic studies in mice, appears to be under the control of a minimum of three genes. The clinical course of autoimmune disease is accompanied by exacerbations and remissions but eventually progresses in most patients in the absence of therapy. Organ-specific diseases frequently are associated with a marked influx of mononuclear cells, whereas the hallmark of the non-organ-specific collagen or connective tissue diseases is fibrinoid necrosis surrounded by much less pronounced accumulations of mononuclear cells. On the other hand, any given autoimmune disease may include lesions that resemble those associated with contact dermatitis, delayed hypersensitivity, cytolytic and cytotoxic reactions, serum sickness, and Arthus reactions (Chap. 8).

Induction of Autoimmune Disease in Man

The available evidence, inconclusive as it is, suggests that autoimmune disease may be precipitated as the result of any of the following events.

1. Tissue injury may lead to initial immunogenic exposure of immunocompetent cells to late-developing endogenous, sequestered antigens (spermatozoa and a lens protein).
2. Tissue injury may lead to initial immunogenic exposure of antigen-responsive (nontolerant) B cells to an increased concentration of semisequestered endogenous antigen to which the T cells are tolerant or partially tolerant (thyroglobulin and many other antigens).
3. Tissue injury or administration of drugs may lead to the chemical and/or conformational alteration of any endogenous antigen, whether sequestered or not, thereby creating or exposing new antigenic determinants while retaining other native determinants, i.e., giving rise to a cross-reacting antigen. Exposure of nontolerant T or B cells to the cross-reacting antigen may result in sensitized cells or antibody formation to both the new and the native antigenic determinants.
4. Cross-reacting exogenous antigens introduced along with or synthesized within the host by microorganisms may lead to the formation of sensitized T cells or the production of antibody by B cell derivatives. In the latter case, autoantibody can cross-react with accessible endogenous antigens and complement within the vascular compartment to mediate tissue damage or may neutralize, for example, the ability of intrinsic factor to mediate the absorption of vitamin B_{12} from the gastrointestinal tract (pernicious anemia). However, autoantibody is unlikely to have a deleterious effect on endogenous antigens located within solid organs or tissues unless there is preexisting pathology in the target organ or tissue. On the other hand, sensitized T cells can attack solid organs or tissues, as noted in allograft rejection (Chap. 10). Thus, with the exception of the first item, which is an extremely rare event, autoimmune disease is precipitated by a breakdown of natural tolerance to endogenous antigens that is established during embryogenesis and presumably functional at the level of T cells, not B cells.

Theoretically, autoimmune disease could be precipitated as the consequence of somatic mutation, leading to a population of T lymphocytes capable of producing an immunogenic response to an endogenous antigen. Unfortunately, there is neither strong experimental data nor conclusive evidence to disprove the somatic mutation theory of autoimmune disease. Further discussion of this possibility will be considered in the context of speculations on cancer.

Table 11-2 Immunological Features of Some Human Autoimmune Diseases

Syndrome	Pathology	Immunological features
Thyroiditis (primary myxedema, Hashimoto's disease)	Enlarged thyroid; normal acinar tissue replaced by massive infiltrate of lymphocytes and plasma cells; fragmentation of epithelial basement membrane of thyroid	Almost universal presence of autoantibodies to thyroglobulin; autoantibodies to other thyroid antigens, parietal cells, intrinsic factor also present; in thyroiditis patients incidence of pernicious anemia is 20 times higher than in random population; delayed hypersensitivity to thyroglobulin and other thyroid antigens present; peripheral lymphocytes destroy target cells coated with thyroid-associated antigens; transformation of patient's lymphocytes by antigen and inhibition of macrophages by antigen in presence of patient's lymphocytes
Pernicious anemia	Neutralization of ability of parietal cells to mediate vitamin B_{12} absorption by combination with intrinsic factor; atrophic gastritis with achlorhydria; dense infiltrate of lymphocytes and plasma cells	High incidence of antibodies to parietal cells and intrinsic factor; autoantibodies to thyroglobulin common; in patients with pernicious anemia, the incidence of thyroiditis is much higher than in random population
Myasthenia gravis	Lymphoid nodules in thymic medulla; collections of lymphocytes in muscle fibers around blood vessels; thymoma in 20 percent of patients	Autoantibodies to muscle fibers and thymic reticular cells

Table 11-2 Immunological Features of Some Human Autoimmune Diseases (CONTINUED)

Syndrome	Pathology	Immunological Features
Systemic lupus erythematosus (SLE)	Widespread lesions in connective tissue characterized by fibrinoid necrosis in skin, glomeruli, joints, serous membranes, and blood vessels; typical LE neutrophils with phagocytized nuclear material; often associated with hemolytic anemia, leukopenia, thrombocytopenic purpura, dry conjunctivitis and salivary gland disease (Sjögren's syndrome), rheumatoid arthritis, and dermatomyositis	Autoantibodies to nuclei, DNA, histones, RNA, mitochondria, microsomes, leukocytes, platelets, and IgG; immune complexes in glomeruli, skin, spleen; depressed serum complement during active phase of disease; cutaneous reactivity to autoantigens; drug-induced form (diphenylhydantoin, isoniazid, hydralazine, procainamide) may cause mild disease which disappears on removal of drug or may lead to fulminant manifestations in preexisting SLE
Rheumatoid arthritis	Inflammation of joints and periarticular tissues with macrophages and lymphocytes; may be associated with hemolytic anemia, splenomegaly, subcutaneous nodules with fibrinoid necrosis; serositis, myocarditis, vasculitis occasionally observed	Hypergammaglobulinemia; autoantibodies to IgG, nuclei, DNA, histones, RNA, mitochondria, microsomes, erythrocytes; immune complexes with lowered content of complement in synovial fluid; release of lysosomal enzymes from macrophages may be involved in arthritis

Once initiated, autoimmune disease tends to be self-perpetuating and is associated with remissions and exacerbations. Stated another way, an immunogenic response to endogenous or cross-reacting antigens initiates tissue damage which causes the release of more endogenous or cross-reacting endogenous antigen. The inflammatory reaction reaches a peak and then subsides, only to start over again after an interval of time.

Each of the preceding events and theories is based on the premise that autoimmune disease stems from immunological hyperactivity. However, the prevalence of autoimmune disease is highest among persons with generalized immunological deficiency or agammaglobulinemia. To account for these observations some investigators postulate that autoimmune disease is the result of generalized or selective immunological deficiency or hypoactivity. On the basis of these observations, it is painfully obvious that autoimmune reactions and disease remain unexplained immunological phenomena.

Therapy

Therapeutic efficacy varies widely with the particular autoimmune disease or group of associated autoimmune diseases occurring in the patient, the severity of the clinical manifestations, and the stage of the disease and is limited by the chronic and slowly progressing nature of most autoimmune diseases. In blood dyscrasias and SLE induced by drugs, recovery ensues but may be somewhat delayed when administration of the drug is halted. In many organ-specific diseases replacement therapy is usually adequate (thyroxine in thyroiditis, vitamin B_{12} in pernicious anemia). In myasthenia gravis the muscle weakness is readily reversed by choline esterase inhibitors. Selected patients with organ-specific disease, however, may require and be benefited by corticosteroids, and in the case of thyroiditis and myasthenia gravis, surgery may be desirable.

Not surprisingly, treatment is frequently complicated and often challenges the ingenuity, judgment, and patience of the physician who must always be alert to the likelihood of multiple autoimmune diseases in the same patient, to their development during the course of therapy, and to the hazards of prolonged therapy with corticosteroids and other immunosuppressive agents and procedures.

For example, treatment of patients with SLE and rheumatoid arthritis may require the use of analgesics, antimicrobial agents, blood transfusions, digitalis, sodium restriction, limited activity, avoidance of undue exposure to sun or drugs that might precipitate fulminating manifestations, antimalarials (chloroquine), corticosteroids, other forms of immunosuppression, application of orthopedic principles, and when needed, corrective surgery. Some physicians recommend the combined use of azathioprine and corticosteroids in selected patients with SLE and rheumatoid arthritis. While judicious treatment of SLE with corticosteroids (drug selection, initiation, dosage, duration) offers reasonable relief to most patients, it does not significantly prolong life and frequently requires gradually increasing dosage with concomitant risks.

SPECULATIONS CONCERNING CANCER

Experimental Observations

Intensive study of oncogenesis in animals has amply documented a number of readily reproducible phenomena that may be relevant to human cancer.

1 Spontaneously arising cancer cells or those induced by chemicals or viruses retain most of the surface antigenic determinants possessed by the cells from which they originated. Thus, the cancer cells will regularly be accepted by isogeneic and rejected by allogeneic members of the same species.
2 The growth of allogeneic cancer transplants can be facilitated by immunological enhancement (Chap. 10), and consequently, the recipient probably becomes tolerant to the malignant allograft.
3 Many RNA and DNA viruses can induce cancer in a wide variety of animals (Chap. 2).
4 Carcinogenic chemicals are potent immunosuppressive (Chap. 10) and mutagenic agents.
5 Most immunosuppressive drugs (Chap. 10) were originally developed as cancer chemotherapeutic agents. Paradoxically, however, immunosuppressive drugs and other forms of immunosuppression sharply increase the incidence of cancer in previously healthy animals.
6 Cancer may occur in 33 percent of animals experiencing preceding spontaneous autoimmune disease.
7 Graft-versus-host reactions (GVHR, Chap. 10) may result in autoimmune disease, and cancer may develop subsequently in 33 percent of the animals.

Clinical Observations

As evident from the data included in Table 11-3, many of the same factors operative in animals exert similar effects in man. Whether immunological enhancement is an important mechanism for establishing tolerance and whether viruses cause cancer in man as they do in animals remains uncertain. Human cancer cells are promptly rejected when transferred to healthy volunteers but do survive and invade the tissues of individuals with similar malignancies.

Despite the bewildering and conflicting experimental and clinical observations there have been numerous attempts to influence the course of autoimmune disease and cancer through the application of immunological procedures. Paradoxically, both immunosuppressive and immunostimulating agents are used in therapy. For example, stimulation of T lymphocytes by BCG vaccine (Chap. 8), endotoxins (Chap. 8), *Corynebacterium parvum,* and of contact dermatitis to DNCB and similar agents has considerable therapeutic value in the treatment of leukemia and malignancies of the skin and other tissues. Presumably, the beneficial effect is mediated by the synthesis and release of lymphokines from the sensitized T cells and the release of lysosomal enzymes from activated macrophages (Chap. 8) in the vicinity of cancer cells. Best results are achieved when the number of cancer cells is reduced to a minimum by surgery, radiation, or chemotherapy prior to the production of delayed hypersensitivity. These observations are generally in accord with the improved prognosis associated with infiltration of solid tumors

Table 11-3 Conditions Predisposing to Cancer in Man

Condition	Type of cancer	Incidence
Generalized immunological deficiency	Lymphoreticular	7–22 %
Selective immunological deficiency		
Agammaglobulinemia	Acute lymphatic leukemia	7–10 %
IgA deficiency	Gastric carcinoma	?
Possession of HL-A2 antigen	Acute lymphatic leukemia	?
Autoimmune diseases	Lymphomas, leukemias	Up to 12 % or more
Sustained lymphoid stimulation		
Myeloma	Acute lymphatic leukemia Acute myelocytic leukemia Acute myeloblastic leukemia	About 1.5 %
Other causes	Lymphomas, leukemias	?
Immunosuppressive drugs	Variable	0.7 %
Other forms of immunosuppression	Mostly lymphoreticular	?
Tolerance	Most tumors	Up to 100 %

with mononuclear cells and with failure to remove or irradiate regional lymph nodes showing paracortical lymphocytic hyperplasia in early breast cancer when the primary tumor is ablated.

Autoimmune Disease, Graft-versus-Host Reactions, and Cancer

The pioneering studies of Little, Strong, and other investigators have revealed the fine details of genetic control of cancer in mice. While the observations are complicated in many cases by the presence or activation of oncogenic viruses, how strongly genetic structure influences the spontaneous development of autoimmune disease is clearly evident from recent findings in mice.

Hemolytic anemia occurs spontaneously in an increasing proportion of inbred New Zealand black (NZB) mice after the age of 5 months. Coombs' and LE tests are positive, hypergammaglobulinemia and antinuclear autoantibodies appear, and immune complex glomerulonephritis is common. Bizarre lymphoid nodules and germinal centers, not normally present, are found in the thymic medulla. Splenomegaly and lymphadenopathy are regularly present. Malignant lymphoma develops in one-third of the mice and probably would show a higher incidence if some of the mice had not died earlier from membranous glomerulonephritis. The disease can be transferred with spleen cells from affected adult mice to young unaffected mice. Rather than preventing autoimmune disease, neonatal thymectomy accelerates the appearance of hemolytic anemia and LE cells.

Closely related NZW (white) mice are resistant to spontaneous autoimmune disease. However, crossing NZB with NZW mice yields F_1 hybrids that die in 8 to 10 months with positive LE cells, antinuclear autoantibodies, and the typical renal lesions of SLE, but with a low incidence of hemolytic anemia. Appropriate $F_1 \times F_1$ and backcross experiments reveal that autoimmunity in these mice is regulated by a minimum of three genes and that the production of hemolytic anemia and antinuclear autoantibodies is probably under separate genetic control.

GVHR in mice are frequently associated with autoimmune disease and cancer. Two examples are cited to illustrate the phenomena. When C_{57} spleen cells are injected into F_1 progeny of $C_{57} \times$ DBA mice, the recipients successively develop a high incidence of hemolytic anemia and progressive disorganization of lymphoid tissues, and malignant lymphomas appear in one-third of the mice. Injection of Balb/c spleen cells into F_1 progeny of Balb/c $\times$ A/J mice leads to the development of glomerulonephritis and malignant lymphomas.

In man, as previously noted, autoimmune disease frequently precedes the appearance of lymphomas and leukemias. The higher incidence of cancer in patients with preexisting hemolytic anemia, thrombocytopenic purpura, SLE, rheumatoid arthritis, Sjögren's sialadenitis, primary amyloidosis, and other autoimmune diseases is well authenticated. In addition, it is recognized that warm and cold types of hemolytic anemia occurring in man show homogeneity of autoantibodies and thus are of monoclonal origin. A recently reported case illustrates the possible sequence of these phenomena in man. Over a period of 7 years a patient successively experienced (1) asymptomatic hypergammaglobulinemia with a monoclonal component; (2) an autoimmune phase with arthritis, pulmonary fibrosis, glomerulitis, hemolytic anemia, leukopenia, antinuclear autoantibodies, and LE cells; and (3) Bence Jones proteinuria and a terminal acute leukemia.

Hodgkin's disease is a lymphoproliferative granulomatous neoplastic disease involving the invasion of many organs by lymphocytes, plasma cells, eosinophils, neutrophils, monocytes, fibroblasts, and giant cells. Characteristically, patients with Hodgkin's disease have normal immunoglobulin concentrations but develop progressive impairment of cell-mediated immunity, as indicated by responses to dinitrochlorobenzene (DNCB), phytohemagglutinin (Chap. 10), and allogeneic leukocytes (Chap. 10). For example, contact dermatitis to DNCB can be induced in more than 90 percent of normal persons and patients with inactive Hodgkin's disease, but none of 25 patients with active Hodgkin's disease could be sensitized to DNCB. Furthermore, skin allografts persist substantially longer in Hodgkin's patients than in normal persons (in one study 17 of 20 grafts survived for 30 days or more). While there are many recognized differences between experimental and human GVHR and Hodgkin's dis-

Table 11-4 Some Immunological Theories of Cancer

Theory	Probable type of tolerance	Unresponsive cells	Description
Somatic mutation	Low zone	T	A series of appropriate and sequential somatic mutations, each involving a single antigenic determinant on the cell surface to which the host becomes successively tolerant.
Virus	High zone	T, B	Replication of viral genes in synchrony with cellular genes coding for new and massive exposure to virus-specific transplantation antigen on cell surface.
Tolerance	Low zone	T	Essentially a variant of somatic mutation theory but could involve reestablishment of tolerance to embryonal antigens as in carcinoembryonic antigen in cancer of the intestine and fetal α-glycoprotein in hepatic carcinoma.
Enhancement	High zone	T, B	New surface antigenic determinants lead to production of IgG2 which depresses T cell surveillance. Not incompatible with virus or exhaustive differentiation theories.
Generalized immunological deficiency	Neither	None present	Total inability of host to inhibit growth of cancer cells arising as a series of appropriate and sequential somatic mutations. The mutant cells, because of their more rapid growth, have a selective survival advantage over normal cells.
Selective immunological deficiency	Low zone	T	In agammaglobulinemia, B cells are absent and cytolytic or cytotoxic antibody is missing and perhaps cannot check metastases of cancer cells that arise by somatic mutation after T cell tolerance has developed.

Table 11-4 Some Immunological Theories of Cancer (CONTINUED)

Theory	Probable type of tolerance	Unresponsive cells	Description
Selective immunological deficiency (Cont.)	High zone	T, B	In IgA deficiency, the absence of secretory IgA may result in exhaustive differentiation of IgG cells lining mucous membranes. Not incompatible with virus or enhancement theories.
Loss of immunological surveillance	Low zone	T	Temporary or prolonged immunosuppression or its absence due to a genetic defect permits uninhibited growth of cancer cells arising as a consequence of somatic mutation.
	High zone	T, B	Gradual return of immunocompetence after halting immunosuppression may be followed by tolerance in B cells due to enhancement and subsequently by destruction of T cells by cytolytic or cytotoxic antibody when they return to the competent state. Exhaustive differentiation unlikely, but high zone tolerance could be established by virus infection.
Exhaustive differentiation	High zone	T, B	Activation of all potential antibody-producing cells leads to their subsequent exhaustion following formation of plasma cells and complement-mediated destruction of T cells by cytolytic or cytotoxic antibody. Not incompatible with virus or enhancement theories.

ease, invasion of many organs by lymphocytes, splenic amyloid, wasting, and terminal depletion of lymphocytes represent common features.

Paradoxes and Theories

Recapitulation of a few of the many paradoxes will serve to illustrate the difficulty of constructing theories to reconcile the close association between autoimmunity and cancer. For example, autoimmune disease and cancer

1 Are prevalent in persons exhibiting hyperactivity, hypoactivity, or generalized deficiency of the immune system.
2 May be enhanced or inhibited by or indifferent to antibody.
3 May be prevented or facilitated by sensitized cells.
4 May be associated with the requirement, loss, reacquisition, or nonexistence of tolerance.
5 May require the presence or absence of complement.
6 May require the presence or absence of lysosomal enzymes.
7 May or may not be the result of exposure to freely accessible, sequestered, semisequestered, chemically, or conformationally altered endogenous antigens, exogenous haptens, or cross-reacting exogenous antigens.
8 May involve tissues that are or are not surrounded by basement membrane, have or do not have lymphatic drainage, or have or do not have access to lymphocytes.

9 May be transferred by sensitized cells or antibody or may be nontransmissible.

10 Are inhibited or facilitated by or indifferent to immunosuppressive drugs and other forms of immunosuppression.

Speculations rather than conclusions are demanded by the present state of knowledge. On the one hand, autoimmune disease, graft-versus-host reactions, and cancer appear to merge in a continuum of overlapping events, the end result of which is cancer. On the other hand, the close association between immunological disorders and lymphoreticular malignancy does not necessarily imply cause and effect. Both, in fact, may be due either to a common cause (genes, viruses, or perhaps both) or to totally independent, but coincidental, events. Admittedly, the answers are presently unknown. A few of the many possible immunological theories of cancer are sketched in outline form in Table 11-4, and as noted in the description of the theories, many are compatible with each other and may be complementary.

BIBLIOGRAPHY

Bretscher, P.: "Hypothesis: A Model for Generalised Autoimmunity," *Cell. Immunol.,* 6:1-11, 1973.

Burnet, F. M.: "A Reassessment of the Forbidden Clone Hypothesis of Autoimmune Disease," *Aust. J. Exp. Biol. Med. Sci.,* 50:1-10, 1972.

Burnet, M.: *Autoimmunity and Autoimmune Disease,* Philadelphia: F. A. Davis Company, 1972.

Chiller, J. M., and Weigle, W. O.: "Termination of Tolerance to Human Gamma Globulin in Mice by Antigen and Bacterial Lipopolysaccharide (Endotoxin)," *J. Exp. Med.,* 137:740-750, 1973.

Dent, P. B.: "Immunodepression by Oncogenic Viruses," *Progr. Med. Virol.,* 14:1-35, 1972.

Lavrin, D. H., Rosenberg, S. A., Connor, R. J., and Terry, W. D.: "Immunoprophylaxis of Methylcholanthrene-induced Tumors in Mice With Bacillus Calmette-Guérin and Methanol-extracted Residue," *Cancer Res.,* 33:472-477, 1973.

Louis, J., Chiller, J. M., and Weigle, W. O.: "Fate of Antigen-binding Cells in Unresponsive and Immune Mice," *J. Exp. Med.,* 137:461-469, 1973.

Mathé, G.: "Immunological Approaches to the Treatment of Acute Leukemia," *Clinics Hematol.,* 1:165-188, 1972.

Möller, G. (ed.): "Immunological Tolerance," *Transplant. Rev.,* 8:3-136, 1972.

Notkins, A. L., and Koprowski, H.: "How the Immune Response to a Virus Can Cause Disease," *Sci. Am.,* 228(1):22-31, 1973.

Paterson, P. Y.: "Multiple Sclerosis: An Immunologic Reassessment," *J. Chronic Dis.,* 26:119-126, 1973.

Perkins, E. H., Makinodan, T., and Seibert, C.: "Model Approach to Immunological Rejuvenation of the Aged," *Infect. Immun.,* 6:518-524, 1972.

Rothfield, N., Ross, H. A., Minta, J. O., and Lepow, I. H.: "Glomerular and Dermal Deposition of Properdin in Systemic Lupus Erythematosus," *N. Engl. J. Med.,* 287:681-685, 1972.

Spitler, L. E., Levin, A. S., and Fudenberg, H. H.: "Agammaglobulinemia, Absent Delayed Sensitivity and Lymphopenia without Infections: A Demonstration of Immunologic Unknowns," *Am. J. Med.,* 54:371-377, 1973.

———, von Muller, C. M., Fundenberg, H. H., and Eylar, E. H.: "Experimental Allergic Encephalitis. Dissociation of Cellular Immunity to Brain Protein and Disease Production," *J. Exp. Med.,* 136:156-174, 1972.

"Symposium. Cell-mediated Immunity to Tumor Antigens," *Fed. Proc.,* 32:153-179, 1973.

"Symposium. Models Used for the Study and Therapy of Rheumatoid Arthritis," *Fed. Proc.,* 32:131-152, 1973.

Teitelbaum, D., Webb, C., Meshorer, A., Arnon, R., and Sela, M.: "Protection against Experimental Allergic Encephalomyelitis," *Nature,* 240:564-566, 1972.

Vossen, J. M., deKoning, J., van Bekkum, D. W., Dicke, K. A., Eysvoogel, V. P., Hijmans, W., van Loghem, E., Radl, J., van Rood, J. J., vander-Waay, D., and Dooren, L. J.: "Successful Treatment of an Infant with Severe Combined Immunodeficiency by Transplantation of Bone Marrow Cells from an Uncle," *Clin. Exp. Immunol.,* 13:9-20, 1973.

Weigle, W. O.: "Recent Observations and Concepts in Immunological Unresponsiveness and Autoimmunity," *Clin. Exp. Immunol.,* 9:437-447, 1971.

Wells, J. V., Michaeli, D., and Fudenberg, H. H.: "Antibodies to Human Collagen in Subjects with Selective IgA Deficiency," *Clin. Exp. Immunol.,* 13:203-208, 1973.

Williams, R. C., Jr., DeBoard, J. R., Mellbye, O. J., Messner, R. P., and Lindström, F. D.: "Studies of T- and B-Lymphocytes in Patients with Connective Tissue Diseases," *J. Clin. Invest.,* 53:283-295, 1973.

Woodruff, M.: "Cancer—The Elusive Enemy," *Proc. R. Soc. Med.,* 183:87-104, 1973.

Chapter 12

Introduction to the Study of Infectious Disease

Bernard A. Briody

PERSPECTIVE

The preceding text has been concerned with (1) the structure and function of prokaryotic and eukaryotic parasites; (2) the general characteristics of bacteria, viruses, rickettsiae, chlamydiae, fungi, protozoa, and helminths with emphasis on those associated with pathogenicity for man, with the origin of new genotypes, and with response to chemotherapy; (3) the attributes of the host that enable it to resist infection and selected factors that lower that resistance; (4) immunological interactions between haptens, antigens, parasites, and man; and (5) the basis of the immunological uniqueness of the individual and its significance in clinical medicine.

Emphasis in the balance of the text will be placed on the disease rather than the parasite and on similar pathogenetic patterns and epidemiological phenomena rather than on the pathogenic potential and epidemiology of a specific parasite in isolation from many other parasites that can cause almost identical disease in man. Such an approach constitutes a sharp break with traditional texts in microbiology but, on the other hand, corresponds to the conventional presentation of subject matter in most medical texts (anatomy, physiology, pathology, pharmacology, medicine, pediatrics, surgery). In addition, an approach based on pathogenesis conforms to the natural diagnostic sequence followed by medical clerks, house officers, and practitioners in evaluating the clinical manifestations of patients.

The intents of this introductory chapter are stated in the following outline:

1 To indicate the standard sequence that will be followed in the balance of the text, namely, a consideration of the following:
   a Biological properties and antigenic structure of the causative agent
   b Pathogenesis of the disease
   c Methods used to establish a laboratory diagnosis
   d Epidemiological features of the disease
   e Methods employed to prevent and control the disease
2 To illustrate by the use of selected examples how a knowledge of these aspects can provide a basis for preventing and controlling the disease or for understanding why there is a limited possibility for developing practical methods of prevention and control
3 To indicate some of the more commonly encountered situations with respect to
   a Growth of the parasite
   b Natural habitat of the parasite
   c Antigenic characteristics of the parasite
   d Reservoir of the parasite
   e Seasonal, sex, age, and geographical incidence of the disease
   f Sporadic, endemic, or epidemic occurrence of the disease
   g Portal of entry of the parasite
   h Portal of exit of the parasite
   i Immunization procedures
   j Interrupting the spread of the disease
4 To emphasize the changing patterns of infectious disease

THE CAUSATIVE AGENT

Biological Properties

The answers to the following questions will usually provide useful information. Where is the organism found? Is it normally a saprophyte or a parasite present as part of the normal microbial flora, or is it only encountered as a pathogen? What is its natural habitat? Is man a reservoir? Are other animals reservoirs? What arthropods, if any, can function as reservoirs? Is soil the reservoir? Is the causative agent free-living or is its survival in nature dependent primarily upon a parasitic existence, or is it an obligate intracellular parasite that cannot replicate apart from living cells? What are the few most important properties of the parasite? How can the parasite be grown in the laboratory?

Antigenic Structure

The answers to the following questions will usually provide worthwhile data. Is it important to know anything about the antigenic structure of the parasite or its metabolic products? If so, what is important? Why is it important? If there is more than one antigen on the surface of the parasite, which one, if any, can be correlated with pathogenicity or with the production of protective antibody? Does the parasite constitute a single antigenic group or are there multiple antigenic types of the causative agent?

General Observations and Illustrative Examples

Most human infectious disease is caused by pathogens that are transmitted directly from man to man or by parasites that are part of the normal flora of the skin and mucous membranes and express their pathogenic potential only after the resistance of the host has been abrogated. In both cases, man is the reservoir. Less frequently, the parasite may be a natural pathogen of animals that can be transmitted to man either as a result of direct contact or through the intervention of an arthropod vector. In the case of mites and ticks, the arthropod can serve as a reservoir of infection as well as a vector because the agent can be passed vertically from generation to generation by transovarial transmission.

While man is an accidental host when the causative agent has an animal reservoir, the frequency of the accidents can be extremely high, as in the case of salmonellosis. Occasionally, an animal reservoir may exist, as in shigellosis, but is of no consequence because the parasite is perpetuated by man himself. In a few unusual situations, man may pass an infection on to primates as in hepatitis, measles, and tuberculosis, and the animals can subsequently act as a source of infection for man.

The soil can function as a reservoir of infection for man after contamination with the parasite from human or animal sources (many helminth infections, anthrax, Q fever). In other cases, the source of soil contamination is not obvious (many fungal infections, tetanus, botulism).

The few most important properties of the parasite are those that determine pathogenicity (M protein of group A streptococci, capsular polysaccharides of a number of bacteria, diphtheria and tetanus toxins, enterotoxins produced by staphylococci, cholera vibrios, *Escherichia coli*) or are characteristic of pathogenic organisms (coagulase production by staphylococci, extreme susceptibility to bacitracin of group A streptococci) and those that permit isolation and identification or have survival value for the parasite (growth requirements, surface antigens, colonial morphology, hemolysis, resistance to selected antibiotics, dyes and disinfectants, morphology of the parasite especially in the case of fungi, protozoa, and helminths, motility, spore formation, carbohydrate fermentations, and enzymatic reactions).

Knowledge of the surface structure of parasites in many cases has practical implications. One of the key facts is whether the parasite has a single antigenic type or multiple antigenic types. With a few important exceptions, including poliomyelitis, effective immunizing preparations involve causative agents that have a single antigenic type (smallpox, measles, mumps, rubella, yellow fever, pertussis, BCG vaccine for tuberculosis) or, in the case of diphtheria and tetanus toxoids, are derived from organisms that produce a single antigenic type of toxin. A significant number of parasites have multiple antigenic types ranging from a few (meningococci, poliovirus, parainfluenza virus, dengue virus), to 50 or more (rhinoviruses, echoviruses, streptococci, pneumococci, and gram-negative enteric bacilli), to more than 1,300 in the case of salmonellae. Multiple antigenic types are associated with type-specific immunity, complicate serological identification, and seriously limit the possibility of prevention of disease by immunization.

PATHOGENESIS

Patterns of Pathogenesis

In Chapter 5 pathogenetic patterns, factors, and mechanisms were considered without regard to the entrance and exit of the parasite, which are also integral aspects of pathogenesis. In order to develop an understanding of the pathogenesis of infectious disease, therefore, it is essential to have accurate information concerning the following questions: What is the usual portal of entry of the parasite? Are there alternate portals by which the parasite can gain access to the host? Does the organism remain more or less localized to the portal of entry, or is its extension limited at the level of the regional lymph nodes? Is parasitemia a regular feature of the disease? If so, when does it occur, and what are the usual consequences? If the causative agent is spread systemically, does it attack a particular target tissue, or are its effects manifest in many tissues? What factors operate to cause fulminating infections? In other words, what is the sequence of events (pathogenesis) occurring between contact with the parasite and the initial appearance of clinical manifestations, i.e., during the incubation period? Why is the incubation period as short as 24 hr. or as long as several years? What types of infection are associated with short or long incubation periods? How does the infecting dose of the parasite affect the incubation period and the subsequent course of the disease? Is the course of the disease acute or chronic? What factors are involved in determining whether the disease is acute or chronic? Why do no individuals become long-term carriers of the parasite in some diseases, a few individuals in several diseases, and 100 percent of those infected in other cases? In what types of infection is the parasite likely to persist for a long time? In those cases in which the parasite persists for the life of the individual, as in many latent infections, what factors precipitate periodic or sporadic reappearance of clinical manifestations? In what situations is an allergic response pertinent to the pathogenesis and natural history of the disease? Are there any infectious diseases of man in which the parasite cannot exit from the host? In what types of infections does the parasite enter and exit from the host through the same portal of entry? In what types of infections can the parasite exit from a portal other than the one used for entry? In what types of infections do the parasites develop multiple portals of exit?

General Observations and Illustrative Examples

About two-thirds of the causative agents of infectious disease enter and exit by way of the respiratory tract and the balance are largely acquired through other mucous membranes (small intestine, conjunctiva, urethra) and the skin. In many cases, parasites have alternate portals of entry. For example, the causative agent of tularemia may infect man by the dermal, conjunctival, oral, and respiratory routes or may be transmitted by arthropods. In diphtheria, the parasite is normally transmitted from man to man via droplet infection but can be acquired by the dermal route, in which case the course of the disease is totally different from respiratory diphtheria. Even rabies, which is invariably transmitted by the bite of a rabid animal, can be acquired by the respiratory route under appropriate conditions (inhalation of contaminated droppings of infected bats in caves). A number of agents which are regularly transmitted by other routes (venereally, by arthropod vectors, by the respiratory route) can be acquired by placental transfer, blood transfusion, or in utero infection in the case of syphilis, malaria, and rubella, respectively.

Parasitemia While the vast majority of infectious disease is localized to the mucous membranes or the skin, there are a number of human diseases in which the parasite is present in the blood at some phase in the disease (Chaps. 22 to 26). The presence of the causative agent in the blood is an integral part of its ability to survive as a parasite in the case of some diseases that are transmitted by arthropod vectors (dengue, sandfly fever, epidemic typhus, bartonellosis, leishmaniasis, trypanosomiasis, malaria, urban yellow fever, relapsing fever, loiasis). In other cases of arthropod-transmitted diseases, however, the concentration of the pathogen in human blood is below the critical amount required to infect the arthropod when it takes a blood meal (most of the viral encephalitides and rickettsial diseases). In addition, there are a large number of other diseases in which parasitemia occurs, but as long as the parasite is present only in the blood there is no danger to susceptible individuals. On the other hand, many of these pathogens have developed effective means of exiting from the infected host. For example, smallpox, vaccinia, herpes, varicella, and rubella exit primarily from the respiratory tract, whereas typhoid bacilli, Coxsackie viruses, echoviruses, and polioviruses can exit by way of the stools.

Parasitemia may be a fulminating episode as in gram-negative endotoxin shock, meningococcemia, staphylococcal and streptococcal septicemias, anthrax, *Clostridium perfringens* septicemia following attempted abortion, or almost any pathogen if the resistance of the host is compromised by acute leukemia or by a deficiency of complement, defective lysosomes in neutrophils or macrophages, neutropenia, or an inability to produce immunoglobulins or cell-mediated immunity.

Incubation Period The incubation period is usually short when the disease is localized to the respiratory or gastrointestinal tracts, as in the common cold, influenza, streptococcal pharyngitis, salmonellosis, shigellosis, cholera, and other acute diarrheal diseases. There are, however, a few exceptions which occur in the respiratory tract, including pertussis and mycoplasma infections. In the case of the respiratory viruses, the probable reason for the short incubation period is that within a few days all the susceptible cells of the mucosal epithelium have been infected and destroyed. In cholera and other nonexudative acute diarrheal diseases, the enterotoxins produce their effects rapidly. Infections of the eye and the urethra caused by the gonococcus and other organisms similarly have short incubation periods.

With few exceptions, such as yellow fever, in which the incubation period is about 4 days, most systemic infections have a longer incubation period, often 1 to 3 weeks. Included in this category are the common exanthematous diseases (smallpox, varicella, measles, rubella), mumps, the rickettsial diseases, typhoid, and syphilis. In these diseases, there is frequently local multiplication of the pathogen, systemic distribution to target organs and tissues, a redistribution of the pathogen, and local multiplication before the incubation period is completed. The pathogens may then exit from the infected host via the respiratory tract and skin (exanthemata); the respiratory secretions (Q fever rickettsiae); the skin (other rickettsiae); the skin, stools, and urine (typhoid); the respiratory tract and secretions (mumps); and the skin and mucous membranes (syphilis). Naturally, time is required to accomplish these events, and dilution of the parasite in the circulation is a factor that probably prolongs the incubation period. In localized infections, on the other hand, the pathogen is concentrated, and the pathological effects quickly become apparent.

Several diseases are associated with variable and frequently long incubation periods. For example, in trypanosomiasis the incubation period may vary between 10 days and 4 years, in serum hepatitis from 2 to 5 months, in leishmaniasis from 2 months to 10 years, in leprosy from 7 months to 5 years, in dracontiasis from 8 to 14 months, in filariasis usually more than 9 months, and several years in loiasis. In the case of the helminths, the long incubation period is directly related to the time required for the development of adult worms or the production of larval forms. In protozoal diseases, the explanation is less apparent and is vaguely ascribed to the time required for intracellular replication of the parasite as conditioned by the inflammatory response of the host. In leprosy, the slow generation time of the bacteria and the requirement for a temperature below 37°C may be factors that are involved in the prolonged incubation period. In lepromatous leprosy, in which there is extensive proliferation of the bacilli with continuous bacteremia, systemic reaction is minimal, and destruction is limited to those tissues in close contact with the environment (skin, subcutaneous tissues, oral and nasopharyngeal mucosa, testes, eye). Perhaps leprosy bacilli, like certain other mycobacteria (Chap. 15), grow readily only at temperatures below 37°C! In serum hepatitis, no reasons are apparent for the long incubation period.

The Dose The number of parasites required to produce disease can vary widely with the particular pathogen. For example, inhalation of one tubercle bacillus or ingestion of one larva of the fish tapeworm is adequate to induce disease in man. At the other end of the scale, the injection of 100,000 staphylococci into the skin or the ingestion of 100,000 or more typhoid bacilli is ordinarily required to produce disease in man. Between these two extremes, it is generally assumed that most of the strictly human parasites and many of the more pathogenic animal parasites that infect man fall at the lower end of the scale, and many of the helminths are at the upper end of the scale. A few examples will illustrate some of the parameters involved. The dose required to produce syphilis in 50 percent of previously uninfected volunteers is 57 organisms. In tularemia, less than 50 bacteria will cause disease in volunteers when given by the dermal or respiratory routes, but more than 10^7 bacteria must be ingested to induce the disease.

In typhoid studies in volunteers, 10^5 bacteria produced disease in 27 percent, 10^7 in 50 percent, and 10^9 in 95 percent. The course of the disease was identical in each group. The only difference noted was a shorter incubation period in those receiving higher doses. Disease could not be induced with 10^3 bacteria. However, if a single oral dose of neomycin or streptomycin preceded the ingestion of 10^3 bacteria, typhoid regularly occurred. By way of contrast, 180 *Shigella* organisms produced disease in 22 percent of volunteers, and 5,000 bacteria produced disease in 57 percent. In many helminthic diseases, on the other hand, the incubation period is inversely proportional to the number of parasites present in the infecting dose, and the resulting disease is directly proportional to the number of adult worms. In intoxications (staphylococcal food poisoning and botulism), the incubation period is also inversely proportional and the severity directly proportional to the dose. Nonetheless, it is generally assumed that the course of the majority of infectious diseases of man is relatively uninfluenced by multiples of the minimal infecting dose that are normally encountered.

The Duration of the Disease Clinical manifestations, once developed, may persist for a few days to 30 years or more. In helminthic infections, disease may continue for 20 years in paragonimiasis, 25 years in schistosomiasis, 30 years in clonorchiasis, and 40 years in taeniasis. Chronicity or progressive infectious disease is generally associated with (1) intracellular location of the parasite, (2) characteristics of the inflammatory response, and (3) failure of the host to mount an effective immune response. In certain cases, each of these factors may be involved. On the other hand, it is important to emphasize that the majority of intracellular parasites are promptly and effectively eliminated by the host.

Chronicity of infectious disease is typical of helminths, whose size precludes phagocytosis and against which the host cannot mount an effective immune response that will eliminate the worms or halt their ability to induce progressive disease. Long-term disease, occasionally interrupted by remissions, often involves intracellular parasites including most protozoa (malaria, leishmaniasis, trypanosomiasis, amebiasis), most systemic fungi (histoplasmosis, blastomycosis, coccidioidomycosis), chlamydiae (trachoma, psittacosis, lymphogranuloma venereum), a few viruses (hepatitis, measles in subacute sclerosing panencephalitis, congenital rubella, and the slow virus disease kuru), and some bacterial diseases (brucellosis, cutaneous diphtheria, granuloma inguinale, gonorrhea, typhoid, tuberculosis, leprosy).

The nature of the inflammatory response exerts a definite influence on the duration of the disease, especially when it is associated with chronic granulomatous reactions, as in the superficial and deep mycoses, many helminthic infections (trichinosis, echinococcosis, dracontiasis, filariasis, loiasis, onchocerciasis), protozoal infections (leishmaniasis, trypanosomiasis), and some bacterial infections (tuberculosis, leprosy, syphilis). In most of these diseases, delayed hypersensitivity or cell-mediated reactions play a key role in minimizing the progress of the disease but at the same time are responsible for much of the pathology. In addition, as noted in Chapter 6, when the humoral or cell-mediated immune responses of the host are impaired, recurrent and progressive infections are invariably encountered.

Latency The perpetuation of the parasite in the absence of progressive disease or in fact any disease (latency) is a feature of several pathogens including bacteria, viruses, rickettsiae, chlamydiae, and protozoa. The persistence of the pathogen may occur in 100 percent of those infected (herpes simplex and varicella-zoster), in many of those infected (adenoviruses, syphilis, gonorrhea in females, tuberculosis), in an unknown number of those infected (pneumocystis, toxoplasma, cytomegalovirus, inclusion conjunctivitis), and in a small percentage of those infected (serum hepatitis, typhoid, epidemic typhus, Q fever, psittacosis). In many cases, the parasite may persist for the life of the individual, but in other situations it is limited to a finite period, usually of several years. The consequences of latent infection may be nil, or the infection may be readily spread to susceptible persons (gonorrhea, syphilis, herpes simplex, typhoid, inclusion conjunctivitis); clinical manifestations of limited extent may occur with considerable regularity (recurrent herpes) or only in unusual circumstances (zoster, tuberculosis, serum hepatitis, epidemic typhus, Q fever, psittacosis, pneumocystis, toxoplasmosis, cytomegalovirus disease). In the case of epidemic typhus, the long-term persistence of the rickettsiae is essential for the perpetuation of the disease in man, and in all cases the latent state makes elimination of the parasite virtually impossible.

Human Infectious Disease As a Dead End for the Parasite Disease in man is often a dead end for the parasite which cannot exit from the host at all or in sufficient concentration to be transmitted directly or indirectly to other susceptible persons. Included are the causative agents of trichinosis, echinococcosis, and larva migrans which cannot exit from man; many of the fungi which are rarely passed directly or indirectly to others; most of the encephalitides and most of the rickettsiae (except for epidemic typhus) in which the concentration of the causative agent in the blood is insufficient to infect the arthropod vector; and in many diseases in which man-to-man transmission does not occur (anthrax, brucellosis, lymphocytic choriomeningitis, melioidosis, glanders). Note that with the exception of the fungi, most of the causative agents are primarily diseases of animals. Finally, it is important to emphasize that all the infectious diseases associated with parasites that are part of the normal flora represent organisms that are not transmitted from a diseased person to a susceptible person.

LABORATORY DIAGNOSIS

Isolation and/or Identification

Whenever practical, the first step in attempts to establish a laboratory diagnosis should be the prompt microscopic examination of the appropriate clinical specimen (pus, sputum, swabs, membranes, stools, urine, cerebrospinal fluid, serous fluid, synovial fluid, blood, bone marrow, tissue imprints, scrapings, and biopsies). For bacteria, the standard procedure is the Gram stain, but acid-fast staining is useful for tubercle bacilli, and dark-field microscopy is of limited value in the case of spirochetes. For fungi, wet unfixed specimens treated with 10 percent potassium hydroxide, India ink, or lactophenol cotton blue are employed, and acid-fast staining is useful in the case of *Nocardia.* For rickettsiae, chlamydiae, blood flagellates, and malarial parasites, Gimenez and Giemsa stains are utilized. For intestinal protozoa and helminthic eggs, wet mounts of stool specimens are examined.

Attempts at isolation of the causative agent should be performed immediately. If this is not possible, the specimen should be placed in transport medium (a buffered, reduced, nonnutritive survival medium) until cultures can be inoculated. In addition, cultural procedures must take into account the source of the specimen which may regularly contain other parasites that are part of the normal flora. In some cases, the presence of members of the normal flora is less troublesome than might be anticipated because the pathogen is often found in much higher concentration (nasopharyngeal secretions, urine, skin lesions) or may have recognizable characteristics (acid-fast tubercle bacilli in sputum, amebic cysts, trophozoites, and helminthic eggs in stools). In other cases, the examination of sputum from patients with pneumonia presents greater difficulty because many of the causative agents are also members of the normal flora. In the case of enteric bacterial pathogens, the members of the normal flora usually greatly outnumber the pathogens, and special selective methods must be used.

Identification of certain pathogens in body fluids can be achieved by microscopic examination alone (trypanosomal flagellates and asexual forms of malaria in blood, cryptococci in cerebrospinal fluid). In most cases, however, a definitive laboratory diagnosis requires that the causative agent be cultured and then identified. With few exceptions, such as syphilitic treponema and leprosy bacilli, bacteria and fungi can be readily isolated in the laboratory and cultured on blood agar plates incubated aerobically and anaerobically. In certain situations, primary isolation is facilitated by the addition of an atmosphere of 5 to 10 percent CO_2 and the use of other media (Sabouraud's glucose agar at 25°C and 37°C for fungi, chocolate agar containing antibiotics for gonococci, agar incorporating inhibitory dyes, glycerol, high salt concentrations or heavy metals for enteric bacterial pathogens, tubercle bacilli, staphylococci, and *Mycoplasma*). Blood cultures also require special procedures (Chap. 14), and the causative agents are usually isolated on blood agar plates after a period of growth in liquid culture. Viruses, rickettsiae, and chlamydiae require living cells, and cultures are not routinely attempted in the diagnostic laboratory but when carried out usually include antibiotics to inhibit the bacterial or fungal contaminants that might be in the clinical specimen.

Serological Tests

While definitive identification can be achieved on the basis of morphology alone in the case of fungi, protozoa, and helminths, other methods must be employed for bacteria, viruses, rickettsiae, and chlamydiae. A battery of biochemical reactions is of great assistance in the presumptive identification of bacteria, but definitive identification in almost all cases involving bacteria, viruses, rickettsiae, and chlamydiae is based on their antigenic structure. The serological methods employed for this purpose usually involve either the serum of the patient tested against known microbial antigens or a clinical specimen from the patient tested against known microbial antibodies. When the test employs the patient's serum to detect antibodies, paired specimens are routinely evaluated, one obtained early in the acute phase of the disease and the other 1 to 6 weeks later, depending upon the suspected causative agent, for rises in antibody titer.

The specific tests designed to identify the microorganism include those utilizing precipitation, agglutination, passive hemagglutination and passive hemagglutination inhibition, hemadsorption inhibition, hemagglutination inhibition, complement fixation, neutralization, and direct and indirect immunofluorescence. Each of these procedures has advantages and disadvantages in terms of sensitivity, specificity, and reliability. Currently, the complement-fixation test is probably the most widely used.

"Nonspecific" tests, because of their practical convenience, have also proved to be useful diagnostic tools. Included in this category are flocculation and complement-fixation tests for syphilis, the agglutination of sheep erythrocytes in infectious mononucleosis, the agglutination of human group O red blood cells in the cold (cold hemagglutination) in *Mycoplasma* pneumonia, and the agglutination of *Proteus* species (Weil-Felix test) in rickettsial diseases.

EPIDEMIOLOGY

The Study of Epidemiology

While some aspects of epidemiology were included in the preceding discussions of pathogenesis and the causative agent, there are many other factors encompassed within the framework of epidemiology. Naturally, the relative importance of epidemiological features of specific infectious diseases will vary widely, but awareness of the secular trends occurring in different situations will provide greater insight into the overall problems of infectious disease in the last quarter of the twentieth century.

Epidemiology, as it pertains to human infectious disease, asks and seeks answers by describing phenomena that occur not in the individual but in the population group, by monitoring on a limited scale the current behavior of infectious diseases, and by analyzing epidemics in progress in order to halt further spread of the disease and to prevent recurrences. The types of data sought include the following: What has been the natural history of the disease in human populations? Is a characteristic illness associated with a specific parasite, can multiple antigenic types induce the same disease, or can the same pathogen produce a multiplicity of syndromes? What is the ratio of subclinical to clinical infection? How can this ratio be determined? Is the method reliable? What is the prevalence of the disease (the number of cases in a specific population at a given point in time), and what factors influence the prevalence? What is the incidence of the disease (the number of cases in a specific population during a specified period of time, e.g., annually), and what factors influence the incidence? How, for example, is the incidence of a particular disease influenced by age, sex, season, geography, occupation, socioeconomic status, residence, composition and density of the household, school, travel, avocational interests, sanitary facilities, malnutrition, household pets, vaccination status or previous contact, personal habits (cleanliness, the types of food eaten, the use of alcohol, cigarettes, and drugs, sexual contacts), genetic background, the carrier state, the ability of the parasite to survive in soil, water, food, or on fomites (clothes, bed linen, eating utensils, dust particles, and other inanimate objects), the habits, behavior, and climatic conditions that affect arthropods and environmental pollution?

General Observations and Illustrative Examples

The Natural History of the Disease Many serious infectious diseases, spread from man to man by respiratory droplets, reached their highest intensity during the Industrial Revolution and progressively declined thereafter. The secular trend is evident from the few figures included in Table 12-1 and was well established before effective immunization procedures or chemotherapy became available. These data are not cited as arguments against either immuniza-

Table 12-1 Deaths from Selected Diseases*

	In 1860	When immunization became available	When chemotherapy became available	In 1972
Tuberculosis	300	—	50 (1947)	3
Scarlet fever	195	—	—	0.015
Pertussis	135	20 (1938)	—	0.017
Diphtheria	130	50 (1924)	—	0.015
Measles	110	0.16 (1965)	30 (1935)†	0.012

* Deaths per 100,000 persons under 15 years of age except for tuberculosis, in which all ages are included.
† For treatment of secondary bacterial pneumonia.

tion or chemotherapy but are presented to emphasize that the natural history of infectious disease frequently follows such long-term trends. Currently, the availability of effective vaccines and chemotherapy have greatly accelerated the pattern of declining mortality—witness the more than 100-fold diminution in deaths from pertussis, diphtheria, and measles in the past 25 years. On the other hand, the decline in scarlet fever mortality cannot be thus explained, since immunization has played no part at all, nor has chemotherapy had anything to do with it.

Similarly, the provision of sewage disposal facilities, an adequate supply of safe water, sanitary drainage, refrigeration, the wearing of shoes, and personal hygiene have eliminated many of the epidemic scourges of the preceding centuries. Large-scale milk- and water-borne epidemics have virtually disappeared from developed countries, as have such diseases as cholera, hookworm, urban yellow fever, and malaria. For example, cases of typhoid in Philadelphia declined from 10,000 per year in 1906 to 100 per year in 1926. This period coincided with filtration of the public water supply in 1906 and chlorination in 1913. Typhoid was not entirely eliminated by the provision of safe water because of the existence of the long-term carrier state in man and also because of alternate methods of transmission, principally by contamination of food. While the prospect of eliminating typhoid as a disease in man is not good for this reason, the effectiveness of available control measures is indicated by the fact that there were only 377 cases in the United States in 1972.

The long-term decline in the severity of infectious disease is sometimes accompanied by marked shifts in other parameters. For example, in 1860 the majority of deaths from tuberculosis were concentrated in the age groups under 5 years and between 25 and 35 years (annual death rates of 560 and 420 per 100,000), whereas today the highest number of cases and deaths occur in those over 65 years of age. In addition, at present the incidence of tuberculosis in males is twice as high as in females and five to ten times as high in nonwhites as in whites in the United States.

The Pathogen, Type of Disease, and Immune Status Key factors which greatly influence, if not determine, the epidemiological features of specific diseases include the (1) localized or systemic nature of the disease, (2) incubation period, (3) number of antigenic types, (4) nature of the immune response, and (5) carrier state, whether overt or latent. With the exception of pertussis, the available immunizing procedures acknowledged to be effective involve infections that are systemic (smallpox, yellow fever, measles, poliomyelitis, rubella, mumps) or diseases in which a toxin is systemically distributed (diphtheria, tetanus). With the exception of yellow fever and diphtheria, the incubation period is usually 1 week or more. Except for poliomyelitis, all are caused by microorganisms or toxins of a single antigenic type.

Thus, for example, even though pertussis is a localized infection, the incubation period is 1 week or more and the causative agent has a single antigenic type. The incubation period is adequate to permit an effective anamnestic response in previously immunized individuals. Presumably, on reexposure to the microorganism, minor tissue damage ensues which facilitates (1) the anamnestic response, (2) the pathotopic localization of the greatly increased concentration of antibodies produced in the anamnestic response, and (3) the infiltration of phagocytic cells and complement which together with antibody leads to accelerated disposal of the parasite by complement-mediated reactions before clinical manifestations of the disease can become apparent. In most other localized infections involving mucous membranes the incubation period is 1 to 3 days, and the overt disease occurs before the anamnestic reaction develops. Thus, there is no infectious disease involving a localized infection with a short incubation period for which an effective immunizing agent is available or which is followed by prolonged immunity. In addition, secretory IgA is the only antibody that can prevent infection upon reexposure in such cases, and this class of antibody is not subject to an anamnestic response.

The epidemiological behavior is, of course, greatly conditioned by the number of antigenic types of the causative agent, since immunity to reinfection is type-specific. Curiously, most parasites that exhibit multiple antigenic types are usually associated with infections of mucous membranes and short incubation periods (group A streptococci, salmonellae, and adeno-, rhino-, influenza, Coxsackie, and echoviruses), whereas most systemic infections are caused by pathogens that have a single antigenic type and a longer incubation period. In the latter case, even when immunizing agents are not available, recovery is associated with prolonged immunity to reinfection. Other combinations exist. For example, gonorrhea has a short incubation period, and recovery is accompanied by little, if any, immunity, but the causative organisms belong to a single antigenic type. Poliovirus produces a systemic infection and an incubation period of 1 to 2 weeks, and provided that the immunization procedure incorporates the three antigenic types, immunity to clinical disease on reexposure is prolonged. Herpes simplex is a systemic infection caused by two closely related antigenic types which have a distinct epidemiological pattern and is associated with a high and prolonged degree of resistance to systemic reinfection but little, if any, resistance to localized recurrences which represent reactivation of the latent virus which is carried by all who were infected.

Thus, the current immune status of the individual or the population is a key to the incidence of the disease provided that the incubation period is long enough to permit an effective anamnestic response before the causative agent produces overt pathology. On the other hand, when the incubation period is 1 to 3 days and the infection is localized to the mucous membranes, recovery from a previous infection or prior immunization is irrelevant unless the individual or the population group has a high concentration of secretory IgA at the time of reexposure. The usual time limits for persistence of protective concentrations of secretory IgA are estimated to range from a few weeks to a few months. Consequently, these types of infections present imposing obstacles to the development and practical use of effective vaccines. For too long and for too many localized infectious diseases with short incubation periods, the evaluation of the immune status of the host has been based on an assessment of IgG antibodies; such information is meaningless because protection is associated with secretory IgA antibodies. As noted in the section on prevention and control, vaccines designed to prevent localized infections with short incubation periods are administered by routes which fail to induce the formation of secretory IgA.

Arthropods and Arthropod Transmission of Infectious Disease Arthropods are segmented invertebrates with jointed appendages, are members of the largest phylum of animals, are widely distributed and diversified, and include both aquatic and terrestrial species. The classes that are primarily involved as biological vectors of human parasites are the Insecta (lice, fleas, bugs, mosquitoes, flies) and the Arachnida (ticks, mites), and a few species of the Crustacea (water fleas, crabs, crayfish) can serve as intermediate hosts for some helminths (fish tapeworm, guinea worm, lung fluke). As noted from the data included in Table 12-2, arthropods can function as biological vectors of a number of bacterial (tularemia, plague, relapsing fever, bartonellosis), viral (hundreds of arboviruses including the encephalitides, yellow fever, dengue, sandfly fever), rickettsial (epidemic typhus, murine typhus, scrub typhus, Rocky Mountain spotted fever, rickettsialpox), protozoal (malaria, leishmaniasis, trypanosomiasis), and helminthic diseases (fish tapeworm, guinea worm, lung fluke, filariasis, loiasis). In addition, some of the ticks and mites can serve as a reservoir of infection, since the parasite is passed vertically from generation to generation by transovarial or congenital transmission.

A knowledge of the nature of the arthropod, its ecological distribution, the species upon which it feeds, its feeding habits, and the factors which influence its prevalence is critical to the rational formulation of practical methods for preventing and controlling arthropod transmission of infectious disease to man. Naturally, with such a wide diversity of species, it is not surprising that arthropods exhibit many different patterns of behavior which are reflected in the seasonal and geographical distribution and incidence of the disease.

Table 12-2 Arthropod-transmitted Infectious Diseases of Man

Arthropod	Diseases
Crustacea:	
Water fleas (copepods)	Fish tapeworm, dracontiasis (guinea worm)
Crabs, crayfish (decapods)	Paragonimiasis (lung fluke)
Arachnida:	
Ticks	Rocky Mountain spotted fever, Russian Far Eastern encephalitis, tularemia, relapsing fever
Mites	Scrub typhus, rickettsialpox, possibly western equine encephalomyelitis, St. Louis encephalitis
Insecta:	
Lice	Epidemic typhus, relapsing fever
Fleas	Plague, murine typhus
Triatoma bugs	American trypanosomiasis (Chagas' disease)
Mosquitoes	Malaria, filariasis, hundreds of arboviruses
Flies	Filariasis, loiasis, leishmaniasis, sandfly fever, African trypanosomiasis, bartonellosis

A few examples are cited to illustrate the variety and complexity that can be encountered in diseases transmitted by arthropod vectors. Female black flies *(Simulium)* that transmit the filarial disease onchocerciasis bite during the daytime often in bright sunshine and toward evening in proximity to thick vegetation. Female sandflies *(Phlebotomus)* and triatoma bugs are nocturnal household feeders. Both male and female tsetse flies *(Glossina)* are daytime feeders and, depending upon the particular species, prefer areas surrounding streams or woodlands.

Among the mosquitoes, even within the same genera, there are species that are domesticated, that are abundant only in jungles, that thrive only in tropical areas, that are cosmopolitan in distribution, that are nocturnal or daytime feeders, and that prefer human to animal blood. Ticks feed primarily on wild or domesticated animals, and mites generally parasitize field rodents but can attack man. Lice and fleas are wingless insects that parasitize man (lice) or rodents (fleas), and both males and females are active feeders. When taking a blood meal, lice, fleas, and triatoma bugs deposit infected feces on the skin which is rubbed or scratched into the skin by the individual. In the other Insecta and the Arachnida, the pathogen is injected into the skin or the blood along with the saliva while the arthropod is taking a blood meal.

From the preceding description it is probably apparent that diseases transmitted by arthropod vectors vary according to the distribution, behavior, population dynamics, and movements of the arthropods and their vertebrate hosts and according to meteorological and topographical conditions. For example, human cases of louse-borne epidemic typhus frequently are most prevalent in the winter, tick-borne diseases in the spring, and mosquito-borne diseases in the summer. Other significant factors involved in arthropod transmission include the nature of the parasitemia in the human or animal host, the time required for multiplication of the pathogen in the vector to reach the critical concentration which will permit its transmission to a susceptible host (extrinsic incubation period), and the interval during which the arthropod remains capable of transmitting the pathogen to man. For example, the most efficient hosts are those that have an extensive and prolonged parasitemia. The extrinsic incubation period is greatly influenced by the moisture, rainfall, ambient temperature, abundance of vegetation, and terrain and generally requires about 7 to 14 days but may be shorter (3 to 5 days in epidemic typhus and leishmaniasis) or longer (20 days in trypanosomiasis). The parasite may kill the vector in 10 to 15 days (louse-borne epidemic typhus), may persist in the vector for life (most mosquito-borne diseases), or may survive from generation to generation (most tick- and mite-borne diseases).

While it may not be immediately apparent, arthropod-borne diseases are socioeconomic diseases. For example, malaria is absent from large areas of the world where it was once prevalent because of comprehensive antivector programs involving flood control, drainage, and sanitary engineering combined with the eradication of breeding places, the destruction of larvae, and the reduction of adult mosquitoes, especially in proximity to residential areas. The elimination of urban yellow fever before the cause of the disease became known is testimony to the effectiveness of antivector programs designed to destroy the breeding grounds of the domesticated mosquitoes involved. Residual spraying of dwellings with dichlorodiphenyltrichloroethane (DDT) is effective in preventing sandfly-transmitted disease (leishmaniasis, sandfly fever, bartonellosis). The use of solid wall construction in dwellings eliminates contact with the vectors which accompany their vertebrate hosts in nocturnal incursions in American trypanosomiasis (Chagas' disease). Reduction of the rodent population in proximity to dwellings is highly effective in the control of plague and murine typhus. Accessory measures in many of the arthropod-borne diseases found in urban or domestic situations include the use of sleeping nets and repellents applied to skin and clothing. In addition, special measures are indicated in specific cases (chemoprophylaxis in malarial areas).

Even in those arthropod-borne diseases associated with jungle areas, dense vegetation, rain forests, woodlands, scrub growth, river crossings, and streams which present imposing obstacles to control because of the density of vectors and animal reservoirs (jungle yellow fever, many other arboviruses, Rocky Mountain spotted fever, scrub typhus, African trypanosomiasis), socioeconomic factors are important elements in preventing human disease. In such situations, control of the vector or the reservoir is rarely practical, and reliance must be placed upon protection of the individual primarily by the use of residual repellents applied to clothing and skin and, in certain cases, immunization (jungle yellow fever), the use of head nets, gloves, and high boots (in hyperendemic areas), and the selective clearing of scrub (scrub typhus) or river crossings (Gambian trypanosomiasis).

The Epidemiological Setting Before concluding the section on epidemiology, attention must be directed toward the special problems encountered in particular epidemiological settings. The most universal setting, the household, is importantly involved in terms of its composition, density, location, and construction. Tuberculosis is recognized as a household disease (Chap. 15), and rheumatic fever, the immunological end result of repeated group A streptococcal infections, is almost linearly related to crowding in the home. Young children of school age (5 to 9 years) are adept at acquiring infection in the school environment and transporting it to the home setting where it can spread rapidly to preschool siblings and to adults. When young children are present in the home, the adults experience more frequent respiratory and gastrointestinal infections than would occur in homes with older children or without children.

Infectious disease is prevalent in a number of situations where public sanitary facilities are not available (in whole geographic areas comprising many countries, in rural areas, in camps, and in wartime) or where personal hygiene is likely to break down, where crowding is likely to occur and a continuous influx of new susceptibles are added (orphanages, mental institutions, jails). In these settings, acute diarrheal disease (especially shigellosis) and infectious hepatitis are major problems. Occupational and avocational activities present other opportunities for the acquisition of infectious disease, as can be seen in the incidence of diseases that have an animal reservoir in individuals who process animal products.

In recent years with the assistance of antimicrobial agents, immunosuppressive drugs and procedures, and the use of mechanical inhalators, nosocomial or hospital-acquired infections represent one of the more important epidemiological settings. Prominent pathogens include staphylococci, gram-negative enteric bacilli, and to a lesser extent, fungi and serum hepatitis. In many respects the hospital provides a fertile environment for the spread of infections, since it involves a group of individuals whose resistance is lowered by underlying disease or necessary surgical intervention, a continuous influx of susceptibles, a high population density, and a high employee turnover rate. The problem of nosocomial infections is further complicated by the fact that the common causative agents are generally resistant to a number of potent, relatively nontoxic antibiotics and are susceptible to the more toxic antibiotics.

Another important epidemiological setting, considered in Chapters 6, 14, 19, and 20, develops when the integrity of the mucous membranes of the upper respiratory tract are abrogated as a consequence of viral or bacterial infection or allergic rhinitis. Acute otitis media is an epidemiological complication of streptococcal pharyngitis or respiratory viruses. Acute bacterial conjunctivitis follows preceding viral infection or allergic rhinitis. When the respiratory mucous membranes are destroyed or their mucociliary, secretory, and mechanical functions impaired, especially when the causative agents can produce large-scale epidemics (influenza, measles, smallpox), the incidence and mortality of bacterial pneumonia rise sharply and exhibit a parallel secular trend. When the preceding epidemic wanes, the incidence and mortality of bacterial pneumonia return to the pre-epidemic pattern.

PREVENTION AND CONTROL

Without question the goal of medical microbiology is to provide a sound basis for the prevention and control of infectious disease. Achievement often falls short of the goal. In many cases, this is due to failure to apply accepted principles of prevention and control (Table 12-3), but in other cases lack of success is the result of biological factors inherent in host-parasite interactions and socioeconomic factors that currently overwhelm the developing countries of the world (Tables 12-3 and 12-4).

Infectious disease may be prevented or controlled by a variety of procedures and methods (Table 12-3). Generally, some of the basic questions for which answers must be sought include the following: Is a suitable vaccine available? If so, what is its nature? How and when should it be used? If a vaccine is not available, what factors preclude its development and use? What advantage, if any, can be taken of other methods of controlling the disease by interrupting the spread, by chemoprophylaxis, by sanitary procedures, by chemotherapy, by case detection, and by other methods (some of which are included in Table 12-3)? What are some of the more important factors that limit or seriously hamper efforts to prevent and control infectious disease (Table 12-4)?

The Major Problems: Localized Infections

As noted earlier, the morbidity of infectious disease is overwhelmingly due to localized infections of the respiratory and gastrointestinal tracts. It is appropriate to add that in the developing nations of the world digestive and respiratory infectious diseases are the major cause of death in those under 5 years of age. Regrettably, this situation could be eliminated by the application of accepted principles of prevention and control (Table 12-3) which currently are beyond the resources of the nations involved.

Admittedly, the problem of localized infections of the respiratory tract is complicated by the short incubation periods of the diseases and the multiplicity of antigenic types of the causative agents, but resolution is unlikely to occur as a consequence of the continued use of vaccines that induce the formation of little or no secretory IgA, the antibody that appears to be clearly implicated in protection against infections involving the mucous membranes. Fortunately, several recent ingeniously conceived and executed studies designed to provoke maximal production of secretory IgA are encouraging.

The concept of mucous membrane immunization depends upon the physical state of the antigen, the route by which it is administered, and whether it is living or dead. For example, a soluble antigen administered either subcutaneously, intramuscularly, or intranasally results in the production of secretory IgA, whereas the same antigen adsorbed onto alum or present on the surface of a microorganism fails to induce secretory IgA by any route unless the living parasite multiplies in the mucous membranes of the host or in close proximation to the mucous membranes. Evaluation of the use of soluble antigens capable of forming protective secretory IgA is being explored in connection with a number of pathogens that cause localized infections (influenza, adenovirus, cholera). The use of live enteric-coated adenovirus type 4 vaccine in young children and military recruits induces subclinical infection, a high degree of immunity, and a potent production of secretory IgA which is not limited to the intestinal tract but involves the respiratory tract as well. Distribution of secretory IgA in the respiratory tract is critical for protection against adenovirus type 4 pneumonia.

Table 12-3 Practical Methods for the Prevention and Control of Selected Infectious Diseases

Method	Diseases
Active immunization	Important in diphtheria, tetanus, pertussis, smallpox, yellow fever, poliomyelitis, measles, mumps, and rubella Limited use in tuberculosis, cholera, pneumococcal pneumonia, rabies, plague, tularemia, anthrax, epidemic typhus, Rocky Mountain spotted fever, and adenovirus pneumonia Marginal in influenza and typhoid Under evaluation in meningococcal meningitis, influenzal (bacterial) meningitis, and shigellosis
Passive immunization	Important, but of limited use in diphtheria, tetanus, botulism, pertussis, infectious hepatitis, measles, rabies, poliomyelitis, smallpox, generalized vaccinia, varicella, zoster
Chemoprophylaxis	Important in rheumatic fever, tuberculosis, malaria, and urinary tract infections Important, but of limited use in meningococcal meningitis, gonorrhea, syphilis, shigellosis, smallpox, endocarditis, contacts of patients with poststreptococcal glomerulonephritis, gas gangrene, chronic obstructive pulmonary disease, cystic fibrosis, burns, skull fractures with CSF rhinorrhea, leprosy, trachoma, and scrub typhus
Chemotherapy	In any disease for which effective drugs are available
Sanitary procedures	
Sanitary disposal of human excreta	Amebiasis, typhoid, shigellosis, salmonellosis, cholera, schistosomiasis, hookworm, taeniasis, strongyloidiasis, trichuriasis, clonorchiasis, giardiasis, balantidiasis, and infectious hepatitis
Sanitary disposal of dog and cat feces	Larva migrans
Protection, purification, and chlorination of public water supplies	Cholera, typhoid, shigellosis, salmonellosis, and amebiasis
Provision of safe private water supply	Cholera, typhoid, shigellosis, salmonellosis, amebiasis, infantile diarrhea, and giardiasis
Adequate cooking of contaminated food	Trichinosis, infectious hepatitis, acute diarrheal disease due to *Clostridium perfringens* and *Vibrio parahemolyticus,* clonorchiasis, and fish tapeworm
Refrigeration	Staphylococcal food poisoning, enteric pathogens, milk-borne diseases including diphtheria, streptococcal pharyngitis, blood containing syphilitic spirochetes, and taeniasis
Pasteurization	Milk-borne diseases including enteric pathogens, tuberculosis, diphtheria, Q fever, streptococcal pharyngitis, and brucellosis
Drainage	Malaria
Wearing of shoes	Tetanus, hookworm, chromomycosis, and mycetoma
Control of flies (mechanical vectors)	Enteric pathogens
Supervision of food processing, distribution, preparation, serving, and storage	Enteric pathogens, staphylococcal food poisoning, and botulism
Application of sound principles of personal hygiene	Enteric pathogens, staphylococcal food poisoning, conjunctivitis, trachoma, vulvovaginitis, otitis externa, yaws, pinta, and dermatomycoses
Chlorination of swimming pools	Enteric pathogens, inclusion conjunctivitis
Boiling and chlorination of water under emergency situations	Enteric pathogens

Table 12-3 Practical Methods for the Prevention and Control of Selected Infectious Diseases (CONTINUED)

Method	Diseases
Disinfection of contaminated materials	Numerous diseases that can be spread from man to man by inhalation or ingestion
Control of biological vectors or protection against vectors	Arthropod-transmitted diseases
Control of animal reservoirs	Many arthropod-transmitted diseases, rabies, plague, tuberculosis, brucellosis, murine typhus, psittacosis, rickettsialpox, rat-bite fever, lymphocytic choriomeningitis, and relapsing fever
Detection, treatment, and monitoring of cases and carriers	Typhoid, tuberculosis, staphylococcal disease, cholera, shigellosis, meningococcal meningitis, serum hepatitis, diphtheria, syphilis, and gonorrhea
Isolation of cases	Smallpox, cholera, diphtheria, plague, typhoid, and meningococcal meningitis
Prevention of prematurity	Many neonatal diseases of the respiratory and intestinal tracts, oral cavity, and CNS
Case reporting and/or recognition of source	Numerous diseases including tuberculosis, typhoid, shigellosis, cholera, amebiasis, smallpox, diphtheria, serum hepatitis, infectious hepatitis, syphilis, gonorrhea, meningococcal meningitis, malaria, botulism, staphylococcal food poisoning, rabies, pertussis, rubella, poliomyelitis, and leprosy
Surgical drainage, debridement, or excision	Abscesses, osteomyelitis, empyema, tetanus, gas gangrene, wound infections, and onchocerciasis
Aseptic technique	Numerous hospital-acquired diseases and serum hepatitis
Specialized forms of treatment	
Fluid and electrolyte replacement	Cholera, shigellosis, salmonellosis, and infantile diarrhea
Hyperbaric oxygenation	Gas gangrene
Control of underlying disease (diabetes)	Staphylococcal disease, urinary tract infection, candidiasis, trichomoniasis, phycomycosis, and erythrasma
Correction of anatomical defects	Numerous diseases depending upon the location of the defect (urinary tract infections, respiratory and intestinal tract, and CNS infections)
Replacement of C3 and C5 components of complement	Numerous gram-negative enteric infections and staphylococcal disease
Replacement of immunoglobulin in agammaglobulinemics	Diseases caused by staphylococci, streptococci, pneumococci, meningococci, and influenza bacilli
Transfer factor	Disseminated candidiasis and vaccinia
Moist air	Croup and bronchiolitis
Tracheostomy	Croup, bronchiolitis, and diphtheria
Antidust measures (grass, oil)	Coccidioidomycosis
Decontamination of infected materials	Anthrax
Mass therapy	Trachoma, yaws, bejel, and pinta
Central heating plus residential plumbing and regular washing	Epidemic typhus
Cautery	Molluscum contagiosum, warts
Laws against feeding raw garbage to swine	Trichinosis

Table 12-4 Major Problems in Prevention and Control of Infectious Disease

Biological factors
Localized infections
Short incubation periods
Number of antigenic types
Frequency of subclinical or unrecognized cases
Long-term persistence of the causative agent
Extent of the animal reservoir and/or arthropod vectors
Prolonged survival of causative agent in nature
Ubiquitous distribution of causative agent
Underlying cardiopulmonary and metabolic disease
Failure of the natural defense of the host
Dissemination of the pathogen before overt disease is evident
Cross-reactions of pathogen with host components
Frequency of unrecognized obstruction
Trauma
Waning of naturally acquired or induced immunity
Therapeutic difficulties or lack of effective antibiotics
Socioeconomic factors
Failure to apply accepted principles of prevention and control (Table 12-3)
Social habits: sexual promiscuity; use of cigarettes, alcohol, or drugs; poor diet
Educational efforts limited by age, personnel, economics, lack of interest, mildness of disease, remoteness of serious consequences

Control of shigellosis in man is possible through the use of live oral vaccines. Two types of live oral vaccines are safe and effective in man, one containing streptomycin-dependent mutants and the other a hybrid derived from mating between an avirulent shigella mutant and an *Escherichia coli* K 12 Hfr isolate. The level of immunity resembles that seen after recovery from active infection, especially with the streptomycin-dependent vaccine. Two other live oral vaccines, although safe and effective in monkeys, were unsuitable for human use. A hybrid obtained from mating virulent shigellae with *E. coli* K 12 produced an acute febrile illness unlike dysentery, with vomiting and watery diarrhea. A spontaneously derived, nonpenetrating shigella mutant reverted in vivo when a dose of 10^{10} was administered to volunteers. As a result of these ingenious experiments, the important biological requirements of live oral *Shigella* vaccines are that the causative agent must not penetrate the intestinal mucosa and must be stable without reverting to virulence at the dosage used. In the human studies, to induce resistance it is necessary first to alter gastric function with oral sodium bicarbonate, and then to administer multiple doses of attenuated *Shigella* organisms. Information concerning the use of enteric-coated capsules and the production of secretory IgA is not available, but it seems reasonable to assume that a potent secretory IgA response is achieved, since specific protection persists for at least 6 months and since humoral antibody is formed.

Hopefully, studies similar to those outlined will be expanded to many other causative agents. The investigations should not be restricted to parasites that produce localized infections but should encompass organisms whose portal of entry is a mucous membrane and for which effective vaccines are not available (typhoid, meningococcal meningitis, gonorrhea). Another potential approach that merits further exploration is the use of nonpathogenic organisms that can colonize mucous membranes and result in the formation of cross-reactive protective antibody. For example, a nongroupable meningococcus carried in the oropharynx induced protective antibody against group B and group C meningococci in a significant number of military recruits.

A serious problem was encountered a few years ago in connection with field studies of respiratory syncytial (RS) virus vaccine. One to three intramuscular doses of a killed vaccine produced uniformly good titers of complement-fixing antibody in infants 2 to 7 months of age. On this basis, field studies were carried out with disastrous results. Potent antibody responses were achieved, but when the annual outbreak of RS infection arrived in the respective communities, the vaccinees suffered much more severely than unvaccinated controls. For example, pneumonia occurred seven times as frequently in vaccinees as in controls, hospitalization was required 16 to 18 times as often, and there was a sharp rise in the severity of the disease among older infants and children (63 percent of vaccinees developed illness between 7 to 18 months of age, whereas among the control group 65 percent of illness occurred in the first 6 months. Taking into account the age incidence of the natural disease, the induction of potent antibody responses in the vaccinees, the severity of the disease in the vaccinees, and the sharp rise in severity among older vaccinees (hospitalization was at least 18 times more frequent among vaccinees 9 to 23 months of age as among controls), the most logical conclusion to draw is that RS disease is an immune complex disease and that the production of IgG antibody following intramuscular vaccination increased the frequency and severity of the disease. The data probably also provide another compelling argument for the concept of mucous membrane immunization with the consequent production of secretory IgA which cannot form immune complexes that are damaging to the host but which is protective.

Similar paradoxical disease-enhancing effects of vaccination have been recognized with other killed vaccines administered subcutaneously or intramuscularly (trachoma, mycoplasma, measles, and rickettsial vaccines), but fortunately the consequences have not been as disastrous.

THE CHANGING PATTERN OF INFECTIOUS DISEASE

Despite the long-term secular trends in a number of infectious diseases, some of which were indicated in Table 12-1, the morbidity of infectious disease in the world today is probably little different from what is was a century ago. The prime reason for the continued high incidence of infectious disease is almost entirely due to the prevalence of infections of the respiratory and intestinal tracts. In the developed countries, however, there has been a marked reduction in mortality due to parasites that once were considered a lethal challenge and the virtual elimination of all deaths due to gastrointestinal and respiratory infections between the ages of 1 and 4 years. Concomitantly, the expected life span at birth now exceeds 70 years.

Changing patterns of infectious disease, always occurring, appear to have accelerated and become more evident with the advent of the antibiotic era, the use of corticosteroids, new modalities of immunosuppressive and cancer chemotherapy, the increased incidence of cardiopulmonary and cardiorenal disease, and a rising proportion of older, more susceptible individuals in the population. Many facets of the shifting alterations in infectious disease are mentioned in Chapters 5, 6, and 11 and in earlier sections of this chapter but are covered in more detail in much of the balance of the text, especially in Chapters 14, 18, 20, and 24. Consequently, only the general outline of some of the changing patterns is indicated below.

In the preantibiotic era, the serious life-threatening situations—reflected by bacteremia, endocarditis, and meningitis—were predominantly caused by gram-positive bacteria (approximately 90, 90, and 68 percent, respectively). In the postantibiotic era of current medical practice, there has been a remarkable shift so that gram-negative bacteria account for approximately 75 and 55 percent of the cases of bacteremia and meningitis. For unaccountable reasons, the marked increase in gram-negative etiology of bacteremia has not been reflected in a proportionate increase in cases of endocarditis or meningitis. However, there has been a modest increase in pneumonia caused by gram-negative enteric bacteria. The principal factors involved in these changing patterns are the (1) remarkable sensitivity of the common gram-positive pathogens to penicillin (pneumococci and group A streptococci), (2) increasing frequency of urinary tract infections with advancing age of the population which are caused predominantly by gram-negative enteric bacteria, (3) resistance of gram-negative enteric bacilli to the commonly used antibiotics, (4) more extensive atherosclerosis which accompanies advancing age, and (5) sensitivity of gram-negative gonococci to penicillin (gonococci formerly caused up to 10 percent of cases of endocarditis, but this is extremely rare today).

Accompanying these shifts, there has been a reversal of the case fatality ratios caused by gram-positive bacteria to gram-negative bacteria from 5 to 1 in the preantibiotic era to 1 to 5 in the postantibiotic era. In addition, in the postantibiotic era, there has been a striking shift in the incidence and case fatality ratios in those over 60 years of age (two and one-half times) and a fivefold reduction in the proportion of deaths in those from 10 to 40 years old.

The changes noted above do not, however, accurately reflect the accelerated pace which has been observed, and as a matter of fact, the trend is not always unidirectional. In staphylococci, for example, there was a steady increase in frequency of bacteremia from about 20 percent in the preantibiotic era to a peak of 40 percent in 1957, followed by a return to about 20 percent of all cases currently. The case fatality ratio varied from close to 50 percent in the preantibiotic era to a low of less than 20 percent in 1947 to a high of 48 percent in 1961 and has been declining again since then. The changes in the relative incidence and mortality are related sequentially to the appearance of penicillin-resistant organisms, the appearance of certain specific phage patterns 52/42B/81, followed by 80/81, and most recently by a decline in 80/81 organisms.

Other important changes have been noted in connection with the widespread use of antibiotics, the increasing use of immunosuppressive procedures, and the advancing age of the population with its accompanying increased incidence of immunosuppression (Chap. 10). These include the sharply increased incidence of serious infections caused by members of the normal flora, especially by those that are adapted to intracellular survival and growth (fungi such as *Candida,* bacteria such as *Listeria,* viruses that are latent such as cytomegalovirus, and protozoa such as *Pneumocystis*).

BIBLIOGRAPHY

Barclay, W. R., Busey, W. M., Dalgard, D. W., Good, R. C., Janicki, B. W., Kasik, J. E., Ribi, E., Ulrich, C. E., and Wolinsky, E.: "Protection of Monkeys against Airborne Tuberculosis by Aerosol Vaccination with Bacillus Calmette-Guérin," *Am. Rev. Resp. Dis.,* 107:351-358, 1973.

Blaese, R. M., Weiden, P., Oppenheim, J. J., and Waldmann, T.: "Phytohemagglutinin As a Skin Test for the Evaluation of Cellular Immune Competence in Man," *J. Lab. Clin. Med.,* 81:538-548, 1973.

Charles, D., and Finland, M. (eds.): *Obstetric and Perinatal Infections,* Philadelphia: Lea & Febiger, 1973.

Chin, J., Magoffin, R. L., Shearer, L. A., Scheible, J. H., and Lennette, E. H.: "Field Evaluation of a Respiratory Syncytial Virus Vaccine and a Trivalent Parainfluenza Virus Vaccine in a Pediatric Population," *Am. J. Epidemiol.,* 89:449-463, 1969.

DuPont, H. L., Hornick, R. B., Snyder, M. J., Libonati, J. P., Formal, S. B., and Gangarosa, E. J.: "Immunity in Shigellosis: I. Response of Man to Attenuated Strains of *Shigella,*" *J. Infect. Dis.,* 125:5-11, 1972.

Farrand, R. J., and Williams, A.: "Evaluation of Single-use Packs of Hospital Disinfectants," *Lancet,* 1:591-593, 1973.

Fulginiti, V. A., Eller, J. J., Sieber, O. F., Joyner, J. W., Minamitani, M., and Meiklejohn, G.: "Respiratory Virus Immunization. I. Field Trial of Two Inactivated Virus Vaccines; An Aqueous Trivalent

Parainfluenza Virus Vaccine and an Alum-precipitated Respiratory Syncytial Virus Vaccine," *Am. J. Epidemiol.,* 89:435-448, 1969.

Gardner, P., and Charles, D. G.: "Infections Acquired in a Pediatric Hospital," *J. Pediatr.,* 81:1205-1210, 1972.

Hambraeus, A.: "Studies on Transmission of *Staphylococcus aureus* in an Isolation Ward for Burned Patients," *J. Hyg. (Camb.),* 71:171-183, 1973.

———, and Sanderson, H. F.: "The Control of Ventilation of Airborne Bacterial Transfer between Hospital Patients, and Its Assessment by Means of a Particle Tracer. III. Studies with an Airborne-particle Tracer in an Isolation Ward for Burned Patients," *J. Hyg. (Camb.),* 70:299-312, 1972.

Hattis, R. P., Halstead, S. B., Herrmann, K. L., and Witte, J. J.: "Rubella in an Immunized Island Population," *J.A.M.A.,* 223:1019-1021, 1973.

"Immunity and Infection," (a symposium) *Postgrad. Med. J.,* 48:325-350, 1972.

Janicki, B. W., Good, R. C., Minden, P., Affronti, L. F., and Hymes, W. F.: "Immune Responses in Rhesus Monkeys after Bacillus Calmette-Guérin Vaccination and Aerosol Challenge with *Mycobacterium tuberculosis,*" *Am. Rev. Resp. Dis.,* 107:359-366, 1973.

Kapikian, A. Z., Mitchell, R. H., Chanock, R. M., Shvedoff, R. A., and Stewart, C. E.: "An Epidemiologic Study of Altered Clinical Reactivity to Respiratory Syncytial (RS) Virus Infection in Children Previously Vaccinated with an Inactivated RS Virus Vaccine," *Am. J. Epidemiol.,* 89:405-421, 1969.

Kass, E. H.: "Infectious Diseases and Social Change," *J. Infect. Dis.,* 123:110-114, 1971.

Kim, H. W., Canchola, J. G., Brandt, C. D., Pyles, G., Chanock, R. M., Jensen, K., and Parrott, R. H.: "Respiratory Syncytial Virus Disease in Infants Despite Prior Administration of Inactivated Vaccine," *Am. J. Epidemiol.,* 89:422-434, 1969.

Lidwell, O. M.: "The Control of Ventilation of Airborne Bacterial Transfer between Hospital Patients, and Its Assessment by Means of a Particle Tracer. II. Ventilation in Subdivided Isolation Units," *J. Hyg. (Camb.),* 70:287-298, 1972.

Lodmell, D. L., Newa, A., Hayashi, K., and Notkins, A. L.: "Prevention of Cell-to-Cell Spread of Herpes Simplex Virus by Leukocytes," *J. Exp. Med.,* 137:706-720, 1973.

Louie, J. S., and Goldberg, L. S.: "Lymphocyte-Monocyte Defect Associated with Anergy and Recurrent Infections," *Clin. Exp. Immunol.,* 11:469-474, 1972.

MacLeod, C. M.: "Relation of the Incubation Period and the Secondary Immune Response to Lasting Immunity to Infectious Diseases," *J. Immunol.,* 70:421-425, 1953.

Meiklejohn, G.: "Control of Smallpox and Influenza," *J. Infect. Dis.,* 127:215-219, 1973.

Miller, M. E.: "Uses and Abuses of Plasma Therapy in the Patient with Recurrent Infections," *J. Allergy Clin. Immunol.,* 51:45-56, 1973.

Mims, C. A., and Blanden, R. V.: "Antiviral Action of Immune Lymphocytes in Mice Infected with Lymphocytic Choriomeningitis Virus," *Infect. Immun.,* 6:695-717, 1972.

Minden, P., McClatchy, J. K., and Farr, R. S.: "Shared Antigens between Heterologous Bacterial Species," *Infect. Immun.,* 6:574-599, 1972.

Nye, F. J.: "Social Class and Infectious Mononucleosis," *J. Hyg. (Camb.),* 71:145-150, 1973.

———, and Lambert, H. P.: "Epstein-Barr Virus Antibody in Cases and Contacts of Infectious Mononucleosis; A Family Study," *J. Hyg. (Camb.),* 71:151-161, 1973.

Potter, C. W., Oxford, J. S., Shore, C. L., McLaren, C., and Stuart-Harris, C.: "Immunity to Influenza Virus in Ferrets. I. Response to Live and Killed Virus," *Br. J. Exp. Pathol.,* 53:153-167, 1972.

Raubitschek, A. A., Levin, A. S., Stites, D. P., Shaw, E. B., and Fudenberg, H. H.: "Normal Granulocyte Infusion Therapy for Aspergillosis in Chronic Granulomatous Disease," *Pediatrics,* 51:230-233, 1973.

Smith, H.: "Opportunistic Infection," *Br. Med. J.* 2: 107-110, 1973.

Stites, D. P., Levin, A. S., Lauer, B. A., Costom, B. H., and Fudenberg, H. H.: "Selective 'Dysgammaglobulinemia' with Elevated Serum IgA Levels and Chronic Salmonellosis," *Am. J. Med.,* 54:260-264, 1973.

Sullivan, N. M., Sutter, V. L., Mims, M. M., Marsh, V. H., and Finegold, S. M.: "Clinical Aspects of Bacteremia after Manipulation of the Genitourinary Tract," *J. Infect. Dis.,* 127:49-55, 1973.

Top, F. H., Jr., Buescher, E. L., Bancroft, W. H., and Russell, P. K.: "Immunization with Live Types 7 and 4 Adenovirus Vaccines. II. Antibody Response and Protective Effect Against Acute Respiratory Disease Due to Adenovirus Type 7," *J. Infect. Dis.,* 124:155-160, 1971.

———, Grossman, R. A., Bartelloni, P. J., Segal, H. E., Dudding, B. A., Russell, P. K., and Buescher, E. L.: "Immunization with Live Types 7 and 4 Adenovirus Vaccines. I. Safety, Infectivity, Antigenicity, and Potency of Adenovirus Type 7 Vaccine in Humans," *J. Infect. Dis.,* 124:148-154, 1971.

"Vector Ecology. Report of a WHO Scientific Group," *WHO Tech. Rep. Ser.,* no. 501, 1972.

Worthington, M., Rabson, A. S., and Baron, S.: "Mechanism of Recovery from Systemic Vaccinia Virus Infection," *J. Exp. Med.,* 136:277-290, 1972.

Chapter 13

Bacterial Food Poisoning and Diseases in Which Toxins Play a Decisive Role

Bernard A. Briody

BACTERIAL FOOD POISONING

Perspective

Bacterial food poisoning is the term applied to acute gastroenteritis which follows the ingestion of bacteria or their products. Staphylococcal food poisoning and botulism result from the ingestion of *preformed toxin* and are classic examples of how a specific bacterial product can cause disease in man. Acute gastroenteritis due to *Salmonella* species, entertoxin-producing *Escherichia coli, Vibrio parahemolyticus, Bacillus cereus,* and *Clostridium perfringens (Clostridium welchii)* develops following multiplication of the ingested bacteria within the intestinal tract.

There has been an approximately threefold increase in bacterial food poisoning in each 5-year interval over the past 30 years. In the United States alone, an estimated 1 million cases occur each year. Of these, staphylococci are assumed to be responsible for 60 to 70 percent, salmonellae for 15 to 20 percent. On the other hand, in England and Wales 95 percent of food poisoning outbreaks have been associated with salmonellae, 3 percent with staphylococci, and 2 percent with clostridia. In this chapter, the discussion of food poisoning will be limited to that caused by staphylococcal entertoxins and botulinus toxins. The other causative agents will be considered in Chapter 18.

Staphylococcal Food Poisoning

Production of Enterotoxins Ability to produce enterotoxin, and consequently staphylococcal food poisoning, is a property of certain coagulase-positive strains of *Staphylococcus aureus* (Chap. 14) within phage groups III and IV. These particular staphylococci have been isolated from the noses of healthy persons (34 of 155 staphylococcal isolates in one study) and from the noses and hands of food handlers who contaminated the food. The organism grows well at temperatures above 18°C and produces enterotoxin under aerobic and anaerobic conditions. Milk and meat products provide excellent media for the synthesis of enterotoxin by the organism. Although the initial number of staphylococci in the food influences the extent of enterotoxin production, the more important determining factor is the length of storage of the food at temperatures which permit extensive multiplication of the organism and concomitant synthesis of enterotoxin.

Antigenic Types of Enterotoxin As revealed by gel diffusion studies, there are several antigenically distinct types of enterotoxin of which type A is the most common. It is the only enterotoxin produced by 90 percent of the strains of staphylococci isolated from outbreaks of food poisoning. Type B was synthesized by 8 percent of the strains, and 2 percent produced both Type A and Type B enterotoxins. There have only been five enterotoxigenic staphylococcal isolates which synthesize neither A nor B enterotoxins.

Predominance of Type A Enterotoxin The predominance of Type A enterotoxin as a cause of staphylococcal food poisoning is a reflection of the wide distribution of organisms capable of producing this enterotoxin in the noses of healthy persons (80 percent of the strains isolated). The explanation may also be partly due to the ease with which 42D strains of staphylococci are lysogenized by temperate phage (Chap. 3) carrying the gene responsible for production of type A enterotoxin.

Properties of Enterotoxin Chemically, the enterotoxins are basic proteins of low molecular weight (around 24,000). They are resistant to acid, proteolytic enzymes, and can withstand boiling for more than 30 min. Although there is considerable variation in individual susceptibility, man is uniquely sensitive to the enterotoxin. Few people will escape the disease after ingesting enterotoxin. In most outbreaks the incidence approaches 100 percent.

Pathogenesis The incubation period is inversely related to the amount of preformed enterotoxin ingested and the susceptibility of the individual, but usually averages about 3 hr. with a range of 1 to 6 hr. The severity of the disease is directly proportional to the amount of toxin ingested. Symptoms persist for about 6 hr., and recovery is usually complete in 24 hr. In extremely rare instances death may occur in infants and debilitated adults. Increased salivation, nausea, vomiting, retching, abdominal pain, prostration, and diarrhea occur in varying intensity.

The site of action of the enterotoxin is uncertain. Results have been cited to indicate that the effects of the toxin are mediated by peripheral and central neurons, but in other studies gastroscopic changes complemented by histological evidence recorded in patients suffering from the disease have suggested a more direct toxic action on the intestinal mucosa.

Diagnosis A short incubation period and the brief course of the disease suggest a staphylococcal etiology. This can be confirmed by recovery of the organism from the suspect food and demonstrating that it produces enterotoxin by performing gel diffusion tests with antibody against types A and B enterotoxins. Although the patient will have recovered from the disease within 24 hr., it is important from the standpoint of the future welfare of his family, friends, and associates to trace the source of the infection. This can be accomplished by phage typing the organism isolated from the food and matching the phage type with the food handler carrying the staphylococci of the same phage type (Chap. 14).

Prevention and Control The disease occurs everywhere and is most prevalent during the summer months when the ambient temperature is more suitable for growth of the organism and production of enterotoxin. Every effort should be made to keep persons with open lesions from preparing food and to instruct food handlers in the rudiments of food hygiene. Since it is virtually impossible to prevent nasal carriers from contaminating food with enterotoxin-producing staphylococci, the best and most practical method of control is the prompt refrigeration of milk and meat products. This will prevent the growth of staphylococci and synthesis of enterotoxin. Since the enterotoxin survives boiling for more than 30 min., heating of food containing the enterotoxin is of little value in preventing the disease. No specific treatment is available, and there is little evidence that any significant level of immunity accompanies recovery from the disease.

Botulism

The Organism Producing Botulinus Toxin Botulism is an intoxication due to the ingestion of minute amounts of the most potent toxin known. *Clostridium botulinum,* the organism which produces botulinus toxin, is a gram-positive rod with rounded ends, measuring about 6 μm in length by 0.6 μm in width. The organism is an anaerobic spore former that exists in soil as a saprophyte. Bacilli which produce type E toxin are commonly found in fresh and salt water. The spores are oval and located near the end of the bacillus (subterminal). The spores are extremely resistant to heat and may survive boiling for prolonged periods but are inactivated in the pressure cooker or autoclave when heated at 120°C for 20 min. In improperly canned or preserved foods, the spores survive, and under anaerobic conditions they germinate, and botulinus toxin is produced by the vegetative forms.

Antigenic Types of Botulinus Toxin As demonstrated by specific neutralization tests, different strains of *C. botulinum* produce antigenically distinct toxins which have been designated types A, B, Cα, Cβ, D, E, and F. Types A, B, and E are primarily involved in human disease. Only a few human cases have been due to types C, D, and F. Types C and D are responsible for botulism in herbivores.

Properties of Botulinus Toxins Botulinus toxins appear to be produced as inactive protoxins which are converted to active toxins by proteolytic enzymes. The size of the toxin molecules varies from particles of molecular weight (M. W.) less than 70,000 to about 1,000,000. Crystalline type A toxin with a M. W. of about 1,000,000 and a sedimentation constant (S) of 15.5S is highly resistant to proteolysis by pepsin. On the other hand, at pH 9.2 the intact toxin is irreversibly dissociated into toxic fragments with the formation of a principal component with a sedimentation constant of 7S and a M. W. of about 158,000. The dissociated or 7S fragment is extensively degraded by pepsin with retention of a considerable amount of its toxicity. The molecular size range of the toxic fragments formed by peptic cleavage of the 7S toxin has not yet been determined, but in some experiments significant diffusion of toxic fragments (M. W. about 3,800) through dialyzing membranes was observed. Similar findings of diffusible toxic fragments have been reported for type E protoxin (sedimentation constant 5.6S) activated by trypsin.

After ingestion it is probable that type A botulinus toxin is present in the intestinal tract of man either as the 7S toxin or in a form that is susceptible to cleavage by pepsin or trypsin. In any event, in orally posioned rats or intravenously injected rabbits the toxin appearing in the lymph and plasma of the animals was shown to consist of smaller toxic fragments in the range of 4.4 to 11.4S. These data may partly explain the unique effectiveness of botulinus toxin following ingestion. For example, type A toxin is 50,000 times more lethal for the mouse by the oral route than by the intraperitoneal route.

The extreme toxicity of botulinus toxins is indicated by the demonstration that crystalline type A toxin contains 45 million MLD per mg N for the mouse and by the finding that liquid cultures of *C. botulinum* can yield 200 million mouse LD_{50} per ml. Although all types of botulinus toxins have the same pharmacologic action, they differ greatly in relative lethality for animals. For example, the potency of types A and B toxins for monkeys, and presumably for man, is 10 to 3,000 times that for types C, D, E, and F. The lethal dose of type A toxin for man is probably less than 1 μg.

Pathogenesis Preformed botulinus protoxin is highly resistant to acid and after ingestion traverses the stomach undamaged. In the small intestine the protoxin is activated by proteolytic enzymes and dissociates into toxic fragments of smaller size which are readily absorbed. The toxin circulates in the bloodstream and eventually reaches its site of action in the peripheral nervous system where it suppresses the output of acetycholine from the endings of cholinergic motor nerves at the neuromuscular junction. The toxin acts at the tips of the nerve endings where it causes a reduction of the frequency of miniature end plate potentials without changing their mean amplitude. Experimentally, the rate of paralysis induced by the toxin has been shown to vary with factors that influence the release or metabolism of acetycholine such as increased nerve ending activity, anticholinesterase drugs, atropine, and guanidine, the latter being of limited value in treatment.

The incubation period is inversely proportional and the case fatality rate directly proportional to the amount of protoxin ingested. The incubation period usually averages 12 to 36 hr., but may be as short as 6 hr. or as long as 8 days. With incubation periods of 1, 3, and 8 days in type A intoxications, the case fatality rates were 84, 55, and 20 percent, respectively. The signs and symptoms of the disease include mild intestinal manifestations, fatigue, diplopia, and difficulty in swallowing and speech. In about two-thirds of the cases, death occurs in 3 to 6 days due to respiratory failure. In general, mortality is higher in type A than in type B or type E intoxications.

Laboratory Diagnosis Definitive laboratory diagnosis is best accomplished by performing a protection test in mice. Suspected items of food are injected intraperitoneally into untreated mice and into mice protected by antitoxin specific for types A, B, and E toxins. If botulinus toxin is present in the food, mice receiving the appropriate antitoxin will be protected. Occasionally, the test may be positive when 1 ml of the blood of the patient is used as the source of toxin.

Epidemiology The frequency of a particular type of botulinus toxin as the cause of human disease is related to the distribution of the organisms in soil, the potency of the toxins, and the eating habits of the people. In the United States where home-canned vegetables are commonly implicated, outbreaks due to type A toxin are more common than those due to type B or E toxins. In Europe, types A and B are found in outbreaks primarily associated with sausages, hams, preserved meats, and meat pastes. Type E is predominant in regions bordering the sea, especially where there is a local preference for raw fish, as in British Columbia, Alaska, Japan, and the Baltic area.

Fortunately, the annual number of cases of botulism reported in this country is low. From 1899 to 1972 there have been 1,731 cases with 86 percent (1,489) associated with home-prepared food and 14 percent (242) with commercial food products. As is apparent from Figure 13-1 there have never been more than 89 cases reported in any year since 1899, and in only 5 years has the number exceeded 50. The 47 reported in 1963 was the highest number recorded since 1935. It marked the most serious outbreak associated with commercial products since appropriate control measures were instituted in 1922. The commercial products involved were smoked whitefish, smoked whitefish chubs, tuna fish, and liver paste. The contaminated home-prepared foodstuffs responsible for cases of botulism included chili peppers, green beans, corn, mushrooms, figs, beets, and home-smoked whitefish. Almost all the cases associated with commercial products were due to type E toxin, while most of the home-canned foodstuffs contained type A toxin. There have been only 17 outbreaks of type E intoxication recorded in the United States (of which 7 were in Alaska) with the largest occurring in 1963. In 1964 none of the 22 cases were due to type E, and none were associated with commercial products. In general, there are a greater number of cases in the winter months when home-canned foods are consumed.

Prevention and Control There are two practical ways in which botulism can be controlled. The first and most important is to kill the spores by using a pressure cooker or autoclave in commercial and home canning of foods. The second way takes advantage of the fact that botulinus toxins can be inactivated by boiling for 10 min.

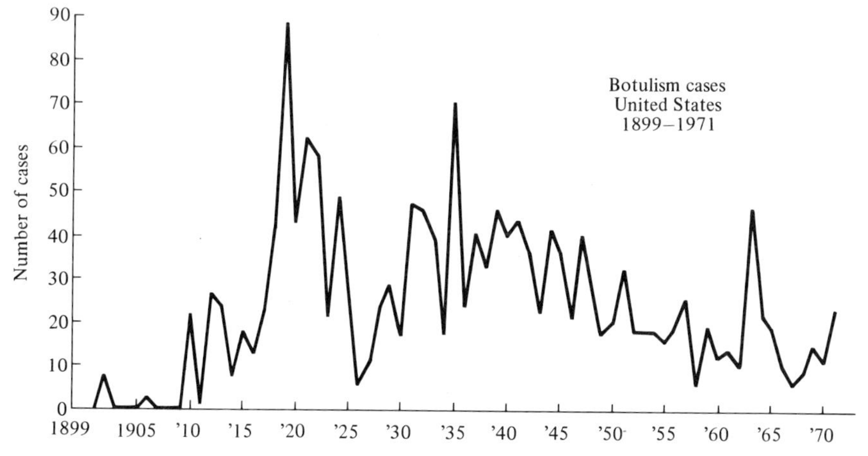

Figure 13-1 Reported cases of botulism in the United States, 1899-1971. [(1899-1949) *From K. F. Mayer and B. Eddie, Fifty Years of Botulism in the United States and Canada: Report from George Williams Hooper Foundation, July 1950;* (1950-1971) *from Morbidity Mortality Weekly Report, 20 (53):63, 1972.*]

Home-prepared food should never be tasted prior to boiling. Treatment is of little value due to the irreversible combination of toxin with tissue components and failure to promptly recognize the disease. Nonetheless, 50,000 or more units of polyvalent antitoxin should be given to all persons suspected of eating the contaminated food. The disease is so rare and sporadic that prophylactic immunization is impractical, although laboratory workers engaged in studies with botulinus toxins should be immunized with the toxoids.

Prospective

The use of proper commercial and home-canning procedures has largely eliminated the danger of botulism. Although staphylococcal food poisoning can be prevented by prompt refrigeration of perishable foods, failure to apply this measure has resulted in a steady increase in the disease over the years.

Part of the explanation for the rising prevalence of food poisoning is associated with the affluent society, its demand for food, and its penchant for dining out. A few pertinent statistics will serve to illustrate the logistics of the problem in the United States. The food industry is the country's leading employer. At more than $18 billion per year it is the fourth largest industry. There are an estimated 750,000 food establishments, of which 95 percent are single units—independently owned. The industry employs unskilled transitory labor and management that has limited concepts of food hygiene and inadequate skill in supervision. Many outbreaks are associated with failure to thoroughly cook contaminated foods, failure to refrigerate perishable foods, poor personal hygiene of employees, ineffective food processing and storage practices, and failure to clean and disinfect kitchen machines and equipment.

With all of their other essential duties, it is difficult to visualize how existing public health departments can cope with a problem of this magnitude by licensing and frequent inspection of the facilities of food establishments. An effective alternative would be a more vigorous educational approach concentrating on food processors, manufacturers, retailers, and restaurateurs who would in turn accept responsibility for the instruction of their employees in the essentials of food hygiene. Concomitantly, families must be educated and instructed in the methods which are known to prevent food poisoning in the home.

Diseases in Which Toxins Play a Decisive Role

DIPHTHERIA

Perspective

Although epidemics of diphtheria have unquestionably occurred for many centuries, the specific clinical features of the disease were first recognized in 1826 by Bretonneau. Understanding of the disease developed quickly after 1883 when Klebs observed the causative agent in smears from diphtheritic pseudomembranes. A year later Loeffler reproduced a similar disease in animals with cultures of diphtheria bacilli. In 1888 Roux and Yersin discovered diphtheria toxin and showed that the toxin alone produced a fatal disease in animals with lesions similar to those caused by the viable bacteria. The production of antitoxin was reported in 1890 by von Behring and Kitasato, and a year later antitoxin was successfully used in the treatment of diphtheria. In 1913 von Behring showed that immunity could be induced with toxin neutralized by antitoxin, and Schick developed a test for detecting immunity which involved the intradermal injection of minute amounts of toxin. Large-scale immunization of children with toxin-antitoxin mixtures was begun by Parks in 1922. A year later Ramon demonstrated that formalin-treated toxin (toxoid) was a more desirable immunizing agent than toxin-antitoxin mixtures. The subsequent widespread use of diphtheria toxoid for the prevention and control of diphtheria represents one of the most outstanding achievements in the history of microbiology.

The Causative Agent

Biological Properties *Corynebacterium diphtheriae,* the causative agent of diphtheria, is a characteristically pleomorphic, gram-positive, club-shaped bacillus that stains unevenly, resulting in a beaded or barred appearance. The deeply staining beads (metachromatic granules or Babés-Ernst bodies) are composed mainly of high molecular weight polyphosphates. Diphtheria bacilli are obligate parasites of man that are found in the upper respiratory tract and occasionally on the skin. Bacilli that are lysogenic for phage β, or certain mutants of phage β, are toxigenic and consequently capable of producing diphtheria in man.

Cultivation Aerobically, the organism grows well on most laboratory media. Loeffler's coagulated serum-egg-glucose medium and blood agar containing potassium tellurite have proved to be particularly valuable for the isolation of the organism from clinical specimens which often contain many other bacteria including nonpathogenic species of *Corynebacterium* (*C. hofmannii* and *C. xerosis*). Diphtheria bacilli grow moderately well on Loeffler's medium, forming small, granular, gray colonies with irregular edges, while streptococci and pneumococci grow poorly. Although tellurite inhibits the growth of most bacteria, diphtheria bacilli grow readily, producing rough (gravis), smooth (mitis), or dwarf (minimus or intermedius) gray to black colonies due to the reduction of tellurite. It should be emphasized that the connotation implied by the terms gravis and mitis in relation to clinical severity is no longer valid since typical rough (gravis) colonies have been isolated which are nontoxigenic.

Antigenic Structure Diphtheria toxin is the most important antigen produced by the organism. It is responsible for both the local cellular injury and the systemic manifestations of the disease. Conversely, protection against diphtheria is related to the level of antitoxin.

Toxigenicity and Lysogenicity When nontoxigenic strains of *C. diphtheriae* are infected with temperate β phage derived from toxigenic diphtheria bacilli, the lysogenic survivors acquire the hereditary ability to synthesize toxin (phage conversion). Kinetic analysis of the phenomenon reveals that conversion is due to the lysogenic state per se and not to selection by the phage of toxigenic survivors. Integration of β phage DNA with the bacterial genome is completely correlated with toxigenicity. Conversely, whenever the phage is lost, the diphtheria bacilli revert to a nontoxigenic state. Furthermore, genetic crosses between β phage and related phages which lack converting ability may yield recombinant phage particles which cannot confer toxigenicity. Thus, it is apparent that genetic control of toxin production resides in lysogenic β phage rather than in the diphtheria bacillus.

Toxin Production Toxin production by strains of diphtheria bacilli lysogenic for β phage begins at the end of the exponential growth period and continues at a linear rate until bacterial growth stops. During this period, the iron content of the culture medium is reduced, the cellular content of cytochromes falls, and equivalent amounts of toxin and coproporphyrin II are released into the medium. These findings suggest that diphtheria toxin may be structurally related to the protein moiety of cytochrome b.

Kinetic studies with labeled amino acids indicate that toxin is synthesized *de novo* and that its release is not accompanied by lysis of significant numbers of cells.

Properties of Diphtheria Toxin Crystalline diphtheria toxin is a heat-labile protein which has a M. W. of 62,000, contains about 3,000 flocculating doses of toxin (Lf) per milligram of nitrogen and is lethal for susceptible animals in doses of less than 0.1 μg/kg of body weight. There is some uncertainty as to whether the crystalline toxin is a single molecular species with several antigenic determinants or a mixture of several molecular species bound together in a complex that is immunologically and kinetically homogenous.

From a practical standpoint, the most important property of diphtheria toxin is that when treated with 0.3 to 0.5 percent formalin (pH 8.0 at 37°C) its toxicity is lost, but its antigenicity is retained. The detoxified but antigenic product of the interaction of toxin with formalin is *toxoid.* Immunization with toxoid induces the formation of diphtheria antitoxin and forms the basis for the prevention of diphtheria.

Mode of Action of Diphtheria Toxin Most preparations of diphtheria toxin consist predominantly of mixtures of various proportions of two proteins, each with a M. W. of about 62,000. Intact toxin consists of a single polypeptide chain, while nicked toxin is composed of fragment A (M. W. 24,000) and fragment B (M. W. 38,000) linked by a disulfide bond. Presumably, nicked toxin arises as a derivative of intact toxin following the action of proteases from the bacterial culture in which the toxin is produced.

It is assumed that either intact toxin or nicked toxin fixes to receptors on the eukaryotic cell membrane by means of fragment B. The adsorbed toxin dissociates following reduction of disulfide bonds, the enzymatically active component (fragment A) is released into the interior of the cell by a cellular peptidase, and fragment B is left behind at the cell membrane. Within the cell, fragment A catalyzes a reaction between adenine-ribose-P-P-ribose-nicotinamide (NAD) and aminoacyltransferase II (transferase II, translocation factor, or T2) to form a covalently linked, enzymatically inactive adenosine phosphoribosyl derivative of transferase II. This reaction inhibits protein synthesis by inactivating transferase II which is required for elongation of polypeptide chains in eukaryotic cells. Fragment A alone is not toxic. Linkage to fragment B is required for toxicity, presumably to permit adsorption to the plasma membrane and facilitate entry of fragment A into the cells. Toxin has no effect on the analogous elongation factor in prokaryotic cells.

Cells resistant to the lethal effects of diphtheria toxin have been isolated from the toxin-sensitive human KB cell line. Interestingly, the toxin-resistant cells are also resistant to several viruses, including poliovirus. Perhaps, the release of fragment A of diphtheria toxin into the interior of the cell is a process analogous to that associated with the eclipse of some viruses, such as poliovirus, at or near the cell membrane and may involve similar surface receptors on the plasma membrane.

Pathogenesis and Natural History of the Disease

Basically, diphtheria is a localized superficial infection of the upper respiratory tract which is associated with the formation of a pseudomembrane, composed of fibrin and necrotic tissue, and with *toxemia.* The organisms ordinarily gain entrance to the upper respiratory tract by droplet infection from a case or a carrier. Localization of diphtheria bacilli most commonly occurs in the tonsils and faucial pillars and less frequently in the nasopharynx or the larynx. After an incubation period of 1 to 4 days the patient usually develops fever and a sore throat, followed by formation of a pseudomembrane.

The Pseudomembrane Growth of diphtheria bacilli in the upper respiratory tract is accompanied by the production of toxin which is absorbed into the superficial layer of cells and destroys them in a few hours. Further growth of the organisms results in the formation of more toxin, and the process extends both laterally and more deeply into the tissue. Concomitantly, there is an inflammatory response leading to the accumulation of leukocytes, extravasation of red blood cells, and deposition of fibrin which together with the local necrotic tissue forms a layer of exudate. As the process continues, the layer becomes thicker, and the characteristic pseudomembrane forms. Initially, the membrane resembles a raw egg white, then coagulated egg white, and finally it takes on a rubbery consistency with color shades from gray to reddish brown. During the early stages, the membrane is tough, closely adherent, and leaves a raw surface when torn away. After a few days, the membrane separates and disappears, usually with minimal ulceration of the underlying tissue.

The association of the anatomical site of the primary lesion with the severity of the disease is undoubtedly a reflection of the quantity of toxin produced. In faucial diphtheria the process is limited essentially to the tonsillar area, and the disease is of moderate severity. In nasopharyngeal diphtheria the process extends from the faucial area to the uvula, soft palate, posterior pharyngeal wall, and nasal mucosa. When the cervical lymph nodes are greatly enlarged and accompanied by massive edema of the neck and chest, the term bullneck diphtheria is applied. Toxemia is a prominent feature of nasopharyngeal diphtheria. If the patient recovers, sequelae are common. In laryngeal diphtheria, infection spreads downward from the nasopharynx or may initially involve the larynx. Because the pseudomembrane and the accompanying edema may produce mechanical obstruction of the airway *(diphtheritic croup)*, this is a particularly dangerous form of the disease. Death by suffocation ensues unless the airway is restored by intubation or tracheostomy.

Toxemia In the course of producing the local cellular injury, a variable quantity of toxin enters the vascular system. If the causative strain of *C. diphtheriae* produces a large amount of toxin within a short time, death may occur within 72 hr. after onset of symptoms as a result of massive toxemia affecting mainly the heart. A less profound toxemia may cause death in the first 2 weeks as a result of cardiac damage. When smaller quantities of toxin enter the circulation, paralytic manifestations are prominent with involvement of the soft palate, the ciliary muscles of the eye, or the extremities. Both the cranial and peripheral nerves are affected.

Skin or Wound Diphtheria Although rarely seen in temperate climates, skin or wound diphtheria is commonly observed in the tropics. The infection appears at the site of wounds or abrasions and persists as a chronic, nonhealing ulcer which may cover an area several centimeters in diameter. A dirty, grayish membrane gradually appears over the base of the lesion. Absorption of toxin from the lesion is minimal, and the disease is consequently mild. On the other hand, absorption of toxin is adequate to produce immunity to the respiratory form of the disease.

Laboratory Diagnosis

Presumptive Diagnosis Because early specific treatment of the disease with antitoxin is essential, the presumptive diagnosis of diphtheria must be made on clinical grounds without waiting for laboratory confirmation.

Isolation and Identification of Toxigenic Diphtheria Bacilli The first step in establishing a laboratory diagnosis of diphtheria is to obtain a specimen from the pseudomembrane and to inoculate without delay a Loeffler slant, a tellurite plate, and a blood plate. In 18 hr. the microscopic morphology and staining reactions of *C. diphtheriae* on Loeffler's medium are typical. Growth of diphtheria bacilli on the selective tellurite medium requires 36 to 48 hr. before characteristic colonies appear. The blood plate is examined for the presence of hemolytic streptococci which can cause tonsillitis often confused with diphtheria. A stained smear of the specimen is usually adequate to determine if Vincent's infection is involved (Chap. 17).

In view of the possibility that diphtheria bacilli may be nontoxigenic and consequently incapable of producing diphtheria, it is imperative that the organisms isolated on culture be shown to produce toxin. This can be demonstrated by an intradermal test in a guinea pig or by an in vitro gel diffusion test.

Guinea Pig Intradermal Test The growth on a Loeffler slant is emulsified and 0.1 ml of the suspension injected into one (shaved) side of a guinea pig. Four hours later 500 units of antitoxin is given intraperitoneally, and 30 min. later 0.1 ml of the suspension is injected into a different area of the skin. If diphtheria toxin is produced by the organism, an inflammatory lesion which progresses to necrosis in 48 to 72 hr. develops only at the site injected before antitoxin was given.

Double Gel Diffusion Test In this test a strip of filter paper saturated with antitoxin is placed on an agar plate containing 20 percent horse serum. The suspected toxigenic culture is streaked in a single line across the plate at a right angle to the strip. After 48 hr. antitoxin diffusing from the strip precipitates with toxin diffusing out from the growing culture and forms lines that radiate out from the point at which the bacterial growth crosses the strip.

Epidemiology

Incidence: Morbidity and Mortality ***Before Immunization Procedures Were Developed*** For unknown centuries diphtheria in epidemic form was the leading cause of death among children. It is estimated that more than 20 percent of the population under 15 years of age in New England and the Middle Atlantic States died of diphtheria between 1735 and 1740. In New York City between 1880 and 1889 the diphtheria death rate for children under 10 years of age was 825 per 100,000 per year. In Omaha, Nebraska between 1890 and 1899 the annual case fatality rate was 32.4 per 100 and the yearly mortality rate per 100,000 (all ages) was 118.5.

The age incidence was always highest in preschool children. Diphtheria was uncommon during the first year of life, reached a maximum incidence between the ages of 2 and 5, gradually declined in the age group 5 to 10, and thereafter fell rapidly. As a rule, adult cases were seen only in the most widespread and severe epidemics (Fig. 13-2). In accordance with these findings, epidemic peaks in urban areas occurred every 6 to 7 years.

After Immunization Procedures Were Developed Within 10 years after the introduction of antitoxin in treatment the diphtheria death rate per 100,000 New York children under 10 years of age fell to less than 200. In Omaha in the same interval the case fatality rate dropped to 11.4 per 100 and the mortality rate per 100,000 (all ages) decreased to 15.7.

Additional progress in reducing the case and death rates was limited until the introduction and widespread use of artificial immunization. As has become dramatically evident, diphtheria has been brought under effective control in the United States. The case rate has fallen from 201.4 to 0.10 per 100,000 and the mortality rate from 17 to 0.01 per 100,000. In 1972, there were only 124 cases of diphtheria compared with 207,000 in 1921. The case fatality rate (6 to 11 percent) has remained relatively constant since 1921. However, the case fatality rate increased to 14 percent in 1963, 1964, and 1967.

With artificial immunization of a high proportion of preschool children, the incidence of diphtheria has shifted to the higher age groups (Fig. 13-2). In 1964, 40 percent of diphtheria

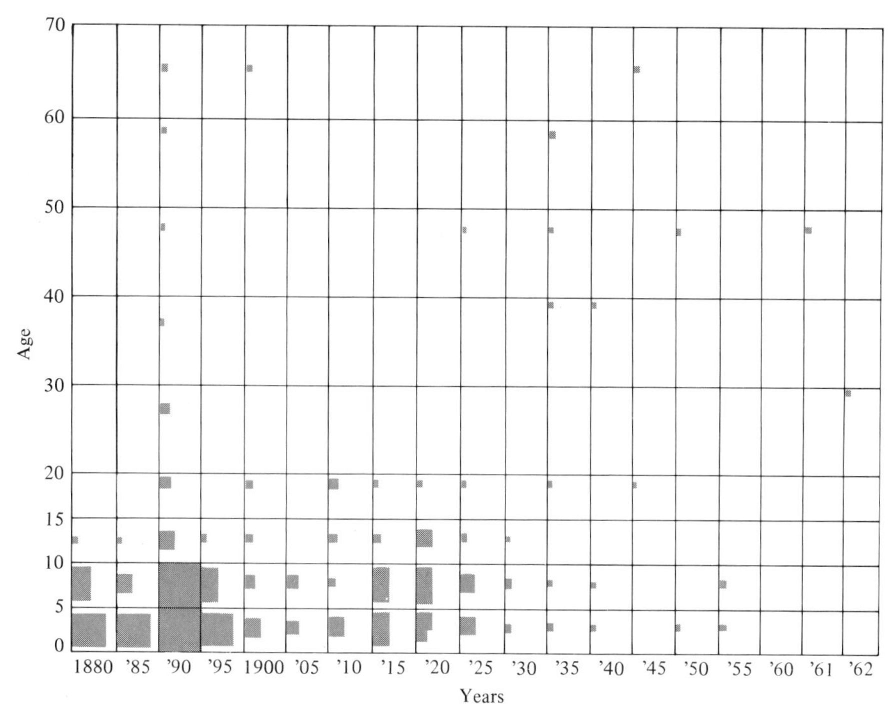

Figure 13-2 Age distribution of diphtheria deaths every fifth year, between 1880 and 1960, and epidemic years 1961-1962, Omaha-Douglas County, Neb. (*R. C. Eelkema and E. D. Lyman, Nebr. State Med. J., 49:612-621, 1964.*)

cases in the United States occurred in those over 15 years of age.

Schick Test When a minute amount of diphtheria toxin (1/50 MLD or minimal lethal dose in 0.1 ml) is injected intradermally in a susceptible person, it produces a local damage which develops in 24 hr. and reaches a maximum in 4 to 7 days. A Schick positive reaction consists of erythema in an area a few centimeters in diameter, usually with a more deeply colored central area, and may show some swelling. A positive test indicates little or no circulating antitoxin and probable susceptibility to diphtheria.

Negative Schick Test If the same dose of diphtheria toxin is injected into a person whose level of antitoxin is sufficient to protect him against ordinary exposure to diphtheria, the toxin is neutralized and produces no reaction. In general, a negative reaction is associated with 0.01 or more of a unit of antitoxin per milliliter. The degree of immunity possessed by Schick-negative persons, however, is not absolute. On the other hand, the occasional negative reactor who does develop clinical illness usually has a mild attack.

Allergic Reactions Because some persons show delayed hypersensitive reactions to diphtheria toxin which may be confused with the reaction due to the toxicity of the toxin, diphtheria toxoid (0.01 Lf in 0.1 ml) is included as a control in carrying out the Schick test. Inflammatory reactions at the sites of injection of both toxin and toxoid which reach a maximum within 48 or 72 hr. and then fade are known as pseudoreactions. Persons who show pseudoreactions are almost always immune to diphtheria but are hypersensitive to toxin, toxoid, or other materials in the preparations of toxin and toxoid. Furthermore, pseudoreactors almost invariably show a booster-type antitoxin response.

If the reaction at the toxin site persists as a positive reaction after the allergic inflammation has subsided, the result is known as a combined reaction. In persons showing a combined reaction circulating antitoxin is either absent or present in low titer; however, such persons regularly respond to the Schick test by forming antitoxin.

Delayed hypersensitive reactions to diphtheria toxin or toxoid are seldom observed in young children, but their frequency increases with age. Consequently, in older children and adults it is best to perform a Schick test prior to attempting artificial immunization. Individuals reacting to toxoid used in the Schick test should not be immunized further, since they respond to the test itself with an effective antitoxin response. Delayed reactions are highest in populations that have not been actively immunized and where diphtheria is prevalent.

The Carrier Although contact with toxigenic bacilli may be followed by clinical disease, more commonly the organism multiplies in the upper respiratory tract for a short period of time without causing signs of illness. Such a person is termed a *healthy carrier.* In most cases the carrier is Schick-negative, indicating possession of a good level of immunity. When toxigenic bacilli persist in the nasopharynx of carriers for several weeks, as they may in rare instances, the organism is difficult to eradicate. For these long-term carriers, tonsillectomy and corrective surgery for deviated septa or draining sinuses may be effective in eliminating the organism, but immunization and antibiotics fail to alter the carrier state.

Patients convalescing from diphtheria usually eliminate the organism in 2 to 4 weeks, more rapidly from the throat than the nose, but 2 to 4 percent may carry the organism in the nose for 2 months (convalescent carriers). In the majority of patients recovering from diphtheria, the toxigenic bacilli quickly become nontoxigenic presumably due to the effect of antiphage antibodies in causing the organism to lose the lysogenic phage β which exerts genetic control over toxin production. In a few patients the toxigenic bacilli persist and are as difficult to eradicate as in the case of the long-term carriers discussed above.

Cutaneous Carriers In epidemics in tropical areas cutaneous diphtheria is seen in approximately half the cases, 10 percent of whom also have pharyngeal diphtheria. Although Schick-negative individuals exhibit definite protection against pharyngeal diphtheria, cutaneous diphtheria is found with equal frequency in Schick-negative and Schick-positive individuals. Since patients with cutaneous diphtheria may harbor the organism for months, they represent an important source of infection for their own respiratory tracts as well as the respiratory tract and skin of others. In areas where cutaneous diphtheria is endemic, it is instrumental in producing immunity to the more serious respiratory forms of the disease.

Prevention and Control

Immunization of Infants and Young Children In many countries including the United States, prevention and control of diphtheria are based on the universal immunization of infants and young children with purified diphtheria toxoid usually combined with tetanus toxoid and pertussis vaccine. The toxoid is purified by alcohol fractionation at low temperatures or by ammonium sulfate fractionation followed by dialysis. The toxoid is usually injected as an alum precipitate or absorbed on aluminum phosphate gel as adjuvant and diluted so as to contain 10 to 20 Lf per immunizing dose of 0.5 or 1.0 ml with 1:10,000 Merthiolate added as a preservative.

At the age of a few months infants are given two doses of diphtheria toxoid combined with tetanus toxoid and pertussis vaccine at an interval of one month. A booster dose of the triple antigen is injected one year later and a second booster dose of diphtheria and tetanus toxoids is given at school age. Prior Schick testing is not necessary.

Children so immunized develop a high level of immunity to diphtheria through adolescence and are completely protected for life against death due to diphtheria but not against clinical diphtheria. Ideally, however, effective prevention and control of diphtheria should include one or more booster injections of diphtheria toxoid for older children or adults.

Immunization of Older Children and Adults Because delayed hypersensitive reactions of varying severity occur in a significant proportion (as high as 40 percent) of older children and adults, either a Schick test should be performed prior to immunization or, if this is not feasible, a minute amount of diphtheria toxoid (0.5 to 1 Lf), usually combined with tetanus toxoid, should be used for each immunizing dose. In the former situation, individuals who react to the Schick control toxoid require no further immunization because they respond to the test itself with the rapid and effective production of antitoxin. When 0.5 to 1 Lf of toxoid is employed for immunization, severe hypersensitive reactions are rarely observed, and most individuals will form antitoxin.

Current State of Immunization in the United States Results of the 1964 nationwide immunization survey in the United States show that 11.4 percent of children aged 1 to 4 years and 5.5 percent of children aged 5 to 9 years are not immunized with diphtheria toxoid. While 9.3 percent of white children aged 1 to 4 years are not immunized, 22.9 percent of nonwhite children in this age group are not immunized. The comparable figures for the 5- to 9-year-olds are 4.4 percent for white children and 12.3 percent for nonwhite children. Concurrent findings in other countries where universal immunization of children is practiced reveal a similar situation. For example, 6 to 18 percent of Australian school children 6 years of age are Schick-positive.

In the various geographical areas of the United States there is significant variation in the numbers of children who have not been immunized with diphtheria toxoid. For example, in the New England and Middle Atlantic states less than 9 percent of children between the ages of 1 and 4 are not immunized, whereas more than 21 percent of children in this age group in the East South Central and West South Central states are not immunized.

Treatment When there is strong clinical suspicion that a patient has diphtheria, a single large intravenous dose of antitoxin (10,000 to 100,000 units) must be administered as soon as sensitivity to the protein in the antitoxin preparation can be ruled out. If the patient is sensitive, desensitization must be undertaken before giving antitoxin. The earlier the diagnosis is made and antitoxin used, the lower the chance of mortality and the fewer the complications.

At best, antimicrobial therapy is a secondary consideration. After specimens have been obtained for culture in order to confirm the presumptive diagnosis, in many cases penicillin is of value in eliminating the organisms from the nose and throat and in preventing the establishment of the carrier state. In order to exert its optimal effect, penicillin must be given early in the course of the disease. However, it must be emphasized that treatment of diphtheria is dependent solely on the early administration of antitoxin.

Control of Epidemic Diphtheria Apart from prompt and effective treatment of the patient with diphtheria, there are a number of steps which should immediately be taken to prevent the further spread of the disease. The patient should be isolated until such time as he no longer carries toxigenic diphtheria bacilli. After hypersensitivity to serum has been ruled out, close contacts should immediately receive a prophylactic intramuscular injection of 500 to 1,000 units of antitoxin. Cultures should be obtained from the nose and throat, chemoprophylaxis with penicillin instituted, and active immunization with toxoid completed.

Institutional Epidemics If an epidemic occurs in a school, hospital, or other institution, a combination of active and passive immunization represents an effective method of halting the disease. This procedure involves the simultaneous injection into opposite arms of diphtheria toxoid and diphtheria antitoxin (500 to 1,000 units), followed in 2 to 4 weeks by a second dose of toxoid. Nose and throat swabs of the entire population group should be taken at weekly intervals until 2 weeks after the second dose of toxoid. By this time a high level of immunity will have developed and the risk of further cases will be negligible.

Urban Epidemics If an epidemic of diphtheria develops in an urban community, close contacts are managed as indicated above. Another important measure of preventing the spread of the disease is to institute without delay a mass immunization campaign with priority assigned to those who have never been immunized. In communities and countries where immunization of infants and young children is widely practiced, diphtheria is characteristically concentrated in those areas where the proportion of susceptible preschool children and adults has risen to a critical level, as in the case with poliomyelitis (Chap. 24). The problem areas frequently consist of the lower socioeconomic groups in overcrowded and substandard housing. In these areas special teams for home immunization are of great value, and all members of the family should be immunized.

Prospective

Freedom from diphtheria is virtually guaranteed by a universal program of immunization of infants and young children with toxoid, reinforced by two or more booster doses of toxoid later in life. No other serious infectious disease has been more diligently and effectively controlled than diphtheria. Prevention of diphtheria truly represents the most outstanding achievement in the history of microbiology.

TETANUS

Perspective

Tetanus (lockjaw) is a disease known since antiquity to occur as a dreaded sequel to wounds sustained in combat. In the preantitoxin era the fatality rate was 85 per 100 cases. The production of antitoxin in 1890 by von Behring and Kitasato and, more importantly, the introduction of tetanus toxoid for active immunization in 1925 by Ramon closely paralleled similar developments in diphtheria and provided an effective basis for prevention and control of tetanus. The 50,000 deaths caused annually by tetanus throughout the world could be avoided if universal immunization with tetanus toxoid were a reality.

The Causative Agent

Biological Properties In young cultures, *Clostridium tetani,* the causative agent of tetanus in man (and horses), is a gram-positive rod measuring about 6 μm in length by 0.5 μm in width. The organism is an anaerobic spore former. The tetanus bacillus is one of the few pathogens that can be identified on morphology alone because the spore is rounded or slightly oval and located terminally, giving a drumstick or squash racket appearance. The spores are extremely resistant and may survive boiling or prolonged contact with antiseptic agents but are inactivated by autoclaving. The vegetative forms of the organism are vigorously motile and usually fail to ferment any carbohydrates. Toxigenic bacilli are found in most samples of soil. Although the organism can frequently be isolated from animal feces, about half the strains are atoxic. Following ingestion of raw foods the organism may be transiently present in human feces.

Cultivation Growth of *C. tetani* requires a low oxidation-reduction (OR) potential which is achieved only when the concentration of free oxygen is low. The organism will grow in nutrient broth to which chopped meat or brain has been added and on the surface of blood agar plates incubated in an anaerobic jar. The colonies on blood agar are rough, hairlike, and swarming.

Antigenic Structure Although tetanus bacilli can be divided into a number of antigenic types on the basis of specific agglutination of flagellar antigens, all types produce an identical toxin which causes the systemic manifestations of the disease. Conversely, protection against the disease is related to the level of tetanus antitoxin.

Toxin Production Under optimal conditions for toxin production cultures of *C. tetani* may yield 2 million LD_{50} per ml for mice (the lethal dose or the dose that will kill half of the animals), but clones from individual bacilli in a culture may vary widely in toxigenic capacity. Little is known concerning the mode of formation of toxin or its release into the culture medium. It is apparent, however, that intracellular toxin is formed early during the growth of the organism because young washed cells are toxic for mice treated with penicillin to prevent bacterial growth. The toxin reaches a maximum within a few days, just before autolysis of the bacteria; with autolysis, the toxin is released into the culture fluid.

Properties of Toxin In potency, tetanus toxin is second only to botulinus type A toxin. When obtained in a highly purified, electrophoretically homogeneous, crystalline state, the toxin is a heat-labile protein with a M. W. of 67,000 containing 70 million mouse LD_{50} per mg. The toxin combines with and is neutralized by tetanus antitoxin, and is readily converted to toxoid when treated with formalin.

Mode of Action of Toxin Tetanus toxin is specifically and avidly fixed by the gray matter of nervous tissue (Wasserman-Takaki phenomenon). The substance responsible for this fixation is a ganglioside, a water-soluble lipid containing residues of stearic acid, sphingosine, glucose, galactose, N-acetylgalactosamine, and N-acetylneuraminic acid. The fixation is toxin-specific and also ganglioside-specific. Tetanus toxoid is much less avidly fixed than tetanus toxin, and recent evidence indicates that choleragen (Chap. 18) also binds to tissue gangliosides. Ganglioside can bind up to 20 times its weight of toxin, but this is increased considerably when complexed with water-insoluble cerebroside in a ratio of 1 part ganglioside to 3 parts cerebroside. There is no evidence that ganglioside is changed by tetanus toxin, and its role, if any, in the action of the toxin is not yet known.

The ganglioside is differentially localized in microsomal and mitochondrial-lysosomal fractions of rabbit brain homogenate. These fractions can remove 9 mouse MLD of toxin, whereas nuclear and cell sap fractions fail to fix toxin. However, increased leakage of lysosomal enzymes (acid ribonuclease and acid phenophthaleinphosphatase) does not occur in the presence of 1,200 mouse MLD.

Tetanus toxin acts on the central nervous system by suppressing synaptic inhibition, but it is not known whether it acts pre- or postsynaptically at the inhibitory synapse or whether fixation of toxin by ganglioside is essential for the lethal action of the toxin. Influence of the toxin on peripheral nerves, as for example in paralyzing the cholinergic sphincter pupillae of the eye, appears to be secondary to the central effects.

The mechanism whereby a previous injection of 0.01 MLD shortens by 24 hr. the survival time of mice subsequently injected with 1 MLD of toxin is unknown but may be related to the mode of action of the toxin. Efforts to obtain an endogenous toxic principle from the mice pretreated with 0.01 MLD have failed.

Pathogenesis

Introduction of Spores The essential elements for the development of tetanus are the introduction of spores, germination of the spores, production of toxin, transfer of the toxin to its site of action in the central nervous system, and suppression of synaptic inhibition.

The ubiquitous distribution of tetanus spores in soil and dust provides ample opportunity for the entry of the organism whenever the integrity of the skin is broken. Entry of spores may be accomplished in a variety of ways. For example, the spore may lodge in tissue following combat and puncture wounds, puerperal infections and infections of the umbilical stump associated with unsanitary midwifery and the use of animal dung as an umbilical dressing, contaminated needles especially in narcotic addicts and occasionally in vaccination procedures, burns, contusions, lacerations, and surgery with contaminated sutures, dressings, and plaster.

Germination of Spores Tetanus spores may remain dormant for long periods in the tissues unless a low OR potential is present. Among the factors which decrease the OR potential and favor the germination of tetanus spores are devitalized or necrotic tissue, calcium ions in soil introduced with the spores, trauma, hemorrhage, foreign bodies, and other microorganisms which often contaminate the injured area. If the spores survive in the tissues, they can be induced to germinate and may cause fatal tetanus. When injected into the tissue site where the spores are located, a variety of agents including aerobic bacteria, calcium salts, filtrates of *Clostridium perfringens* and *Clostridium septicum,* quinine, lactic acid, and trimethylamine will induce tetanus. Undoubtedly, these agents favor the germination of spores by lowering the OR potential.

The Role of Toxin After germination of the spores, the vegetative forms multiply locally and liberate toxin. The organism has limited powers of invasion which are not reinforced by toxin, as in the case with diphtheria toxin. After centripetal spread via regional nerve trunks, the toxin acts on the motor cells of the spinal cord. By suppressing synaptic inhibition the toxin causes hyperactivity and spasticity in the appropriate muscles. The clinical manifestations include generalized neuromuscular disturbance, spasms of the masseter muscles (trismus) and the facial muscles, and stiffness and rigidity of the neck, back, abdomen, and extremities. In fatal cases, death is preceded by tetanic spasms, faulty respiration, anoxia, and cyanosis. In nonlethal cases full recovery occurs.

The severity of the disease is inversely related to the length of the incubation period which is ordinarily 5 to 10 days but may be as short as 3 days and as long as 4 weeks or more. Despite the dramatic clinical effects induced by the toxin there are no recognizable pathologic lesions in the central nervous system or elsewhere in the body.

Laboratory Diagnosis

Tetanus represents an emergency situation. Treatment must be initiated without delay. Consequently, a presumptive diagnosis must be made on the clinical picture and a history of injury.

Bacteriological diagnosis is a secondary consideration. Demonstration or recovery of the organism is often difficult because the site of infection may be inconspicuous, because the tetanus bacilli are occasionally present in small numbers, because other spore-forming bacilli frequently greatly outnumber *C. tetani,* or because the patient has received antibiotic treatment. Another complication is introduced by the fact that *C. tetani* may be isolated from wounds in which there is no evidence of tetanus.

Stained smears prepared from the wound may sometimes reveal typical tetanus bacilli with terminal spores and a squash racket appearance. Recovery of the organism from the wound is best accomplished by first heating the obtained specimen at 70°C for 20 min. to kill nonsporulated bacteria and inoculating the material at the base of a blood agar slant incubated in an anaerobic jar. Because of their vigorous motility tetanus bacilli may be isolated from the advancing edge of the slant culture by subinoculation onto a blood plate containing 4 to 8 percent agar to minimize swarming. If half of the blood plate contains tetanus antitoxin, hemolytic colonies on the untreated half and nonhemolytic colonies on the antitoxin half are almost certainly toxigenic tetanus bacilli. Further confirmation may be obtained by performing a neutralization test in mice.

Epidemiology

Tetanus Neonatorum (Tetanus of the Newborn) In this disease the umbilical stump is infected as a result of unsanitary midwifery which in some countries involves the use of animal dung as an umbilical dressing. Tetanus of the newborn is a leading cause of death in many countries of Asia, Africa, and Latin America. The data included in Table 13-1 provide a shocking demonstration of the ravages of this disease in selected countries of Latin America.

In the United States in 1972, there were 118 cases of tetanus. The highest incidence was observed in the South among nonwhites under 1 year of age. More deaths occurred in those under 1 year of age than in any other age span covering a period of 40 years.

Older Children and Adults Compared with the unusually great prevalence of tetanus in children under 1 year of age, tetanus in older children and adults is infrequent in occurrence. It is more common in those countries where medical services are inadequate (puerperal infections and postoperative tetanus) and where shoes are not worn. The disease is also more prevalent among agricultural workers, narcotic addicts, and soldiers in time of war.

Prevention and Control

Immunization Prevention and control of tetanus are based on universal immunization of infants and young children with tetanus toxoid usually combined with diphtheria toxoid and pertussis vaccine, along with appropriate booster doses.

Despite its general decline throughout the

Table 13-1 Deaths Due to Tetanus among Children under 1 Year of Age in Selected Countries of Latin America, 1961–1962

Country	Rank as a cause of death	Death rate per 100,000	Percent of all deaths	Percent of all deaths of children 1–4 years old
Colombia	Fifth	243	2.7	0.2
El Salvador	Third	338	4.8	0.1
Nicaragua	Third	423	7.7	1.5
Panama	Fourth	369	8.7	0.3
Trinidad-Tobago	Fifth	53	1.4	0.9
Venezuela	Fifth	92	1.9	0.4

Source: Health Conditions in the Americas 1961–1962, Pan American Health Organization, Scientific Publication no. 104, 1964.

United States, tetanus persists within pockets of the population in which levels of immunization are low and obstetrical care is inadequate. Today, the disease, especially neonatal tetanus, is concentrated largely among nonwhite population groups in the South and among Latin Americans in Florida, Texas, and the Southwest. Sustained and intensive immunization efforts directed at these population groups are required if the incidence of tetanus is to be effectively reduced in the future.

In those Latin American countries where tetanus neonatorum is prevalent and only minimal medical services are available, field trials have shown that maternal immunization with tetanus toxoid prevents the neonatal disease.

Prophylaxis

In Nonimmunized Persons There can be no doubt that prompt surgical cleansing of the wound and prophylactic use of 5,000 to 10,000 units of tetanus antitoxin has greatly reduced the incidence of tetanus. In nonimmunized patients the use of antitoxin is best reserved for those with serious injury or for those with less extensive injury who are not seen for 48 hr. Any person receiving tetanus antitoxin should be subsequently immunized with tetanus toxoid. When the wound was surgically cleansed, the patient given 50 million units of penicillin, and a full course of active immunization with tetanus toxoid begun within 4 hr. after injury, excellent results have been obtained in preventing tetanus without using antitoxin.

In Immunized Persons Prompt surgical care and a booster dose of fluid tetanus toxoid are effective in preventing the disease in previously immunized persons. If the patient is not seen for 48 hr. after injury, penicillin is used in combination with surgery and toxoid. There is no need to employ antitoxin in the prophylaxis of tetanus in injured persons who have been previously immunized.

Treatment Specific therapy of tetanus requires the intravenous administration of 100,000 to 200,000 units of tetanus antitoxin as soon as possible. Human tetanus antitoxin is available in the event that the patient is senstive to the proteins in horse antitoxin.

Excellent results have been obtained when antitoxin is accompanied by the induction of paralysis with curare and by positive-pressure respiration. In a recent series 36 tetanus patients were treated by this method without a single death—a dramatic improvement on previous mortality figures where antitoxin alone was employed in treatment. Upon recovery the patient should receive a full course of active immunization with tetanus toxoid.

In view of the pathogenesis of the disease it is unlikely that the use of hyperbaric oxygenation would be beneficial for patients with tetanus.

Prospective

Tetanus is an entirely preventable disease. Universal immunization of infants with tetanus toxoid along with appropriately spaced booster doses of toxoid can eliminate the disease.

GAS GANGRENE AND OTHER INFECTIONS ASSOCIATED WITH *Clostridium perfringens (Clostridium welchii)*

Perspective

Except for tetanus, most clostridial infections of man are usually associated with a mixed flora in which *Clostridium perfringens* is the chief pathogen. In addition to *C. perfringens,* bacteria commonly found in the lesions include *C. novyi. C. septicum,* other clostridia, gram-negative enterics, anaerobic streptococci, and aerobic cocci.

Apart from its role in food poisoning (Chap. 18), *C. perfringens* is infrequently responsible for anaerobic cellulitis, gas gangrene, septicemia, and necrotic enteritis secondary to trauma, carcinoma, surgery, criminal abortion, and difficult parturition. Infection with the organism may be essentially self-limiting as in food poisoning and anaerobic cellulitis or fulminating as in gas gangrene and postoperative and uterine infections.

The Causative Agent

Biological Properties *C. perfringens* is an anaerobe that is part of the normal intestinal flora of man and animals. On occasion it may be present on epithelial surfaces of the vagina and the lower extremities. It is also found in soil, raw milk, dust, and sewage. The organism is a stout bacillus with dimensions of 6μm × 1 μm. It grows well on chopped meat media and on blood plates incubated anaerobically. Spores are seldom seen in cultures. but large capsules are found in infected tissues. *C. perfringens* is unique among the pathogenic clostridia in being nonmotile. The organism produces a double zone of hemolysis on blood agar due to the action of β- and α-toxins.

When *C. perfringens* is grown in human serum or egg yolk agar, an opalescence develops due to the breakdown of lecithin containing proteins by α-toxin, or lecithinase (Nagler reaction). A number of carbohydrates including glucose, lactose, and sucrose are actively fermented with the formation of acid and gas. In milk, *C. perfringens* produces an acid clot which is torn by gas (stormy clot or stormy fermentation).

Antigenic Structure *C. perfringens* is divided into types A, B, C, D, and E on the basis of the main lethal toxins produced. Most human infections are associated with type A organisms that synthesize α-toxin as their major lethal component. However, the type A organisms that cause food poisoning (Chap. 18) produce little α-toxin. Necrotic enteritis, a rare clinical entity, is induced by type C bacilli (formerly designated type F) that synthesize lethal β-toxin as well as α-toxin. Types B, C, D, and E are primarily associated with enterotoxemia in sheep and cattle.

Lecithinase (Alpha Toxin) Alpha toxin (α-toxin) is a calcium-dependent enzyme (phospholipase or lecithinase C) that catalyzes the hydrolysis of phosphate bonds with the liberation of phosphorylcholine and a diglyceride from lecithin. It is the most important toxin produced by *C. perfringens.* In experimental infections antibody against the toxin is protective and toxoid is effective in prevention. Partially purified preparations contain about 10,000 mouse LD_{50}/mg. Other clostridia and *Bacillus cereus* also produce lecithinases. However, except for the lecithinase synthesized by *C. bifermentans,* all are immunologically distinct from the α-toxin of *C. perfringens.*

Although the chemical basis of its interaction with lecithin is precisely known, the mechanism whereby α-toxin exerts its lethal effect remains obscure. The substrate lecithin is present in the membranes of every tissue cell. The toxin not only can lyse erythrocytes, leukocytes, and other cells but can inactivate enzyme systems dependent on lecithin such as the adenosine triphosphatase of muscle, which has a lecithin prosthetic group, and the succinic dehydrogenase system, which requires lecithin.

Collagenase (Kappa Toxin) Kappa toxin (κ-toxin) is a powerful proteolytic enzyme which specifically attacks collagen and its breakdown product gelatin. When injected into laboratory animals, collagenase causes the disintegration of muscle by breaking down collagen and reticulin and favors the production of hemorrhage and thrombosis by removing the supporting reticulin around the capillaries and small vessels. Collagenase may be readily distinguished from other products of *C. perfringens* by immunological techniques.

The lethal effect of partially purified κ-toxin (500 mouse LD_{50}/mg) is much less than that of α-toxin, and the action of collagenase is ancillary to that of the organism and its α-toxin. For example, antibody against collagenase neither prevents nor modifies the course of the experimental or clinical disease.

Other Toxins and Metabolic Products In addition to lecithinase and collagenase, type A strains of *C. perfringens* synthesize a number of products of secondary importance referred to as toxins or designated as enzymes. The oxygen-labile σ-toxin is lethal, hemolytic, necrotizing, and cardiotoxic and is antigenically related to the hemolysins of *C. tetani, Streptococcus pyogenes, Diplococcus pneumoniae,* and other bacteria. The μ-toxin (hyaluronidase) is an enzyme that hydrolyzes the cementing mucopolysaccharide (hyaluronic acid) of the tissues. Culture filtrates also contain a deoxyribonuclease (ν-toxin), a fibrinolysin, and a neuraminidase or receptor-destroying enzyme which destroys myxovirus receptors on red blood cells.

Lethal and necrotizing β-toxin is synthesized in large quantity by the type C (formerly type F) strains of *C. perfringens* involved in necrotic enteritis.

Pathogenesis

Gas Gangrene (Anaerobic Myonecrosis) The most important prerequisite for clostridial infection is an area of tissue with a reduced OR potential, for only then can the anaerobic bacteria begin to multiply. Characteristically, the lowered OR potential is brought about as a consequence of mechanical injury due to reduced blood supply, the presence of foreign bodies, the occurrence of necrotic tissue and hemorrhage, or the multiplication of other bacteria. In such areas of reduced oxygen tension muscle pyruvate is reduced to lactate, the pH falls, and endogenous cathepsins are activated with the consequent release of amino acids into the lesion. In this favorable milieu, growth and toxin production by *C. perfringens* proceeds rapidly, healthy muscle tissue is destroyed, and the infection spreads through the tissue spaces.

In addition to causing the necrosis of cells by disrupting the lecithin-containing cell membrane and inhibiting cellular metabolism, α-toxin increases capillary permeability and produces the gross edema so characteristic of gas gangrene. Myonecrosis is prominent and involves the disruption of the sarcolemma and fragmentation of the muscle fibers. Collagen and reticulin virtually disappear in the infected muscle, presumably as a result of the action of collagenase; and the loss of hyaluronic acid in the lesion is probably related to the action of hyaluronidase.

These massive necrotizing infections of muscle usually develop within 24 hr. after a deep and lacerating wound. Invariably the infections are associated with pain which increases in severity but remains localized to the affected area. These symptoms are accompanied by edema, hypotension, profuse serous discharge, a "mousy" smell, swollen and discolored tissues, severe shock, and collapse. In untreated cases death results. Gas is often manifest in the late stage of the disease but is rarely as extensive as the involvement of the underlying muscle.

Although there is ample evidence to indicate the importance of toxin in the production of myonecrosis, the mechanism responsible for shock and death remains obscure. No direct evidence for the presence of a circulating toxin has ever been obtained. If such a toxin is involved, then it is almost certainly not the α-toxin. The prevailing theory designed to account for the rapid and profound toxemia found in gas gangrene patients postulates the production and absorption of an unknown toxic factor in the muscles of the host as a result of clostridial activity.

Anaerobic Cellulitis (Gas Abcess) Anaerobic cellulitis is a comparatively benign clostridial infection involving necrotic tissue which is produced as a result of ischemia or direct trauma. Intact, healthy muscle is not invaded. Typically, several days following injury there is a gradually increasing foulness of the wound with the appearance and increase of gas in the tissues. As a rule there is no local pain or edema and little general toxemia. Gas is far more evident than in gas gangrene but is limited to the wound and the tissue spaces and is never found intramuscularly. Why the infection fails to invade healthy muscle and fails to induce shock is not understood.

Uterine Infections (Clostridial Septicemia) Following attempts at criminal abortion or less commonly following spontaneous abortion or during labor or the puerperium (prolonged labor, instrumental delivery, or unhygienic conditions), *C. perfringens* may invade the healthy, intact, uterine muscle and produce a rapidly fatal outcome. Unlike gas gangrene, clostridial septicemia often develops following uterine infection and is associated with jaundice, intravascular hemolysis, hemoglobinemia, and hemoglobinuria. Even though the patient may apparently recover from the acute septicemic phase of the disease, relapse frequently occurs, a uremic syndrome ensues, and death results.

Necrotic Enteritis The ingestion of foodstuffs contaminated with type C strains of *C. perfringens* may be followed by extensive but patchy hemorrhagic necrosis of the small intestine, accompanied by bloody diarrhea, collapse, and not infrequently, death. This infection corresponds closely to various clostridial enterotoxemias of animals. Type C strains produce little α-toxin but large quantities of β-toxin.

A few human cases have been reported to be caused by type D strains which produce large quantities of the lethal and necrotizing ε-toxin.

Laboratory Diagnosis

Because treatment must be initiated without delay, a presumptive diagnosis of infection with *C. perfringens* must be made clinically on the basis of pain, edema, and the general condition of the patient without waiting for laboratory confirmation. In some cases, direct microscopic examination of stained smears prepared from the lesion provides important diagnostic information, i.e., when typical gram-positive bacilli with well-marked capsules are seen in large numbers.

Bacteriological confirmation is obtained by culturing the organism on blood agar plates incubated anaerobically. Colonies which show a double zone of hemolysis are strongly suggestive of *C. perfringens.* Further identification is based on sugar fermentation reactions, formation of a stormy clot in milk, a zone of opacity around colonies on egg yolk agar, and toxin production and neutralization.

Epidemiology

Because of the ubiquitous distribution of the organism, infections with *C. perfringens* secondary to deep and lacerating wounds are found throughout the world and in all age groups. In time of war, there are between 200 and 1,000 cases of gas gangrene per 100,000 soldiers wounded, and anaerobic cellulitis is two or three times as common as gas gangrene. The incidence of gas gangrene varies with the extent of contamination of the soil, the speed and efficiency of evacuation, and the adequacy of surgical debridement.

Although there are no really accurate figures on the incidence of gas gangrene in civilian life, it has been estimated that there may be between 2 and 50 cases per 100,000 serious injuries (anaerobic cellulitis occurs less frequently). However, in major civilian disasters gas gangrene may be a great problem. For example, in the Texas City explosion 15 cases of gas gangrene developed among the 850 casualties that were hospitalized (this is equivalent to a rate of 1,765 per 100,000 casualties). The incidence of uterine infection varies with the quality of maternal care and the frequency of criminal abortion from less than 100 to more than 300 per 100,000 abortions.

Among civilian groups more likely to develop

clostridial myonecrosis or septicemia are patients subjected to gastrointestinal, biliary, or genitourinary surgery; diabetics who receive intramuscular injections; and cancer patients. In cancer patients, the incidence may approach 500 per 100,000. In contrast to noncancer patients, patients with carcinoma usually have clostridial septicemia with jaundice and rapid and persistent circulatory collapse refractive to the usual treatment for shock.

The actual incidence of clostridial infection is more frequent than is usually realized, since patients who recover from spreading peritonitis following perforated appendix show significant amounts of antitoxin produced by *C. perfringens* in a large percentage of cases. This antitoxin is absent in the serum of control patients.

Prevention and Control

Because of its rare and unpredictable occurrence in the general population, no effort has been made to prevent and control *C. perfringens* infection by universal immunization with α-toxoid, which experimentally has been shown to prevent the disease.

Although 10,000 units of α-antitoxin against *C. perfringens,* and antitoxin against *C. novyi,* and 5,000 units of *C. septicum* antitoxin have been used prophylactically, and three times these quantities employed therapeutically, the value of polyvalent antitoxin in the prophylaxis and treatment of gas gangrene is questionable.

Treatment Until recently, the therapy of gas gangrene and other clostridial infections was the prompt and complete debridement of all necrotic tissue, leaving the wound open and installing catheters for the instillation of penicillin and peroxide, and giving high doses of penicillin intramuscularly or intravenously. This treatment has been modified by the use of hyperbaric oxygenation. In this procedure the patient is placed in a compression chamber and exposed to 3 atm of air pressure while breathing 100 percent oxygen under general anaesthesia. A few treatments at elevated atmospheric pressure for 1 to 2 hr. have produced dramatic results.

Both surgical debridement and hyperbaric oxygenation are designed to raise the OR potential of the tissues, to stabilize the pH, and to prevent the growth of the clostridia. Exposure to 3 atm of air pressure causes 15 to 18 times as much oxygen to be forced into physical solution, makes the blood able to oxygenate the tissues adequately even in the absence of red blood cells, and thus halts the progression of the infection.

Prospective

Early and accurate clinical diagnosis, prompt and adequate surgical debridement, hyperbaric oxygenation, and penicillin form the basis for the effective management of cases of gas gangrene. How effective and practical these methods will prove to be in any major civilian catastrophe with its increased complement of cases of gas gangrene is problematical.

OTHER CLOSTRIDIA INVOLVED IN HISTOTOXIC INFECTIONS OF MAN

Next to *C. perfringens,* the most important of the histotoxic clostridia in human traumatic disease are *C. novyi (C. oedematiens)* and *C. septicum.*

C. novyi is difficult to grow, produces a lecithinase C as its major toxin (antigenically distinct from the α-toxin of *C. perfringens*), causes no change in milk, and ferments glucose but not lactose or sucrose. Some strains produce penicillinase. Infections with *C. novyi* have a much longer incubation period (3 to 6 days) than those caused by *C. perfringens,* edema is especially pronounced, and there is a profuse golden yellow discharge from the wound.

C. septicum is easy to grow but difficult to isolate because of its tendency to form continuous films of growth on solid media rather than discrete colonies. The major toxin of the organism is an oxygen-stable hemolysin the precise nature of which is not known. Stormy fermentation occurs in milk but is less pronounced than in the case of *C. perfringens.* The organism ferments glucose and lactose but not sucrose. Infections with *C. septicum* have an incubation period of 1 to 3 days and follow an acute course. The wound exudes large quantities of bright red hemorrhagic fluid, and gas is usually a prominent feature even early in the disease.

Mixed infections are considerably more severe than monoclostridial infections, particularly when *C. septicum* and *C. histolyticum* are involved. Mixed infections with *C. perfringens* and *C. septicum* are the most acute, with death within 10 hr. of the appearance of symptoms the usual outcome. *C. histolyticum,* an organism with marked proteolytic power and no fermentative ability, can rarely initiate infection by itself. In combination with other clostridia, however, *C. histolyticum* can frequently produce a fatal outcome before digestion of tissue is obvious.

BIBLIOGRAPHY

Bazaral, M., Goscienski, P. J., and Hamburger, R. N.: "Characteristics of Human Antibody to Diphtheria Toxin," *Infect. Immun.,* 7:130-136, 1973.

Cherington, M., and Ryan, D. W.: "Treatment of Botulism with Guanidine," *N. Engl. J. Med.,* 282: 195-197, 1970.

Collier, R. J. and Kandel, J.: "Structure and Activity of Diphtheria Toxin. I. Thiol-dependent Dissociation of a Fraction of Toxin into Enzymatically Active and Inactive Fragments," *J. Biol. Chem.,* 246: 1496-1503, 1971.

Gill, D. M., and Pappenheimer, A. M., Jr.: "Structure-Activity Relationships in Diphtheria Toxin," *J. Biol. Chem.,* 246:1492-1495, 1971.

Ittelson, T. R., and Gill, D. M.: "Diphtheria Toxin: Specific Competition for Cell Receptors," *Nature,* 242:330-332, 1973.

MacLennan, J. D.: "The Histotoxic Clostridial Infections of Man," *Bacteriol. Rev.,* 26:177-276, 1962.

Macrae, J.: "Tetanus," *Br. Med. J.,* 1:730-732, 1973.

National Communicable Disease Center: "Botulism in the United States," U.S. Department of Health, Education and Welfare, 1969, 30 pp.

Pappenheimer, A. M., Uchida, T., Jr., and Harper, A. A.: "An Immunological Study of the Diphtheria Toxin Molecule," *Immunochemistry,* 9:891-906, 1972.

Shinefield, H. R., and Ribble, J. C.: "Current Aspects of Infections and Diseases Related to *Staphylococcus aureus,*" *Annu. Rev. Med.,* 16:263-284, 1965.

Stanfield, J. P., Gall, D., and Bracken, P. M.: "Single-dose Antenatal Tetanus Immunisation," *Lancet,* 1:215-219, 1973.

Wiester, M. J., Bonventre, P. F., and Grupp, G.: "Estimate of Myocardial Damage Induced by Diphtheria Toxin," *J. Lab Clin. Med.,* 81:354-364, 1973.

Zabriskie, J. B.: "Viral-induced Bacterial Toxins," *Annu. Rev. Med.,* 17:337-350, 1966.

Chapter 14

Infections Caused by Gram-positive Cocci

Bernard A. Briody

STAPHYLOCOCCAL INFECTIONS

Staphylococci are gram-positive cocci that are arranged in irregular grape-like clusters on solid media when stained. By definition, staphylococci that produce coagulase are designated *Staphylococcus aureus (S. pyogenes).* Coagulase-negative staphylococci are termed *S. epidermidis (S. albus).* Man is both the primary reservoir and the primary target of pathogenic *S. aureus. S. epidermidis* is also a part of the normal flora of man, but it produces disease much less frequently than *S. aureus.* Anaerobic staphylococci, which are sometimes found in lung abscesses, are referred to as *peptococci.*

The Causative Agent

Biological Properties

Natural Habitat From birth to death man lives in an environment that is rarely free of *S. aureus.* The human nose is the natural reservoir of the organism. The skin and the large intestine represent additional sources for the contamination of the atmosphere with *S. aureus.*

Morphology and Growth In the presence of oxygen, the organism grows abundantly on most conventional nutrient media. Surface colonies on blood agar are usually large (1 to 4 mm), round, convex, pigmented, and surrounded by a clear zone of hemolysis (beta hemolysis).

Stained smears from a colony contain gram-positive cocci, 0.8 to 1.0 μm in diameter, arranged in irregular grape-like clusters.

Growth of staphyloccoci is readily inhibited by many of the aniline dyes, such as crystal violet. In general, however, staphylococci are among the more resistant of the vegetative (nonsporing) bacteria. For example, the organisms grow in the presence of 10 percent sodium chloride and in concentrations of tellurite, phenol, mercury, and other heavy metallic ions that inactivate other bacteria. Staphylococci readily survive drying and are resistant to heat, serum bactericidins, fatty acids, lysozyme, and a number of antibiotics. As indicated below in the discussion of penicillinase production, many of these properties may be controlled by an extrachromosomal collection of genes known as a plasmid.

Variation Staphylococci vary widely in their biological properties. Small gonidial or G colonies may be encountered which are nonpigmented and nonhemolytic. The pigment produced may vary from the typical golden yellow of *S. aureus* to pale yellow or fawn to white. *S. aureus* synthesizes a large number of enzymes and toxins, but marked differences are found when several cultures are compared. Important variations are encountered in susceptibility to phage and to antibiotics.

Pathogenicity and Virulence Except for the production of enterotoxin (Chap. 13), and possibly for the role of exfoliative toxin in dermatologic disease, no specific staphylococcal product or component can be directly correlated with pathogenicity for man. While all coagulase-positive staphylococci are pathogenic, the amount of coagulase produced is not proportional to virulence.

In addition to producing coagulase and enterotoxin, many pathogenic staphylococci are lysogenic, can be typed by virulent phage (phage typing), are resistant to antibiotics, and synthesize a considerable number of antigenic toxins and enzymes. These include penicillinase, alpha toxin (alpha hemolysin), other hemolysins, leukocidins, staphylokinase, hyaluronidase, nucleases, proteases, phosphatase, lipase, and phospholipase. Because of their importance in pathogenicity, diagnosis, epidemiology, or treatment, a detailed discussion of coagulase, alpha toxin, penicillinase, exfoliative toxin (exfoliatin), and phage typing will be presented.

Coagulases

Free Coagulases During the logarithmic phase of growth *S. aureus* produces extracellular enzyme-like proteins, free coagulases, or staphylocoagulases. Before fibrinogen is converted to fibrin, coagulase interacts with a prothrombin-like coagulase reacting factor (CRF) in plasma to form a coagulase-CRF complex resembling thrombin. The coagulase-CRF complex acts on fibrinogen to form fibrin releasing peptides comparable to those produced when thrombin converts fibrinogen to fibrin. However, formation of the coagulase-CRF complex is not dependent on calcium ions and is relatively insensitive to heparin, thus differing from thrombin.

Although different cultures of *S. aureus* produce at least seven antigenically distinct extracellular coagulases, the clotting of plasma by each coagulase proceeds according to the mechanism outlined above.

Bound Coagulase In addition to extracellular coagulases, many cultures of *S. aureus* synthesize an antigenically distinct bound coagulase attached to the bacterial cell that converts fibrinogen directly to fibrin without CRF. Bound coagulase is not present in culture filtrates but can be liberated from staphylococci by autolysis. When staphylococci are mixed with plasma or fibrinogen on a glass slide, thick clumps containing the bacteria and fibrin are rapidly formed.

Coagulase Tests In the slide test for bound coagulase, organisms from a colony on a blood agar plate are mixed with a drop of 1 to 5 dilution of plasma (or fibrinogen). A positive test is indicated by the microscopic clumping of the bacteria by the fibrin and occurs within 30 sec. Cultures that are positive for bound coagulase almost always produce free coagulase, but cultures that are negative for bound coagulase may be positive for free coagulase.

In the tube test for free coagulase a loopful of organisms from a blood agar plate (or 0.5 ml of a broth culture) is mixed with 0.5 ml of a 1 to 5 dilution of citrated rabbit (or human) plasma and incubated at 37°C. A positive test is indicated by the formation of a macroscopic clot within 24 hr. Most positive tests, however, develop within 3 hr. Because of the possible presence of antibodies or inhibitors that might block the test, each lot of plasma should be checked with a culture known to produce coagulase.

α-Toxin (Alpha Hemolysin) α-Toxin is a heat-labile protein with a molecular weight of 44,000. The toxin can be converted to a toxoid by treatment with formalin and antitoxin can neutralize the biological activities of the toxin. Toxic activity can be demonstrated by hemolysis of rabbit but not human erythrocytes, by cytotoxicity for rabbit but not human leukocytes, and by dermonecrosis and lethality for animals. The amount of toxin required to produce the observed effect in rabbits varies from 0.08 μg for hemolysis to 4 μg for lethality. The precise mechanism of action, however, is unknown.

Formation of α-toxin in broth develops slowly and does not reach a peak for about 10 days. However, if the broth is incubated in 20 percent carbon dioxide and gently shaken, or if 0.8 percent nutrient agar is incubated in 20 percent carbon dioxide and extracted with saline, potent preparations of alpha toxin can be obtained in 24 hr.

The role of α-toxin in human staphylococcal disease was suspected following the unfortunate experience in Bundaberg, Australia, in 1928. One lot of diphtheria toxin-antitoxin which had become contaminated with *S. aureus* was inoculated into 21 children. Within several hours 16 children became acutely ill and within 2 days 12 died of staphylococcal septicemia and toxemia probably due to the action of α-toxin. In the surviving children staphylococcal abscesses appeared at the site of injection.

Except for its possible role in acute staphylococcal toxemia, an extremely rare manifestation of infection, there is no convincing evidence that α-toxin is significantly involved in producing disease in man. For example, the clinical use of α-toxoid and antitoxin has no proved value, and the intradermal injection of α-toxin along with *S. aureus* does not increase the severity of the local lesion.

Penicillinase One of the important realities associated with staphylococcal infection is the fact that the bacteria are resistant to penicillin, especially the organisms in phage groups I and III. Penicillin resistance of staphylococci is associated with the inactivation of penicillin by penicillinase which opens the β-lactam ring of the penicillin molecule. Penicillinase is a genetically constitutive enzyme whose phenotypic expression is enhanced by the presence of the penicillin substrate.

Recent evidence suggests that synthesis of penicillinase by most staphylococci isolated from lesions is controlled by a plasmid, an extrachromosomal set of genes which can often be eliminated as a unit by treatment of staphylococci with acriflavine. In addition to the genes regulating the formation of penicillinase, other genetic loci in the 10 recognized plasmids govern resistance to heavy metallic ions, to tetracyclines, and occasionally to erythromycin. Specific genes within the plasmid have been transferred by transducing phage. In this way, penicillinase, and consequently penicillin resistance, can be transferred to organisms which lack the enzyme and are sensitive to penicillin.

Operation of the plasmid and its selection as a unit by exposure of staphylococci to penicillin provide a genetic basis for the finding that penicillin-resistant strains of staphylococci are also resistant to other antibiotics and to heavy metals. In this connection, it is important to note that staphylococci that synthesize penicillinase were detected prior to the advent of penicillin therapy. Thus, the current prevalence of penicillin-resistant staphylococci is a function of both plasmid formation in the prepenicillin era and the subsequent selection of the plasmid by the widespread use of penicillin.

Exfoliative Toxin (Exfoliatin) Coagulase-positive staphylococci of phage group II have the capacity to produce a soluble protein which can induce exfoliation or intraepidermal separation in newborn mice after intraperitoneal, oral, or subcutaneous administration. Infections with these organisms in infants and young children are associated with a spectrum of dermatologic disease that includes generalized exfoliation (Ritter's syndrome or toxic epidermal necrolysis), localized bullous impetigo, and generalized scarlatiniform eruption. On the basis of clinical similarities and common causative agents, the term "staphylococcal scalded-skin syndrome" has been proposed to describe these clinical manifestations. The data suggest that exfoliative toxin is the cause of the skin changes in affected children.

Phage Typing Phage typing is based on the observation that most pathogenic staphylococci are lysogenic and that the phage carried by one culture frequently is virulent for other cultures of staphylococci. Utilizing a set of 25 phages which can cause their lysis, staphylococci have been shown to exhibit many hundreds of different phage patterns; i.e., they can be typed according to their susceptibility to various phages. Phage typing has proved a useful epidemiological tool in tracing the source of staphylococci within the hospital environment and the source of staphylococci involved in outbreaks of food poisoning (Chap. 13).

Certain combinations of phages that attack staphylococci occur much more frequently than others. On this basis, staphylococci have been placed into phage groups. A staphylococcus that is lysed by one of the typing phages within a group is more likely to be lysed by one or more phages within the same group than by phages associated with other groups (Table 14-1). Most staphylococci that produce infection in man fall into phage groups I, II, and III. Organisms in phage group IV produce enterotoxin and are involved in food poisoning (Chap. 13).

In determining the phage type of a staphylococcus, the organism is spread heavily over the surface of a nutrient agar plate. After drying, 25 or more fine drops each containing an appropriate concentration of a different phage are placed at suitable distances from each other on the plate. After incubation for 18 hr. at 30 to 32°C, the culture is examined for plaques, clear areas where the bacteria have been lysed, and the plaques correlated with the lytic phage. In this way, the phage pattern is found. For exam-

Table 14-1 Phage Groups of Coagulase-positive Staphylococci

Group	Phages in the group								
I	29	52	52A	79	80				
II	3A	3B	3C	55	71				
III	6	7	42E	47	53	54	75	77	83A
IV	42D								
Miscellaneous	81	187							

ple, a staphylococcus lysed by phages 7, 47, 53, and 77 is designated as phage type 7/47/53/77.

Antigenic Structure Although serological analysis of staphylococci represents an active area of research, classification of staphylococci on the basis of their antigenic structure is not definitive or practical. Staphylococci do, however, contain a battery of polysaccharide and protein antigens in the cell wall and produce a number of extracellular proteins, toxins, and enzymes which are antigenic. Except for enterotoxin (Chap. 13), the function of these antigenic components in the pathogenesis of staphylococcal disease is unknown.

Pathogenesis

Because of the ubiquitous distribution of staphylococci in the environment, precise knowledge concerning the relative importance of the various means of spreading the organisms is lacking. Many infections are endogenous, while others are exogenous.

In the majority of human staphylococcal infections the healthy nasal carrier is the source, and the skin is the portal of entry. Human skin, however, exhibits a high degree of natural resistance to pathogenic staphylococci. More than a million organisms are required to produce a pustule in man. Natural infection is preceded by injury, often of superficial extent. The usual outcome is a trivial, localized skin lesion.

Localized Skin Lesions Infection with staphylococci is characterized by the formation of a circumscribed suppurative, inflammatory lesion of the skin known as an abscess. Depending upon the location and extent of the inflammatory process, the abscess may be termed a pustule or pimple which is often limited to a hair follicle (folliculitis), a furuncle or boil which involves the adjacent subcutaneous tissue, or a carbuncle which is a furuncle with multiple foci involving the thick, collagenous tissue of the back of the neck.

In the development of the abscess, bacterial multiplication leads to a rapid influx of numerous granulocytes and the exudation of plasma. Staphylococci are ingested and may be destroyed quickly with the rapid resolution of the pustule. On the other hand, the inflammatory process may continue for 3 to 5 days or more, accompanied by the accumulation of more phagocytes and fluid. At this time, there is a central necrotic core of dead leukocytes and bacteria surrounded by a fibroblastic wall containing viable bacteria and phagocytes. Necrosis increases, liquefaction (pus formation) sets in, pressure within the abscess rises, pain and tenderness appear, the skin at the apex of the furuncle thins, and the lesion opens and drains, relieving the pain. Healing occurs spontaneously over a period of several days without scarring.

Efforts have been made to account for the pathogenesis of staphylococcal infections in terms of the cell-bound components and extracellular products elaborated by the bacteria. For example, the initial spreading of the lesion is said to be due to hyaluronidase, the necrosis is stated to be due to alpha toxin, the walling off of the lesion is ascribed to coagulase, the survival of the bacteria is thought to be due to the action of coagulase which deposits fibrin around the organisms thus enabling them to resist phagocytosis, while breakdown and spread of the lesion is accounted for by staphylokinase which lyses the fibrin. Although these attempts provide an attractive explanation, convincing, supporting evidence is totally lacking.

Systemic Infections On rare occasions, staphylococci may escape from the local lesion, usually in the form of infected thrombi, and spread hematogenously. When this occurs a number of serious infections may result, each involving the formation of typical abscesses. In young children the bacteria may localize in the metaphysis of bone (characteristically a bone of the lower extremity), producing acute osteomyelitis. Before the introduction of antibiotics, most cases of acute osteomyelitis were caused by staphylococci, resulted in the necrosis of bone, often served as a focus for further hematogenous spread, and were associated with a case fatality rate of about 25 percent. Since the introduction of antibiotics, the incidence and the mortality of staphylococcal osteomyelitis have declined sharply.

If the staphylococci localize on previously damaged heart valves, or less frequently on a normal valve, acute bacterial endocarditis with metastatic abscess formation, destruction of the valve, and death usually result.

Staphylococcal bacteremia is accompanied by the almost continuous presence of numerous organisms in the blood, the formation of successive crops of metastatic abscesses, profound toxemia, and a high mortality (90 percent before and 30 to 50 percent after the introduction of antibiotics). The abscesses in fatal cases are found in the heart, lungs, kidneys, spleen, liver, adrenals, and brain. In patients who survive more than a few days, the metastatic abscesses are found most frequently in the skin, subcutaneous tissues, and lungs.

Staphylococcal Pneumonia Although staphylococcal pneumonia may result from bacteremia, it more commonly occurs as a complication of epidemics of influenza, measles, and pertussis. With the development of effective vaccines for measles and pertussis, the incidence in young children has declined. It remains, however, as an important hazard of epidemic influenza particularly in individuals over 55 years of age or in those who have underlying cardiopulmonary disease (Chap. 20). The patchy pneumonia which develops is characterized by the presence of abscesses and empyema and often terminates fatally.

Staphylococcal Pseudomembranous Enterocolitis Staphylococcal pseudomembranous enterocolitis is a serious disease characterized by diarrhea, dehydration, fever, nausea, abdominal pain, vomiting, and in some cases shock and death. The disease is an infrequent but major hazard of broad-spectrum antibiotic therapy, often preceding major bowel surgery. The normal intestinal flora are inhibited by the antibiotics, but the growth of some staphylococci is unaffected because of their resistance. Under these circumstances, which favor the growth of staphylococci, pseudomembranous enterocolitis may develop.

Chronic Staphylococcal Infections Recurrences of staphylococcal infections are relatively common. This is especially evident in osteomyelitis in which recurrences may occur over a period of many years and in which the individual is exposed to certain predisposing factors. A small number of patients are afflicted with chronic furunculosis. The same phage type that caused the initial lesion is frequently involved in these cases of chronic osteomyelitis and chronic furunculosis.

Predisposing Factors In addition to the considerations mentioned above, there are a number of other factors which predispose to staphylococcal infections. These include friction; pressure; trauma; wounds; contact with oil, grease, coal dust, dirt, and other skin irritants; hormones; and underlying disorders such as diabetes, malignancy, cystic fibrosis, hypogammaglobulinemia, and agranulocytosis. Many of these situations are associated with recurrent staphylococcal infection.

Laboratory Diagnosis

Laboratory diagnosis of infections caused by pathogenic staphylococci is based on (1) isolation of the organism from the specimen (pus, swab, sputum, etc.), by dilution streaking of a blood agar plate, (2) detection of irregular grape-like clusters of gram-positive cocci in stained smears prepared from large pigmented colonies appearing on the plate, and (3) demonstration that the isolated organisms produce coagulase. Although other organisms, including gram-negative bacilli and enterococci, can coagulate plasma, they are unlikely to be confused with staphylococci.

Attempts to recover staphylococci and other bacteria as well from blood are based on aerobic and anaerobic culture of 5 ml of blood in bottles containing 45 ml of broth. If organisms grow in the blood broth, they are then isolated and identified as indicated above.

Efforts to recover staphylococci from stool specimens usually involve the use of nutrient agar containing 7.5 percent sodium chloride as well as the standard blood agar plate. In this case, the sodium chloride agar is employed as a selective medium.

Epidemiology

The Carrier State

Sites Healthy persons carry pathogenic staphylococci in the nose, on the skin, and in the large intestine. In terms of the frequency and duration of the carrier state as well as the numbers of organisms present and their dispersal in the environment, the nose is the most important site. The back of the hands, the fingers, and the face receive their quota directly from the nose. Thus, it is not surprising that the phage type of staphylococci in the nose and on the skin are identical. The perineum may also represent a significant carrier site after acquiring staphylococci from the fingers or indirectly from organisms shed from the nose. The chief relevance of the large intestine as a carrier site is in connection with the alteration of the flora by antibiotics, leading to an increase in staphylococci and occasional development of staphylococcal pseudomembranous enterocolitis.

Incidence The highest carrier rates are found in the nose and on the umbilicus of newborn infants in a hospital environment. The nasal carrier rate approaches 100 percent at the age of 1 week. Thereafter, the nasal carrier rate declines to about 25 percent during the first two years of life and then rises until at 6 years it reaches 30 to 50 percent, the rate associated with adults. Approximately one-third to one-quarter of nasal carriers also carry the organisms on the hands.

Many factors apart from age influence the carrier rate. These include the closeness of association with nasal carriers and cases with skin lesions, population density, hygienic habits, and the presence of predisposing factors, some of which were listed above.

Duration The duration of the carrier state in any particular individual is unpredictable. The majority of nasal carriers harbor staphylococci for a few weeks, are free of the organism for an equivalent period, and once again become carriers of staphylococci of a different phage type. As many as 20 percent of normal adults carry the same phage type over a period of months or years. Other individuals rarely carry staphylococci.

Transmission Since most staphylococcal infections are preceded by injury and result in localized skin lesions, it is pertinent to determine the source of the invading bacteria. Although the problem is complex and the answer may vary somewhat with the particular environment and the specific circumstances, the balance of evidence in the majority of instances favors an endogenous source. The injured person who is a nasal carrier and who may also be carrying the same phage type on his skin, or who can readily contaminate the wound with organisms from his nose, is the endogenous source. Thus, it is apparent that the nasal carrier occupies a central role in the epidemiology of staphylococcal infections. This is not intended to deny the fact that staphylococci can spread exogenously by direct contact, by droplet infection, by airborne infection, or indirectly by contact with fomites.

Incidence Considering the fact that staphylococcal infection is endemic in our species and that the organism survives well under the usual atmospheric conditions, the incidence of disease is low and is usually associated with a localized skin lesion that heals spontaneously. In other words, the staphylococcus is a successful parasite well adapted to survive in most of its encounters with its human host.

The annual incidence of infection involves as much as 10 percent of the population and few persons escape staphylococcal disease in their lives. As with the carrier state, the incidence of infection is a function of the closeness of association with nasal carriers and persons with skin lesions, population density, and other factors. Infection is more common in family cohorts with an index case than in the general population and is a particularly difficult problem in the hospital environment. Fortunately, serious staphylococcal disease is a rare event and no reliable estimates are available concerning its incidence. Despite antibiotics, however, staphylococcal bacteremia, endocarditis, pneumonia, and psuedomembranous enterocolitus are associated with a significant mortality.

Hospital Infections The problem of hospital staphylococcal infections begins with selection outside the hospital environment and is greatly exaggerated by conditions within the hospital. One survey revealed that 68 of 1,172 patients were infected on admission and an additional 113 acquired infection in the hospital. Of the total of 181 infections 16 were serious.

Among the many factors within the hospital environment that favor the acquisition of the nasal carrier state and the high incidence of staphylococcal infection are those listed below.

Factors Facilitating Staphylococcal Infections in the Hospital

1 The widespread use of antibiotics that selectively favor staphylococci with multiple antibiotic resistance and a greater capacity for epidemiological spread
2 The population density
3 The constant influx of new susceptible individuals—personnel as well as patients
4 The prevalence of highly susceptible patients—those with surgical and obstetrical wounds, with underlying predisposing disease; nursing mothers

The staff as well as the patients are at greater risk in the hospital. This is particularly true of student nurses and orderlies who have closer contact with infected patients. As many as 10 percent of clean surgical wounds may become infected with staphylococci. Within the nursery as many as 15 percent of the neonates may develop staphylococcal skin lesions. Breast abscesses, usually acquired from nursing infants who are nasal carriers, are common. Outbreaks of furunculosis occasionally occur. Staphylococcal pneumonia and pseudomembranous enterocolitis are especially dangerous infections that have a higher incidence in hospitals.

If widespread unsatisfactory aseptic technique is present in the hospital, staphylococcal infection with many phage types is prevalent. If aseptic technique is rigorously enforced, infections are usually associated with a single phage type. Although these infections may be traced to a single nasal carrier, an outbreak is generally associated with a single phage type that is widely distributed among the staff and the patients. Staphylococci of phage type 80/81, for example, have been responsible for many hospital epidemics.

Prevention and Control

Immunization In the past, and to a lesser extent today, many staphylococcal preparations including alpha toxoid, killed vaccines, culture filtrates, and phage lysates were used in an effort to prevent and control chronic infections. Although immunization with alpha toxoid results in the production of a high concentration of serum antitoxin, there is no convincing evidence that it exerts any beneficial effect on the course of chronic or recurrent infections. Similar conclusions can be drawn for all of the other immunizing materials that have been employed.

Control Although certain general principles are of importance in reducing the spread of pathogenic staphylococci both in the community and the hospital, there is no practical way of controlling staphylococcal infections. The major factor involved in this failure is the widespread prevalence, especially in hospitals, of healthy nasal carriers who continuously seed themselves, their contacts, and their environment with pathogenic staphylococci. Despite intensive efforts to apply diligently all the procedures listed below, infection with staphylococci remains a major infectious disease problem within the hospital environment.

Procedures Designed to Reduce the Incidence of Staphylococcal Infections in the Hospital Environment

1 Isolate persons with lesions.
2 Use germicidal soaps to reduce opportunity for endogenous spread in those subject to recurrent skin lesions and to prevent the establishment of the umbilical carrier state in newborn infants.
3 Provide maximal asepis for all operations, for the dressing of wounds, and in the newborn nursery.
4 Sterilize all materials known to be heavily contaminated with the organisms (dressings and bedclothes of patients with lesions).
5 Eliminate, whenever practical, the factors that predispose to infection and, when impractical, protect those who are highly susceptible (Chap. 6).
6 Establish a hospital surveillance committee to evaluate the risks of infection and to take prompt action in the event of an epidemic.
7 Detect and remove nasal carriers from especially dangerous areas such as operating rooms and newborn nurseries.
8 Explore thoroughly the value of utilizing penicillin-sensitive organisms to establish a carrier state in the nose or on the umbilicus of newborn infants in order to temporarily prevent colonization with staphylococci prevalent in the hospital.
9 Avoid the indiscriminate use of antibiotics.

Treatment Most staphylococcal infections do not require antibiotic therapy, but spontaneous healing may be facilitated by promoting adequate drainage through the use of moist hot compresses. Carbuncles frequently do not drain satisfactorily and may require surgical drainage and a local antibiotic (bacitracin, neomycin). Lysostaphin may be useful in topical or spray treatment of staphylococcal infections and carriers. Lysostaphin is an extracellular factor produced by staphylococci which lyses other staphylococci by acting on the cell wall mucopeptide.

Serious staphylococcal disease requires the prompt use of an effective cidal antibiotic in therapeutic dosage and often must be continued for a prolonged period. As soon as possible, the antibiotic sensitivity of the organism must be determined as a guide to therapy. If the organism is susceptible, penicillin is the drug of choice. Unfortunately, more than 80 percent of hospital infections and as many as 40 percent of community infections are caused by penicillin-resistant organisms. Consequently, in serious staphylococcal disease it is desirable to use a drug that is most likely to be effective such as a penicillinase-resistant penicillin (oxacillin, methicillin, cloxacillin), until the sensitivity of the organism is determined. Vancomycin and the cephalosporins are useful drugs in treating patients who are allergic to penicillin. In many infections, antibiotic therapy must be supplemented by surgical drainage in order to effect a cure, since antibiotics do not readily penetrate walled-off lesions.

Alpha antitoxin and virulent phage have been used in treatment but without success.

Infections due to *Staphylococcus epidermidis*

Coagulase-negative staphylococci (*S. epidermidis* or *S. albus*) are a part of the normal mucocutaneous flora of man. In general, they resemble *S. aureus* in microscopic and colonial morphology. The pigmented colonies are almost invariably white. Many cultures of *S. epidermidis* produce penicillinase and are resistant to other antibiotics. On rare occasions, they cause minor skin lesions (pustules and stitch abscesses). Much less frequently, they produce serious systemic infection, such as endocarditis or bacteremia. These serious infections usually develop in persons with underlying disease and in patients who have had cardiac surgery. Despite the most effective methods of treatment these systemic infections are associated with a mortality of about 20 percent.

STREPTOCOCCAL INFECTIONS

Streptococci are gram-positive cocci that are arranged in chains of varying length, usually 10 or more. The organisms are subdivided in a practical way on the basis of the presence or absence of hemolysis on blood agar plates and on whether the hemolysis is partial or complete. Streptococcal colonies that are surrounded by a sharply defined, clear, colorless zone of hemolysis within which the erythrocytes are lysed completely are designated beta-hemolytic streptococci. If the colony is surrounded by a zone of greenish discoloration having an indefinite margin within which the erythrocytes are partially lysed, it is said to contain alpha-hemolytic streptococci. If no change is produced in the blood agar surrounding the colony, the organisms are referred to as nonhemolytic streptococci.

The beta-hemolytic streptococci have been further subdivided into a number of distinct serological groups on the basis of group-specific antigens usually found in the cell wall and known as the C carbohydrates. Because beta-hemolytic streptococci belonging to a single group, group A, are responsible for 90 to 95 percent of acute streptococcal infections in man and for the sequelae of rheumatic fever and acute hemorrhagic glomerulonephritis as well, serological grouping is of primary inportance in the recognition of pathogenic streptococci. Although they are sometimes referred to as *Streptococcus pyogenes*, the more descriptive term, group A beta-hemolytic streptococci, will be used throughout this text. The characteristic infection produced by group A beta-hemolytic streptococci in man is pharyngitis, and the natural habitat is the nasopharynx.

Included within the group D beta-hemolytic streptococci are the enterococci, organisms which are occasionally involved in urinary tract infections, subacute bacterial endocarditis, wound infections, and less frequently, in food poisoning. The designation enterococci will be used throughout this text because it is descriptive of the natural habitat of the organisms and because they are usually nonhemolytic, and only occasionally exhibit alpha or beta hemolysis. All enterococci, however, possess the group-specific antigen of the group D beta-hemolytic streptococci.

The viridans (green) group represents a heterogeneous collection of streptococci that produce alpha hemolysis. Viridans streptococci are part of the normal flora of the human mouth. Their chief relevance is that they are the major cause of subacute bacterial endocarditis and are involved in oral disease (Chap. 17). In addition, they must be distinguished from pneumococci which also produce alpha hemolysis.

Anaerobic streptococci, which are part of the normal flora of the mouth and of the female genital tract, represent a heterogeneous group. They are occasionally involved in endocarditis, in suppurative and gangrenous wounds, and formerly were implicated in some cases of puerperal fever. On blood agar, most cultures of anaerobic streptococci are nonhemolytic. Currently, anaerobic streptococci are referred to as *peptostreptococci.*

GROUP A BETA-HEMOLYTIC STREPTOCOCCAL INFECTIONS

The Causative Agent

Biological Properties

Natural Habitat The human nasopharynx, especially that of the child, is the natural reservoir of group A beta-hemolytic streptococci. In this site, the organisms may cause pharyngitis, or subclinical infection, they may be temporarily carried by a person who has had a recent pharyngitis or subclinical infection, or they may be present without clinical, historical, or serological evidence of streptococcal infection or disease (carrier state). From the nasopharynx the organisms are spread to the skin and into the environment. Injury to the skin may be followed by infection and further dissemination of the organisms.

Morphology and Growth Group A streptococci are fastidious in their growth requirements. On blood agar, organisms isolated directly from lesions produce small (1 mm) mucoid or glossy colonies surrounded by a zone of beta hemolysis. Stained smears reveal the presence of chains of gram-positive cocci of varying length and less than 1 μm in diameter. The unusual sensitivity of group A organisms to bacitracin (inhibition by disks containing 0.1 unit), as compared with other beta-hemolytic streptococci, provides a presumptive method for their recognition. Group B and some other streptococci occasionally have been shown to be sensitive to bacitracin.

Pathogenicity and Virulence The primary factor associated with the virulence of group A streptococci is the M protein, present in the cell wall, which inhibits phagocytosis. As noted earlier (Chap. 5), the M protein enables group A streptococci to adhere to the epithelial cells of the oropharynx. Specific secretory IgA antibodies can coat the M protein and prevent adherence. A secondary factor in pathogenicity is the production of erythrogenic toxin, which is associated with the rash in scarlet fever. Phage plays an important role in the synthesis of erythrogenic toxin, but the genetic mechanisms involved are not understood. The role of the nonantigenic hyaluronic acid capsule in the virulence of group A streptococci is less certain, although capsular material can inhibit phagocytosis to a slight extent under experimental conditions.

There is ample evidence, however, that group A streptococci are virulent in proportion to the amount of M protein they produce. On the other hand, ability of group A organisms to spread from person to person under natural conditions is not correlated with synthesis of M protein or any known factor.

Poststreptococcal disease may be associated with other streptococcal components. An antigen present in the cell (protoplast) membrane of all group A streptococci is immunologically related to an antigen in the sarcolemma of human cardiac muscle. This streptococcal protoplast antigen can induce the formation of antibodies that can combine with the sarcolemma. Another antigen, the group-specific C carbohydrate, can produce antibodies that can cross-react with structural glycoproteins of human heart valves. The presence of these two streptococcal antigens may be significant in the pathogenesis of rheumatic fever, although the finding of antibodies against these antigens in patients with rheumatic fever may represent the outcome of the disease and not its cause. In addition, crude sonic extracts of group A streptococci produce chronic inflammation of all layers of the heart after intraperitoneal inoculation in mice. Microscopically, the lesions in the mice resemble those in rheumatic fever, i.e., Aschoff-like bodies.

A somewhat similar, but as yet undefined, immunological mechanism may operate in the pathogenesis of acute hemorrhagic glomerulonephritis. In this case, however, the unknown component involved is largely restricted to a specific type (type 12) of group A beta-hemolytic streptococci.

In addition to M protein, erythrogenic toxin, the protoplast antigen, and the group-specific carbohydrate, group A streptococci elaborate an appreciable number of other components. These include the T and R antigens, the hyaluronic acid capsule, streptolysins S and O, streptokinase, hyaluronidase, diphosphopyridine nucleotidase, deoxyribonucleases, proteinase, amylase, and esterase. Because of their importance in pathogenicity, diagnosis, epidemiology, prevention, or control, further consideration will be given to group-specific carbohydrate, the M and T proteins, the protoplast antigen, erythrogenic toxin, and the streptolysins.

Antigenic Structure

Group-specific Carbohydrate C Antigen The group carbohydrate or polysaccharide antigen is the major component of the bacterial cell wall. It is a polymer whose constituents are rhamnose and N-acetylglucosamine in a ratio of approximately 2 to 1. The dominant determinant group is a terminal beta-N-acetylglucosamine residue. Variant cultures, in which this determinant group is absent, do not react with antiserum against group A organisms.

The group carbohydrate is firmly bound to the cell wall but can be released by a variety of procedures which partially hydrolyze the cell wall. These include extraction of cells at pH 2 and 100°C, extraction with formamide at 160 to 180°C, autoclaving cells at 15 lb pressure for 15 min., lysis of cells by enzymes derived from *Streptomyces albus*, and lysis of cells by phage lysates of group C streptococci. Serological reactivity of the group carbohydrate is usually assayed by precipitin tests but can be detected in intact cells by its ability to react with fluorescein-labeled antibody. In the diagnostic laboratory, serological reactions and fluorescent antibody tests rather than the bacitracin method should be relied upon for the definitive identification of group A streptococci.

Group A carbohydrate shows little or no cross-reaction with heterologous group antisera. On the other hand, purified preparations of group A carbohydrate induce the formation of antibody that can cross-react with the structural glycoproteins of human heart valves as demonstrated by precipitin tests, passive hemagglutination, immunofluorescence, and removal by adsorption. Similar antibodies are found in the serum of patients with rheumatic disease and, as previously mentioned, may be involved in the pathogenesis of rheumatic carditis.

From 2 to 14 days after intradermal injection of rabbits, purified carbohydrate-peptide complexes prepared from groups A and C streptococci cause relapsing nodular lesions of the skin as long as 80 days later. The complex appears to have a direct toxic action, since tissue damage can be detected microscopically 3 hr. after initial inoculation. Neither whole streptococcal cells nor group A carbohydrate can produce these nodular lesions.

Following intraperitoneal inoculation in mice, crude sonic extracts of group A streptococci containing a high concentration of rhamnose (probably in the form of group A carbohydrate) cause chronic inflammation of all layers of the heart. Like rheumatic fever, the lesions are more prominent on the left side of the heart, and microscopically, Aschoff bodies are present.

Type-specific M Protein Antigen Firmly attached on the surface of the cell wall of pathogenic group A streptococci are the M proteins which determine type specificity, virulence, and the formation of protective antibodies. There are about 50 recognized types of group A streptococci, each type possessing an antigenically distinct M protein. The role of the M protein in virulence is based on the fact that it inhibits phagocytosis. Protective immunity in group A streptococcal infection is a function of antibodies against the M protein and is type-specific, a concept of fundamental significance. In the presence of type-specific M antibodies streptococci are readily phagocytized.

The M protein is resistant to heat in acid solution and readily destroyed by trypsin without killing the streptococci. The antigen may be released from the cell wall by boiling at pH 2 or by treatment with group C streptococcal phage lysates. Precipitin tests are of limited value in the detection of antibody to M protein and reliance has been placed on the ability of specific antibody to enhance phagocytosis of group A streptococci, to significantly increase the chain length of organisms containing M antigen when grown in blood broth, or to agglutinate tanned erythrocytes treated with M antigen (passive hemagglutination).

The T Protein Antigen In addition to the M antigens, group A streptococci contain a large number of antigenically distinct T antigens. The T antigens are firmly attached on the surface of the cell wall, readily demonstrated by agglutination, resistant to proteolytic enzymes, and quickly destroyed by heat at acid pH. The T antigens are unrelated to the virulence of the organism, and their specific antibodies do not protect against infection. However, the T antigens are occasionally useful in the identification of streptococci that produce little or no M antigen or M antigen that is poorly antigenic (e.g., type 49). A common T antigen may be found in streptococci containing different M antigens, or streptococci with a single M antigen may contain one of a number of different T antigens.

The Cell Membrane (Protoplast) Antigen Purified group A streptococcal cell (protoplast) membranes are antigenic. The antibodies produced react not only with the protoplast antigen, but cross-react with the sarcolemma, the complex membrane structure, of human cardiac muscle as revealed by immunofluorescence. Such antibodies are also found in patients with uncomplicated streptococcal infections and in patients with rheumatic fever. Antibodies against the protoplast antigen may be removed by adsorption with group A membranes or with the sarcolemma of human cardiac muscle. Thus, the possibility exists that antibody against group A streptococcal membranes may be involved in the pathogenesis of rheumatic carditis by virtue of the fact that it reacts with the sarcolemma.

All types of group A streptococci contain the protoplast antigen that is antigenically related to the sarcolemma. In addition, groups C and G streptococcal membranes are antigenically related to group A membranes and some group C antisera contain the heart-reactive antibody. Antisera to membranes from other groups of beta-hemolytic streptococci are nonreactive.

Erythrogenic (Scarlatinal) Toxins and Lysogenicity Potentially, all types of group A streptococci have the capacity to synthesize an extracellular erythrogenic toxin which is responsible for the rash in scarlet fever, but the amount of toxin elaborated by different cultures may vary greatly. Of erythrogenic toxin-producing cultures, approximately 80 percent synthesize a particular type designated *erythrogenic toxin A*. Most of the remaining 20 percent produce one of two additional antigenically distinct erythrogenic toxins. In the case of erythrogenic toxin A, production of the toxin is associated with the lysogenic state.

Approximately 25 to 30 per cent of randomly selected group A streptococci are lysogenic. During streptococcal epidemics the proportion of lysogenic strains may rise to 70 percent. Phage isolated from lysogenic erythrogenic toxin A-producing cultures can lysogenize nontoxigenic cultures of group A streptococci which acquire the capacity to synthesize both phage and toxin (conversion). Ultraviolet irradiation of the lysogenized cultures stimulates the production of phage and enhances by 10- to 20-fold the production of erythrogenic toxin A. After ultraviolet irradiation the peak burst of phage occurs in 2 to 3 hr., while maximal yields of toxin are found in 8 to 10 hr. Obviously, phage plays an important role in the synthesis of erythrogenic toxin A, but the genetic mechanisms involved in toxin production are not understood.

Erythrogenic toxin causes an erythematous, often edematous, area of more than 10 mm in diameter appearing in 6 to 24 hr. following intradermal injection in a susceptible individual (a positive Dick test). In individuals who have antitoxin by virtue of a previous infection, a similar injection of erythrogenic toxin usually results in a negative skin test. If antitoxin is injected intradermally early in the course of scarlet fever, the rash will blanch *(Schultz-Charlton blanching reaction)*.

Streptolysin O Most cultures of group A streptococci produce an oxygen-labile hemolysin, streptolysin O, which can be activated by sulfhydryl-reducing agents. Streptolysin O is antigenic; its action can be neutralized by specific antibody, and it is readily inactivated by trypsin and cholesterol.

Under experimental conditions, streptolysin O induces a large and rapid increase in the permeability of mammalian cells, has a cytolytic action on lysosomes, causes mitochondrial swelling, and exerts a cardiotoxic effect, leading to an irreversible loss of myocardial contractility and death. It is probable that degranulation of leukocytes by streptolysin O represents a nonspecific response of the neutrophil to injury. Despite the multitude of effects that streptolysin O can produce experimentally, there is no evidence to suggest that it exerts a significant role in the pathogenesis of streptococcal infection or rheumatic fever.

On the other hand, most patients with group A streptococcal infection show an antibody response to streptolysin O (ASTO) during convalescence. A rise in ASTO titer has proved more useful than any other test in providing serological evidence of a preceding streptococcal infection in the pathogenesis of rheumatic fever. Furthermore, as the magnitude of the ASTO response increases, the incidence of rheumatic fever rises.

Streptolysin S Streptolysin S is a cytolytic streptococcal growth product responsible for the zone of beta hemolysis surrounding surface colonies on blood agar plates. The active moiety of streptolysin S appears to be a polypeptide with a molecular weight of approximately 2,800, frequently attached to an oligoribonucleotide carrier. Streptolysin S is nonantigenic, hemolytic under anaerobic conditions, and resistant to trypsin and cholesterol. Under experimental conditions, it has a cytolytic action on the lysosomes of mammalian cells and interacts with phospholipids or long-chain polar lipids to release anions or glucose from artificial lipid spherules with or without cholesterol. However, it has no known function in the pathogenesis of human infections.

Pathogenesis

Human contact with group A streptococci primarily involves the upper respiratory tract. The invading streptococci are usually limited to the mucous membranes and lymphatic tissue of the pharynx. Occasionally, however, the organisms may spread from this focus to involve almost any tissue of the body. In addition, their products may be disseminated from this site to initiate other manifestations of disease in the skin (the rash in scarlet fever or the nodules in erythema nodosum), the heart, joints, and central nervous system (rheumatic fever) and the kidneys (acute hemorrhagic glomerulonephritis).

The outcome of contact with group A streptococci is chiefly determined by the amount of M antigen synthesized by the bacteria and by the presence or absence of type-specific M antibodies in the host. Other factors that may affect the outcome are (1) the amount of erythrogenic toxin elaborated by the bacteria, (2) the concentration of antitoxin in the host, (3) the number of previous streptococcal infections experienced by the host, (4) the specific antigenic type of the organism, (5) the presence of a recent viral infection of the host, and (6) the age and, perhaps, the genetic constitution of the host.

Streptococcal Infections of the Pharynx Group A streptococci are usually acquired by direct contact with droplets disseminated by an infected person or a carrier. If the organisms become established in the upper respiratory tract, the result may be that (1) the person will become a carrier without clinical or serological evidence of streptococcal infection (carrier state), (2) the individual will produce antibodies without clinical manifestations and will carry the organism temporarily (subclinical or inapparent infection), or (3) within 2 or 3 days the person will develop a pharyngitis, will subsequently form antibodies, and will carry the organism temporarily (clinical infection). It is estimated that between one-half and two-thirds of group A streptococcal infections are subclinical.

Streptococcal Pharyngitis The characteristic clinical infection associated with group A streptococci is a pharyngitis (tonsillitis or sore throat) involving mucous membranes and lymphatic tissue, especially the tonsils and the cervical nodes. Group A streptococci have a special predilection for the lymphatic system and localize initially in the tonsils. In 2 to 3 days swelling and reddening of the tonsils and other pharyngeal lymphatic tissue are accompanied by focal or confluent accumulation of exudate on the affected areas. The adjacent mucous membranes are commonly involved, and systemic manifestations of fever and toxicity are usually present.

This relatively superficial infection may be associated with cervical lymphadenitis. The cervical lymph nodes at the angle of the jaw drain the tonsillar area and often become swollen and tender as a result of group A streptococcal infection.

Recovery is usually prompt and uneventful. However, because immunity is type-specific, recurrent attacks are not uncommon. In addition, more serious events may ensue. These include, as indicated below, the spread of infection or the development of poststreptococcal sequelae (rheumatic fever or glomerulonephritis).

Age It has long been recognized that the clinical manifestations of streptococcal infections vary with the age of the host. For example, in infants and young children infection frequently follows a protracted and indeterminate course. Rhinorrhea, cervical lymphadenitis, and otitis media (Chap. 19) are common. In older children and adults, a sore throat, exudative tonsillitis, and pharyngitis are prominent. The incidence of cervical lymphadenitis and otitis media (Chap. 19) declines with age. There is, however, no satisfactory explanation to account for the increasing tendency for the infection to localize with advance in age.

Scarlet Fever Scarlet fever is a streptococcal pharyngitis with an accompanying exanthematous (scarlatinal) rash. The rash is caused by systemic distribution of erythrogenic toxin and not by dissemination of streptococci. The rash is characterized by diffuse reddening of the skin, most prominently seen on the trunk. The skin lesions usually desquamate during convalescence.

All types of group A streptococci can cause scarlet fever. However, recurrent attacks are extremely rare because 80 percent of group A streptococci that produce toxin synthesize the same antigenic type (erythrogenic toxin A) and because antitoxin frequently develops in the absence of a rash. It is probable that what are thought to be subsequent attacks of scarlet fever are actually due to other causative agents (Chap. 22).

Streptococcal Infections of the Skin Streptococcal infections of the skin usually follow a typical pattern and often present a greater threat to the individual than upper respiratory infection. The bacteria are introduced into the injured skin by direct exogenous or endogenous contact with infected material from the upper respiratory tract. The lymphatic vessels are quickly involved with minimal reaction at the site of the local lesion or the portal of entry. Advancing lymphadenitis (red streaks) and swollen and tender nodes are prominent features. In its most dramatic form, the infection may result in bacteremia, septicemia, and death in 24 to 48 hr.

In infants and young children superficial, spreading, vesicular lesions of the skin (pyoderma, impetigo) also produced by staphylococci, are relatively common, and may occur in epidemic form. Epidemics of impetigo are often associated with certain types of group A streptococci (i.e., type 49). Their chief threat and their major importance is that they may be followed by glomerulonephritis. For example, glomerulonephritis associated with type 49 has been found more often as a sequel to pyoderma than to infection of the respiratory tract. As previously indicated, however, glomerulonephritis is most commonly preceded by infection with type 12.

Puerperal Fever In puerperal fever group A streptococci may enter the bloodstream directly through the damaged endometrium, or hematogenous spread may follow rapid passage through the draining lymphatics and the thoracic duct. Minimal local reaction is seen in the uterus. The most frequent result of endometrial infection with group A streptococci is an overwhelming fatal septicemia with death occurring in 24 to 48 hr. Fortunately, the disease has been controlled by careful attention to aseptic technique in obstetrical practice.

Other Streptococcal Infections Most of the more serious manifestations of streptococcal infections encountered in the preantibiotic era are rarely seen today. These include erysipelas, peritonsillar and retropharyngeal abscesses, cellulitis and abscesses at the base of the tongue and on the floor of the mouth, mastoiditis and osteomyelitis secondary to chronic or recurrent otitis media, and meningitis, cerebral sinus thrombosis, and endocarditis following entry of the organisms into the blood. The rarity of these serious complications of streptococcal pharyngitis is primarily a function of the effective use of penicillin in therapy.

Extension of streptococcal pharyngitis into the paranasal sinuses via the anatomical openings or into the middle ear via the eustachian tube (Chap. 19) are encountered all too frequently. However, judicious use of penicillin in treatment of these conditions has prevented the development of more serious complications.

Bronchitis, interstitial bronchopneumonia, and pleurisy secondary to pulmonary infection remain major serious manifestations of streptococcal infections. Infection of the lower respiratory tract with group A streptococci is almost always preceded by a recent viral infection. Especially dangerous in this connection are influenza, measles, and smallpox. The mechanisms involved probably are associated with damage to the ciliated epithelial cells lining the upper respiratory tract (influenza and possibly also measles and smallpox) and destruction of lymphatic tissue (measles and smallpox). The best method of preventing streptococcal infections of the lower respiratory tract is through the effective use of vaccines to prevent the preceding viral infections (influenza, measles, smallpox).

Rheumatic Fever The connection between group A streptococci and rheumatic fever has been firmly established on the basis of epidemiological, serological, and prophylactic evidence. The incidence of rheumatic fever clearly follows the rise and fall in streptococcal antibodies (ASTO, antihyaluronidase, or antistreptokinase) in almost 100 percent of patients with acute rheumatic fever and confirms the epidemiological observation. The unquestioned value of penicillin therapy in the prevention of initial attacks of rheumatic fever after proved infection with group A streptococci, as well as the success of penicillin or the sulfonamides in preventing recurrent attacks of rheumatic fever, strengthens the presumption that the streptococcus is the protagonist of this disease. However, group A streptococci are not found within the lesions of rheumatic fever, and the mechanisms involved in the initiation of rheumatic fever by streptococcal infection await clarification.

Initial or Primary Attack The initial or primary attack of rheumatic fever is preceded by streptococcal pharyngitis and commences after an average latent period of 19 days (Fig. 14-1). The incidence of primary attacks of rheumatic fever varies between 0.3 and 3 percent depending in large part upon the severity of the streptococcal infection and the magnitude of the antibody response. For example, in one large series the attack rate of rheumatic fever in nonexudative pharyngitis was 0.33 percent while the attack rate in exudative pharyngitis was 0.9 percent. In another study, the incidence per streptococcal infection rose from 0.8 to 3.4 to 5.5 percent when the ASTO response increased from 0 to 120, 121 to 250, or over 250 units per milliliter, respectively.

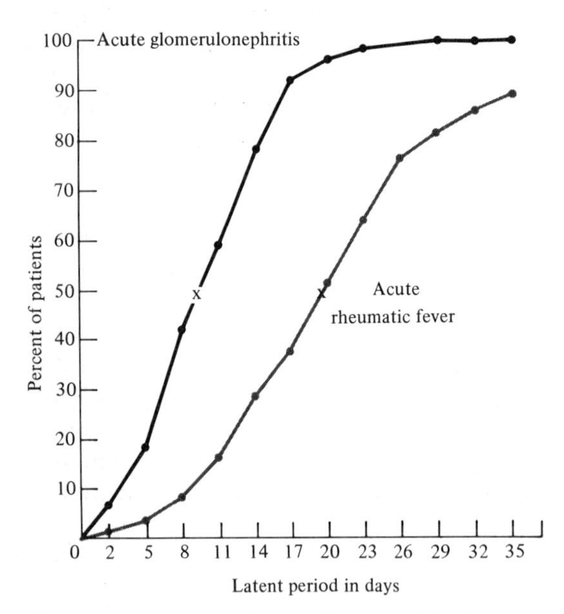

Figure 14-1 Cumulative distribution of latent periods in acute glomerulonephritis and acute rheumatic fever. [*From C. H. Rammelkamp, Jr., in J. W. Uhr (ed.), The Streptococcus, Rheumatic Fever and Glomerulonephritis, Baltimore: The Williams & Wilkins Company, 1964, pp. 289–300.*]

The clinical manifestations, as well as their severity and persistence, vary widely. The most prominent features are fever, migratory polyarthritis, and carditis. Uncoordinated and spasmodic movements (chorea) are encountered less frequently and often appear after a longer latent period. The arthritis regularly heals without residual damage to the joint. Rheumatic carditis develops in about one-third of patients experiencing their first attack and represents the most significant feature of the disease. The severity of the acute rheumatic attack and the production of permanent change are determined by the extent of the carditis. Most attacks of acute rheumatic fever subside within 6 months, but recur with succeeding streptococcal infections.

All layers of the heart may be involved. The histological hallmark of active rheumatic carditis is the finding of Aschoff bodies or nodules in the myocardium. The Aschoff bodies are the result of chronic focal inflammatory changes. They are formed in the center by granular fragmentation of collagen bundles with peripheral accumulation of large mononuclear and multinuclear cells with basophilic and irregular cytoplasm. The lesions usually heal by fibrosis within 6 months.

Recurrent or Secondary Attacks In sharp contrast to the initial attack, the incidence of recurrent rheumatic fever from streptococcal infection is high and two-thirds of recurrences follow asymptomatic infections. This incidence of recurrent attacks increases with the magnitude of the antibody response, the existence and extent of previous cardiac damage irrespective of the ASTO rise, the proximity of the last recurrence, and the number of previous attacks.

In one study, a recurrent attack rate of 16 percent was recorded when the ASTO titer increased 25 to 100 units per milliliter but was 50 percent when the ASTO increase amounted to 334 or more units. In another study, recurrent attacks increased from 15 percent to 24, 30, 38, and 70 percent with increasing ASTO response.

Recurrent attacks of rheumatic fever have a tendency to repeat the clinical manifestations seen in the primary attack. This is especially serious in the case of rheumatic carditis. In one series, for example, rheumatic carditis increased from 33 to 60, 75, 80, and 100 percent with none, one, two, three, and four previous attacks, respectively.

The increased incidence of heart disease in patients with numerous attacks is associated with an increased tendency to recurrences in patients with heart disease. In one study, for example, in patients with no previous heart disease, the recurrent attack rate was found to be 9 percent. However, in patients with heart disease with no or slight cardiomegaly, the rate rose to 28 percent and increased to 43 percent in patients with heart disease and marked cardiomegaly.

Thus, the patients who develop rheumatic carditis have been shown to be prime candidates for recurrent attacks of rheumatic carditis and chronic rheumatic valvular disease. The latter occurs as a result of involvement of the endocardium with deformative scarring of the valves and adjacent structures as the lesions heal by fibrosis. It is primarily in and on heart valves damaged by rheumatic carditis that the vegetative lesions of subacute bacterial endocarditis appear later in life.

Mechanism Preceding infection with all types of group A streptococci is clearly implicated in initial and recurrent attacks of rheumatic fever, but the mechanisms by which the disease develops await clarification. The group A streptococcus type involved in recurrent attacks is different from the type that initiated the primary attack and the previous recurrent attacks. The disease initially strikes only 0.3 to 3 percent of the persons infected with a group A streptococcus, and the organisms cannot be recovered within the rheumatic lesions.

The latent period between infection with the streptococcus and the onset of rheumatic fever together with the rising incidence of the disease with increasing antibody response led to the prevalent theory that rheumatic fever was an immunological or autoimmune disease (Chap. 11). Until recently, efforts to elucidate the underlying nature of the disease have been unrewarding.

The demonstration of antigenic cross-reactions between protoplast membranes of group A streptococci and the sarcolemma of human cardiac muscle and between the group-specific carbohydrate antigen of group A streptococci and the structural glycoproteins of human heart valves and the finding of antibodies in the serum of patients with rheumatic disease that cross-react with sarcolemma and cardiac glycoprotein have placed the immunological theory on a much firmer foundation. However, either or both of these cross-reacting antibodies may be the outcome of the disease, not its cause; i.e., they may be formed as a result of the release of a modified antigen from cardiac tissue damaged by one or more streptococcal products. On the other hand, there is no need to postulate preceding cardiac damage when antibodies regularly produced in the course of streptococcal infection have the potential for combining with, and perhaps damaging, cardiac tissue. Established immunological relationships between group A streptococci and heart tissue may be significant in the pathogenesis of rheumatic carditis, but much more information is required before the precise mechanism can be understood.

It would prove most interesting to determine if either the protoplast antigen or the group A carbohydrate antigen (or both) has the capacity to reproduce in mice the chronic inflammation of all layers of the heart and the Aschoff-like bodies induced by crude sonic extracts of group

A streptococci. Such a model might serve as a useful guide to further elucidation of the development of rheumatic carditis in man.

Acute Hemorrhagic Glomerulonephritis (Poststreptococcal Glomerulonephritis) The connection between certain nephritogenic group A streptococci and acute hemorrhagic glomerulonephritis has been firmly established on the basis of epidemiologic and serologic evidence. The vast majority of attacks, 90 percent or more, are preceded by infection with type 12 group A streptococci and the balance following infection with types 1, 4, 18, 25, and 49. Streptococci, however, cannot be recovered from the renal lesions. The glomerulonephritis commences with an average latent period of 10 days (Fig. 14-1). The incidence following type 12 infections varies between 1.7 and 13 percent. The majority of cases of glomerulonephritis are preceded by streptococcal pharyngitis. With type 49, however, glomerulonephritis occurs more often as a sequel to streptococcal pyoderma than to streptococcal pharyngitis.

Penicillin therapy after onset of nephritogenic streptococcal infections does not prevent the development of acute hemorrhagic glomerulonephritis. The finding of hematuria during the acute stage of the streptococcal infection may reflect the rapid onset of the disease and has prognostic significance. For example, of 44 patients with type 12 infections and hematuria, 12 subsequently developed nephritis, whereas in 140 patients in whom hematuria was absent during the acute infection only 9 went on to develop nephritis.

In contrast to the failure of penicillin therapy, in epidemics due to type 12 group A streptococci, chemoprophylaxis with penicillin or sulfonamides has a marked effect in reducing the incidence of glomerulonephritis.

In young children, in whom the majority of cases are found, recovery occurs in 85 to 98 percent, is invariably complete, and recurrences are rare. For example, of 61 survivors who had poststreptococcal nephritis in the same epidemic, none showed evidence of chronic renal disease over the course of the next 10 years. In adults, however, 25 percent of the cases following acute hemorrhagic glomerulonephritis may develop chronic renal disease.

In poststreptococcal glomerulonephritis the glomeruli are enlarged, bloodless, and excessively cellular. The genesis of the glomerulonephritis is unknown but may be associated with the deposition of antigen-antibody complexes in endothelial cells and between these cells and the basement membrane.

Erythema Nodosum Some cases of erythema nodosum, a disease characterized by red, tender, nodular swellings on the extensor surface of the extremities, are preceded by group A streptococcal infections. The lesions tend to recur with subsequent attacks of streptococcal infection. The disease usually occurs in the absence of rheumatic lesions, and recovery occurs without residual damage. It is not known if carbohydrate-peptide complexes are involved in the human disease, but they can produce relapsing nodular lesions of the skin in rabbits after a latent period.

Laboratory Diagnosis

Since most cases of pharyngitis are caused by viruses (Chap. 20) and since streptococcal pharyngitis cannot be distinguished on the basis of clinical manifestations, the diagnosis must be established on laboratory findings.

The presumptive diagnosis of group A streptococcal infections is based on (1) the isolation of characteristic colonies showing beta hemolysis on blood agar plates and short chains of gram-positive cocci, and (2) the demonstration that the organisms are members of group A streptococci by the use of the 0.1 μg bacitracin disk. Streptococci which do not show beta hemolysis, but which are isolated from lesions frequently associated with group A streptococci, should be checked for their sensitivity to bacitracin. Nephritogenic type 12 streptococci are often found to be nonhemolytic. Determination of the antigenic type is reserved for epidemiologic studies.

Antibody studies have been used extensively in rheumatic fever and in acute hemorrhagic glomerulonephritis to demonstrate that the patient has had a recent streptococcal infection. The ASTO test, based on the ability of antibody to inhibit hemolysis, is the test of choice, although antihyaluronidase and antistreptokinase tests have also been employed. The absence of ASTO antibodies does not rule out the clinical diagnosis of rheumatic fever or glomerulonephritis, but the demonstration of a rise in ASTO titer is of value in confirming the clinical diagnosis.

Epidemiology

Source The nasopharynx of the child, and to a lesser extent the adult, is the natural reservoir of group A streptococci. From their primary site in the nasopharynx of an infected person or carrier, the streptococci are spread by droplets to the respiratory tract of other individuals. From the nasopharynx the organisms are also spread to the skin and into the environment. In some cases, as for example in epidemics of type 49 pyoderma in infants and young children, the skin and direct contact with skin lesions may be of importance in the spread of infection. Before pasteurization, milk-borne epidemics of streptococcal sore throat were prevalent. Before commercial and home refrigeration, food-borne epidemics were not uncommon. However, all available evidence points to direct contact with infected droplets as the major source of infection.

If the skin or mucous membranes of the lower respiratory tract are injured, group A streptococcal infections may follow. In these instances, the invading organisms may be endogenous or exogenous.

Carrier State Some individuals may carry group A streptococci in the upper respiratory tract in the absence of clinical, historical, or serological evidence of streptococcal infection (carrier state). When the organisms are carried in the nose, the carrier is more likely to transmit streptococci to others than when the organisms are found only in the throat. The carrier state is most prevalent in preschool children during the winter and early spring (the respiratory season). The carrier state varies widely between about 10 and 60 percent, but usually rises prior to an epidemic. During a single respiratory season the majority of the population may carry the organism for a short period. Approximately 25 to 30 percent of group A streptococci selected at random are lysogenic, but the proportion of lysogenic organisms may rise to 70 percent during epidemics.

In addition, following clinical or subclinical infection group A streptococci are usually carried for a period of several weeks. However, with time the number of organisms in the nose and throat decreases, less and less M antigen is produced, and as a result, the frequency of nontypable group A streptococci increases.

Incidence The incidence of clinical streptococcal infections varies with the age and family status of the individual, the geographical area, the season of the year, crowding, and many other factors. Highest attack rates are found in children between 5 and 15 years of age. Approximately 25 percent of household contacts of index cases will become infected, siblings more commonly than parents. In this context, an *index case* is the individual who introduces the infection into the household unit. The peak incidence is found in the winter and early spring in colder climates. Higher attack rates are associated with crowded conditions as are found in tenements, classrooms, dormitories, and military barracks. In addition to children, the risk of exposure and infection is high in mothers of young children, school teachers, pediatricians, pediatric nurses, dentists, and military personnel.

The incidence of rheumatic fever parallels the rise and fall of streptococcal infections. It is highest in children between 5 and 15 years of age and, under civilian conditions, declines significantly thereafter. In military recruits, epidemic exudative streptococcal pharyngitis is followed by rheumatic fever in about 3 percent independent of the age group, the area of the country from which the recruits came, the serological type, and the initial ASTO titer at the time of infection. The epidemiology of glomerulonephritis, on the other hand, only parallels streptococcal infections when nephritogenic streptococci (primarily type 12) are involved.

Prevention and Control

The Goals The primary goals in streptococcal prevention and control are (1) to limit the duration and the extent of the infection in all individuals and (2) to prevent infection in rheumatic subjects. Remarkable success has been achieved through the therapeutic use of penicillin and through the prophylactic use of penicillin or sulfadiazine.

Treatment Acute streptococcal disease requires prompt and vigorous treatment with a cidal drug in order to eliminate the streptococcus and to prevent primary and recurrent attacks of rheumatic fever. Penicillin is the drug of choice preferably administered as long-acting repository benzathine penicillin G in one intramuscular injection (600,000 to 900,000 units in children and 900,000 to 1,200,000 units in adults). An alternate method involves oral therapy with buffered penicillin G (200,000 to 250,000 units three or four times daily for 10 days). This method is dependent upon the cooperation of the patient, but is preferred by some physicians and by many patients. For patients who are allergic to penicillin, erythromycin is effective when given for 10 days.

Sulfonamides and other static drugs are not used for treatment because they fail to achieve prompt bacteriological cure and because they have no influence in reducing the rheumatic fever attack rate because of the persistence of streptococcal antigens.

Therapy is begun as soon as possible, but almost always after receiving the result of the throat or other culture. Even when treatment is delayed for 9 to 10 days, the administration of adequate doses of penicillin significantly reduces the incidence of rheumatic fever. The inference is that streptococcal infection must persist for at least 9 or 10 days for rheumatic fever to be initiated with greatest frequency (Table 14-2 and Fig. 14-1).

The physician's responsibility should not end with early and adequate treatment of the patient with streptococcal pharyngitis. Since approximately 25 percent of household contacts of the patient will also be infected, efforts should be made to detect infections in other members of the family by history, inspection, and throat cultures. Family contacts who have clinical manifestations of streptococcal pharyngitis, large numbers of group A streptococci on throat culture, or streptococcal infection within the past 10 days should receive effective treatment with penicillin. Since treatment with penicillin prevents the development of type-specific immunity, failure to encompass the family unit in the management of streptococcal pharyngitis often leads to reinfection of the treated patient with the same type of group A streptococcus that caused his initial infection.

In sharp contrast to its value in the prevention of rheumatic fever, as indicated previously, penicillin therapy does not prevent the development of acute hemorrhagic glomerulonephritis following infection with nephritogenic streptococci (Table 14-2 and Fig. 14-1).

Chemoprophylaxis

In Rheumatic Subjects All patients with a well-documented history of rheumatic fever or definite evidence of rheumatic heart disease should receive penicillin or sulfadiazine prophylactically. Since about two-thirds of recurrent attacks of rheumatic fever follow subclinical infection, chemoprophylaxis should be continued throughout life, especially if rheumatic heart disease is present. In view of the significant reduction in streptococcal infection beyond the age of 15 years, exceptions may be considered in the case of selected adults without heart disease who have had no attacks for many years, and reliance should be placed wholly on prompt and vigorous treatment with penicillin. Exceptions would not be made, however, for those with a high risk of exposure to streptococcal infection (military personnel, mothers of young children, school teachers, hospital nurses).

For chemoprophylaxis, monthly intramuscular injections of benzathine penicillin G give the most consistently reliable results, but oral medication is preferred by most patients. Oral sulfadiazine and oral penicillin G are equally effective. Sulfadiazine is taken in one dose of 0.5 Gm daily in patients under 60 lb and 1 Gm in patients over 60 lb. Penicillin is taken in a dose of 200,000 and 250,000 units once or twice a day.

Table 14-2 Differences between Rheumatic Fever and Glomerulonephritis

Property	Rheumatic fever	Glomerulonephritis
Initiated by	All types of group A streptococci	Primarily type 12 group A streptococci, occasionally types 1, 14, 18, 25, 49
Incidence	0.3 to 3 percent of all group A infections	1.7 to 13 percent of type 12 infections
Latent period		
Average	19 days	10 days
In 8 days or less	9 percent	42 percent
Value of penicillin therapy in prevention	Highly effective	Not effective
Chemoprophylaxis (penicillin or sulfadiazine)	Continuous use recommended	Used only in nephritogenic epidemics or in mass chemoprophylaxis in military recruits
Permanent healing	Does not develop	Occurs in 85 to 98 percent of children who survive, but in adults 25 percent may develop chronic glomerulonephritis
Recurrences in absence of chemoprophylaxis	Frequent	Extremely rare

Two daily doses are probably more effective than one, and higher blood levels are achieved if the drug is taken ½ hr. before a meal.

The efficacy of sulfadiazine in chemoprophylaxis of streptococcal infections and consequently in the prevention of rheumatic fever is in sharp contrast to its failure in the treatment of attacks of rheumatic fever. In both instances sulfadiazine acts to inhibit the multiplication of streptococci. However, in chemoprophylaxis the drug is confronted with a small number of streptococci, while in treatment large numbers of streptococci are involved. Despite the fact that sulfadiazine effectively limits the spread of streptococcal infection, the persistence of streptococcal antigens is sufficient to initiate the immunological responses associated with initial and recurrent attacks of rheumatic fever.

In Epidemics Under epidemic conditions or in the face of a sharp increase in the carrier state preceding epidemics, mass prophylaxis with sulfadiazine or penicillin exerts a marked effect in reducing the incidence of streptococcal infections and, thus, rheumatic fever and acute hemorrhagic glomerulonephritis. Penicillin is preferred, however, because its effect is more rapid, since it eradicates the streptococcus.

The mass use of benzathine penicillin in military recruits at the onset of their training program eliminates streptococcal epidemics, rheumatic fever, and acute hemorrhagic glomerulonephritis in this highly susceptible population for the duration of their basic training period. In civilian life mass chemoprophylaxis is generally reserved for use in closed communities of children (orphanages, homes for the retarded, mental institutions, and hospital nurseries) when streptococcal infections become prevalent.

The Impact of Chemotherapy and Chemoprophylaxis The introduction of sulfonamides and, especially, penicillin has had a tremendous impact in minimizing the damage induced by group A streptococci in their human hosts. Because of prompt and vigorous treatment of streptococcal infection with penicillin, most of the more serious manifestations of streptococcal infection are rarely seen today (bacteremia and its consequences, erysipelas, peritonsillar and retropharyngeal abscesses, cellulitis and abscesses at the base of the tongue and on the floor of the mouth, mastoiditis). Otitis media (Chap. 19), paranasal sinusitis, and infections of the lower respiratory tract (following recent viral infection) do occur but can be effectively treated with penicillin, as mentioned previously.

Early and adequate treatment of streptococcal pharyngitis with penicillin has also had a dramatic effect in preventing initial and recurrent attacks of rheumatic fever. Rheumatic fever is quickly becoming a rare disease limited to patients with untreated exudative streptococcal pharyngitis.

Equally significant has been the effect of penicillin and sulfadiazine in continuous chemoprophylaxis of streptococcal infection in rheumatic subjects. Its impact has been especially significant in preventing recurrent attacks of rheumatic carditis which inevitably led to chronic valvular disease and in many cases to subacute bacterial endocarditis.

Penicillin has had little influence on the incidence of scarlet fever. Fortunately, however, the severity of scarlet fever began to decline long before the introduction of penicillin and has since continued to abate.

Other Control Measures The multitude of antigenic types, the difficulty of preparing potent vaccines containing M antigen, the potential risk of inducing rheumatic fever or glomerulonephritis, and the efficacy of penicillin have precluded attempts to control streptococcal infection and disease by immunization. Immunization with erythrogenic toxoid was never widely employed in prevention of the rash in scarlet fever, and antitoxin was not routinely used in treatment, probably because the severity of scarlet fever was already declining when toxoid and antitoxin became available in 1924.

Efforts aimed at epidemiological control are complicated by the respiratory route of transmission of the infection, the prevalence of the carrier state, and subclinical infections. The failure of ultraviolet light and glycol aerosols to reduce the incidence of streptococcal infection emphasizes the fact that group A streptococci are spread from person to person as a result of direct and intimate contact with infected droplets.

Historically, pasteurization of milk has eliminated milk-borne epidemics of streptococcal sore throat, and home and commercial refrigeration has minimized food-borne outbreaks. Aseptic obstetrical practice has proved effective in the prevention of puerperal fever, and asepsis in other hospital areas has greatly reduced the incidence of group A streptococcal infections following surgery.

INFECTIVE ENDOCARDITIS (BACTERIAL ENDOCARDITIS)

Infective endocarditis is a microbial infection of the heart valves or of the endocardium occurring in persons who have chronic rheumatic valvular disease, aortic valvular disease, congenital cardiac defects, or no underlying heart disease. The infection may develop abruptly or slowly, may pursue a fulminant or protracted course, and is invariably fatal unless treated. The majority of infections are caused by microorganisms that are part of the normal flora. The most frequent physical and laboratory findings are fever, positive blood cultures, cardiac murmurs, increased erythrocyte sedimentation velocity, cardiomegaly, petechiae, and anemia. Embolic phenomena are late manifestations of the disease.

The differentiation of bacterial endocarditis into subacute bacterial endocarditis (SBE) and acute bacterial endocarditis (ABE) is debatable but has been widely used. Generally, SBE is caused by indigenous microorganisms of low pathogenicity, develops in patients with rheumatic or congenital cardiac lesions, and pursues a prolonged course. ABE, on the other hand, generally is caused by microorganisms of relatively high pathogenicity in the absence of underlying heart disease and follows a fulminant course. Most of the causative agents, however, can initiate either SBE or ABE. Different investigators have used varying criteria to classify the disease as acute or subacute. For example, less than 4 weeks and less than 50 days have been termed acute.

The term infective endocarditis is preferable because it emphasizes the increasingly evident fact that microorganisms other than bacteria may cause the disease and because differentiation of the disease into acute and subacute is largely academic since the advent of effective treatment. A more meaningful approach would be to classify the disease on the basis of the infecting organism.

Historically, and continuing to the present day, infective endocarditis has been a disease of changing patterns. Before 1910 more cases were classified as acute than subacute, probably due to the prevalence of septic disease (beta-hemolytic streptococci, gonococci, meningococci, pneumococci). In the 1920s the ratio of subacute to acute cases was estimated at 2:1. This ratio increased in the period from 1944 to 1958 to about 3:1. Between 1920 and 1958 the vast majority of cases were caused by viridans streptococci and occurred in patients with rheumatic heart disease. Between 1962 and 1964, and continuing to the present day, the subacute/acute ratio is about 0.8:1.

Since the introduction of antibiotics, not only has the proportion of acute cases increased, but there has been a marked shift in most of the other parameters of the disease. Many of the classic manifestations of the disease—emboli, petechiae, splenomegaly, clubbing of the fingers, purplish or erythematous tender papules in the pulp of the fingers (Osler's nodes)—are rarely seen today. Enterococci and staphylococci have moved up to become the principal causative agents along with viridans streptococci. A greater proportion of the cases are occurring in the absence of rheumatic or congenital heart disease. A significantly higher proportion of cases develop in older individuals. Congestive heart failure has replaced infection as the leading cause of death in patients with endocarditis.

Early recognition of the disease is currently the single most important factor influencing the survival of the patient. Consequently, the diagnosis should be considered and blood cultures promptly taken in patients with persistent fever of a week or more, with or without underlying heart disease. Cultures usually are positive in 80 to 90 percent of the cases. A substantial majority of patients early in the course of the disease have no evidence of many of the classic features of the disease, and an increasing number have no history or presenting evidence of underlying heart disease.

The Causative Agents

Relative Prevalence and the Normal Flora Infective endocarditis may be caused by bacteria, fungi, rickettsiae, chlamydiae, viruses, protozoa, and other parasites. The greatest number of cases are caused by gram-positive bacteria, primarily by viridans streptococci, staphylococci, and enterococci. Today these bacteria are responsible for about 70 to 80 percent of proved cases. An appreciable, but as yet somewhat undefined, proportion are associated with microaerophilic and anaerobic streptococci. The balance of the cases are due to a large number of saprophytic and pathogenic bacteria and fungi and less frequently to rickettsiae, chlamydiae, viruses, protozoa, and other parasites

Table 14-3 The Causative Agents of Infective Endocarditis

Frequency	Causative agents*
Most prevalent	Viridans streptococci, staphylococci, enterococci
Prevalent	Microaerophilic and anaerobic streptococci
Occasionally found:	
Gram-positive bacteria	*Listeria*, *Bacillus* species, micrococci, *Erysipelothrix*, diphtheroids, pneumococci, group A streptococci
Gram-negative bacteria	*Escherichia*, *Enterobacter*, *Klebsiella*, *Proteus*, *Mima*, *Pseudomonas*, *Alcaligenes*, actinobacilli, streptobacilli, flavobacterium, *Bacteroides*, gonococci, meningococci, saprophytic *Neisseria*, *Serratia* *(Chromobacterium)*, *Vibrio* fetus, *Brucella*, *Pasteurella*, *Salmonella*, *Hemophilus influenzae*, *H.* parainfluenzae, and others
Fungi	Especially *Candida* and *Histoplasma* but also *Blastomyces*, *Coccidioides*, *Aspergillus*, *Cryptococcus*, and *Mucor*
Rarely encountered	Rickettsiae *(Coxiella burnetii)*, chlamydiae, viruses (enteroviruses), protozoa *(Trypanosoma)*, and parasitic helminths

* Microorganisms underlined are generally considered part of the normal flora of the mouth. However, enterococci, *Escherichia*, *Proteus*, and *Bacteroides* are more commonly found as part of the normal flora of the large intestine.

(Table 14-3). Mixed infections are occasionally encountered and often include one of the prevalent gram-positive bacteria.

As indicated in Tables 14-3 and 14-4, the majority of the causative microorganisms are part of the normal flora of the mouth and frequently enter the blood following dental manipulations. Many of the same organisms are found as part of the normal flora of the nose (staphylococci, diphtheroids, viridans streptococci, saprophytic *Neisseria*), the nasopharynx (viridans streptococci, saprophytic *Neisseria*, pneumococci, *Hemophilus influenzae*), the skin (staphylococci, micrococci, *Candida*, *Aspergillus*, *Mucor*, and gram-negative bacteria that are more commonly found in the large intestine), and the large intestine (enterococci, *Bacillus* species, *Escherichia*, *Enterobacter*, *Klebsiella*, *Proteus*, *Pseudomonas*, *Alcaligenes*, *Mima*, *Bacteroides*, *Candida*). Further discussion of the role of these microorganisms in infective endocarditis will be found in the section on pathogenesis.

With respect to the 10 to 20 percent of cases of infective endocarditis with negative cultures, it is probable that the causative agents might be recovered by improved cultural methods (note the results in Table 14-4), including methods favorable for the growth of fungi. The magnitude of the role played by viruses in endocarditis awaits clarification.

Relative Mortality Following Chemotherapy Since untreated cases are invariably fatal, regardless of the causative agent, it is not quite accurate to speak of pathogenicity or virulence of the organism. There are, however, differences in the duration of survival in untreated cases depending upon the infecting microorganism. Infections due to group A streptococci, staphylococci, pneumococci, and meningococci usually are more fulminating.

Following therapy with appropriate antibiotics the mortality rate varies appreciably depending upon the causative agent. Even with ideal treatment, the mortality in enterococcal and staphylococcal endocarditis may approach 50 percent. On the other hand, the mortality in viridans streptococcal endocarditis may be only 10 to 15 percent. The differences in mortality are generally ascribed to the sensitivity of the

Table 14-4 Isolation of Bacteria from the Blood after Dental Extractions without Chemoprophylaxis

Group	Organism and number of times isolated	Total
Aerobic bacteria	Viridans streptococci (34), corynebacteria (21), saprophytic *Neisseria* (4), *Staphylococcus aureus* (2), beta-hemolytic streptococci (2), *S. epidermidis* (1), *Micrococcus* (1), enterococcus (1), *Klebsiella* (1)	67
Anaerobic bacteria	*Bacteroides* (22), anaerobic streptococci (17), fusiform bacilli (3), *Veillonella* (2), corynebacteria (2)	46
Anaerobic bacteria (+5% CO_2)	Corynebacteria (16), viridans streptococci (9), anaerobic streptococci (7), fusiform bacilli (5)	37
Aerobic bacteria (+5% CO_2)	Corynebacteria (3), viridans streptococci (1), fusiform bacilli (1)	5
		155

Source: Adapted from O. Khairat, *J. Clin. Pathol.*, 19:561–566, 1966.

Note: The isolations were obtained from 100 normal patients. No cases of endocarditis were associated with the bacteremias.

Table 14-5 Incidence of Microorganisms in Cases of Infective Endocarditis before and after the Introduction of Antibiotics

Causative agent	Percent of cases during preantibiotic era	Percent of cases during antibiotic era
Viridans streptococci	60 to 88	19 to 51
Coagulase-positive staphylococci	1.5 to 6	15 to 39
Enterococci	0 to 6.5	8 to 30
Pneumococci	8 to 12	1
Gonococci	4 to 10	Extremely rare
Microaerophilic and anaerobic streptococci	Unknown	1 to 13

microorganism to antibiotics and the duration of the disease prior to the initiation of treatment but may reflect in part the pathogenicity and virulence of the microorganism in certain cases (i.e., staphylococci).

The Changing Nature of the Causative Agents

Some of the major shifts in the etiology of infective endocarditis are indicated in the data included in Table 14-5. The trends that have become apparent are continuing and may well be extended. For example, within the antibiotic era, viridans streptococci are less commonly encountered (Table 14-5) even though they remain the principal causative agent in endocarditis occurring in patients with rheumatic heart disease. For example, in one series, between 1944 and 1958, 71 percent of patients had rheumatic heart disease whereas only 46 percent did between 1958 and 1964. During these two periods, viridans streptococci accounted for 51 and 39 percent of all cases, respectively. With the accelerated decline in the incidence and severity of rheumatic carditis, viridans streptococci will undoubtedly continue to decline as causative agents in infective endocarditis. On the other hand, coagulase-positive staphylococci have become more and more prevalent as causative agents since the introduction of antibiotics, and the trend shows no sign of leveling off. The increasing incidence of enterococci in infective endocarditis, especially in older men following urinary catheterization and infection or surgery of the urinary tract, has been amply documented. As the population at risk becomes older, enterococci will probably continue to increase in importance in the etiology of endocarditis.

The sharp decline in the incidence of pneumococcal and gonococcal endocarditis within the antibiotic era is largely due to the efficacy of penicillin in the treatment of pneumococcal pneumonia and gonorrhea which precede the endocarditis in most cases.

Several recent reports have commented on the rising proportion of endocarditis associated with infection by microaerophilic and anaerobic streptococci, but no satisfactory explanation that would account for this observation has been provided.

There has been, in addition, increasing recognition of the role of coagulase-negative staphylococci and opportunistic, as well as pathogenic, fungi in infective endocarditis. Coagulase-negative staphylococcal endocarditis is prominent as a complication of cardiac surgery. Mycotic endocarditis due to opportunistic *Candida, Aspergillus, Rhodotorula,* and *Mucor* is found in patients receiving protracted antibiotic or steroid therapy, immunosuppressive drugs, those subjected to cardiac surgery and "main-line" (using heroin or morphine intravenously) narcotic addicts. In the case of *Histoplasma, Blastomyces, Coccidioides,* and *Cryptococcus,* endocarditis may occur as a manifestation of disseminated mycotic disease.

The infrequent association of the common Enterobacteriaceae with endocarditis is surprising in view of the increased frequency with which bacteremia caused by these organisms occurs following urinary tract infections (Chap. 18) and because such persons often have thrombotic, nonbacterial valvular lesions considered to be the site in which endocarditis often develops. Gram-negative bacteria (Enterobacteriaceae and others) are the causative agents in about 1 to 3 percent of cases of endocarditis at present.

Biological Properties of Viridans Streptococci Viridans streptococci in addition to producing alpha hemolysis are not inhibited by bacitracin or optochin and are not virulent for mice. They are prominent as members of the normal flora of the human mouth.

Biological Properties of Enterococci Enterococci are normal inhabitants of the human intestinal tract. The group-specific D antigen is a glycerol teichoic acid composed of alpha glycerophosphate polymers with additional substituents of sugars and D-alanine. In addition to possession of the group D antigen and showing variable hemolysis, enterococci can grow at 10 and 45°C and in 6.5 percent sodium chloride broth, are not inhibited by bacitracin or optochin, and are not virulent for mice. Recently, hydrolysis of esculin (a glucoside) has replaced other tests in the preliminary identification of enterococci.

Pathogenesis

Predisposing Factors Infective endocarditis frequently occurs in patients with rheumatic, congenital, arteriosclerotic, or syphilitic valvular disease. In the preantibiotic era it was estimated that 10 to 20 percent of patients with rheumatic heart disease would sooner or later acquire endocarditis and die of the infection. Before the advent of cardiac surgery an equivalent proportion of patients with congenital heart disease developed infective endocarditis. With the rapid decline in the incidence and severity of rheumatic and syphilitic valvular disease in the antibiotic era and with the surgical correction of congenital valvular lesions, arteriosclerotic valvular disease may well become the major underlying factor in the pathogenesis of infective endocarditis in the near future.

As indicated by the information included in Table 14-6, a variety of major and minor surgical procedures as well as extracardiac infections and severe trauma are commonly associated with the initiation of infective endocarditis.

Portal of Entry Although the portal of entry is often not apparent, there can be little doubt that in the majority of cases microorganisms enter the blood following injury in the oral cavity, the skin, the large intestine, and the urinary tract. The normal flora of the mouth, the skin, and the large intestine are the principal sources of the infecting organisms (Tables 14-3 and 14-4). The urinary tract is normally sterile, but in infected persons the microorganisms are derived predominantly from the large intestine (Chap. 18). Thus, of the prevalent causative agents, viridans streptococci enter the blood from the oral cavity where they are present in large numbers, staphylococci enter by way of the skin or skin lesions, and enterococci are derived from the large intestine or from infections of the urinary tract. Illustrative of the various portals of entry is the frequency of endocarditis due to viridans streptococci in children and in adults with underlying rheumatic valvular disease following dental manipulation, the incidence of staphylococcal endocarditis in "main-line" narcotic addicts (15 of 16 were caused by staphylococci in one series), and the proportion of cases caused by enterococci in older men following urinary catheterization or infection of the urinary tract.

The Development of Endocarditis and Other Manifestations The deposition of microorganisms usually occurs at the site of structural change or abnormality probably as a consequence of altered hemodynamics which cause marked changes in the vascular endothelium. Infection primarily involves the left side of the heart and the mitral valve more commonly than the aortic valve. The importance of preceding valvular lesions in the pathogenesis of endocarditis may be illustrated indirectly by the fact that no cases of endocarditis occurred in 100 normal young patients from whom 155 microorganisms were isolated from the blood following dental extractions (Table 14-4).

Table 14-6 Predisposing Factors in Infective Endocarditis

Major underlying factors	Chronic rheumatic valvular disease
	Congenital cardiac lesions, especially intraventricular septal defects and patent ductus arteriosus
	Aortic valvular disease (arteriosclerosis)
Less common underlying factor	Syphilitic valvular disease
Common initiating factors	Tooth extractions, oral surgical procedures, manipulation of periodontal tissue
	Surgical removal of tonsils and adenoids
	Bronchoscopy
	Urinary catheterization, infection, or surgery
	Extensive abdominal and skin surgery for cancer
	Extracardiac infections
	Cardiac catheterization and surgery
	Severe trauma
Occasional initiating factors	Parturition or abortion
	Protracted use of antibiotics, steroids, immunosuppressive drugs, radiotherapy, intravenous infusions
	Hemodialysis
	Burns
	"Main-line" narcotic addiction (intravenous use of heroin or morphine)
	Insect bites

The lodgement and growth of the microorganism on the damaged valve is followed by the deposition of fibrin and platelets at the site, producing a vegetation. There may be marked destruction of the valve substance with perforation, or large friable or polypoid vegetation may develop with only slight cellular reaction. The infection may extend from the valve to the endocardium. The healing process after successful therapy is slow and consists of gradual fibrosis, calcification, and endothelialization after many months.

If the disease progresses, emboli derived from the vegetations may be propelled throughout the bloodstream and lodge in the spleen, kidneys, brain, and other tissues. Petechial lesions (acute vasculitis) may develop anywhere on the skin and in the mucosa of the mouth, pharynx, or conjunctiva. Cardiac murmurs may develop or there may be major changes in the cardiac murmurs noted at onset. Myocardial infarction may occur. Perforation may result in profound valvular insufficiency.

In untreated cases death is due to infection in 64 percent, to emboli in 14 percent, and to congestive heart failure following perforation in 12 percent. In treated cases in whom the infection has been eradicated congestive heart failure is the leading cause of disability and death (61 percent). Only 16 percent of the deaths in treated patients are associated with infection, and 8 percent are associated with emboli. When perforation occurs, the aortic valve is involved about twice as frequently as the mitral valve.

In treated cases relapses (less than 6 months after completion of treatment) are extremely rare. Recurrences (more than 6 months after completion of treatment), however, are relatively common and may develop in 2 to 4 percent.

Laboratory Diagnosis

Recognition of infective endocarditis in the laboratory depends upon recovery and identification of the microorganism from the blood. Three to five samples of blood (10 ml), obtained at hourly intervals or intervals of several hours, are cultured as 5 percent suspensions in broth incubated aerobically and anaerobically in 5 to 10 percent carbon dioxide both at room temperature and at 37°C. The cultures should be examined at periodic intervals and kept for 3 weeks before discarding as negative. Addition of polyanethol sulfonate (0.05 percent) to blood broth is widely used because it significantly increases the ability to obtain positive cultures and may be supplemented by 30 percent sucrose when attempts are made to recover spheroplasts, protoplasts, or L-forms.

Although the cultural procedure will lead to recovery of certain fungi *(Candida)* from the blood, it is unsuited to the isolation of other fungi. Despite their limited involvement it might be desirable to inoculate media more suitable to the isolation of fungi (glucose agar) as a routine procedure. Certainly, however, fungal cultures should be employed in patients with endocarditis following protracted use of antibiotics, steroids, immunosuppressive drugs, those subjected to cardiac surgery, in "main-line" narcotic addicts, and in patients with associated systemic mycotic disease. At present, attempts to isolate other agents are limited to those who have concomitant disease along with the endocarditis.

Epidemiology

Incidence In the preantibiotic era infective endocarditis was invariably fatal. Consequently, autopsy data provided an accurate indication of the prevalence of the disease. However, the incidence in the antibiotic era is difficult to determine because endocarditis is not a reportable disease. Since many patients with the disease are treated by the family physician in the community hospital, comparison of the incidence of endocarditis in university hospitals before and after the introduction of antibiotics should be interpreted with caution.

Two conflicting trends are affecting the incidence of the disease. On the one hand, the sharp decline in the incidence of rheumatic and syphilitic valvular disease together with the surgical correction of congenital cardiac defects are operating to significantly reduce the incidence of endocarditis; on the other hand, the steady increase in the age of the population at risk is paralleled by a significant increase in arteriosclerotic aortic valvular disease and a higher incidence of endocarditis in older individuals.

Age The age distribution of endocarditis in the preantibiotic era revealed that between 2 and 13 percent of the cases occurred in those over 60 years of age. In the antibiotic era, there has been an increasing shift to older individuals with 12 to 60 percent of the cases in those over 60 years of age, and the trend shows no sign of leveling off. The average age of patients with endocarditis has increased to 40 to 55 years compared with 30 to 39 years in the preantibiotic era.

Mortality Since the introduction of antibiotics there has been a significant decline in the total number of deaths due to endocarditis, but a significant increase in both the number and the proportion of deaths in those over 60 years of age (Table 14-7). In Great Britain between 1954 and 1963, when the number of deaths remained constant at 350 per year, the number of deaths in those over 60 years of age rose from 105 to 165 per year, and the proportion rose from 30 to 47 percent. The median age of death has increased from 39 to 55 years, and deaths in older persons are primarily associated with valvular perforation leading to valvular insufficiency and congestive heart failure (Table 14-7), often occurring after the microorganism causing the endocarditis has been eradicated.

Factors Affecting Prognosis The prognosis of infective endocarditis in the antibiotic era is determined by a complex of many independent and dependent factors. With ideal treatment, the survival of the patient is influenced by the date of recognition, the nature of the infecting organism, the age of the patient, the nature and extent of valvular damage, and the nature and extent of extracardiac disease (Table 14-8).

Early recognition of endocarditis is the single most important factor affecting the survival of the patient. Blood cultures should be taken on each patient with persistent fever of a week or more, whether explained or not. It is unfortunate that between 5 and 25 percent of cases are unrecognized during life. The common pitfalls in failing to establish the clinical diagnosis of endocarditis are the presence of an unrelated disease thought to be the only disease present, the absence of heart murmurs or embolic phenomena, and failure to understand the significance of a complication of the disease such as the frequent occurrence of mental aberration in the older patient. The most common cause of delay in diagnosis, especially in subacute cases, is the similarity of the early stage of endocarditis to everyday illness ("virus" infection) and, to a lesser extent, to the finding of low-grade fever in disseminated cancer which may be present concomitantly. If the physician's level of suspicion is raised by the persistence of fever to the extent that cultures are taken (especially in the older patient without cardiac murmurs), earlier recognition of the disease will be achieved, and the prognosis will be improved.

Prevention and Control

General Aspects Prevention and control of infective endocarditis are based primarily on (1) the prevention of the major underlying factors that predispose to the disease, (2) prompt and effective treatment of those acute infectious diseases which may be complicated by endocarditis, and (3) chemoprophylaxis of persons most likely to develop the disease. With one excep-

Table 14-7 Changes in Mortality Due to Infective Endocarditis

Finding	Preantibiotic era	Antibiotic era	Trend
Great Britain			
Reported deaths per year			
Total	1,000	350	Declining (65%)
Under 60 years of age	870	185	Declining (80%)
Over 60 years of age	130	165	*Increasing* (27%)
Philadelphia General Hospital			
Deaths per 1,000 autopsies	16.9	9.2	Declining (45%)*
Cause of death			
Infection	64%	16%	Declining
Emboli	14%	8%	Declining
Perforation	15%	64.5%	*Increasing*
Congestive heart failure	12%	61%	*Increasing*
Median age at death	39 years	55 years	*Increasing*

* $P < 0.001$.

Source: Adapted from data (editorial), *Lancet*, 1:605–606, 1967; and from M. J. Robinson and J. Ruedy, *Am. J. Med.*, 32:922–928, 1962.

tion (arteriosclerotic aortic valvular disease), remarkable progress has been achieved in the antibiotic era.

Endocarditis as an immediate or remote consequence of acute infectious disease (group A streptococci, pneumococci, gonococci, syphilis) has been, or is increasingly being, brought under control. Effective treatment and chemoprophylaxis of group A streptococcal infections has led to a sharp decrease in rheumatic heart disease and infective endocarditis. Prompt treatment of syphilis, gonorrhea, and pneumococcal pneumonia has prevented the development of endocarditis as a complication. Surgical repairs of congenital cardiac defects has removed another of the factors which predispose to endocarditis. Arteriosclerotic aortic valvular disease alone remains as the major problem in the pre-

Table 14-8 Survival of Patients with Infective Endocarditis Following Ideal Antibiotic Treatment

	Approximate percent of patients surviving	
Causative agent		
Viridans streptococci	85	
Microaerophilic and anaerobic streptococci	80	
Staphylococci	50	
Enterococci	50	
Fungi	25	
Type of heart disease		
Congenital	83	
Without congestive failure	70	
Sclerosing aortitis in narcotic addicts	50	
Congestive failure	37	
Arteriosclerotic and syphilitic	17	
All types	54	
Presence of emboli	40	
Duration of symptoms (all cases)		
More than 4 weeks*	68	
Less than 4 weeks	39	
Duration of symptoms	SBE*	All cases
Less than 2 weeks	90	75
Between 2 and 8 weeks	83	75*
More than 8 weeks	74	75*
Age of patient		
Under 20 years	76	
Over 20 years	49	
Under 60 years	84	
Over 60 years	50	
Five years after discharge from hospital	82	

* A significant proportion of these cases are caused by viridans streptococci.

Source: Based on a number of sources, including W. R. Vogler, E. R. Dorney, and H. A. Bridges, *Am. J. Med.*, 32:910–921, 1962; M. M. Uwaydah and A. N. Weinberg, *N. Engl. J. Med.*, 273:1231–1234, 1965; E. S. Cooper, J. W. Cooper, and T. G. Schnabel, Jr., *Arch. Intern. Med.*, 118:55–61, 1966 (copyright 1966, American Medical Association); P. I. Lerner and L. N. Weinstein, *N. Engl. J. Med.*, 274:199–205, 1966.

vention and control of endocarditis as well as one of the most important problems confronting medicine today.

When endocarditis develops, the main props of effective control are (1) early diagnosis, (2) prompt and effective treatment with cidal antibiotics, and (3) careful attention to the early recognition and surgical correction of valvular insufficiency or mycotic vegetations.

Chemoprophylaxis As currently employed by the physician, chemoprophylaxis is based on the prevention of endocarditis in individuals with rheumatic or congenital heart disease. The purpose of antibiotics is (1) to prevent bacteremia, (2) to reduce its magnitude and duration should it occur, and (3) to eradicate organisms that may implant on damaged heart valves before a vegetation is formed.

Chemoprophylaxis preceding dental manipulation, oropharyngeal surgery, or bronchoscopy is designed largely to prevent endocarditis due to viridans streptococci and involves the use of penicillin before and subsequent to the surgical procedure. Procaine penicillin (600,000 units) plus crystalline penicillin G (600,000 units) are administered 1 to 2 hr. before surgery, and 600,000 units of procaine penicillin are given intramuscularly for 2 days after surgery. An alternate method involves the use of oral penicillin [alphaphenoxyethyl penicillin V, alphaphenoxyethyl penicillin (phenethicillin) or buffered penicillin G] five times in doses of 0.25 Gm on the day of surgery and four times daily for 2 days after surgery. In patients who are sensitive to penicillin, erythromycin is recommended, 250 mg by mouth four times daily for 3 days for adults and older children and 20 mg per pound of body weight divided into three or four doses for young children (not exceeding a total of 1 Gm per day).

Chemoprophylaxis preceding urinary catheterization, lower abdominal surgery, and childbirth is designed largely to prevent endocarditis due to enterococci. The dose of penicillin used for viridans streptococci is not adequate to prevent enterococcal endocarditis and must be supplemented by 1 to 2 Gm of streptomycin on the day of and for 2 days after the procedure in adults (50 mg/kg of body weight in children not to exceed 1 Gm per day). In sensitive patients, erythromycin is substituted for penicillin.

Chemoprophylaxis preceding and following other procedures must be based largely on clinical judgment. There would, for example, appear to be less danger associated with failure to use chemoprophylaxis for patients undergoing cardiac surgery due to the prevalence of staphylococcal and fungal superinfection than with the use of antibiotics to which these microorganisms are resistant.

Treatment Treatment must be based on the sensitivity of the causative microorganism and on the use of a cidal antibiotic, whenever possible, and must be of sufficient duration to prevent relapse and recurrence of the disease. For viridans streptococci, 6 to 12 million units of penicillin daily for 28 days or longer (intramuscularly or intravenously) are associated with a cure rate approaching 90 percent. In enterococcal endocarditis, most cases respond to a combination of penicillin and streptomycin but the dose of penicillin may have to be raised to 60 million units or more per day along with 1 Gm of streptomycin, or "tailor-made" drug combinations may be required possibly by adding erythromycin or bacitracin to the basic regimen. The treatment of staphylococcal endocarditis presents special problems. If the staphylococcus is sensitive, penicillin is the drug of choice. Since most staphylococci are resistant to penicillin (and other antibiotics as well), treatment must be based on sensitivity of the causative culture as determined by adequate laboratory tests. Penicillinase-resistant penicillins (oxacillin, methicillin, cloxacillin), cephalothin, lincomycin, and combined therapy have all been successful in selected cases.

For gram-negative microorganisms, mixtures

of drugs are occasionally required (streptomycin and polymyxin along with a broad-spectrum antibiotic), but treatment should be based largely on the sensitivity of the causative agent. Treatment of fungal endocarditis is generally unsatisfactory, but amphotericin B is useful in selected cases. Surgery is often indicated, and successful, in removing large fungal vegetations, especially those following cardiac surgery or intravenous use of heroin or morphine. Mixed infections require the use in most instances of combinations of drugs to which the organisms are sensitive. Microaerophilic and anaerobic streptococci are usually effectively treated by the same drugs and dosages that are used in the treatment of viridans streptococci. In all cases, however, the clinical response determines the future course of treatment.

In clinically diagnosed cases of endocarditis in which cultures remain negative, the treatment program must be based on the use of drugs that will be likely to produce an effective response to staphylococci or enterococci as well as to viridans streptococci and should be based on the preceding course of the disease. If the onset of the disease is acute, initial treatment should be based on the use of penicillinase resistant penicillins, cephalothin, or lincomycin. If the disease is more insidious in onset, penicillin (50 to 60 million units) and streptomycin (2 Gm/day) are recommended before changing treatment on the basis of the clinical response.

PNEUMOCOCCAL PNEUMONIA

Despite the remarkable progress achieved in the past 30 years (Table 14-9), pneumococcal pneumonia remains one of the major causes of morbidity and mortality in the United States today and throughout the world as well. It is estimated that between 9,000 and 18,000 deaths occur annually in the United States as a result of infection with the six most prevalent types of pneumococcus (types 1, 7, 8, 4, 3, 12).

The pneumococcus is a normal inhabitant of the nasopharynx. Following damage to the anatomical and physiological barriers that normally protect the lungs from microorganisms, pneumococci may be carried to the alveoli in droplets of saliva or mucus and initiate infection. Having reached the lungs, pneumococci produce disease by virtue of their possession of a type-specific polysaccharide capsule which inhibits phagocytosis and thus permits the organisms to grow without restriction until the defenses of the host are mobilized, until type-specific antibodies are produced, or until penicillin therapy is begun (Table 14-9).

The Causative Agent

Biological Properties The pneumococcus (*Diplococcus pneumoniae* or *Streptococcus pneumoniae*) is a gram-positive, encapsulated, ovoid or lancet-shaped coccus, arranged in pairs or short chains when stained. On blood agar, pneumococcal colonies are usually smooth or mucoid and surrounded by a zone of alpha hemolysis. Pneumococci are inhibited by optochin (a synthetic detergent, ethylhydrocupreine hydrochloride) disks in a concentration of 1:500,000 or 1:100,000 and are virulent for mice.

Antigenic Structure The capsular substances of the pneumococci are complex polysaccharides which are responsible for virulence, for type-specific immunity, and for differentiation of the organisms into about 80 serotypes. Chemically, the capsular polysaccharides (soluble-specific substances) are high molecular weight compounds (140,000 to 500,000) containing galacturonic acid, N-acetylglucosamine, and acetic acid (type 1); D-glucose, D-glucuronic acid, and L-rhamnose (type 2); glucuronic acid and glucose (type 3). They are potent antigens in man but act as haptens in the rabbit.

The classical series of experiments that demonstrated that synthesis of capsular polysaccharides was under the control of DNA established

Table 14-9 Bacteremia and Mortality According to Age, Therapy, and Complications in Pneumococcal Pneumonia

Age (years)	Therapy (percent mortality) in positive blood cultures (all types)			Penicillin therapy (percent mortality)		Percent mortality (all types)			
						With complications		Without complications	
	Untreated	Serum	Penicillin	Positive blood cultures*	Negative blood cultures*	Untreated	Penicillin	Untreated	Penicillin
12–29	66	26	6	8	0.6				
30–49	75	49	8	9	3.0				
50+	93	64	20	30	20.0				
Totals	80	45	17	13	9.6	92	27	79	6

* Only the most prevalent types (types 1, 7, 8, 4, 3, 12).
Source: Adapted from R. C. Tilghman and M. Finland, *Arch. Intern. Med.*, 59:602–619, 1937; and from R. Austrian and J. Gold, *Ann. Intern. Med.*, 60:759–776, 1964.

the molecular basis of genetics (see section on transformation in Chap. 3). Encapsulated pneumococci are virulent because the capsular polysaccharide mechanically inhibits phagocytosis. Pneumococci that have lost their capsules are avirulent, but retain their viability.

Under special circumstances where phagocytes can pin the pneumococci against a rough surface, phagocytosis may occur in the absence of specific antibody (see discussion of surface phagocytosis in Chap. 6). Phagocytosis is greatly enhanced in the presence of specific antibody. Thus, immunity is type-specific since phagocytosis is the primary way in which encapsulated pneumococci are killed.

Pathogenesis

At any given time virulent (encapsulated) pneumococci may be present in the nasopharynx of 5 to 60 percent of the population without causing disease. Pneumococcal pneumonia may occasionally occur following viral infection of the upper respiratory tract (especially influenza) which apparently modifies the anatomical and physiological barriers that normally prevent the pneumococci from reaching the lung. Virus infection may exert its effect by destroying the ciliated epithelial cells of the respiratory tract, by decreasing the viscosity of the mucus, by impairing the cough reflex, or by a combination of these factors. The frequency of pneumococcal pneumonia in patients with underlying cardiac disease, cirrhosis, carcinoma, or nephritis, especially in those over 50 years of age, suggests that other unknown factors may be involved in pathogenesis.The development of pneumococcal pneumonia is associated with marked edema of the alveolar walls, rapid spreading of the edema fluid containing the multiplying pneumococci through the bronchioles and bronchi, filling of the alveoli with a fibrinous exudate in which bacterial multiplication is limited by surface phagocytosis (Chap. 6), and consolidation which may involve large segments of one or more lobes but is not accompanied by necrosis. During the stage of spreading pulmonary infection pneumococci enter the blood by way of the lymphatics, producing a transient or a continued bacteremia. Persistence of pneumococci in the blood occurs in about 25 percent of cases (529 out of 2,000 in a recent series), reflects poor localization of the pneumonic process, and is a poor prognostic sign (Table 14-9).

The outcome is dependent upon the rate at which pneumococci multiply and spread to new areas and the ability of the host to immobilize and destroy them by surface phagocytosis or, later on, by greatly enhanced phagocytosis in the presence of specific antibody. If the infection is arrested by the natural forces of the host or by the intervention of penicillin therapy, the alveolar exudate undergoes liquefaction, the process resolves presumably by lymphatic removal of the inflammatory debris, and the lung returns to normal within a few days.

Clinically, the disease characteristically has an abrupt onset with a sudden shaking chill, sharp pleuritic pain, and cough, productive of blood-tinged (rusty) mucoid sputum within a few hours. In untreated cases that recover, there is sustained fever, pleuritic pain, cough, and sputum for 7 to 10 days followed by abrupt and dramatic improvement (crisis). In fatal cases, extensive pulmonary involvement, dyspnea, cyanosis, and tachycardia are prominent. Circulatory collapse is common.

Serious complications prior to the initiation of therapy may be present in about 7.5 percent of bacteremic cases, two-thirds of whom subsequently die. In order of frequency, the complications associated with increased mortality are meningitis (Chap. 24), endocarditis (this chapter), pulmonary embolus, arthritis, and peritonitis. Meningitis is present in about 1 percent of all cases of pneumococcal pneumonia and in 4 percent of bacteremic cases prior to therapy; endocarditis in 0.4 percent of all cases and 1.7 percent of bacteremic cases. Extrapulmonary infection after the start of penicillin therapy is virtually unknown.

Laboratory Diagnosis

A laboratory diagnosis of pneumococcal pneumonia depends upon (1) demonstration of large numbers of typical organisms in Gram-stained smears of emulsified sputum, (2) a positive capsular swelling (Quellung) test on unstained sputum in the presence of type-specific antibody, (3) isolation and identification of the organism on blood agar plates, and (4) demonstration of pathogenicity for mice.

Blood cultures should be routinely employed as a useful guide to prognosis.

Epidemiology

Source Pneumococci are normal inhabitants of the human nasopharynx and are regularly present in 5 to 60 percent of the population at any given time, more commonly in the winter. The types most commonly found in the nasopharynx are usually the most prevalent in causing pneumococcal pneumonia. In adults, types 1, 3, 4, 7, 8, and 12 are prevalent, with type 3 being most prevalent. In children, types 1, 5, 6, 7, 14, and 19 are often found.

Incidence In the absence of exact data, it is difficult to assess the morbidity and mortality of pneumococcal pneumonia. It is estimated that there may be 150,000 to 300,000 cases of pneumococcal pneumonia annually in the United States with as many as 15,000 to 30,000 deaths, 60 percent of which are due to types 1, 7, 8, 4, 3, and 12. In one careful study between 1952 and 1962, 2,000 cases of pneumococcal pneumonia were found in a 225-bed county hospital affiliated with an urban university medical service.

The age distribution of morbidity and mortality follows a U-shaped curve that falls sharply in the first year of life, remains in a low trough for 3 decades, and gradually rises with increasing age to a much higher level. The two most prevalent types present striking contrasts. Type 1 is associated with a mortality of 3 percent, while type 3 causes a mortality of 22 percent. Only one-third of type 1 infections occur in persons over 50 years of age, but two-thirds of type 3 infections occur in persons over 50 years of age.

The seasonal peak of morbidity and mortality in pneumococcal pneumonia can best be explained by its dependence upon preceding viral infection of the upper respiratory tract during the winter. The association of morbidity and mortality of pneumococcal pneumonia with epidemics of influenza is a striking and predictable finding (Chap. 20).

Prevention and Control

Treatment Prevention and control of pneumococcal pneumonia are based largely on penicillin therapy and to a lesser extent on the use of vaccines to prevent the occurrence of influenza (Chap. 20), measles and smallpox (Chap. 22), and other viral infections involving the respiratory tract (Chap. 20). As indicated by the data included in Table 14-9, remarkable progress has been achieved. Nonetheless, despite penicillin therapy, pneumococcal pneumonia remains as a frequent and serious disease in those over 50 years of age (Table 14-9).

Pneumococcal pneumonia is best treated with 600,000 units per day of injectable penicillin which is continued until the patient has been afebrile for 2 to 3 days. The response is rapid, and relapse does not occur. For pneumococcal meningitis (Chap. 24) and pneumococcal endocarditis (this chapter) massive doses of penicillin are required over an extended period.

Immunization A strong case can be made for the use of a vaccine containing purified pneumococcal polysaccharides (types 1, 7, 8, 4, 3, and 12) in persons over 50 years of age with systemic disease (cardiac disease, cirrhosis, carcinoma, or nephritis). Pneumococcal polysaccharides are potent antigens in man and in the past have been shown to significantly reduce morbidity and mortality of pneumococcal pneumonia in those over 50 years of age. For example, 33 cases of pneumococcal pneumonia (types 1, 2, 3) occurred in 5,153 unvaccinated persons, while only 3 cases (types 1, 2, 3) occurred in 5,750 persons immunized with types 1, 2, and 3 polysaccharides.

If a vaccine containing the six pneumococcal polysaccharides (types 1, 7, 8, 4, 3, 12) is employed, capsular typing of pneumococcal isolations will be imperative to monitor any change in the spectrum of types causing clinical disease.

BIBLIOGRAPHY

Austrian, R., and Gold, J.: "Pneumococcal Bacteremia with Especial Reference to Bacteremic Pneumococcal Pneumonia," *Ann. Intern. Med.*, 60:759-776, 1964.

Bernheimer, A. W., Kim, K. S., Remsen, C. C., Antanavage, J., and Watson, S. W.: "Factors Affecting Interaction of Staphylococcal Alpha Toxin with Membranes," *Infect. Immun.*, 6:636-642, 1972.

Berry, F. A., Jr., Yarbrough, S., Yarbrough, N., Russell, C. M., Carpenter, M. A., and Hendley, J. O.: "Transient Bacteremia during Dental Manipulation in Children." *Pediatrics*, 51:476-479, 1973.

Bisno, A. L., Nelson, K. E., Waytz, P., and Brunt, J.: "Factors Influencing Serum Antibody Responses in Streptococcal Pyoderma," *J. Lab. Clin. Med.*, 81:410-420, 1973.

Dajani, A. S.: "The Scalded-Skin Syndrome: Relation to Phage-Group II Staphylococci," *J. Infect. Dis.*, 125:548-551, 1972.

Douglas, R. M., and Devitt, L.: "Pneumonia in New Guinea. II. Pneumococcal Serotypes and the Possible Utility of Polyvalent Vaccines of Capsular Polysaccharides," *Med. J. Aust.*, 1:49-52, 1973.

Dowling, J. N., Sheehe, P. R., and Feldman, H. A.: "Pharyngeal Pneumococcal Acquisitions in 'Normal' Families: A Longitudinal Study," *J. Infect. Dis.*, 124:9-17, 1971.

Finland, M.: "Excursions into Epidemiology: Selected Studies during the Past Four Decades at Boston City Hospital," *J. Infect. Dis.,* 128:76-124, 1973.

Ginsburg, I.: "Mechanisms of Cell and Tissue Injury Induced by Group A Streptococci: Relation to Poststreptococcal Sequelae," *J. Infect. Dis.,* 126: 294-340, 419-456, 1972.

Hapte-Gabr, E., January, L. E., and Smith, I. M: "Bacterial Endocarditis: The Need for Early Diagnosis," *Geriatrics,* 28(3):164-170, 1973.

Maxted, W. R., Widdowson, J. P., Fraser, C. A. M., Ball, L. C., and Bassett, D. C. J.: "The Use of the Serum Opacity Reaction in the Typing of Group-A Streptococci," *J. Med. Microbiol.,* 6:83-90, 1973.

Robinson, M. J., Greenberg, J. J., Korn, M., and Rywlin, A. M.: "Infective Endocarditis at Autopsy: 1965-1969," *Am. J. Med.,* 52:492-498, 1972.

Rosenblatt, J. E., Dahlgren, J. G., Fishbach, R. S., and Tally, F. P.: "Gram-negative Bacterial Endocarditis in Narcotic Addicts," *Calif. Med.,* 118(2): 1-4, 1973.

Sheehe, P. R., and Feldman, H. A.: "Streptococcal Epidemics in Two Populations of 'Normal' Families," *J. Infect. Dis.,* 124:1-8, 1971.

Singh, G., Marples, R. R., and Kligman, A. M.: "Experimental *Staphylococcus aureus* Infections in Humans," *J. Invest. Dermatol.,* 57:149-162, 1971.

van der Vijver, J. C. M., van Es-Boon, M., and Michel, M. M.: "Lysogenic Conversion in *Staphylococcus aureus* to Leucocidin Production," *J. Virol.,* 10:318-320, 1972.

Wannamaker, L. W.: "Perplexity and Precision in the Diagnosis of Streptococcal Pharyngitis," *Am. J. Dis. Child.,* 124:352-358, 1972.

Chapter 15

Mycobacterial Infections

Bernard A. Briody

Tuberculosis
Other Mycobacteria Pathogenic for Man

TUBERCULOSIS

Perspective

No disease is more interwoven into the development of Western civilization than tuberculosis. In fact, the impact created by tuberculosis in the nineteenth century was pervasive. It has become an intimate part of our heritage, permanently recorded in many of our favorite operas, poems, and novels. In the nineteenth century, tuberculosis was a way of life—a sign of genius and ethereal beauty. Tuberculosis lent itself well as a theme for the creative artist, for despite the tragic outcome, tubercular patients were gay and optimistic to the end. It was truly "captain of the men of death."

Although its clinical features and communicability were known before 1000 B.C., the disease was not designated as tuberculosis (small nodule) until 1834 when Laennec recognized the basic pathology. Hippocratic physicians called the disease phthisis. In the Middle Ages and for centuries thereafter the disease had been known as consumption.

While little precise information was available until the nineteenth century, all evidence indicates that deaths due to tuberculosis reached a peak during the Industrial Revolution when large numbers of people moved from rural areas to cities. Since then there has been a steady decline in tuberculosis mortality in urban countries which was clearly evident before the advent of chemotherapy and preventive measures.

The Causative Agent

Biological Properties *Mycobacterium tuberculosis,* the organism causing tuberculosis, is a thin bacillus measuring about 0.4 μm in diameter and 3 μm in length. At times it may appear to be slightly curved and may exhibit granular staining.

M. tuberculosis is a strict parasite which as a

rule does not multiply naturally outside the infected host.

Cultivation Although egg yolk agar containing 5 percent glycerol is commonly employed for the isolation of the organism from clinical specimens, an oleic acid–albumin medium is equally effective. The generation time is long, 14 to 24 hr. Growth appears in about 2 weeks. The tubercle bacillus is a strict aerobe whose growth is enhanced in 2 to 10 percent carbon dioxide. Although smooth colonies may be encountered, typical colonies are rough, granular, and irregular in outline, resembling dry bread crumbs. Microscopically the stained organisms tend to adhere to each other in haphazard arrangements or in dense clumps.

When grown in oleic acid–albumin liquid media, *M. tuberculosis* characteristically forms long serpentine cords or parallel adherent chains of bacilli. This is probably a result of the presence of a toxic glycolipid *(cord factor)* which has been identified as trehalose-6,6′-dimycolate.

Staining The microorganism does not stain readily, but basic dyes are taken up after prolonged contact, after heating, or in the presence of surface-active agents. Once stained, tubercle bacilli are characteristically acid-fast; i.e., they resist decolorization by ethanol containing 3 percent hydrochloric acid. Acid-fastness is dependent on the integrity of the bacterial cell and on the presence of mycolic acid, a chloroform-soluble wax present in the cell wall.

Chemical Composition *M. tuberculosis* has a high lipid content (24 percent) and a low polysaccharide content (less than 1 percent). Partly because of their high lipid content, tubercle bacilli show a high degree of resistance to acids, alkalis, dyes, and antiseptics. The purified protein derivative (PPD), used in the tuberculin test, is actually a mixture of heat-stable proteins having molecular weights of 2,000 to 9,000. Wax D (mycolic acid-arabinogalactan-peptidoglycan complex), mycolic acid, and sulfolipids are important components of mycobacterial cell walls. Wax D enhances the immunogenicity of a variety of antigens (see Chap. 7).

Disinfection of materials containing tubercle bacilli can be effected by exposure to 70 to 80 percent ethanol, anionic detergents, heat, or radiation.

Types Today, almost all clinical cases of tuberculosis in the United States are caused by the human type of *M. tuberculosis.* In other countries *M. bovis,* formerly *M. tuberculosis* var. *bovis,* is responsible for a variable proportion of human infections following ingestion of unpasteurized milk. There are also other types that regularly produce disease in animals, and the avian type may rarely infect man. There are also saprophytic *Mycobacterium* species which may be mistaken for the human type of *M. tuberculosis.* An extensive literature describes the multiplicity of methods and tests that have been designed to distinguish between the various saprophytic and pathogenic mycobacteria. The usual criteria include ability to grow at 20°C, formation of niacin when grown on glycerol egg medium, and pathogenicity for guinea pigs (Table 15-1).

The rate of growth, the pigmentation of the colonies, and the response to glycerol serve as additional guides in identifying the particular *Mycobacterium* species. For example, the saprophytes grow much more rapidly than the pathogens (*M. fortuitum* excepted), the atypical mycobacteria are more brightly and deeply pigmented, and in the presence of glycerol the growth of the human type is much more luxuriant than *Mycobacterium bovis* which is inhibited by glycerol.

Antigenic Structure The antigenic structure of *M. tuberculosis* is not characteristic. *M. tuberculosis* and *M. bovis* are indistinguishable, and

Table 15-1 Some Reactions of Different Species of Pathogenic Mycobacteria

Type	Growth at 20°C	Formation of niacin	Pathogenicity for guinea pigs
M. tuberculosis	−	+	+
Isoniazid-resistant human	−	+	−
Other human mycobacteria	−	−	−
M. bovis	−	−	+
Saprophytes *(M. smegmatis)*	+	−	−

they show extensive cross-reactions with avian and murine mycobacteria. Many antigens of all these types are shared with other pathogenic and saprophytic species of mycobacteria as well as with organisms of the *Nocardia, Streptomyces,* and *Corynebacterium* groups. Failure to detect significant serological differences among the various mycobacteria is, thus, an exception to the rule that immunological reactivity is a much more sensitive method of differentiating closely related microorganisms than cultural procedures.

Pathogenesis and Natural History of the Disease

The Role of Bacterial Products Although it is held by some investigators that cord factor, neutral red-binding capacity, and catalase production are associated with virulence of tubercle bacilli for guinea pigs, definitive knowledge of the nature of virulence is both uncertain and incomplete. Among the biologically reactive components of tubercle bacilli, there are several which may function in the pathogenesis of the disease. For convenience these are listed in Table 15-2.

Pathology Following infection with *M. tuberculosis* the characteristic microscopic lesion seen is an avascular granuloma *(tubercle)* with associated caseation necrosis. The organism itself is characteristically located intracellularly in monocytes, reticuloendothelial cells, and giant cells. The tubercle consists of scattered Langhans giant cells, a midzone of epithelioid cells, and a peripheral zone of infiltrating fibroblasts, monocytes, lymphocytes, and plasma cells. When the reaction is predominantly cellular, as in chronic pulmonary tuberculosis, the lesion is said to be productive, or proliferative. When the alveolar spaces contain an exudate, the lesion is said to be exudative.

Exudative lesions proceed rapidly to caseation necrosis, which consists of a mixture of coagulated proteins and fatty materials with a cheesy appearance. Productive lesions progress much more slowly by enlargement, coalescence, caseation, softening, liquefaction, and eventually cavitation. The solid caseous material may persist for a long time without damage or may become surrounded by fibrous tissue. For obscure reasons, the lesion may soften and liquefy centrally or peripherally. The result of this process is the expulsion of the liquid contents through the bronchi, leaving a pulmonary cavity with a caseous lining and opening the way for bronchogenic spread of the disease as well as the excretion of the organism into the environment.

Intracellular Multiplication in Alveolar Phagocytes Infection is acquired by the inhalation of *droplet nuclei* that are coughed or sneezed into the air. Droplet nuclei are desiccated or semi-

Table 15-2 Biological Activity of Components of *Mycobacterium tuberculosis*

Component	Experimentally demonstrated biological activity
Cell walls	Induce resistance to infection, induce delayed hypersensitivity, increase reactivity of mice to endotoxin, and can replace whole organisms in Freund's adjuvant.
Proteins	Elicit the tuberculin reaction and when bound to a lipid fraction can induce delayed (tuberculin) hypersensitivity. Induce the formation of monocytes, macrophages, epithelioid cells and giant cells.
Polysaccharides	Induce immediate hypersensitivity, adsorb on to normal red blood cells, and cause exudation of neutrophils from the blood vessels into the tissues.
Lipids	Induce the formation of macrophages and cause exudation of neutrophils from the blood vessels into the tissues.
Phosphatides	Induce tubercles consisting of epithelioid cells and giant cells, sometimes accompanied by caseation necrosis.
Cord factor or toxic glycolipid (trehalose-6,6′-dimycolate)	Inhibits leukocytic migration. Lethal for mice when repeatedly injected in minute amounts (a single large dose is much less toxic).

desiccated particles about 1μm in diameter in which the organism is trapped. These particles have the capacity to reach the pulmonary alveoli. Larger particles are trapped by the ciliated epithelial cells, and particles that are smaller than 1μm are unlikely to contain tubercle bacilli.

The microorganisms lodge in the pulmonary alveoli, are quickly ingested by one or a few fixed mononuclear phagocytes in the alveolar duct, slowly begin intracellular multiplication, and eventually cause the infected cells to rupture. The organisms released are thus free to be engulfed by additional phagocytes, which accumulate in the area along with edema fluid. The cycle is repeated.

Specific Resistance After reaching the alveoli, the tubercle bacilli multiply slowly over a period of weeks, inducing allergy to tuberculin but without, as a rule, producing overt disease. In about 6 to 8 weeks, the multiplication of the organism is interrupted by the development in the host of a level of specific resistance; a few tubercle bacilli, however, manage to survive for the life of the individual without causing disease. This pattern is observed in about 95 percent of those infected with the organism.

Primary Infection in Children The age of the patient at the onset of infection exerts a strong influence on subsequent developments. In children, a single parenchymal focus of tuberculous pneumonia develops, usually in the lower lobe of the lung or the lower part of the upper lobe. Tubercle bacilli pass through the lymph channels to the regional hilar lymph nodes, multiply, and cause caseating lesions and enlargement of the lymph nodes. The parenchymal lesion and the lymph node focus are known as the *primary complex*, or *Ghon complex*.

Before spontaneous cure of the primary infection can ensue, two critical host responses develop more or less concomitantly: (1) altered reactivity to the proteins of the tubercle bacillus (tuberculin allergy) and (2) the development of a level of specific acquired resistance. This acquired resistance causes multiplication of the tubercle bacilli to halt. At this stage the primary complex becomes encapsulated by fibrous tissue. Calcification follows. It must be emphasized that primary infection of children ordinarily takes place without causing symptoms, and throughout the life of the individual the primary complex is essentially a radiological concept.

Primary Infection in Adults In primary infection of adults, the parenchymal lesion is located at the apex of the lung, possibly because when an upright posture is maintained the partial pressure of oxygen is higher at the apex than in other parts of the lung. Cavitation develops within the lesion, but there is no visible hilar node enlargement. The lesion commonly undergoes rapid healing without calcification. The primary lesion is often so similar to that seen in reinfection that only a history of recent conversion of the tuberculin reaction serves to distinguish it as a first infection.

Primary Disease In the rare instances when the level of specific acquired resistance is unable to retard the growth of tubercle bacilli in infected children, progression to clinical disease is rapid and uninterrupted. Primary tuberculosis in children under 5 years of age is characterized by hematogenous spread which results in scattered foci in the upper portions of the lungs and in the meninges, occasionally producing meningitis. Solitary or multiple lesions may also develop in the bones, kidneys, and other organs. In adults, clinical disease as a consequence of primary infection is very rare. When it does occur, the usual result is chronic pulmonary tuberculosis such as is seen following reinfection. When clinical disease follows immediately upon primary infection the incubation period is ordinarily 6 to 12 weeks.

Reinfection As a rule, after recovery from primary infection, tuberculin allergy and partial specific resistance remain, and a few tubercle bacilli may even survive for the life of the patient without causing disease. The balance, however, is precarious. Months or years after the primary infection has been considered quiescent or healed, there may be extension or reactivation of the disease (*postprimary progression* or *endogenous reinfection*). About 75 percent of all new cases of clinical tuberculosis result from postprimary progression. Less frequently, clinical disease may result from exogenous infection in a patient with a healing or healed older lesion, and extremely rarely it may follow exogenous infection in a patient with an active lesion (superinfection).

Regardless of the mechanism by which reinfection occurs, the lesion consists of one or more foci located most commonly in the subapical region. In most cases, the pulmonary lesion in adults heals by resorption or fibrosis and occasionally by calcification. If progression results, it occurs through contiguous spread, caseation, softening, liquefaction, and cavitation. The contents of the cavity are discharged, and the organisms spread through the bronchial tree to other parts of the lungs (bronchogenic spread). Access to oxygen in the cavity enables the tubercle bacilli to multiply readily. The organisms are liberated into the environment and may spread to the bronchi, trachea, larynx, oral cavity, and when they are swallowed, the intestine. Chronic pulmonary tuberculosis develops slowly over a period of years in a clinical course characterized by exacerbations, remissions, and relapses.

Summary

Primary infection
- Spontaneous cure: rapid — Common
  - Characterized by
    - Allergy to tuberculin in 3 to 10 weeks
    - A level of specific acquired resistance in 6 to 8 weeks
    - Calcification of the primary parenchymal pulmonary lesions and the involved lymph nodes usually occurs in children
    - Healing commonly proceeds without calcification and lymph node enlargement in adults

Tuberculous disease: rapid course	Rare
Characterized by	
Hematogenous spread	
Miliary tuberculosis	
Meningitis	
Greater frequency in children than in adults	
Reinfection: postprimary progression (endogenous) months or years after healing; exogenous infection in a patient with a healing or healed lesion; superinfection (exogenous infection in a patient with an active lesion)	
Spontaneous cure: slow	Common
Heals by resorption, fibrosis, and occasionally calcification	
Chronic pulmonary tuberculosis	Rare
Characterized by	
Exacerbations, remissions, and relapses	
Prominent, minor, or absent symptoms	
Bronchogenic spread	
Caseation, softening, liquefaction, and cavitation	
Liberation of tubercle bacilli into the environment	
Involvement of the bronchi, trachea, larynx, oral cavity, and, when organisms are swallowed, the intestine	
Acute with fatal outcome in a few months	Extremely rare

Laboratory Diagnosis

Surprisingly, more than 75 percent of the cases of clinical tuberculosis are moderately or far advanced when detected because of the absence or the minimal extent of symptoms. This is a particularly critical problem in the prevention and control of the disease. Without specific chemotherapy, 21 percent of patients with chronic pulmonary tuberculosis will be dead within 1 year after the diagnosis has been established, 54 percent will continue to excrete tubercle bacilli into the environment, and only 25 percent will be noninfectious at that time.

Isolation of Bacilli The demonstration of tubercle bacilli in clinical specimens is the one essential criterion in the definitive diagnosis of tuberculosis. The organism is found most commonly in the sputum of persons who have chronic pulmonary tuberculosis with a draining cavity. Occasionally, it may be isolated from pleural and spinal fluids, gastric washings, urine, and more rarely from other tissues and tissue fluids.

In practice, demonstration of the organism is accomplished by finding acid-fast bacilli in stained smears or by culturing the organism on glycerol egg yolk agar, or preferably by both procedures. Standard laboratory procedures include attempts to grow acid-fast bacilli at 20°C and to test for the formation of niacin, but efforts to isolate the organisms in guinea pigs are no longer performed. Clinical specimens, such as spinal, pleural, and joint fluids, that are not contaminated with other bacteria are best stained and cultured after sedimentation. When sputum, gastric washings, and other test materials are known to be contaminated, stained smears and cultures are best prepared after preliminary concentration and digestion procedures. Stained films of gastric washings are of little aid because of the frequent presence of saprophytic mycobacteria.

Stained Smears Tuberculosis is one of the few bacterial diseases which can often be diagnosed by microscopic examination alone, provided that certain procedures are followed. Water distilled and stored in glass containers should be employed in the preparation of all stains and reagents because of the presence of saprophytic mycobacteria in tap water. Acid cleaning solution should be employed in the preparation of glassware that is used to hold the stains and reagents. New glass slides should be used for each specimen. Care should be taken not to contaminate the cedar oil, and the oil immersion objective should be cleaned after examining a positive smear. When these precautions are observed, the finding of acid-fast bacilli in stained smears of sputum or spinal fluid is diagnostic in almost every instance.

In the direct microscopic examination of sputum, a purulent or caseous fleck of material is placed on a glass slide, crushed with the aid of a second slide, and a smear is made by drawing the slides apart rapidly.

In the Ziehl-Neelsen acid-fast stain and its various modifications, the procedure is as follows. The smear is fixed by gentle heat. The slide is flooded with carbolfuchsin and heated to steaming for 3 min. It is then rinsed with water and decolorized by ethanol containing 3 percent hydrochloric acid until no more color appears in the washings. After again rinsing with water, the smear is counterstained with methylene blue for 30 sec. Finally, the slide is rinsed, dried, and examined. The addition of phenol or detergent to the carbolfuchsin facilitates penetration of the dye, thus obviating the need for heating.

Digestion and Concentration of Sputum The purpose of this procedure is to homogenize and liquefy the sputum, to sediment it, and to eliminate other bacteria. Digestion and concentration with 3 to 4 percent sodium hydroxide is the most widely used method. After an equal volume of sodium hydroxide is added to the sputum, the mixture is shaken for 10 min. and then incubated at 37°C until homogenization has occurred (15 to 60 min.). After centrifugation at 3,000 rpm for 15 min., the supernatant is decanted and a drop of phenol red indicator added to the sediment; enough normal hydrochloric acid is added to make the sediment neutral. A drop of the sediment is smeared on a slide, which is stained by the Ziehl-Neelsen method and examined for the presence of acid-fast bacilli. Gastric washings are concentrated in the same way as sputum.

An alternative method is to treat the clinical specimen with 2 to 5 percent H_2SO_4 at room temperature for 10 to 40 min. and then neutralize the centrifuged deposit with buffered NaOH prior to inoculating cultures.

Cultures Repeated cultures will detect most of the infectious cases of tuberculosis not found by microscopic examination of stained smears. Ten to 100 organisms per milliliter of sputum yield positive cultures, but 100,000 per milliliter are required for detection in stained smears.

Guinea Pig Inoculation In the past some laboratories inoculated a portion of the material prepared for culture into the groin of young guinea pigs. At intervals of a few weeks the animals were tuberculin tested and examined for tuberculosis when the reaction was positive. However, improvements in culture technique have made it possible to dispense with routine inoculation of guinea pigs. In one recent study 2,000 animal tests added only one useful positive to that obtained by culture when a variety of culture media including pyruvate containing egg medium were employed.

Epidemiology

Incidence: Morbidity and Mortality

In 1910 Following the discovery of the causative agent by Robert Koch in 1882, his subsequent preparation of tuberculin in 1890, and the development of the tuberculin test by von Pirquet in 1907, it was possible for the first time to obtain accurate data on the prevalence of tuberculosis. When a number of tuberculin surveys were completed in 1910, it was apparent that infection with tubercle bacilli was widespread and developed early in life. These surveys indicated that by 5 years of age 30 to 60 percent of the population had become tuberculin-positive and by the age of 14 more than 90 percent were infected.

Recent Trends Since 1930, one of the most significant trends has been the postponement of infection until later in life. As recently as 1932, 90 percent of individuals 20 years of age living in Philadelphia, New York, and London had experienced infection with tubercle bacilli as indicated by positive tuberculin tests, but in rural areas the incidence was usually less than 25 percent. In the United States today, less than 3 percent of the population have been infected with tubercle bacilli by age 20.

When tuberculosis, morbidity, and mortality were at their presumed peak in 1860, young adults between 25 and 45 were predominantly involved. A hundred years later death from tuberculosis occurred primarily in patients over 65 years of age. While the death rate from tuberculosis in 1962 was 4.2 per 100,000 for all white males, the rate for white males over 65 was 36.4. The marked shift in the average age of patients with the disease is clearly evident from Figure 15-1 and Table 15-3.

The Decrease in Mortality The mortality rate has dropped from 400 per 100,000 cases per year in 1860 to 2.7 per 100,000 per year in 1970, a decrease of more than 100-fold. In fact, tuberculosis was the chief cause of death in the United States until 1909 but was seventh in 1947. Since 1949, tuberculosis mortality in the United States has declined more precipitously because of the effectiveness of antimicrobial chemotherapy. However, in many of developing countries today, tuberculosis remains a leading cause of death.

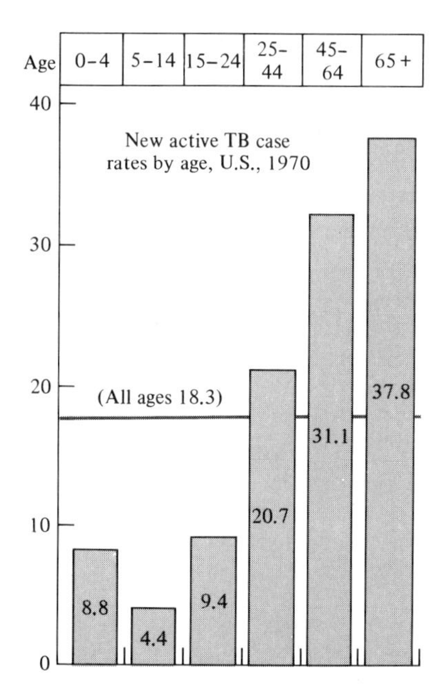

Figure 15-1 New active tuberculosis case rates per 100,000 persons by age in the United States, 1970. [*Morbidity Mortality Weekly Report, 20(53):63, 1972.*]

Reasons for the Decline Many reasons have been put forward to account for this hundredfold decrease in tuberculosis mortality in the past century. Some students of the subject have ascribed the decline to better housing, improved sanitary conditions, decreased drunkenness, earlier diagnosis, segregation of advanced cases, and sanitarium treatment. It is generally conceded, too, that educational and economic status is a factor affecting the disease. In the United States in 1930, for example, the tuberculosis death rate in unskilled laborers was seven times as high as that in professional workers.

In general, the highest rates of tuberculosis are found in areas where there are large concentrations of population (Fig. 15-2) and in places where a low economic status prevails with its accompanying overcrowding and inferior sanitary conditions. For example, in 1968 the death rate in central Harlem was 18.1 per 100,000 versus 1.1 in Flushing, Queens; both areas are located in metropolitan New York City.

Some authorities have placed great emphasis on biological factors, and indeed it is difficult to avoid the impression that a prime factor in the declining mortality from tuberculosis was the natural selection of a more resistant population. With yearly death rates of 200 to 400 per 100,000 cases persisting for several generations, with the majority of deaths occurring during the child-bearing period, and with early death from tuberculosis frequent in children, natural selection must have exerted a great effect in permitting the survival of those who for unknown genetic reasons were more resistant to infection from tubercle bacilli. The presumed role of natural selection in the decline in tuberculosis mortality is in accord with other studies that demonstrate how marked an influence the genetic background exerts on the incidence of

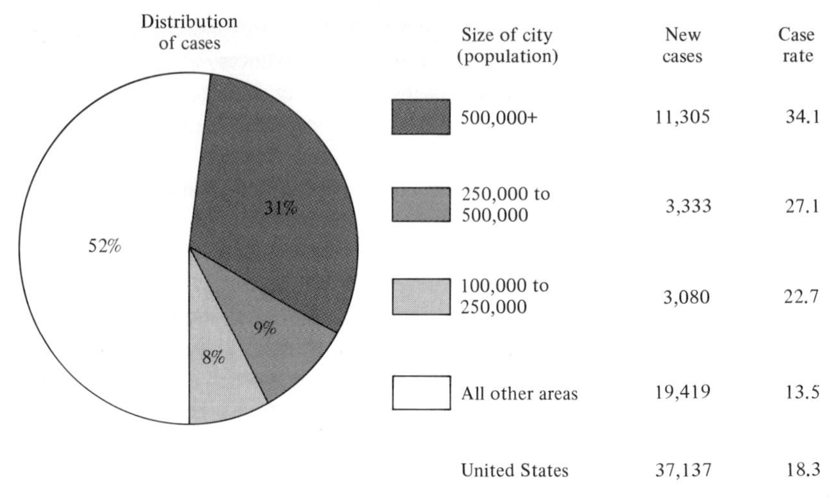

Figure 15-2 Tuberculosis case rates per 100,000 persons in large cities in the United States, 1970. [*United States Public Health Service, Department Health, Education, Welfare Publication no. (HSM) 72-8096, Jan. 1972.*]

clinical tuberculosis. If the disease develops in one member of a pair of monozygotic twins, for example, the incidence of active disease in the other twin has been found to be 2.3 to 3.5 times as high as that in two dizygotic twins.

New Cases In the United States between 1953 and 1970, tuberculosis morbidity and mortality have declined slowly but steadily (Fig. 15-3). The data show that for every death from tuberculosis in 1970 there were 6.7 new active cases reported. The highest rate of new cases was found in those 65 and over; the lowest rate was recorded in the 5- to 14-year-olds. Higher new case rates are found in males than in females and in nonwhites than whites (Table 15-3 and Fig. 15-4).

The morbidity rate in nonwhites is 4.6 times higher than in whites. An extremely important factor in the greater susceptibility of nonwhites to infection with tubercle bacilli is that they have been in contact with the disease for a shorter period (fewer centuries). Hence, natural

Table 15-3 Case Rates for White and Other Races, Males and Females, by Age, United States, 1970

		White			Other		
Age	**Total**	**Total**	**Male**	**Female**	**Total**	**Male**	**Female**
All ages	18.3	12.4	17.4	7.7	59.0	78.2	40.9
0- 4	8.8	4.9	5.2	4.6	29.2	29.1	29.3
5-14	4.4	2.4	2.4	2.4	15.2	15.6	14.8
15-24	9.4	5.6	6.0	5.2	33.6	34.9	32.4
25-44	20.7	11.8	15.6	8.1	86.5	115.8	60.6
45-64	31.1	22.0	35.2	10.0	111.9	170.8	56.6
65+	37.8	30.3	49.8	16.4	115.6	173.6	66.5

Source: Reported Tuberculosis Data, 1970, U.S.P.H.S., D.H.E.W. publ. no. (HSM) 72-8096, Jan. 1972.

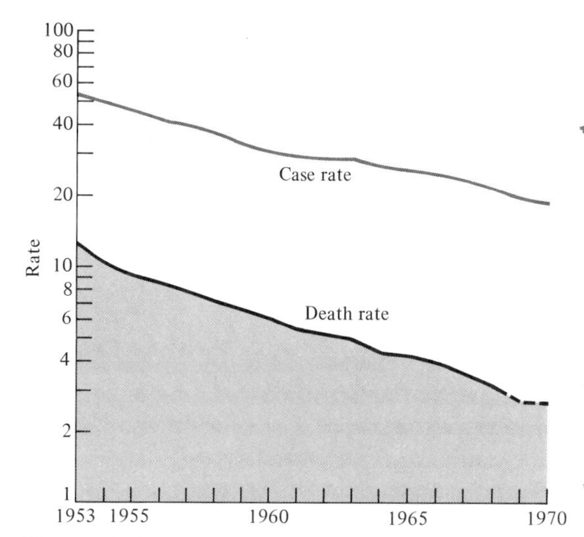

Figure 15-3 Tuberculosis case and death rates per 100,000 persons in the United States, 1953 to 1970. [*United States Public Health Service, Department Health, Education, Welfare Publication no. (HSM) 72-8096, Jan. 1972.*]

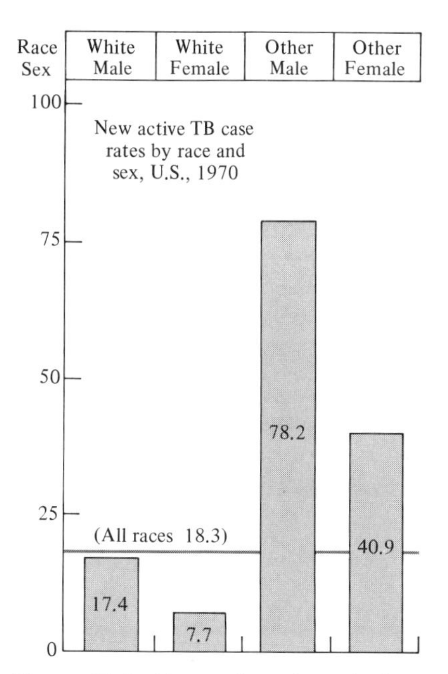

Figure 15-4 New active tuberculosis case rates per 100,000 persons by race and sex in the United States, 1970. [*Morbidity Mortality Weekly Report, 20(53):63, 1972.*]

selection of the more resistant individuals has not yet exerted its full effect.

Predisposing Factors Fatality rates are higher in those under 5 years old and those over 65. Those who have diabetes mellitus are more prone to develop tuberculosis. Tuberculous disease is more common in those with pneumoconioses, particularly silicosis. Medical personnel, including physicians, medical students, and nurses, are more likely to be exposed to infection and have a greater risk of developing active tuberculosis.

The use of corticosteroids increases the hazard of activating a quiescent or healed lesion. Impaired nutrition repeatedly has been noted to increase the incidence of clinical disease, as was recorded in certain countries during World Wars I and II. Tuberculosis is always a possibility to be ruled out in the individual patient who is significantly under normal weight.

The Goal The goal of epidemiologic study is the early detection of active tuberculous disease. At the same time the prevalence of tuberculous infection is revealed. Of particular importance is the identification of patients with chronic pulmonary tuberculosis, who are a threat to the household and the community.

Problems The fact that 80 percent of newly diagnosed cases are already moderately or far advanced has several important implications. It means that the majority of newly diagnosed patients have been periodically or constantly contaminating their household and other close contacts for months or years before detection.

The central problems which preclude case finding prior to the development of a draining cavity are the nature of the disease and the failure to apply the useful and reliable epidemiologic indices. Table 15-4 illustrates the problem.

There are two available case-finding tools: the tuberculin test and the chest x-ray. A third epidemiologic index, finding tubercle bacilli in the sputum, is of no value in detecting early

Table 15-4 Percentage Distribution of New Active Pulmonary Tuberculosis Cases, United States, 1953 to 1970

Stage of disease	1953	1962	1970	Range 1953–1962
Minimal	22.6	20.7	20.0	20.5–22.6
Moderately advanced	40.7	43.9	43.4	40.6–43.9
Far advanced	36.7	35.4	36.6	35.4–37.0
Moderately and far advanced	77.4	79.3	80.0	

Source: United States Public Health Publication no. 638, 1964 edition; and Reported Tuberculosis Data, 1970, U.S.P.H.S., D.H.E.W. publ. no. (HSM) 72-8096, Jan. 1972.

cases because cavitation usually precedes the appearance of the organism in the sputum.

Tuberculosis is not ordinarily detected until it is far advanced because of the frequent absence or minimal extent of symptoms early in its course. The stage of the disease makes a profound difference in the prognosis of the individual case, even when treatment proceeds under favorable conditions, as shown by Table 15-5.

The Tuberculin Test The tuberculin test is based on the fact that infection with tubercle bacilli produces a specific allergy to certain products of the organism that are contained in culture extracts called *old tuberculin* (OT) or in the purified protein derivative (PPD) isolated from filtrates of autoclaved cultures. Both preparations of tuberculin are widely used. Robert Koch in 1891 first prepared OT by heat-killing cultures of tubercle bacilli, filtering off the dead microorganisms, and concentrating the filtrate. PPD is obtained from ammonium sulfate-precipitated filtrates of autoclaved cultures of *Mycobacterium tuberculosis* grown on a synthetic medium.

Table 15-5 Results of Chemotherapy on Previously Untreated Tuberculous Patients

Stage of disease	Death rate per 100,000 under treatment*
Minimal	0
Moderately advanced	
Cavity	220
No cavity	120
Far advanced	
Large multiple cavities (all groups)	3,190
Under 45 years—white	600
Under 45 years—nonwhite	4,700
45 years and over—white	2,810
45 years and over—nonwhite	6,540
All other	1,190

* Occurring during a 40-week treatment period with either isoniazid-PAS or streptomycin-PAS.

Source: United States Public Health Service Publication no. 1036, 1963.

Mantoux Test The preferred method of performing the tuberculin test is the intracutaneous injection of 0.1 ml of the desired concentration of OT or PPD into the skin of the forearm (Mantoux test). The test should be read 48 to 72 hr. after injection. Reactions are classified on the basis of induration as determined by palpation and the largest diameter of induration recorded. A positive reaction is one in which there is an induration of 5 mm or more in diameter.

The amount of OT or PPD ordinarily used is 5 tuberculin units (TU) based on international standards adopted by the World Health Organization. This is equivalent to 0.001 mg of protein for PPD and a 1:2,000 dilution of OT. In persons suspected of hypersensitivity to tuberculin, 1 TU is used for initial testing. As with most other types of delayed hypersensitivity, tuberculin allergy can be passively transferred with leukocytes but not with serum from a tuberculin-positive person.

Use Since tuberculin allergy ordinarily persists for the life of the individual, tuberculin tests have been widely used as a case-finding tool and as a means to define the extent of infection in the community. Only in a few individuals with overwhelming infection, in patients receiving corticosteroids, and in patients with sarcoidosis, Hodgkin's disease, or measles may the tuberculin test be falsely negative and therefore unreliable as an index of infection with the microorganism.

Significance Strictly speaking, a positive tuberculin test indicates past infection with tubercle bacilli but does not distinguish between active and inactive lesions. In countries with low incidence of tuberculous infection, such as Great Britain, Denmark, Canada, and the United States, there is a substantially greater risk of developing clinical tuberculosis with a positive reaction than with a negative tuberculin test. The prognosis is especially grave for those individuals who react strongly to 3 to 5 TU (Table 15-6).

It is evident that persons who react strongly to tuberculin should have priority in follow-up examinations, in receiving treatment if x-rays are positive, and in chemoprophylaxis when the x-ray is negative. Even when not strongly positive, tuberculin reactivity calls for close and prolonged clinical surveillance of all reactors under 5 years of age and in older children and adults with evidence of recent conversion.

Household Infection The tuberculin test has perhaps attained its greatest practical value in finding infection in household and other close contacts of newly reported cases of active tuberculosis. Prompt examination of all household contacts of an infected patient (index case) is of paramount importance because the occurrence of active tuberculosis in household contacts is approximately 100 times greater than in the general population. In one study, at the time of recognition of the index case, 1,900 of every 100,000 contacts had clinical disease and within 1 year another 850 of every 100,000 develop active tuberculosis. The annual incidence in the general population was 29.4 per 100,000. Of the household contacts with active tuberculosis at the time of first examination, almost half were in children under 5 years of age and during the first year after diagnosis of the index case, 26 percent of new active cases were found in this age group. Moreover, tuberculous meningitis is about 10 to 20 times more frequent in children under 5 years of age who have had household contact with a tuberculous patient than in a

Table 15-6 The Hazards Associated with Strongly Positive Tuberculin Tests in Great Britain and the United States

Test dose	Type of reaction	Clinical tuberculosis rate per 100,000 per year
Great Britain		
3 TU	Strongly positive	140
	Moderately positive	31
100 TU	Weakly positive	29
United States		
5 TU	Positive	134
	Negative	9
100 TU	Positive	11
	Negative	7

Source: Adapted from Second Report to the Medical Research Council by their Tuberculosis Vaccines Clinical Trials Committee, *Br. Med. J.*, 2:379–396, 1959; and G. W. Comstock and L. W. Shaw, *Public Health Reports* 75: 583–594, 1960.

control group. Not only do those under 5 within the household acquire active tuberculosis more frequently, but they also acquire the disease earlier. Data such as these indicate why tuberculosis is regarded as primarily a household disease transmitted vertically from generation to generation.

High-risk Groups The tuberculin test also has special value when employed periodically (at intervals of 3 months) in groups with unusual exposure to infection, such as nurses and physicians, and in sanitaria and mental hospitals where chronic pulmonary tuberculosis may be concentrated. In this way, those whose tuberculin reaction has recently become positive (*tuberculin converters*) can be detected and followed by careful clinical study.

With the advent of chemotherapy the conversion rate of student nurses in training has declined from 66 percent in the years 1948 to 1951 to 3.5 percent between 1959 to 1964. Without question the fall is due largely to prompt and adequate chemotherapy of infected patients.

The Chest X-ray In conjunction with tuberculin reactivity, the finding of suspicious x-ray shadows serves as an additional index of the risk of future tuberculous disease. Roentgenographic examination represents the next logical procedure in the evaluation of a person who exhibits tuberculin allergy. Surveys have indicated tuberculin reactors with suspicious x-ray shadows may be as much as 20 times more likely to develop clinical tuberculosis as tuberculin reactors with normal lungs. Thus, the combination of a positive tuberculin test and a compatible x-ray shadow provides ample grounds for instituting specific chemotherapy.

Prevention and Control

Immunity versus Allergy Few topics in the field of microbiology and infectious disease have generated such intense controversy as the mechanism of immunity in tuberculosis and the role of allergy in that immunity. Almost every conceivable partisan conclusion has been drawn. When this happens, it is usually a clear indication that the available data do not permit a definitive answer or that the influence of a given factor will vary with the specific circumstances. From the author's viewpoint, both situations hold true with respect to immunity and allergy in tuberculosis.

In the light of newer knowledge, some of the pertinent findings covering both the protective and injurious aspects of cell-mediated immunity (Chap. 8) in tuberculosis provide an indication of the complexity of the problem.

1 Specific acquired resistance (cell-mediated immunity) is associated with the interaction of sensitized T cells and tubercle bacilli, the release of lymphokines, and the accelerated mobilization of activated macrophages with enhanced bactericidal properties for tubercle bacilli.
2 As a consequence, the tubercles solidify, calcify, and suppress further bacterial multiplication.
3 On the other hand, caseation necrosis, liquefaction, and cavitation (other manifestations of cell-mediated immunity or delayed hypersensitivity) are of definite importance in the pathogenesis of chronic pulmonary tuberculosis. Paradoxically, caseation necrosis produces a local environment unfavorable for the growth of aerobic tubercle bacilli. However, the marked tissue destruction and liquefaction which occur may in turn eventuate in cavitation. In the latter case, the tubercle bacilli gain access to a more aerobic atmosphere essential for their rapid proliferation.
4 In a heavily infectious environment, tuberculin-positive persons are less likely to develop clinical tuberculosis than are tuberculin-negative persons.
5 In a lightly infectious environment (Western Europe, North America), tuberculin-positive individuals are more likely to develop clinical tuberculosis than are tuberculin-negative individuals.

BCG Immunization BCG (bacillus Calmette-Guérin) vaccine contains an attenuated variant of *M. bovis.* It has been widely used in many parts of the world since its introduction in 1922.

After several years of studies of subcultures on a glycerol-bile-potato medium, Calmette and Guérin found that the resulting variant could be injected into animals and man without causing significant lesions. They also established that the vaccine protected calves and heifers against challenge with virulent *Mycobacterium bovis* bacilli capable of killing unvaccinated animals in 2 months.

Since its introduction for human immunization, the protective value of BCG has been the subject of continued controversy. Much confusion was created by failure to compare the vaccinated group with a properly selected control group and by failure to obtain reproducible or standardized preparations of BCG. The use of freeze-dried, heat-stable BCG vaccine has obviated many, but not all, of the standardization problems.

Although many earlier studies indicated that BCG protected against tuberculosis, the English Medical Research Council study in children finishing school between 1950 and 1960 is cited because it is a superb model of experimental design complemented by thorough clinical evaluation. The results convincingly demonstrate that the incidence of tuberculosis in vaccinated children is about one-fifth that in unvaccinated children. Over a period of observation averaging 8.8 years the annual incidence of tuberculosis was 40 per 100,000 in the BCG vaccinated groups as contrasted with 191 per 100,000 in the unvaccinated group. The protective value remained evident throughout the whole observation period. Thus, not only did BCG vaccine offer significant protection against primary tuberculosis, but it also protected against postprimary progression of the infection (Table 15-7).

Currently it is recommended by WHO that BCG be given to tuberculin-negative persons exposed to a high risk of infection, to the entire tuberculin-negative population of a country in which infection is widespread, and to the whole population of some of the developing countries

Table 15-7 Protective Value of BCG Vaccination

Years after vaccination	Percent reduction in clinical tuberculosis
0 to 2.5	80
2.5 to 5.0	86
5.0 to 7.5	71
7.5 to 10.0	61

Source: Adapted from Third Report to the Medical Research Council by their Tuberculosis Vaccines Clinical Trials Committee, *Br. Med. J.*, 1:973–978, 1963.

without regard to their tuberculin reaction. When given by the intracutaneous route to those who are tuberculin-negative, the vaccine will produce a positive tuberculin reaction in almost 100 percent of the persons inoculated.

Chemoprophylaxis Although effective treatment of a newly diagnosed patient almost immediately eliminates further spread of the infection, household contacts (especially those under 5 years of age) who do not already have active disease have a high risk of developing disease during the year after recognition of the index case. This risk may be substantially reduced by the prophylactic administration of isoniazid. When isoniazid is taken daily for 1 year by household contacts of active cases of tuberculosis, the incidence of disease will be reduced by more than 75 percent. Isoniazid exerts its greatest effect in those under 5 years of age who are tuberculin-positive, in those of all ages who have shown a recent conversion to tuberculin reactivity, and to household contacts under 5 years of age who are tuberculin-negative. It is imperative that the drug be taken regularly to achieve the desired effect.

Low Transmission Level Most countries of Western Europe and North America, Australia, and New Zealand have a low level of transmission of tuberculosis infection (not more than 2 percent positive tuberculin tests in children entering school). Tuberculin reactivity among young children is the best indicator of current prevalence.

In such areas, the currently recommended procedures (U.S.P.H.S. Publication no. 1119) assign high priority to the early detection and effective treatment of active cases, with the use of chemoprophylaxis or treatment where necessary or desirable, and to case finding based on the tuberculin testing of all children upon entry to school. Those children who react to tuberculin should have chest x-rays taken. The families should be tuberculin tested, and when indicated, x-ray examination should be carried out. As a part of the program, classmates, playmates, school teachers, and other school employees should have a similar examination. In addition, all children should be tuberculin tested at the age of 14. Another recommended case-finding technique is the routine use of chest x-rays for people hospitalized in cities of over 250,000 population.

Since the continuous supervision of contacts is impossible in slum areas of big cities or among migrant workers, the likelihood of their taking daily prophylactic doses of a drug for 1 year is slight, and BCG should be given to those who are tuberculin-negative.

High Transmission Level Tuberculosis in most other areas of the world is 5 to 100 times as high as that observed in Western Europe and North America. For countries with a high level of transmission, the recommended procedures are entirely different (WHO Expert Committee on Tuberculosis, Eighth Report, 1964).

BCG should be used as widely as possible and as early in life as feasible, and revaccination should be given before children finish school. The initial generation should be vaccinated within the first 2 to 3 years of life, and vaccination should be continued until tuberculosis has been eliminated as a serious public health problem. BCG vaccination is recommended without prior tuberculin testing.

The WHO committee stated that there is no evidence of local, regional, focal, or general complications detrimental to the health of the tuberculin reactors among BCG-vaccinated individuals, nor has vaccination without prior tuberculin testing reduced acceptability of BCG. In developing countries, studies showed prophylaxis intake to be so low as to eliminate entirely the prophylactic effect. On the other hand, the committee thought it necessary to explore the feasibility of short intensive courses of isoniazid for mass use.

Treatment The response to effective chemotherapy rarely, if ever, succeeds in completely eliminating tubercle bacilli from the host. Nonetheless, its use halts the progression of the disease, promptly eliminates the excretion of tubercle bacilli into the environment, promotes the healing of necrotic foci and open cavities, and eventually returns almost every treated individual to normal life. In the past 10 years, the treatment and management of active tuberculosis have undergone a number of changes. The precise choice of drugs for treatment depends on the stage of the disease, the age of the patient, whether the disease was treated before (about 15 percent of clinical cases are previously treated cases that have relapsed), the country where the disease is occurring, and the physician.

The basic and most important drug in the treatment of tuberculosis is isoniazid. In the management of moderately or far advanced disease, isoniazid is combined with another drug, usually ethambutol or para-aminosalicylic acid (PAS). Streptomycin is usually used as the third drug in triple therapy. The combination of isoniazid and PAS with streptomycin has produced excellent results (Table 15-8). More recently, there has been a tendency to utilize ethambutol in place of PAS in combination with isoniazid and streptomycin because ethambutol is more active and more apt to be taken in

Table 15-8 Comparative Efficacy of Antimicrobial Therapy in Tuberculosis: A Few Possible Drug Combinations

Antimicrobial therapy	Percent mortality*	Percent excreting tubercle bacilli*	Percent not excreting tubercle bacilli*
None (1947)	21	54	25
Streptomycin-PAS (1952)	3	32	65
Isoniazid-PAS with streptomycin (1963)	1	4	95

* Results after 1 year.

Source: Adapted from S. H. Ferebee and C. E. Palmer, "The Epidemiologic Bonus," *Am. Rev. Resp. Dis.*, 91: 104–107, 1965.

the prescribed dosage by the patient. Usually after a few months, streptomycin is discontinued, whereas isoniazid and ethambutol (or PAS) are continued for 18 to 36 months. Rifampin is used extensively in Europe, has recently become commercially available in the United States, and when employed along with isoniazid appears to be more effective and less toxic than any other regimen previously utilized.

Isoniazid has the advantage of being readily diffusible and active against intracellular tubercle bacilli. In addition, although mutation of tubercle bacilli to high resistance to isoniazid is common (10^{-4} to 10^{-6}), it is almost always accompanied by decreased pathogenicity. Moreover, neural toxicity of the drug can be largely controlled by giving pyridoxine.

Tubercle bacilli frequently mutate to high resistance to streptomycin while retaining their pathogenicity. This factor, plus the toxicity for vestibular and auditory nerves, frequently irreversible, has limited the use of streptomycin in the treatment of tuberculosis.

Ambulatory Chemotherapy One of the most important recent developments in the treatment and management of active tuberculosis has been the substitution of ambulatory chemotherapy for treatment within the hospital. The WHO committee concluded that in terms of immediate response, of subsequent relapse, and of risk to contacts there was no evidence of special benefits resulting from hospitalization providing the patients actually take the drug regularly throughout the prescribed period. In this country, hospitalization is recommended for close observation during the first several weeks of intensive chemotherapy and in controlling severe pulmonary hemorrhage. Thereafter, isolation of the patient is unnecessary and is usually harmful to the welfare of the patient and his family. With effective antimicrobial therapy there is no evidence that bed rest is beneficial.

Surgery Thoracic surgery is the most important ancillary measure to antimicrobial therapy in the treatment of pulmonary tuberculosis. Unless there are contraindications, all patients with cavitary foci persisting for 6 months or more should have surgical resection. The surgery should be performed without delay in order to avoid the risks of bacterial drug resistance and tuberculous complications of surgery such as bronchopleural fistula and empyema. Thoracoplasty or collapse by extrapleural plombage are occasionally indicated when resectional procedures are not feasible in patients with extensive bilateral disease.

Prospective

The programs adopted and the recommendations made by the WHO and the U.S.P.H.S. (Publication no. 1119) seem unduly conservative and timid in view of the magnitude of the worldwide problem of tuberculosis. The tools for the control of tuberculosis are effective, but the initiative for applying them is weak. At the current pace, it may well be centuries before tuberculosis is brought under control by BCG and other appropriate measures in the developing countries. In the United States the easy way out has been selected. It is convenient to perform tuberculin tests on children who are entering school. But is this the basis for an adequate case-finding program when U.S.P.H.S. data have shown that almost half of all household contact cases of tuberculosis occur in the age group under 5, and when these cases develop earlier and pursue a more rapid downhill course? Is it too much to expect that every child between the ages of 1 and 5 should have an annual tuberculin test so that infection with tubercle bacilli could be detected much sooner? Of course it is not too much to expect.

OTHER MYCOBACTERIA PATHOGENIC FOR MAN

Apart from human tubercle bacilli, *Mycobacterium bovis,* and leprosy bacilli, acid-fast mycobacteria are widely distributed throughout the world. For many years these so-called atypical or anonymous mycobacteria were generally regarded as harmless saprophytes. In 1959, Runyon suggested a practical classification of these bacteria based on pigmentation, colonial morphology, and rate of growth. Subsequent systematic studies have clearly established that many other species of mycobacteria are pathogenic for man, producing chronic pulmonary disease, lymphadenitis, and localized cutaneous and subcutaneous lesions. As noted in Table 15-9, the principal pathogens are *M. kansasii, M. intracellulare* (Battey bacilli), *M. marinum* (*M. balnei*) and *M. ulcerans,* but *M. scrofulaceum* and *M. fortuitum* can occasionally cause disease in man. As a group, these mycobacteria can grow at 20 to 25°C, fail to produce niacin, and are nonpathogenic for guinea pigs. Except for *M. fortuitum,* which is a rapid grower (4 to 5 days), the organisms multiply slowly, forming colonies in 10 to 25 days.

In view of the data included in Table 15-9 as well as other findings, emphasis is given to the following observations.

1 *Mycobacterium kansasii* and *M. intracellulare* are the chief causative agents involved in producing nontuberculous chronic pulmonary disease that is clinically indistinguishable from tuberculosis. Most clinically apparent cases are superimposed on chronic bronchitis, pulmonary emphysema, or pneumoconiosis. As judged by skin tests, subclinical infection with these organisms is more common in certain cases than is infection with tubercle bacilli.
2 Children are rarely subject to chronic pulmonary disease caused by *M. kansasii* or *M. intracellulare,* but do experience cervical adenitis (*M. scrofulaceum*) and, like adults, are susceptible to granulomatous skin lesions (*M. marinum, M. ulcerans, M. fortuitum*).
3 *M. kansasii* usually responds to higher concentrations of the same drugs used in the therapy of tuberculosis, but the other mycobacteria are generally resistant to the same drugs.
4 Diagnosis of infections caused by these bacteria must be approached with caution, particularly when the organism is isolated from sputum. However, repeated isolation of the same bacteria from patients with pulmonary disease or recovery of the organisms from aspirated pus or tissue biopsies are of greater diagnostic significance.
5 Surgical excision may be required in the case of the lesions caused by *M. marinum* or *M. ulcerans.*

Leprosy (Hansen's Disease)

Leprosy is a chronic granulomatous disease of man characterized primarily by the destruction of cutaneous tissues, peripheral nerves, and nasal mucosa. It is one of the oldest known human diseases and was the first against which isolation measures were employed. The disease is mentioned in Indian and Chinese literature about 1400 to 1000 B.C. After its introduction into Europe from the Near East, it flourished from the eleventh to the thirteenth centuries and all but disappeared from that continent in the sixteenth century. In 1973, there were an estimated 10 to 12 million cases, largely found in South Asia, Equatorial Africa, the Pacific Islands, and Brazil. In the United States there are about 2,000 cases of leprosy under treatment concentrated in Texas, Arizona, California,

Table 15-9 Other Mycobacteria Pathogenic For Man

Species and Runyon group	Special characteristics
M. kansasii (I, photochromogens)	Causes chronic pulmonary disease indistinguishable from tuberculosis, especially in middle-aged and older white males who have chronic bronchitis, pulmonary emphysema, or pneumoconiosis; optimal temperature for growth is 37°C; produces yellow pigmented colonies following exposure to light; infected patients cross-react with OT; sporadic infections usually seen, especially in midwestern United States and mining areas of Wales; organism found in raw milk and soil.
M. marinum *(M. balnei)* (I, photochromogens)	Causes chronic granulomatous nodules or ulcers in the skin and subcutaneous tissue; optimal temperature 30 to 33°C; produces intense orange yellow pigmented colonies upon exposure to light; infected patients cross-react to OT; sporadic cases and epidemics occur, especially in association with contaminated swimming pools; natural reservoir in fish.
M. ulcerans (unclassified)	Causes chronic granulomatous nodules and ulcers in the skin and subcutaneous tissue which tend to become extensive; optimal temperature 30 to 33°C; white to pale cream colored colonies; about half of infected patients cross-react to OT; endemic in inhabitants of upper Nile regions; usually found in tropical or subtropical areas; reservoir unknown.
M. scrofulaceum (II, scotochromogens)	Causes cervical adenitis in young children; less commonly involved in inguinal adenitis and conjunctivitis with preauricular adenitis (most scotochromogens, however, are more frequently isolated as saprophytes in sputum); produces yellow orange pigmented colonies in dark; about 50 percent of individuals skin tested with PPD prepared from organisms isolated from cervical nodes developed positive skin tests, but infected patients do not cross-react with OT; reservoir unknown; differs from other scotochromogens in failing to hydrolyze Tween 80.
M. intracellulare (Battey bacilli) (III, nonphotochromogens)	Causes chronic pulmonary disease indistinguishable from tuberculosis, especially in patients with chronic bronchitis and pulmonary emphysema; optimal temperature 37°C; produces translucent, nonpigmented colonies; skin tests performed with PPD prepared from the organism suggest that subclinical infection is common; soil is probable reservoir; together with *M. kansasii* accounts for more than 90 percent of nontuberculosis mycobacterial pulmonary disease.
M. fortuitum (IV, rapid growers)	Most commonly a saprophyte but can cause cutaneous infections, abscesses, and corneal infections following trauma, and pulmonary infections upon preexisting lung disease; grows well between 22 and 37°C in 4 to 5 days; skin tests performed with PPD prepared from the organism are positive in about 8 percent, but cross-reactions with OT do not occur; widespread reservoir in soil, dust, and water.

Louisiana, Hawaii, and Florida. Approximately 100 new cases are detected each year.

The causative agent, *Mycobacterium leprae*, was discovered by Hansen in 1873. The acid-fast bacilli are regularly found in parallel or cigar-shaped bundles, globular masses, or singly in smears, scrapings, or punch biopsies from the skin in lepromatous lesions, rarely from tuberculoid lesions. The organism has never been grown on artificial medium and is an obligate intracellular parasite. Tissue cultures are generally unreliable, but the organism will grow consistently in the footpads of mice, a development that permits experimental evaluation of drugs and vaccines. For example, vaccination of mice with BCG partially suppresses the growth of leprosy bacilli in the footpad.

Pathogenesis Infection is presumably acquired through breaks in the skin following contact with lepromatous or borderline (dimorphous) patients. The incubation period is long, often 3 to 5 years, but may be as short as 6 or 7 months. The disease generally begins with macules that are in no way distinctive, but are frequently anesthetic.

In *tuberculoid leprosy*, skin lesions are usually few and sharply demarcated. Neural involvement occurs early, is pronounced, and may be severe, leading to disfigurement and deformity which is frequently associated with the hand or the foot. Epithelioid cells are prominent, but bacilli are sparse and difficult to demonstrate. The *lepromin skin test* is usually positive and carries a good prognosis. Individuals who are lepromin-positive tend to recover within a few years, and a person with a positive test due to subclinical infection is unlikely to develop disease.

In *lepromatous leprosy*, peripheral sensory nerves are attacked as in the tuberculoid form of the disease, but bacterial multiplication is not limited and disseminated infection occurs. There is a diffuse reaction involving foam cells and globi (globular masses of bacilli) which spreads to contiguous skin areas with invasion of autonomic nerve fibers, dermal appendages, and blood vessels. Bacterial proliferation is extensive (10^9/Gm of affected tissue, 10^7/ml of nasal secretions) and results in almost continuous bacteremia, but tissue destruction is usually limited to the skin and mucous membranes (oral, nasopharyngeal, corneal). Corneal involvement may cause blindness. The lepromin test is generally negative.

Borderline (dimorphous) *leprosy* refers to lesions similar to tuberculoid leprosy as well as lepromatous leprosy occurring in the same patient.

Laboratory Diagnosis In lepromatous leprosy, a laboratory diagnosis is readily established by demonstrating acid-fast bacilli in the lesions. In tuberculoid leprosy, the organism is difficult to demonstrate. A positive lepromin test combined with the clinical picture may prove useful, although it should be noted that immunization with BCG may induce a positive lepromin test.

Epidemiology In areas of the world where the disease is endemic, it characteristically follows a household or village pattern. Infection is most common in childhood and early adult life. As with tuberculosis, the infection rate is high, but the clinical attack rate is low.

Prevention and Control Control of leprosy is based on early detection and treatment with dapsone (4,4′-diaminodiphenyl sulfone, DDS), which interferes with bacterial folic acid synthesis. Therapy must be continued until the organisms are eliminated from the skin (usually 5 years or more). However, within 6 months of therapy, most of the viable bacteria have disappeared from the skin lesions and nasal secretions. Immediate arrest of the disease follows treatment, and except for residual nerve destruction, recovery is complete.

Clinical trials indicate that rifampin is therapeutically effective but is much more costly than dapsone.

Chemoprophylaxis of close contacts, especially children of lepromatous parents, is strongly recommended and should be continued in full therapeutic dosage for at least 1 year. However, separation of children from lepromatous parents who have had effective therapy for several months (and who will continue under ambulatory treatment) is probably no longer necessary.

Some investigators are impressed by the prospective value of immunization with BCG in the control of leprosy and large-scale studies are under way to determine its efficacy.

BIBLIOGRAPHY

Bechelli, L. M., and Martinez, D. V.: "Further Information on the Leprosy Problem in the World," *Bull. W.H.O.*, 46:523-536, 1972.

"Editorial. BCG Tested," *Br. Med. J.*, 1:435, 1973.

Evans, M. J., Newton, H. E., and Levy, L.: "Early Response of Mouse Foot Pads to *Mycobacterium leprae*," *Infect. Immun.*, 7:76-85, 1973.

Furcolow, M. L., and Deuschle, K. W.: "Modern Tuberculosis Control. A Six-year Follow-up in an Appalachian Community," *Am. Rev. Resp. Dis.*, 107:253-266, 1973.

Munt, P. W.: "Miliary Tuberculosis in the Chemotherapy Era," *Medicine*, 51:139-155, 1972.

Rosenblatt, M. B.: "Pulmonary Tuberculosis: Evolution of Modern Therapy," *Bull. N.Y. Acad. Med.*, 49:163-196, 1973.

Schonell, M., Dorken, E., and Grzybowski, S.: "Rifampin," *Can. Med. Assoc. J.*, 106:783-786, 1972.

Shepard, C. C.: "Chemotherapy of Leprosy," *Annu. Rev. Pharmacol.*, 9:37-50, 1969.

"The Tuberculin Skin Test. A Statement by the Committee on Diagnostic Skin Testing," *Am. Rev. Resp. Dis.*, 104:769-775, 1971.

Turk, J. L., and Bryceson, A. D.: "Immunological Phenomena in Leprosy and Related Diseases," *Adv. Immunol.*, 13:209-266, 1971.

Chapter 16

Localized Infections of the Skin and Subcutaneous Tissues

Zigmund C. Kaminski and Bernard A. Briody

PERSPECTIVE

Lesions of the skin are caused by a considerable number of bacteria, viruses, rickettsiae, fungi, protozoa, and helminths. Occasionally, the lesions may reflect an allergic reaction to fungi or damage by a bacterial product (erythrogenic toxin of group A streptococci). The causative agents may produce localized or systemic infections, or both. Systemic infections associated with skin lesions are discussed in Chapters 22 to 26.

Among the parasites that are primarily responsible for localized infections of the skin and subcutaneous tissues, staphylococci occupy the number one position (Chap. 14). Streptococci (Chap. 14) and leprosy bacilli (Chap. 15) are also important causes of skin lesions, and mention has been made of cutaneous diphtheria, anaerobic abscesses, and gas gangrene (Chap. 13). Consequently, in this chapter, emphasis will be given to wound infections, dermatophytes, several other fungal infections including candidiasis, and the treponematoses (yaws, pinta, bejel). In addition, erythrasma, molluscum contagiosum, warts, cutaneous larva migrans, and dracontiasis are mentioned briefly.

WOUND INFECTIONS

Surgical Wounds

Despite careful attention to aseptic technique, available data suggest that 3 to 11 percent of surgical incisions become infected. The use of antibiotics prophylactically prior to surgery to prevent infections that do not exist is without redeeming value and may be detrimental in facilitating colonization of the patient with antibiotic-resistant microorganisms. Infection of the wound generally occurs during the operation with the patient serving as the source of infection. With the exception of group A streptococcal infections, which become apparent within 48 hr., the first signs of infection usually develop 5 days after the operation when there is an increased pulse rate and temperature. By the seventh day, swelling, edema, and tenderness of the wound are apparent. Usually, antibiotics are not required in treatment. The procedure of opening the wound and draining the pus is generally effective. If chemotherapy is employed, it must be based on culture and antibiotic sensitivity testing.

Staphylococci are the principal causative agents accounting for 30 to 50 percent of wound infections. Other important microorganisms producing wound infections include *Enterobacter-Klebsiella* species, *Pseudomonas aeruginosa, Escherichia coli, Proteus* species, *Bacteroides* species, *Clostridium perfringens,* enterococci, anaerobic streptococci (peptostreptococci), anaerobic staphylococci (peptococci), and viridans streptococci. As noted in Table 16-1, the organisms encountered vary with the type of surgery

Table 16-1 Causative Agents in Wound Infections*

General surgery	Gynecologic and obstetric surgery	Tracheostomy
Staphylococcus aureus	Anaerobic streptococci (peptostreptococci)	*Pseudomonas aeruginosa*
Escherichia coli	Nonhemolytic streptococci	*Enterobacter-Klebsiella* species
Enterobacter-Klebsiella species	*Escherichia coli*	*Proteus* species
Pseudomonas aeruginosa	*Staphylococcus epidermidis*	*Escherichia coli*
Proteus species	Anaerobic staphylococci (peptococci)	*Staphylococcus aureus*
Bacteroides species	Viridans streptococci	Fungi

* Listed in order of frequency.

performed. In general surgery, staphylococci and the common gram-negative enteric bacilli are the chief organisms involved, whereas in gynecological and obstetrical postoperative infections anaerobic and other streptococci (excluding group A) are the most frequently encountered bacteria. The differing etiology reflects the normal flora of the skin and the vagina, respectively. In the case of tracheostomy infections, the distribution of the causative microorganisms is probably influenced to a great extent by the prior use of antibiotics and the resistance of the organisms to antibiotics, especially in the case of *Pseudomonas* and *Enterobacter-Klebsiella* which account for the majority of the infections.

Burns

The most common and serious complication of third-degree (destruction of the full thickness of the skin) burns is infection. If a severely burned person survives the first few days, recovery will probably occur if the individual does not develop infection. In the latter event, the mortality rate is approximately 15 percent. The chief pathogens are staphylococci and *Pseudomonas*.

Interestingly, infected burns often follow a predictable sequence. In the first few days, staphylococci are the principal organisms recovered from the damaged tissue. About the fourth or fifth day, gram-negative enteric bacilli frequently predominate, especially if antibiotic therapy is used. By the seventh day, *Pseudomonas, Klebsiella*, and *Proteus* are the chief organisms found in the lesions. The availability of penicillinase-resistant penicillins has made it easier to manage staphylococcal infections. Consequently, *Pseudomonas* bacteria currently present the most difficult therapeutic problem. The most important obstacles are the resistance of *Pseudomonas* to antibiotics, the toxicity of the slime polysaccharide of the organism, and the large number of antigenically distinct types of *Pseudomonas* which make active or passive immunization impractical. When antibiotics are used indiscriminately in the treatment of burned patients, disseminated candidiasis represents a serious hazard (see later in this chapter).

Probably, the most effective method of preventing infections of third-degree burns is debridement of the damaged tissue plus the use of silver sulfadiazine ointment to prevent bacterial multiplication and rigid application of aseptic technique when initially cleansing the wound with a germicidal agent (70 percent ethanol, iodine, or benzalkalonium) and when changing the dressings and reapplying the sulfadiazine ointment daily.

Crush, Penetrating, and Traumatic Wounds

In serious penetrating, gunshot, battlefield, or crush injuries the important causative agents include staphylococci, *Pseudomonas, Escherichia coli*, and *Clostridium perfringens*, but many other members of the normal flora can be etiologically involved. Apart from early debridement of the injured area and cleansing with germicidal agents under aseptic conditions, delayed secondary closure of the lesion on or after the fourth day has reduced the incidence of infections. Indiscriminate prophylactic use of antibiotics is to be avoided, since it facilitates colonization of the wound with resistant microorganisms.

DERMATOMYCOSES (DERMATOPHYTOSES)

The Causative Agents

The dermatophytes are a closely related group of fungi that have the ability to utilize keratin, which partly explains their proclivity for localizing in the skin, hair, and nails. There are three genera—*Trichophyton, Microsporum*, and *Epidermophyton*—and approximately 30 species that infect man. The species most commonly involved in human infections are included in Table 16-2. The dermatophytes are widely distrib-

Table 16-2 The Common Dermatomycoses

Type of tinea	Synonym	Site	Common causative agents*	Geographical localization
Tinea pedis	Athlete's foot	Soles of feet, between the toes	*Epidermophyton floccosum, Trichophyton mentagrophytes,* and *T. rubrum*	Worldwide
Tinea unguium		Nails	*T. mentagrophytes* and *T. rubrum*	Worldwide
Tinea corporis	Ringworm of the body	Glabrous skin	*Microsporum canis, T. mentagrophytes,* and *T. rubrum*	Worldwide
Tinea imbricata	Scaly ringworm	Scattered over the body	*T. concentricum*	Tropical areas
Tinea cruris	Jockey itch	Groin, perineum, and perianal region	*E. floccosum*	Worldwide
Tinea axillaris		Axilla	*E. floccosum*	Worldwide
Tinea barbae	Barber's itch	Bearded areas of face and neck	*Microsporum* and *Trichophyton* species	Europe and rural areas in the United States
Tinea capitis	Ringworm of the scalp	Scalp and hair	*M. audouini,*† *T. tonsurans,* and other *Trichophyton* species	Worldwide
Tinea favosa‡	Favus	Scalp and subcutaneous tissue	*T. schoenleini, T. violaceum,* and *M. gypseum*	Eastern Europe and Mediterranean area
Tinea versicolor		Scattered over the skin	*Pityrosporum orbiculare (Pityriasis versicorlor, Malassezia furfur)*	Worldwide

* Of the species listed, man is the primary source of infection except for *Micosporum canis,* which is found in dogs and cats; *M. gypseum,* which is present in the soil; and *Trichophyton mentagrophytes,* which may be spread by man and animals.

† Can cause epidemic tinea capitis in children.

‡ The most severe infection caused by dermatophytes which destroys the hair papillae causing scarring and baldness.

uted throughout the world and produce infection in animals as well as man. The general name of tinea has been given to the dermatomycoses, and an appellation has been added to describe the site (for example, tinea pedis, tinea capitis).

In infected tissues, the fungi appear as segmented, branching mycelial fragments or as arthrospores arranged in parallel rows inside or outside the hair, or as a mosaic of spores surrounding the hair shaft. On culture at room temperature, the organisms grow slowly in 2 to 3 weeks, forming colonies of varying appearance and pigmentation, and microscopically show different arrangements of macroconidia and microconidia.

Pathogenesis

After contact with infected individuals or animals, objects contaminated by them, or in the case of *M. gypseum,* the soil, the fungi invade the keratinized tissue. The clinical manifestations which appear in about 2 weeks or more range from the most superficial skin infection to one that involves the subcutaneous tissue (tinea favosa). Tinea versicolor differs from the other dermatomycoses in that the causative agent is a lipophilic yeast-like fungus (*Pityriasis versicolor, Pityrosporum orbiculare,* or *Malassezia furfur*) limited to the stratum corneum.

Whatever the nature of the dermatophyte and its site of localization, the infection generally tends to be chronic and is characterized by the presence of sterile vesicles called dermatophytids. The dermatophytids are manifestations of delayed hypersensitivity frequently occurring on the hand in response to fungal infections on the foot. Experimentally, if mycelial elements are deposited on the skin, they incite an allergic response which results in their destruction. In addition, extracts of dermatophytes *(trichophytin)* elicit both immediate and delayed hypersensitive responses in infected or previously infected individuals.

Laboratory Diagnosis

Three methods are available to assist in establishing a laboratory diagnosis. The use of Wood's light (filtered ultraviolet light) on infected skin or hair can detect the presence of infection with *M. audouini* or *M. canis* which are the only common species of dermatophytes that fluoresce a bright or yellow green. If infected hair or scrapings from infected skin or nails are placed on a slide, treated with 10 percent potassium hydroxide, and heated gently, the specimen becomes sufficiently clarified to reveal the presence of mycelial elements (hyphae and arthrospores). Infected hairs may contain parallel rows of arthrospores inside the hair (endothrix) or outside the hair (exothrix) or may show a mosaic of spores surrounding the hair shaft. With the exception of *Epidermophyton,* which does not invade the hair, all genera can invade the hair, skin, and nails, although infection of the nails by *Microsporum* is uncommon.

Definitive identification of the specimen requires culture on Sabouraud's glucose agar containing gentamicin to prevent bacterial overgrowth and cycloheximide to prevent saprophytic fungal overgrowth. Incubation at room temperature for 2 to 3 weeks is required. The color and appearance of the fungal colonies are noted and examined microscopically for macroconidia and microconidia. These observations together with occasional biochemical tests permit the identification of the genus and species.

Epidemiology

Dermatomycoses are worldwide in distribution. Considering the ubiquity of the dermatophytes, it is probable that on numerous occasions contact of infected skin with healthy skin fails to produce infection. Within the family, usually only one or a few members become infected. Presumably, many people are immune. Children are more susceptible than adults to scalp and body infections. The endocrines seem to be involved since tinea capitis usually disappears at puberty. Adults, on the other hand, are more susceptible than children to infections of the hands and the feet.

As noted in Table 16-2, for most of the dermatomycoses man is the source of infection, but others may be acquired from infected animals. With the exception of *M. audouini,* most of the infections are sporadic rather than epidemic. Unlike the systemic or deep mycoses, dermatophytes can be transmitted from man to man or from animals to man. Infection with dermatophytes is so widespread that most persons are infected before reaching adulthood. The high incidence of tinea pedis (athlete's foot) is undoubtedly a reflection of the common use of showers and communal bathing facilities.

Prevention and Control

Prevention and control are based primarily on (1) strict personal hygiene, frequent bathing, the use of clean towels, care in drying areas between the toes, the use of clean socks changed daily, and in communal facilities general cleanliness and the use of fungistatic powders, especially between the toes and on the feet; and (2) treatment of the infection. Therapy of dermatophyte infections of the hair requires the use of oral griseofulvin for 3 to 4 weeks with cutting of the hair in the infected area when new growth appears. Skin infections are usually treated conservatively with tolnaftate, Whitfield's ointment (salicylic acid and benzoic acid), or undecylenic acid. If failure occurs, patients with the skin infections are given griseofulvin for 2 to 4 weeks. Dermatophyte infections of the nail are generally the most refractory to therapy. The use of griseofulvin for 6 to 12 months has proved effective in many cases, but relapses often occur. In many patients, complete removal of the nail along with griseofulvin therapy improves the chances for cure.

The efficacy of griseofulvin in therapy of the dermatomycoses apparently depends on its incorporation and selective localization in the basal cell layer of the skin and its appendages. When these structures are keratinized, their content of griseofulvin prevents the growth of the dermatophytes.

CANDIDIASIS

Candidiasis is the term used to describe a diverse group of clinical syndromes caused by a yeast-like fungus, *Candida albicans*, which is a member of the normal flora of the oral cavity, stool, vagina, and skin. Overt disease primarily involves the skin and mucous membranes but may involve the bronchopulmonary system or may be disseminated, causing endocarditis, meningitis, or renal infection.

Cutaneous manifestations of candidiasis include localized lesions of the nails and skin (onychia, paronychia, intertrigo, pruritis ani); generalized lesions scattered over the smooth, hairless parts of the body often associated with foci of infection in the oral cavity, intestinal tract, or nails; and candidids, or sterile, grouped vesicular lesions found on the hands and body, representing delayed hypersensitivity responses to infection in other parts of the skin. *Onychia* is an inflammation of the matrix which may lead to the loss of the nail. *Paronychia* is an inflammation of the folds of the skin bordering the nails. *Intertrigo* is an inflammation of the webs of the toes, axilla, umbilicus, groin, and gluteal folds. Onychia and paronychia are the commonest forms of cutaneous candidiasis.

Candidiasis of the mucous membranes most commonly involves the oral cavity (thrush) and the vagina (vulvovaginitis). Bronchial candidiasis is generally a subacute or chronic disease that may disappear spontaneously or persist for years with relapses and remissions. Pulmonary candidiasis may follow a similar course but is a much more serious disease that can lead to a fatal outcome. Disseminated candidiasis is always a threat to the survival of the individual and requires expert clinical management.

The Causative Agent

Candida albicans is a small, oval, budding, yeast-like fungus (3 to 5 μm). The organism grows rapidly on blood agar and Sabouraud's glucose agar in 24 to 48 hr. both at room temperature and at 37°C, producing smooth, pasty colonies. Microscopically, pseudomycelia are produced on cornmeal agar, and large thick-walled spherical cells (chlamydospores), 6 to 9 μm in diameter, on a variety of chlamydospore agars.

Pathogenesis

Most *Candida* infections are of endogenous origin, since the organism is present on the skin, on the oral and vaginal mucous membranes, and in the stools. However, infection may be acquired by infants born of mothers with vulvovaginitis, and epidemics of thrush may occur in newborn nurseries.

Probably in no other infection do predisposing factors exert such a strong and determining influence on the incidence of disease. Thrush is encountered in elderly people with tuberculosis or cancer. Cutaneous candidiasis is commonly found in diabetics, in obese individuals, and in persons whose hands are macerated by frequent soakings in water. Vulvovaginitis is a recognized hazard in diabetics, during pregnancy, and in women taking anovulants. Endocarditis occurs in drug addicts. Antibiotics, corticosteroids, cancer chemotherapy, and immunosuppressive drugs predispose to both infections of the mucous membranes and disseminated disease.

A recent study graphically illustrates the increasing incidence of disseminated candidiasis and the difficult problem of the indiscriminate use of antibiotics in the treatment of burned patients. In 427 acutely burned patients *Candida* organisms were recovered from 271. The organism was isolated from the wounds of 233 patients who prior to culture had therapy with 865 chemotherapeutic agents. In addition, *Candida* organisms were isolated from the urine of 131 and from the blood of 22 patients. Sixty-five of the patients died, making the overall mortality rate 15 percent. Of the 22 patients with *Candida* septicemia, 14 died and 11 of them had disseminated candidiasis at autopsy.

The late development of *Candida* septicemia (average day the first positive blood culture appeared was the sixty-first day after burn) clearly reflects the prior use of chemotherapy (an average of 3.7 drugs per patient before the wound was cultured). The data also emphasize the significance of *Candida* in burned patients which accounted for 21 percent of the deaths (14 of 65 patients) and the severity of *Candida* septicemia (case fatality rate of 64 percent, 14 out of 22). Renal involvement in 9 of the 14 autopsied cases of *Candida* septicemia points up another serious complication in disseminated candidiasis.

Laboratory Diagnosis

Because of its presence as part of the normal flora, isolation of *Candida* from the sputum, urine, or skin must be interpreted with caution. Repeated isolation of the organism in large numbers enhances the diagnosis of pulmonary or urinary infection. Lesions in the oral cavity and the vagina are characteristic and together with isolation of the organism usually present no difficulty.

The standard procedure for identifying *Candida* after isolation on blood agar plates or Sabouraud's glucose agar containing gentamicin is to demonstrate the typical pseudomycelia on cornmeal agar and the chlamydospores on special chlamydospore agar. Species other than *Candida albicans (C. stellatoidea, C. parakrusei, C. tropicalis, C. parapsilosis, C. guilliermondii)* can usually be separated and identified on the basis of chlamydospore production and sugar fermentation and assimilation reactions. Other yeasts fail to produce pseudomycelia.

Epidemiology

While candidiasis occurs throughout the world in all age groups and both sexes, it presents in such a variety of forms that it often develops in particular groups of individuals. For example, oral thrush and generalized cutaneous candidiasis occur in infants who acquired infection from mothers with vulvovaginitis. Oral candidiasis is common in elderly individuals with tuberculosis or cancer. Pregnant and diabetic women and those taking anovulants show a higher incidence of vaginal candidiasis. Cutaneous candidiasis is an occupational disease of bartenders, homemakers, bakers, fruit packers, and others whose hands are frequently immersed in water. Drugs addicts may develop endocarditis due to

Candida. Disseminated candidiasis is a disease that is generally associated with lymphoreticular malignancy, diabetes, autoimmune disease, antibiotics, corticosteroids, immunosuppressive drugs, and cancer chemotherapy.

Prevention and Control

Prevention and control of candidiasis present a difficult problem for many reasons. Disease frequently occurs in debilitated individuals with underlying illness or in those who require therapy that predisposes to candidiasis. The organism is regularly present in many individuals as part of the normal flora and need not be introduced from another infected person. The disease is often chronic, and relapses are common.

Therapy involves the use of nystatin for cutaneous, oral, and vaginal candidiasis and amphotericin B 5-fluorocytosine for disseminated candidiasis. Amphotericin B is effective in cutaneous candidiasis, and candicidin or a jelly containing calcium and sodium propionate is used in vaginal candidiasis. Patients with disseminated mucocutaneous candidiasis sometimes have defects in cell-mediated immunity and are refractory to chemotherapy but apparently in some cases have responded to transfer factor obtained from individuals who have recovered from candidiasis.

SPOROTRICHOSIS

Sporotrichosis is usually a chronic, benign, cutaneous lymphatic or localized cutaneous disease caused by a dimorphic fungus, *Sportrichum schenckii*, but occasionally may be pulmonary or disseminated from the skin to involve other tissues, especially the bones and joints. Man acquires infection when the skin is broken and contact occurs with the organism present in the soil or on plants. Consequently, the disease is frequently found in farmers, gardeners, horticulturists, and greenhouse and vegetable-produce workers.

The Causative Agent

Sportrichum schenckii is a dimorphic fungus that grows in the mycelial form on Sabouraud's glucose agar at room temperature but appears as a yeast in tissues of infected patients or when cultured on blood agar containing cystine at 37°C. The organism forms colonies in 2 to 5 days. At room temperature the initial growth involves a creamy white colony which later becomes wrinkled and pigmented (cream, brown, black). Microscopically, the organisms are delicate, branching, septate hyphae bearing groups of pyriform conidia from the ends of lateral hyphae. At 37°C smooth bacterial-like colonies are formed. Microscopically, the organisms are cigar-shaped, oval, or spherical budding yeasts.

The organism is present as a saprophyte in the soil throughout the world and is present on plants, vegetation, and wood. Barberry or rosebush thorns, wooden splinters, and vegetable stalks contaminated with the fungus often serve as inoculating needles for transmitting the disease to man.

Pathogenesis

One week to several months after inoculation of the fungus through the skin, the most common form of the disease (cutaneous lymphatic) develops as a hard nodule which attaches to the skin and eventually presents as a black, necrotic chancre. Thereafter, multiple subcutaneous nodules occur along the draining lymphatics which become thickened and palpable. The extension of the disease process is frequently halted before the larger lymph nodes are reached, but the axillary or inguinal nodes may become involved and may suppurate. The site of infection is most commonly found on the hands or forearm, but infection of the legs often occurs, and no part of the skin covering the body surface can escape infection. If untreated, the primary chancre heals slowly, but the secondary nodules may persist for months or years.

Localized cutaneous sporotrichosis pursues a similar course, but for unknown reasons does not spread to involve the lymphatics. Disseminated sporotrichosis is a rare disease which usually follows the cutaneous lymphatic form, progresses slowly, involves subcutaneous nodules scattered over the body, and eventually spreads to the bones and joints. Pulmonary sporotrichosis is also a rare disease, but pulmonary infection may be much more frequent.

Laboratory Diagnosis

Although the yeast form of the organism can be observed in tissue exudates or biopsies when examined by the fluorescent antibody technique or when stained by the periodic acid Schiff reagent, the laboratory diagnosis is most readily and practically established by culturing the organism and observing its characteristic microscopic appearance. For this purpose, it is preferable to culture the organism on blood agar at 37°C and on Sabouraud's glucose agar at room temperature.

Epidemiology

Sporotrichosis is a disease found throughout the world, especially in persons pursuing agricultural activities. Typically, the disease is sporadic, but outbreaks involving multiple cases do occur. For example, 2,825 South African gold miners developed sporotrichosis following injury to the skin in mines in which the organism was found growing on the timbers. The majority of cases occur in adults, but children are not immune. Recently an outbreak of cutaneous lymphatic sporotrichosis occurred in 9 of 27 children in Kansas who had played in stacks of baled prairie hay.

Subclinical infections greatly outnumber clinical disease. Surveys based on delayed hypersensitivity testing with extracts prepared from the organism indicate that 11 percent of the population had past infection, whereas as many as 58 percent of workers in plant nurseries had positive skin tests.

Prevention and Control

The ubiquitous distribution of the organism and the normal activities of many individuals have precluded the development of any practical measures for preventing the disease. With adequate treatment, however, the prognosis for the infected patient is excellent except in the disseminated form of the disease.

Oral potassium iodide is the drug of choice for the cutaneous lymphatic and localized cutaneous forms of the disease, but must be given for a prolonged period (4 to 6 weeks after apparent complete recovery) in order to prevent relapses.

Amphotericin B has been effective in some cases refractory to iodide therapy and should be used in disseminated sporotrichosis.

CHROMOMYCOSIS

Chromomycosis (or chromoblastomycosis) is caused by three genera of fungi (*Phialophora, Fonsecaea, Cladosporium*). The organisms grow slowly on Sabouraud's glucose agar in 2 to 3 weeks, usually producing black or brown pigmented colonies. The organisms enter through a break in the skin, and in a few days to weeks present as a small papule. Thereafter, the polymorphous granulomatous lesion of the skin and subcutaneous tissue may progress for months or years if untreated. In advanced stages the lesions appear as tumor-like masses, occasionally pedunculated; may cover large areas of the legs or arms; and frequently are secondarily infected by bacteria, giving rise to a goat-like odor. Identification of the causative agent is based on the microscopic features of the conidiophores. Neither the macroscopic appearance of the colonies on Sabouraud's agar nor the tissue phase (round, thick-walled brown bodies about 9 μm in diameter) are of value in distinguishing the fungi.

The fungi are found in the soil in rural areas of the tropics and subtropics. In the United States most of the cases have been reported from the southeastern states among agricultural workers. In the early stages of the lesion surgical excision is recommended. Fully developed lesions are difficult to treat. However, local injections of amphotericin B and administration of thiabendazole are reported to be of value in therapy and warrant further study.

THE NONVENEREAL TREPONEMATOSES: YAWS, PINTA, BEJEL

Apart from syphilis, *Treponema* species cause three chronic, granulomatous infectious diseases of man which are spread from man to man nonvenereally (yaws, pinta, bejel). The causative agents are motile spirochetes, are morphologically indistinguishable from *Treponema pallidum*, cannot be cultured on artificial media, can infect laboratory animals, are present in early lesions as revealed by dark-field microscopy, and can induce some or all of the positive serological tests found in syphilis (VDRL, TPI, fluorescent antibody, and complement-fixation tests). In addition, there appears to be some degree of cross immunity between syphilis, yaws, and bejel. Bejel is so closely related to syphilis that it is often referred to as endemic or nonvenereal syphilis.

As noted in Table 16-3, there are many epidemiological differences between yaws, pinta, bejel, and syphilis. While the clinical manifestations and the pathogenic pattern in yaws and bejel closely resemble those in syphilis, the nonvenereal treponematoses rarely, if ever, produce the serious tertiary manifestations of cardiovascular syphilis or neurosyphilis. On the other hand, the lesions about the nose and mouth and the depigmentation and hyperkeratosis of the skin can lead to social isolation of the individual, and the bone lesions can preclude gainful employment of the individual.

Under the auspices of the World Health Organization, mass penicillin treatment campaigns in the endemic areas have been extremely effective in eradicating the nonvenereal treponematoses. These activities are being assisted by the early use of penicillin in the treatment of individuals and improvements in the increasing use and availability of soap and water.

MYCETOMA

Mycetoma is a localized, chronic, and progressive infectious disease of the skin and subcutaneous tissues and occasionally of bone. The causative agents include bacteria *(Nocardia, Streptomyces)* and fungi *(Allescheria, Madurella, Phialophora)* which are found in the soil. Infection is usually acquired following trauma to the skin of the foot, a result of walking barefoot, especially in tropical areas where the disease is prevalent. Disease is characterized by swelling, the formation of multiple draining sinuses, and the presence of granules (mycelial elements) in the suppurative lesions. In the United States, the principal causative agent *(Allescheria boydii)* produces dark gray colonies on Sabouraud's glucose agar at room temperature which reveal the presence of conidia (5 × 10 μm) when examined microscopically. Prevention of the disease can be accomplished by the use of shoes and protective clothing, a prescription that is beyond the resources of many developing areas of the world. Therapy must be appropriate to the causative agent. Penicillin and sulfonamides are useful in *Nocardia* and *Streptomyces* infections. Oral administration or topical injection of amphotericin B may be of value in therapy of the fungal infections. Estrogens are reported to be effective in the treatment of *Allescheria boydii* infections, which are generally resistant to amphotericin B. Surgical excision may be effective in early infections, but radical surgery may be

Table 16-3 The Nonvenereal Treponematoses: Yaws, Pinta, Bejel

	Yaws	Pinta	Bejel
Causative agent	*Treponema pertenue*	*Treponema carateum*	*Treponema pallidum* (?)
Growth on artificial media	Negative	Negative	Negative
Type of infection	Systemic	Localized to skin	Systemic
Method of transmission	Direct contact through a break in the skin (?)	Same as yaws?	Unknown, spreads within household, perhaps by oral route or direct contact
Target tissues	Skin and bones	Skin	Skin, mucous membranes, bones
Early stage	Primary papillomatous lesion, secondary papules, bone lesions (4 to 5 years)	Red to violet lesions early, secondary lesions slate blue, gray, or black (1 to 3 months)	Similar to syphilis
Latent stage	Three years or more	Variable, several years or more	Similar to syphilis
Late stage	Bone lesions in about 10 percent of patients	Depigmentation, 3 months to 10 years later, and hyperkeratosis of soles and palms	Similar to syphilis
Immunological response	Same as syphilis	Same as syphilis	Same as syphilis
Geographical distribution	Asia, Africa, and the Caribbean, in rural areas	Central and South America, in rural areas	Africa, Southeast Asia, and Western Pacific, in rural areas
Age incidence	Young children	Children and young adults	Young children
Therapy	Penicillin	Penicillin	Penicillin
Prevention and control	Soap and water, regular bathing, mass treatment with penicillin	Soap and water, regular bathing, mass treatment with penicillin	Improved sanitary and personal hygiene within the household, mass treatment with penicillin

required in established infections that prove refractory to chemotherapy.

ERYTHRASMA

Erythrasma is a chronic localized infection of the skin produced by *Corynebacterium minutissimum.* In its clinical manifestations and sites of localization, erythrasma resembles infections caused by dermatophytes. The superficial lesions in the groin, axillae, and gluteal, inframammary, umbilical, and occasionally the intertriginous areas are dry, scaly, pink, or brown serpiginous patches with an erythematous border. The incidence of the disease in diabetics is high and may spread extensively. Presumably, the mechanism of spread involves direct contact with infected lesions. The diagnosis can be established by culturing the organisms from scrapings of the lesions and demonstrating the presence of gram-positive granular rods. The bacterial colonies fluoresce coral red when examined in ultraviolet light (Wood's lamp). The disease occurs throughout the world but is more common and more extensive lesions are found in tropical and subtropical areas. Antibacterial soaps are often effective in therapy, but the use of erythromycin may be desirable or necessary.

MOLLUSCUM CONTAGIOSUM

Molluscum contagiosum is a chronic localized infection of the skin characterized by small (5 mm), firm, waxy, elevated lesions with an umbilicated center. The disease presumably spreads by direct contact from man to man, and the infection may be spread by the infected person from one site to another *(autoinoculable infection)*. The causative agent belongs to the poxvirus group whose host range is limited to man. The disease is common in children, wrestlers, patients with atopic dermatitis, and more recently, in patients attending venereal disease clinics. The lesions are found primarily on the face, trunk, and extremities, but in patients attending venereal disease clinics, the lesions are primarily distributed about the genitalia, inner thighs, and pubic areas. Diagnosis is facilitated by demonstrating intracytoplasmic inclusion bodies in material expressed from the central core of the lesion. Spontaneous regression of the lesion eventually occurs without scarring, but treatment by mechanical removal of the central core of each lesion hastens the healing process and is effective in preventing further spread by autoinoculation. A general eruptive form of the disease may occur in patients receiving immunosuppressive drugs or corticosteroids.

HUMAN WARTS (VERRUCAE)

Warts are extremely common cutaneous infections of man caused by human papilloma virus, which is a member of the papovaviruses, a group of DNA viruses. The disease is present throughout the world, involves children more commonly than adults, and is spread as a result of direct contact with infected lesions. The typical wart is located on the hands and is a solid papillomatous growth which results from viral stimulation of abnormal epidermal proliferation. The tumors generally regress after many months or years, but reinfections occur. Warts on the palms of the hands and soles of the feet are usually flat and often mosaic (in a large cluster beneath the skin). Condylomata acuminatum are nonvenereal warts located in the genital area which may become clustered and cauliflower-like in appearance. Most warts are best treated conservatively by repeated trimming and application of caustic agents such as trichloroacetic acid or salicylic acid.

CUTANEOUS LARVA MIGRANS

The larvae of the dog and cat hookworm, *Ancylostoma braziliense*, can penetrate the skin and produce a self-limited disease of the skin characterized by larval migration above the germinative layer with associated serpiginous, elevated tunnels and indurated, itchy, dry, crusty papules. The disease is an avocational hazard of children who play in sandboxes frequented by cats and an occupational disease of plumbers and other workers who crawl on their backs in areas contaminated by dog or cat feces. Although the disease is self-limited, the lesions may become secondarily infected. Treatment with ethyl chloride causes sloughing of the skin containing the larvae, and thiabendazole administered orally for a few days is useful. Preventing contamination of soil by cats and dogs would eliminate human infections but seems to be too difficult a task for so trivial an infection.

DRACONTIASIS

Guinea worms, *Dracunculus medinensis*, produce human infection of the skin in many tropical areas of the world. The disease is acquired following the ingestion of an arthropod (copepod) water flea *(Cyclops)* containing larval forms of the nematode. Upon digestion of the water flea in the intestine, the larvae are released, penetrate the intestinal wall, migrate through the tissues, and form mature worms. In about a year the fertilized female worm migrates to the skin surface and produces a blister. Upon exposure to water, numerous larvae are discharged. The blister heals until the next immersion in water and the release of more larvae. The chief problem associated with the disease is secondary infection of the blister, but migration of gravid worms may provoke severe hypersensitive reactions. Prevention and control of the disease are based on constructing water sources that cannot be contaminated by infected persons, by chlorination or boiling of drinking water, and by treatment of infected individuals. The most widely used method of treatment is to carefully and slowly wind the worm on a stick (the gravid worm is 2 to 4 ft. in length). Niridazole, metronidazole, and thiabendazole are reported to be effective but are not widely used.

BIBLIOGRAPHY

"Bacteroides in the Blood," (editorial) *Lancet,* 1:27-28, 1973.

Cubie, H. A.: "Serological Studies in a Student Population Prone to Infection with Human Papilloma Virus," *J. Hyg. (Camb.),* 70:677-690, 1972.

Futch, C., Zikria, B. A., and Neu, H. C.: "Bacteroides Liver Abscess," *Surgery,* 73:59-65, 1973.

Gilbert, D. N., Sanford, J. P., Kutscher, E., Sanders, C. V., Jr., Luby, J. P., and Barnett, J. A.: "Microbiologic Study of Wound Infections in Tornado Casualties," *Arch. Environ. Health,* 26:125-130, 1973.

Gilmore, O. V. A., Martin, T. D. M., and Fletcher, B. N.: "Prevention of Wound Infection after Appendectomy," *Lancet,* 1:220-222, 1973.

Knight, A. G.: "A Review of Experimental Human Fungus Infections," *J. Invest. Dermatol.,* 59:354-358, 1972.

Lindell, T. D., Fletcher, W. S., and Krippaehne, W. W.: "Anorectal Suppurative Disease. A Retrospective Review," *Am. J. Surg.,* 125:189-194, 1973.

Louria, D. B., Stiff, D. P., and Bennett, B.: "Disseminated Moniliasis in the Adult," *Medicine,* 41:307-337, 1962.

Lynch, P. J., Voorhees, J. T., and Harrell, E. R.: "Systemic Sporotrichosis," *Ann. Intern. Med.,* 73:23-30, 1970.

Noble, W. C., and White, P. M.: "Isolation for the Control of Infection in Skin Wards," *J. Hyg. (Camb.),* 70:545-550, 1972.

Somerville, D. A.: "Yeasts in a Hospital for Patients with Skin Diseases," *J. Hyg. (Camb.),* 70:667-675, 1972.

Thomas, M. E. M., Piper, E., and Maurer, I. M.: "Contamination of an Operating Theatre by Gram-negative Bacteria: Examination of Water Supplies, Cleaning Methods and Wound Infections," *J. Hyg. (Camb.),* 70:63-72, 1972.

Chapter 17

Microorganisms and Diseases of the Oral Cavity

Francis E. Shovlin and Robert E. Gillis

PERSPECTIVE

Oral infections are excellent illustrations of disease that results from a disturbance of the normal ecological balance. The most important examples of oral disease, *dental caries* and *periodontal disease,* result from disturbances in the relationship of the resident flora to the oral tissues. Infections of the soft tissues are less frequently seen but also result from an alteration of the ecological balance in favor of the endogenous flora.

An appreciation of the pathogenesis of disease in the oral cavity thus requires an understanding of the subtle influences which affect the normal ecological equilibrium as well as those factors which primarily affect the causative organisms.

THE NORMAL FLORA OF THE ORAL CAVITY

The study of the oral microbial flora poses many problems. The mouth is continuously exposed to numerous and varied organisms in the external environment, yet the flora appears to remain relatively stable throughout life. The initial determinant that selects the species which become established is probably environmental. As different organisms are incorporated into the flora, the environmental controls are modified by interrelationships between the organisms.

Establishment

The skin and mucous membranes of the body support an abundant growth of parasites. Within the oral cavity there is an extensive flora with respect to types and numbers of organisms present.

Prior to birth the mouth is sterile. Initial exposure to parasites occurs during passage through the birth canal. Usually, the mouth of the neonate survives this exposure without contamination and remains sterile. However, within hours, the infant begins to develop a flora which reflects that of the mother and also others who may be in close contact with the infant.

Selectivity in the establishment of the flora in the neonatal mouth is evident. The initial flora consists of gram-positive cocci (alpha-hemolytic and nonhemolytic streptococci, staphylococci, and pneumococci). Gram-positive bacilli, gram-negative cocci, and gram-negative bacilli are incorporated slowly into the flora. Once the flora is established, it is believed to remain relatively constant throughout life.

Character

The character of the oral flora is governed by genetic and nongenetic factors. The primary factors may be expressed in outline form:

Oral Microbiota

Genetic	Nongenetic
Saliva	Exposure (parent's flora)
Teeth	Diet
Tissue	Oral hygiene

Genetic Influences

Saliva Saliva plays an important role in the regulation of the flora. Control is brought about by the content as well as the quantity of saliva. The principal components of saliva are water (95 percent); inorganic cations, including calcium, sodium, and potassium; and chloride, phosphate, and carbonate anions. The carbonate ions form the primary buffer system of the saliva, which may be an important control mechanism in selecting organisms in the flora. At mealtime the buffering is maximal, and between meals it is minimal.

The ions present in the saliva are basically the same as those present in plasma, except that the mean values are different. The fluoride ion is found free in saliva, whereas it is conjugated to protein in the plasma. The concentrations found in saliva, however, are below levels necessary to inhibit glycolysis. Several studies have indicated that fluoride concentrations are higher in dental plaque (the noncalcified accumulation of material, composed mostly of bacteria and their products, that adheres to the teeth) than in the saliva but have failed to show specific enzyme inhibition. It is possible that plaque fluoride may inhibit enzyme systems not yet studied in oral organisms, for example, enzymes active in the storage of polyphosphate.

The proteins present in saliva include mucins, enzymes, albumins, and globulin. The mucins form a pellicle on clean surfaces of the teeth, which may give a fisherman's net effect over the tooth surface during the formation of dental plaque. Enzymes in the saliva have been examined in the hope of finding a clue to carious activity, but the study of enzymes, such as amylase, maltase, urease, hyaluronidase, protease, and peroxidase, has failed to reveal any correlation.

The concentration of globulins in saliva is low in relation to the concentration in the plasma. It is doubtful whether specific plasma immunoglobulins can be raised to concentrations high enough to have an effect on a specific microorganism in the oral flora over an extended period of time. The concept of mucous membrane immunization (Chap. 12) leading to the production of secretory IgA may prove more fruitful.

Antibacterial factors have been found in saliva but are of uncertain significance and vary in concentration in different individuals. Included in this category are factors that inhibit streptococci, lactobacilli, and diphtheria bacilli. The antibacterial effect of saliva appears to be partly related to a peroxidase system that is effective against organisms that are unduly sensitive to oxygen.

The quantity of saliva has an important effect on the total number of bacteria in the flora. When the flow of saliva is copious, bacteria are washed away from their place of lodging and swallowed. Assay of the total number of bacteria throughout the day demonstrates the principle. During sleep the salivary flow stops. Consequently, the total flora is at its maximum in the morning. After breakfast, the numbers decrease as a result of the washing action of saliva and the mechanical detergent action of the food dislodging the bacteria that are then swallowed. The flora builds up prior to the noon meal and is again reduced during eating. Because of the change in numbers of bacteria occurring during the day, studies undertaken to investigate the flora and relative numbers of bacteria must consider the time of sampling to avoid a wide margin of error that could be an artifact.

Teeth Before tooth eruption, aerobic and facultative organisms predominate in the flora, since the oral environment is unfavorable for the growth of anaerobes. After tooth eruption, anaerobes appear in greater numbers and persist unless the host becomes edentulous. The flora of edentulous individuals tends to be more aerobic until the insertion of dentures, after which the anaerobes again increase in number.

The comparative number of aerobes and anaerobes is markedly influenced by the number of teeth present, primarily because of the anatomical effect on the oxidation-reduction (OR) potential. Other factors (carious teeth, accumulation of food debris, established aerobic flora) also reduce the OR potential and affect the ratio of aerobic to anaerobic organisms.

Tooth morphology, developmental defects, and alignment in the arch influence the numbers and types of organisms present. The effect is brought about primarily by the presence or absence of increased areas of retention which, in turn, facilitate or hinder the adherence of bacteria and food debris.

Tissue As with the skin and other mucous membranes, the integrity of the oral mucosa is an important factor in controlling the resident flora. Nutritional and debilitating diseases which lead to mucosal breakdown are associated with concurrent overgrowth of bacteria. The extent of bacterial overgrowth is less evident in slowly progressing chronic diseases, such as dental caries or periodontal disease.

Nongenetic Influences

Exposure As mentioned above, the types of organisms presented to the sterile oral cavity of the newborn determine what organisms become established. Morphologically, the organisms that become established in different individuals are relatively constant. However, the species and strains of the different genera that are found in the normal flora reflect those provided by the mother and nursing attendants. Various types of streptococci become established early and remain predominant throughout life, making up almost 50 percent of the total flora.

Diet Since different bacteria have varying nutritional requirements and the intake of food by the host creates the primary source of nutrient for the resident flora, the diet exerts an important effect on the relative numbers of certain bacteria. A good example is the decrease in the number of lactobacilli that occurs when the intake of refined carbohydrate is limited. If the intake is then increased, there is a corresponding rise in the number of lactobacilli present. Other acidogenic bacteria respond similarly to fluctuations in carbohydrate intake.

Oral Hygiene Effective oral hygiene causes a reduction in the total number of microorganisms present in the mouth and affects the particular bacteria that persist in the flora. In clean mouths the aerobes increase and the anaerobes decrease. Continued neglect of oral hygiene leads to an increase in the number of proteolytic and anaerobic microorganisms.

Interaction of Genetic and Nongenetic Influences The interrelationship between genetic and nongenetic effects on the control of the flora is not entirely clear and requires further study. Genetic factors can be modified with fluorides taken internally or applied topically, by the restoration of improperly formed teeth, and by the realignment of malpositioned teeth. Nongenetic factors can be more easily modified by dietary control, medication, and good oral hygiene, which are stressed in most preventive oral health programs.

Limitations

The study of the oral flora presents many problems, most of which are related to the limitations of current techniques. A few of the difficulties encountered and the margin of error introduced by the techniques play an important role in the interpretation of the data. Consequently, in most instances, the available information must be taken as a guide rather than accepted as scientific fact.

Sampling The stability of an individual's flora alluded to above relates to sampling of the flora over a period of time. In this sense, the flora does remain relatively constant. Within short periods, however, it is in a state of flux and is continuously changing in response to the environment. The time of sampling, therefore, is important.

If salivary samples are taken for study, it is important to know whether or not the saliva was stimulated and, if so, what caused the stimulation. As the saliva exits from the salivary duct, it is sterile. The bacteria that are isolated from it are the result of washings from the mucous membranes and the teeth. Few of these organisms can actually grow in the saliva. If the saliva is stimulated to flow, the increase in quantity will decrease the number of organisms per milliliter as compared with nonstimulated saliva. Samples taken from different areas of the teeth are often pooled even though they may be individually different. The samples are sometimes exposed to air in varying degrees during weighing, and this may affect the strict anaerobes that are present; drying of the sample may be injurious to other organisms. Thus, it is apparent that many errors can be introduced by the sampling procedure.

Cultivation and Enumeration Many of the organisms that can be seen under the microscope cannot be isolated on laboratory media. In some instances, this may be due to a change in the morphology of the organism in response to a change in the environment. However, in other instances, it is due to the lack of proper nutrients or the presence of nutrients in concentrations which allow the growth of one organism but inhibit another. The use of selective media not only inhibits the growth of unwanted species but usually is not suited for optimal growth of the desired organism.

Enumeration of isolated bacteria is an additional problem when total numbers and relative types of bacteria are studied. Several methods have been used in attempts to break up clusters and chains of bacteria for counting of individual cells. None of these methods is entirely satisfactory. For example, the most common technique used in recent studies is sonic oscillation. When this method is used in an attempt to break up chains of lactobacilli, the viability of the bacteria is destroyed before the individual microorganisms can be separated.

Identification Many of the organisms isolated from the oral flora have been identified by genus but not by species. Designation of species has been based on comparisons with species identified in other areas of microbiology. However, a number of pioneering investigators have made significant contributions to the classification of oral lactobacilli, spirochetes, and *Bacterionema,* but much remains to be done.

Composition of the Flora

The data included in Table 17-1 indicate the organisms commonly found in the oral cavity and the samples used for isolation (saliva, plaque, calculus). The species designation is included for the commonly studied organisms, and the log counts, where the information is available, give some indication of the numbers present.

Gram-positive Cocci The gram-positive cocci include strains of staphylococci, streptococci, and pneumococci. *Staphylococcus epidermidis* is the species commonly isolated from the mouth. Many different species of streptococci are present, a number of which have not been carefully studied. *Streptococcus salivarius* and *Streptococcus mitis* are frequently found in the flora. *Streptococcus mutans,* a species which has been studied extensively in the production of dental caries in rodents, is also commonly isolated; however, the species designation is not clearly defined, and subgrouping on the basis of antigenic studies is possible. Anaerobic streptococci are currently designated *peptostreptococci.*

Gram-positive Rods *Corynebacterium* species (diphtheroids) are commonly isolated from all areas of the oral cavity. Characteristically, diphtheroids are pleomorphic, anaerobic, or facultative organisms, and many forms can be seen on oral smears. Several species of lactobacilli are commonly isolated, and because of their association with the dairy industry, individual species have been well defined. The relationship of *Lactobacillus casei* and *L. acidophilus* to dental caries represents an area of active research.

Gram-negative Cocci Two types of gram-negative cocci are commonly isolated: *Neisseria catarrhalis,* a facultative, chained coccus; and *Veillonella alcalescens,* or *Veillonella parvula,* an anaerobic, cluster-type coccus that can utilize lactic acid as an energy source, a property that may account for the high numbers of this organism found in gingival crevice plaque.

Gram-negative Rods Most of the gram-negative rods isolated and studied are anaerobic. There are several species of *Bacteroides* present in saliva, as noted in Table 17-1. *B. melaninogenicus* is the species most commonly isolated and has been implicated in periodontal disease by some investigators. The species *Fusobacterium fusiforme* and *F. nucleatum* are frequently present in the oral flora and have been examined because of their potential role in acute necrotizing ulcerative gingivitis. *Spirillum sputigenum* and *Vibrio sputorum* are the members of the Spirillaceae that can be recovered from the oral cavity.

Table 17-1 Indigenous Bacteria in the Oral Cavity of Man

	Saliva (log counts per ml)	Plaque (log counts per Gm)	Calculus
Staphylococcus	+	V	
Streptococcus			
Facultative streptococci	7–8	10	
S. salivarius	6–7	+	
S. mitis	7	+	
Anaerobic streptococci	+	+	
Corynebacterium	+	+	+
Lactobacillus	0–6	0–6	
L. casei	0–5	+	
L. acidophilus	0–4	+	
L. fermenti	0–5	+	
L. brevis	0–4	+	
L. bifidus	+	+	+
Veillonella	7–8	+	+
Neisseria	7–8	10	
Bacteriodes			
B. melaninogenicus	+	–	
B. serpens	+	–	
B. funduliformis	+	–	
B. fragilis	+	–	
Fusobacterium			
F. fusiforme	6	+	+
F. nucleatum	+		+
Spirillum sputigenum	+	+	+
Vibrio sputorum	+	+	
Actinomyces			
A. israelii	+		+
A. naeslundii	+		+
A. odontolyticus	+	–	+
Leptotrichia			
L. buccalis	3	+	+
Bacterionema			
B. matruchotii			
Treponema	+	+	
Borrelia	+	+	

Key to symbols in table: + = regularly present; V = variable; – = not regularly present; blank = no adequate data.

Source: From J. McDonald, "Microbiology of Caries," in R. F. Sognnaes (ed.), *Chemistry and Prevention of Dental Caries*, 1945. Courtesy of Charles C Thomas, Publisher, Springfield, Illinois.

Filamentous Organisms Filamentous organisms are gram-positive, microaerophilic, or anaerobic, and may be involved in the formation of calculus (calcific deposits on teeth) and in periodontal disease. *Actinomyces israelii* is a potential pathogen and is the causative agent of actinomycosis. *A. naeslundii* produces periodontal lesions in laboratory animals, and *A. odontolyticus* has been isolated from deep dentinal caries and from root caries.

Leptotrichia buccalis and *L. dentium (Bacterionema matruchotii)* have been studied with respect to their possible role in plaque and calculus formation. *L. dentium* has morphologic and biochemical properties that distinguish it from *L. buccalis.*

Other Organisms The spirochetes found in the saliva and the gingival crevice belong to the genera *Treponema* and *Borrelia.* Several species have been described, the most common being *T. macrodentium, T. oralis,* and *B. vincentii.* An increased number of spirochetes have been described in gingivitis, and they are present in all cases of acute necrotizing ulcerative gingivitis.

Yeasts are common inhabitants of the oral cavity. Several species of *Candida* have been isolated, but *C. albicans* is the only one of significance in the oral cavity. Oral candidiasis, or thrush, occurs in patients treated with antibiotics or in individuals with ill-fitting or improperly cared for dentures.

Among the mycoplasmas, *Mycoplasma orale* is the species usually present. Protozoa found in the oral cavity include *Entamoeba gingivalis* and *Trichomonas tenax.* While herpesvirus is not considered a member of the normal oral flora, it is present at any given time in the saliva of about 2.5 percent of the population and frequently produces recurrent disease on the mucous membrane of the lips and the adjacent skin.

DENTAL CARIES

The historical background of the microbiology of dental caries is interesting in that it points up the difficulties involved in the study of this disease. At various times, dental caries have been held to be (1) a mixed infection initiated by acidogenic organisms followed by proteolytic bacteria, (2) caused by acidogenic streptococci, (3) caused by lactobacilli, (4) induced by enterococci and filamentous organisms, and (5) produced by *Streptococcus mutans.*

For 40 years, between 1915 and 1955, lactobacilli dominated caries research. A selective medium was held to show the presence of lactobacilli in all carious lesions, specific isolates of lactobacilli were said to produce the disease in vitro, and it was demonstrated that a limited carbohydrate intake decreased the incidence of caries and brought a concomitant reduction in the number of lactobacilli.

Since 1955, findings in germ-free animals have become the main theme in caries research. It became apparent that caries do not develop in germ-free animals and that significant carious lesions cannot be produced by introducing lactobacilli, but that caries can be produced by introducing enterococci and filamentous organisms. Subsequently, it was shown that *Streptococcus mutans* was a potent producer of caries in germ-free animals. This finding led to numerous isolations of caries-producing streptococci both from animals and humans, and the gnotobiotic (defined flora) animal became the preferred test system. Interest in lactobacilli has declined, since only limited success can be achieved in experimentally reproducing caries in animals.

Acidogenic Theory

The acidogenic theory is currently accepted as the best explanation of the etiology of the carious process. Stated briefly, the theory attributes carious lesions to the acid produced by acidogenic bacteria from residual carbohydrates which causes a local increase in hydrogen-ion concentration that lowers the pH below the critical decalcification pH of hydroxyapatite (enamel). The process is constantly repeated until the carious lesion is initiated and progressively enlarges.

Proteolytic Theory

The proteolytic theory visualizes that the carious lesion is initiated through an attack on enamel protein by proteolytic bacteria. The theory proposes that enamel protein is exposed through developmental defects to proteolytic organisms which degrade it. The enamel rods supported by the protein matrix then break off and the carious lesion enlarges. Evidence to support this theory is lacking, since bacteria isolated from the mouth cannot hydrolyze the enamel matrix unless it is first denatured or treated with acid.

Chelation Theory

Chelating agents are held to be formed as metabolic by-products of viable bacteria and to act by decalcifying the enamel. The exposed protein is then degraded by proteolytic organisms. The hypothesis is not unattractive, but to date, only weak chelators in low concentration have been isolated from dental plaque.

General Considerations

The acidogenic theory best explains the carious process; however, it is oversimplified as presently stated and does little to explain the possible mechanisms involved. Superficial in vitro lesions, indistinguishable from in vivo "white spot lesions," can be produced in enamel by exposing the surface to acid. In the absence of bacteria, the lesion does not progress into the dentine. The findings suggest that bacteria may play a more active role than that of acid production.

For example, some cariogenic bacteria produce predominantly the L(+) form of lactic acid and store polyphosphate. Both factors may play a significant role in the mechanism of caries formation. The L(+)-lactic acid dissolves more hydroxyapatite powder than the racemate under identical conditions. The process is characterized by the formation of small amounts of calcium phospholactate and is evidenced by lower calcium- and higher phosphate-ion concentrations in the supernatant of the pure isomer than are found in the racemate supernatant. Calcium complexing with dimers of lactic acid may also occur and may be more prevalent with the pure isomer.

The dissolution of hydroxyapatite crystals by direct acid attack may be expressed by the following equation:

$$Ca_{10}(PO_4)_6(OH)_2 + 8H^+ \rightleftharpoons 10Ca^{++} + 6HPO_4^{--} + 2HOH$$

The build-up of calcium and phosphate ions without interference results in exceeding the solubility product, and a precipitate of acid-insoluble secondary calcium phosphate will form. The presence of aciduric organisms that can remove calcium ions and utilize the metaphosphate ion as substrate for intracellular inorganic phosphate storage would actively partake in the dissolution process. The removal of calcium and phosphate ions would move the equilibrium to the right and favor the continued dissolution of the inorganic portion of the tooth.

Essential Factors

The Susceptible Host A small percentage of the population remains immune to caries throughout life. In some cases, the relative immunity is the result of restricted carbohydrate intake, but in many immune individuals, the diet is unrestricted, and carious lesions do not develop. The reasons for the immunity are uncertain. It has been attributed to saliva, tooth form, and tooth insolubility, but as yet, there is no scientific evidence to support any of these concepts. Elucidation of the mechanisms involved in caries immunity, however, may provide clues that will lead to the prevention of the disease.

Bacteria The introduction of germ-free animals has made it possible to demonstrate that susceptible strains of rats and hamsters do not develop caries in the absence of bacteria when other environmental factors are kept constant. The significance of this finding was the elimination of claims for nonspecific and/or psychogenic causes of dental caries.

Retention Areas The presence of dental plaque is essential for caries to occur. The emphasis here is to indicate that plaque found in retention areas differs from plaque found on exposed smooth surfaces.

Retention areas are defined as pits and fissures, interproximal contact points, and the gingival margins where mechanical forces retain the bacteria on the surface of the tooth. Lesions which develop in interproximal areas are not the result of these surfaces being more susceptible to caries, but are due to the mechanical retention of bacteria and food debris. In the case of rotated teeth, lesions do not develop on the exposed anatomical mesial or distal surface of the tooth. Rather, lesions develop on the anatomical facial or lingual surface where contact is made with the adjacent tooth. Similarly, when the gingival margin recedes, new lesions develop close to the gingival margin, a retention area, and not where the margin was originally on an exposed smooth surface. Dental plaque in a retention area must have specific properties which make it more cariogenic than dental plaque on exposed tooth surfaces.

Carbohydrates Laboratory and epidemiologic studies have shown that carbohydrates must be present in the diet for caries to occur. Experiments with tube-fed rats designed to bypass the oral cavity, avoiding contact with the teeth, demonstrated that tube-fed rats did not develop caries. Rats fed normally on the same diet developed caries. In man, a lowering of the carbohydrate intake leads to a reduction in new carious lesions, whereas patients fed on a sticky, high-carbohydrate diet have an increased incidence of caries. Epidemiologic studies also provide strong support for the importance of carbohydrate in dental caries.

Dental Plaque Because of experimental studies which reveal that caries occur only in the presence of massive accumulation of dental plaque, many researchers believe that dental

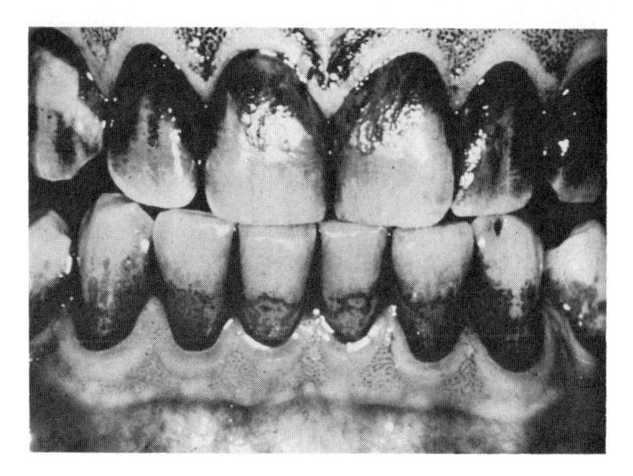

Figure 17-1 Dental plaque accumulation of approximately 6 days' undisturbed growth emphasized by means of F. D. C., No. 3 Green (0.5 percent) disclosing solution. Note how the plaque is limited to the cervical areas above the height of contour of the crowns. The incisal portion of the tooth is cleansed by mechanical abrasion of food. (*Courtesy of A. J. Formicola, College of Medicine and Dentistry of New Jersey, New Jersey Dental School, Newark.*)

plaque is essential for the initiation of caries. If human dental plaque is defined as the adherence of bacteria to the exposed smooth surfaces of teeth, then it is not significant in the production of caries, since "white spots" usually form in these areas, and frank lesions are seldom seen clinically. If the definition of human dental plaque were to include the bacterial accumulation in retention areas, then it should be pointed out that the flora is probably different in these areas from that seen on exposed smooth surfaces.

Smooth surface plaque has been studied extensively. It is initiated by salivary mucin, which forms a pellicle. Gram-positive cocci and filamentous organisms grow and form a network that entraps other bacteria. The gram-positive organisms predominate. The food debris provides carbohydrate substrate that increases the bacterial flora. As the plaque ages, gram-negative organisms become established, and the acidogenic character of the flora decreases.

Retention area plaque has not been studied extensively. Indications from initial studies appear to show that the acidogenic character of

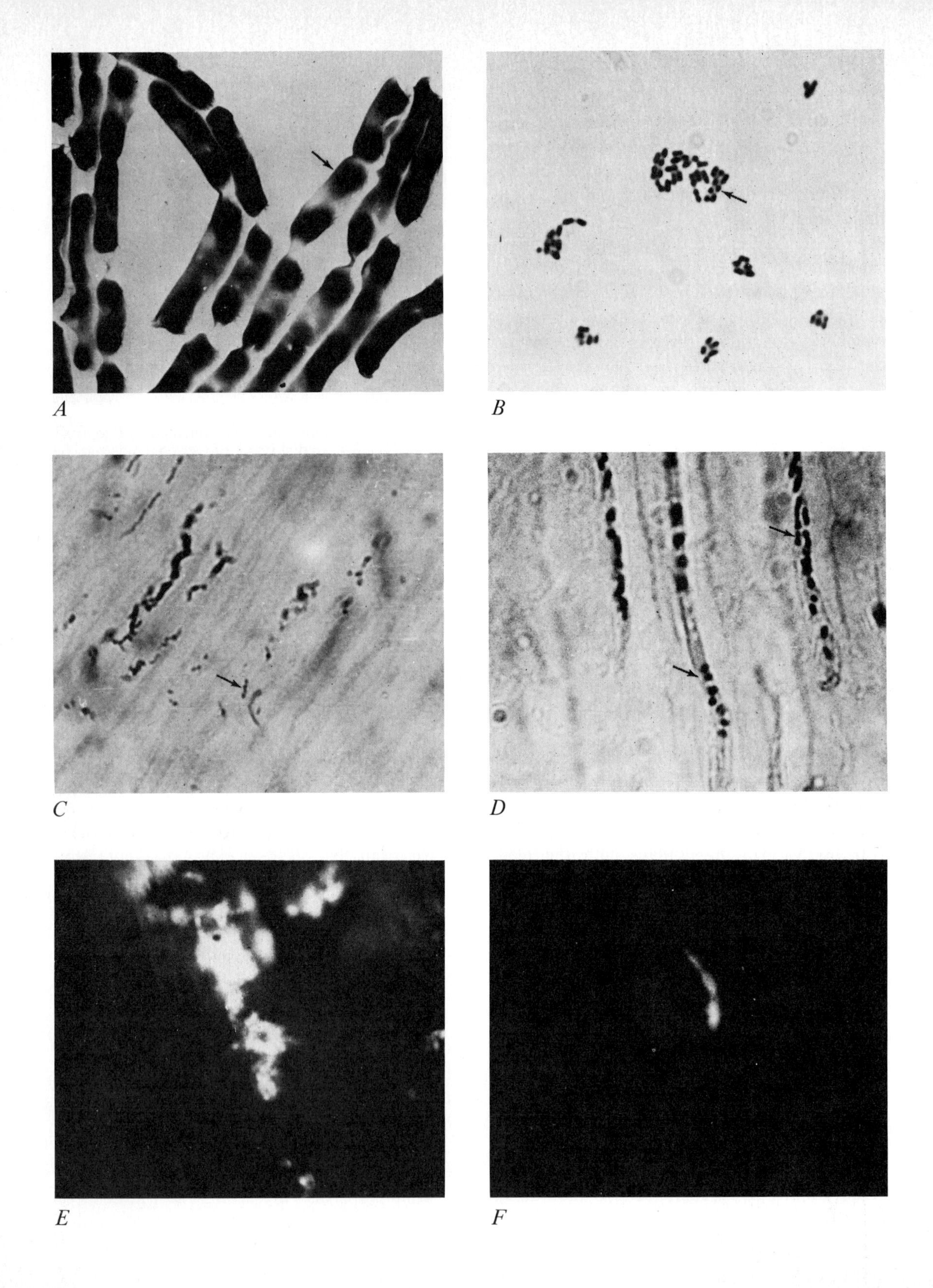
A
B
C
D
E
F

this plaque remains relatively unchanged. Acidogenic organisms (streptococci, lactobacilli) have been isolated from retention areas but the same strains were not found on the exposed smooth surfaces of the adjacent teeth. Therefore, plaque on different areas of the tooth probably contains distinct bacterial floras. The flora in retention areas may tend to remain more acidogenic.

Pathogenesis

In smooth surface lesions, "white spot" formation is the characteristic initial finding and is produced by subsurface decalcification which leaves the enamel surface intact. There are several proposals offered to explain why the enamel surface remains intact: (1) Salivary mucin forms an enamel cuticle that protects the surface; (2) fluoride which is present in greater concentrations in the surface layer of enamel makes the surface less soluble; and (3) the effect of dissolution of enamel is greater along the protein matrix of the enamel than at the surface.

In retention areas in the absence of pits and fissures, the surface lesion progresses laterally and inwardly in spearhead fashion until it reaches the dentinoenamel junction. At the dentinoenamel junction, it again spreads laterally and then inwardly in a spearhead design. It progresses at a more rapid rate in the dentine, probably because of the lower content of inorganic salts and a higher content of organic matrix.

In the case of pits and fissures, the protein matrix is more prominent, and in some cases, it may even extend into the dentinoenamel junction. With the increase in organic material and a corresponding decrease in the inorganic salts, the lesion progresses more rapidly than lesions that are initiated on the outer enamel surface.

Epidemiology

Dental caries is probably the most prevalent disease of civilized man. The bulk of the population in the United States is susceptible to the disease, and collected data indicate that more than 95 percent are affected. The number of teeth attacked varies, but by adolescence, an average of 10 to 14 carious teeth is not unusual.

Certain primitive peoples are resistant to caries, probably as a result of their diet. Contact with and adoption of a modern mode of living in such groups lead to an increased incidence of dental caries. A significant decline in caries was noted in restricted populations during World War II, when refined sugar was unavailable in the diet.

Diagnosis

The best means available for diagnosis is clinical examination, which must include both visual inspection and bitewing roentgenograms.

Figure 17-2 Bacteriological examination of human carious lesion comparing morphology of culture-grown *L. casei* with the morphology of invading organisms and the identification of the organisms using fluorescein-tagged serologic group C antiserum. *A.* Electron micrograph of culture-grown organisms showing intracellular granules of polyphosphate. The granules give a coccoid appearance and usually are dipolar (magnification approx. 40,000 ×). *B.* High-power view of gram-stained preparation of culture-grown organisms showing the dipolar staining and coccoid appearance in many cells (magnification approx. 800 ×). *C.* Brown and Brenn preparation of human dentinal lesion showing organisms along the dentinal tubules with similar morphology to those shown in *B* (magnification approx. 600 ×). *D.* Gram-stained preparation of human dentinal lesion showing intracellular inclusions similar to culture-grown organisms in *A* and *B* (magnification approx. 800 ×). *E.* Medium-power view of fluorescent antibody preparation showing positive staining of organisms in transverse clefts of the dentinal lesion. Individual organisms are also evident (magnification approx. 600 ×). *F.* High-power view of individual bacterial chain along a dentinal tubule showing positive staining with Sharpe's serological group C fluorescein-tagged antiserum.

Laboratory tests to detect or predict the onset of caries in an individual are not available. However, the *Lactobacillus* count and the Snyder test have been shown to be reliable in predicting the caries incidence in a population.

Prevention and Control

The best public health measure available for the control of dental caries is fluoridation of the water supply. The preponderance of evidence indicates that fluoridation of the water supply is an efficacious practice that benefits the whole community. The best explanation for the caries-inhibiting action of fluoride is that the fluoride ion replaces the hydroxyl ion in hydroxyapatite and forms a fluorapatite which is less soluble in acid. Topical applications of fluoride and the incorporation of fluoride in toothpaste have been shown to be helpful in reducing caries.

Patient education in the practice of good oral hygiene and regular dental care is also beneficial. Instructions to the patient regarding the diet, especially the intake of refined carbohydrate, are important, since it has been clearly demonstrated that the intake of sugar and the incidence of caries are directly related. Strict controls on sugar intake would probably eliminate the high incidence of caries, but the modern mode of living eliminates this approach. The addition of phosphates to the diet and the sealing of pits and fissures with polymers are recent practices that may bring about a further reduction in dental caries.

On the other hand, the magnitude of the problem of preventing dental caries can be gauged by the sobering realization that (1) approximately 50 percent of the population in the United States have never had dental care; (2) resistance to fluoridation of water supplies has precluded the initiation of this public health measure in many communities in the country. Thus, dental caries is a socioeconomic and sociopolitical disease.

EXPERIMENTAL CARIES

One of the difficulties in more exactly defining the etiology of dental caries has been the lack of a suitable experimental animal in which the disease can be produced under conditions which approximate those seen in human dental caries. Most experimental investigations have utilized rodents, but their dentition is anatomically and chemically dissimilar to that of humans.

For this reason, it is emphasized that results obtained from animal experimentation must be cautiously interpreted and that extrapolation of the meaning cannot be as directly made for dental caries as for other microbial diseases in which animal models have been used so successfully. On the other hand, these data can be useful in outlining broad avenues to be followed in evaluating the human disease and in suggesting hypotheses for further experimentation. With these limitations in perspective, the implications of the experimental findings for human caries are reviewed.

Comparison of the incidence of caries in germ-free and conventional animals on a cariogenic diet yielded dramatic results. In experiments continuing for 170 days, germ-free animals failed to develop caries. Even when examined histologically, the teeth were unchanged except for a minor number of cuspal fractures. In the conventional animals, caries was widespread and affected 38 of 39 animals. When germ-free animals were challenged with various microorganisms, it was found that caries could be induced with some bacteria but not with others. For example, enterococci in combination with proteolytic bacilli produced caries, but lactobacilli were negative.

The next advance came when it was shown that a streptococcus isolated from a caries-susceptible colony of hamsters could induce caries in stock colonies of hamsters. Subsequently, numerous isolations of cariogenic streptococci were made from both human and animal

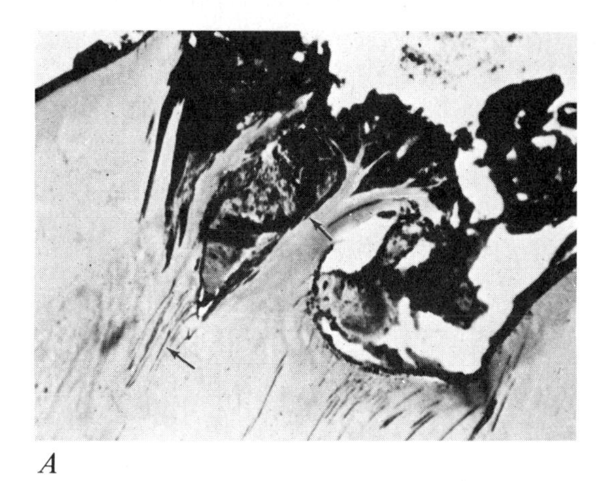

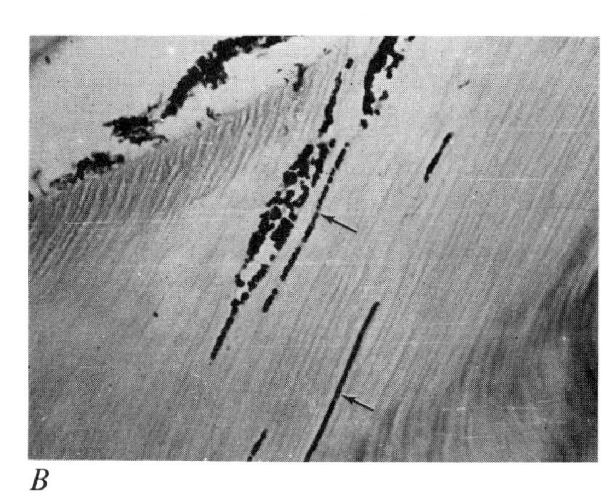

Figure 17-3 Brown and Brenn preparations of carious lesions in gnotobiotic rat molars by bacterial strains isolated from laboratory stock caries-susceptible rats. *A*. Massive accumulation of dental plaque in the occlusal pits (upper arrow) and invasion by bacteria into the subjacent dentin (lower arrow). Lesion was induced by rat streptococcal strain 25QR-4R (magnification approx. 95 ×). *B*. High-power view of bacteria along the dentinal tubules. Lesion was induced by rat lactobacilli strain 108TR. The short coccoid forms of the organism are indicated by the upper arrow; the long, rod forms are indicated by the lower arrow. Similar forms are discernible in culture preparations of lactobacilli species (magnification approx. 400 ×). (*Courtesy of R. J. Fitzgerald, V. A. Hospital, Miami, Fla.*)

sources. Many of these organisms were designated *Streptococcus mutans* on the basis of fermentation of mannitol and sorbitol. Analyses of guanine/cytosine ratios and cell wall antigens indicate that many organisms identified as *S. mutans* are not closely related and that at least four subgroups can be recognized.

Organisms identified as *S. mutans* produce an extracellular dextran that forms heavy plaque over the tooth surface when animals are maintained on a high sucrose diet. The importance of this plaque in the production of dental caries in hamsters was demonstrated by showing that dextranase included in the diet inhibited plaque accumulation and the occurrence of caries. Attempts to utilize dextranase to inhibit human caries have not been successful. Dextran is found in insignificant quantity and probably does not play an important role in the formation of human plaque.

Experimental studies with lactobacilli generally have failed to induce a significant number of carious lesions, but *Lactobacillus casei* (ATCC 4646) has been reported to be cariogenic in gnotobiotic animals. In addition, *L. casei* recovered from deep dentinal caries in man was found to produce a high incidence of caries in conventional rats (Fig. 17-4). In these experiments, *L. casei* was identified in the dentinal tubules at the base of the lesion using fluorescent antibody techniques. The importance of lesions produced in animals using *L. casei* is the absence of heavy plaque. Lesions occur along pits and fissures and interproximally in much the same manner as found in humans.

A serious impediment to the evaluation of etiological agents in dental caries is that the organisms are often identified solely on the basis of morphology (streptococci, bacilli) or genera (*Streptococcus, Lactobacillus*). In many human diseases caused by microorganisms, pathogenicity is a property of a particular species or even of strains within the species (*Corynebacterium diphtheriae, Staphylococcus aureus,* group A

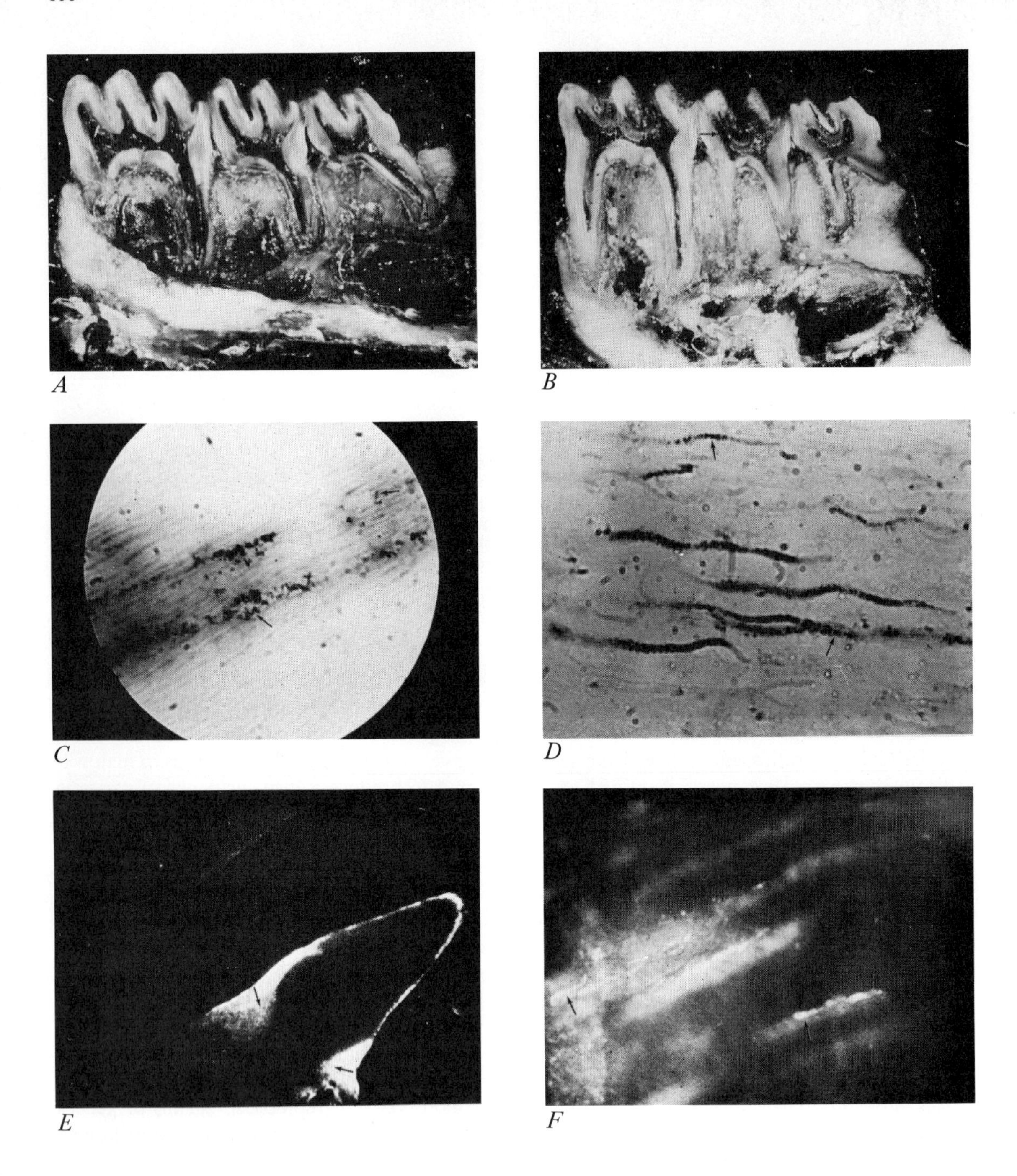
A
B
C
D
E
F

beta-hemolytic *Streptococcus pyogenes, Escherichia coli*). If the principle is applicable to dental caries, it is probable that caries will be found to be produced by specific isolates of *Streptococcus mutans* or *Lactobacillus casei.*

INFECTION OF THE DENTAL PULP AND PERIAPICAL REGION

The dental pulp is the inner vital tissue of the tooth. During early development of the tooth, its function is both formative and nutritive. After the tooth is fully developed, it continues its nutritive function with respect to the dentine but in addition performs a sensory function to indicate injury to the tooth, and to a limited extent, it has defensive properties.

Pathogenesis of Infections of the Dental Pulp

Infections of the dental pulp may develop in a number of ways. Carious pulpal exposure is the most common pathway for bacterial invasion of the dental pulp and the most common cause of pulpal infection is the untreated carious lesion. Bacteria can also invade the pulp through the dentinal tubules from deep carious lesions prior to pulpal exposure. Occasionally, bacteria can be forced through the tubules into the pulp during cavity preparation or taking impressions.

The periodontal lymphatics provide another route for infections of the dental pulp. Vessels that drain the tissue lymph from around the periodontal membrane enter the pulp. When the tooth is traumatically injured and disrupted in the socket, bacteria from the gingival crevice can enter the underlying tissue and cause pulp infection. The result may be acute bacterial infection of the pulp in the absence of pulpal exposure. The pulp may also be infected via the blood *(anachoresis).* In the presence of bacteremia, even when there is slight insult to the pulpal tissue, organisms can migrate from the blood and become established in the pulp.

Along the side of the root surface, there are communications between the pulp canal and periodontal ligament through which blood vessels pass. When a break in the epithelial attachment occurs and a periodontal pocket forms, the bacteria in the pocket may invade the pulp through these lateral canals. The reverse is also true; that is, bacterial infection in the pulp canal can reach the periodontal ligament through these canals.

Causative Agents in Infections of the Pulp

Examination of the pulp cavity for bacteria is done by performing cultures. The specimen obtained from the pulp cavity by means of a sterile

Figure 17-4 Laboratory-induced caries in stock Sprague-Dawley rats inoculated with a strain of *L. casei,* Sharpe's serologic group C organism. *A.* Control group showing the absence of lesions in a Schiff reagent–treated mesiodistal section through the lower molar teeth (magnification 40 ×). *B.* Same preparation of an experimental animal showing the severe retention area lesions that occur adjacent to the pits. The left arrow indicates an area of complete destruction of the underlying dentin with exposure of the pulp tissue. The right arrow indicates an area of lateral spread along the dentinoenamel junction as occurs in human lesions. *C.* Gram stain preparation of transverse section through the dentin showing the peritubular arrangement of the bacteria and the intracellular granules (arrow). Bacterial invasion of the dentin characteristically is adjacent to the tubules, and bacteria do not invade the tubules until there is considerable tissue destruction and bacterial overgrowth (magnification 800 ×). *D.* Gram-stained preparation of vertical section through the dentin showing the morphology of the bacteria. The similarity to culture-grown preparation of *L. casei* and the presence of inclusion bodies are obvious in some areas (see arrows; magnification 800 ×). *E.* Fluorescent antibody preparation of maxillary molar tooth showing fluorescence in retention area lesions, both interproximal and occlusal pit (see arrows; magnification approx. 60 ×). *F.* High-power view of interproximal lesion shown in *E.* The individual bacteria are evident along the dentinal tubules (see arrows; magnification approx. 400 ×).

Table 17-2 Strains Isolated from 4,186 Root Canal Cultures

Organism	A In pure culture	B In mixed infections	C Total
Streptococcus faecalis	240	45	285
Streptococcus mitis	153	130	283
Streptococcus salivarius	5	15	20
Streptococcus hemolyticus	33	22	55
Anaerobic streptococci	54	15	69
Indifferent streptococci	81	71	152
Other streptococci	11	17	28
Total	577	315	892
Staphylococci	161	71	232
Lactobacilli	57	41	98
Diphtheroids	45	13	58
Gram-positive rods	10	11	21
Bacillus species	9	12	21
Actinomyces	17	3	20
Fusobacterium	5	3	8
Sarcina	1	0	1
Neisseria	1	14	15
Gram-negative rods	5	23	28
Yeasts	15	8	23
Mixed infection	238		
Total positive cultures	1,141	Total organisms	1,417
Turbid, no growth	56*		
Negative cultures	2,989		
Total	4,186		

* Slight turbidity on initial culture which could not be subcultured.

Note: Column B gives the frequency of each organism isolated from mixed infection, and column C gives the frequency of isolation for all organisms.

Source: According to K. C. Winkler and J. van Amerogen, *Oral Surg., Oral Med., and Oral Pathol.* 12:857–875, 1959.

paper point is transferred to a suitable broth which is incubated at 37°C and examined for bacterial growth after 24 and 48 hr. Separation of the organisms present in the broth is achieved by preparing streak plates, and preliminary identification is determined by colonial morphology and Gram's stain. Definitive identification of the causative agent, however, presents serious difficulties.

While there is considerable variation in the relative numbers or the proportion of particular bacteria recovered from infected pulp canals, there is general agreement with respect to the groups of bacteria or the specific organisms that can be isolated. The data from one rather exhaustive study are included in Table 17-2. Of 4,186 canals cultured, 3,045 (72.7 percent) were negative and 1,141 (26.3 percent) were positive. If only teeth with necrotic pulps are included, the number of positive cultures approximates 50 percent.

Streptococcus faecalis (enterococci, group D streptococci) which produced α-hemolysis on blood agar was the most common isolate. The *S. mitis* grouping includes α-hemolytic organisms that could not otherwise be classified. *S. salivarius,* although frequently isolated from saliva and dental plaque, is not commonly found in infected pulp canals. The bulk of the cultures yielded streptococci (63 percent). Since streptococci are the most difficult organisms to eliminate from the pulp canal and are the chief cause of endodontic treatment failures, treatment should be directed at the elimination of these organisms.

The remaining data show that staphylococci and lactobacilli are present in 14 and 8.5 percent of the infected patients. Staphylococci can also cause treatment problems, and occasionally, suppurative cases yield gram-negative bacilli that are resistant to treatment.

When the pulpal tissue of a tooth becomes infected, the body defenses cannot eliminate the infection. As a result, the tooth must be extracted or treated endodontically, which involves careful debridement of the pulp canal and the placing of an inert filling material to obliterate the canal space in order to prevent reinfection.

Knowledge of the causative agents involved in pulp canal infections requires special precautions (see Table 17-4) when a patient presents a history of rheumatic heart disease, congenital heart damage, or prosthetic valves. During treatment, precautions must be taken to eliminate bacteremia that may occur by chance, since the infecting organisms are the same as those most commonly associated with subacute bacterial endocarditis. It has been demonstrated that bacteremias do not occur during debridement of cases of vital pulp extirpation but do occur when necrotic cases are treated. Nevertheless, the patient must be protected in all cases because of the serious nature of the possible ensuing infection.

Alpha-hemolytic streptococci and enterococci characteristically develop resistance to penicillin. Although penicillin is the drug of choice in the absence of a history of allergy when a local abscess or diffuse cellulitis develops during treatment, the practitioner should be alert to the fact that antibiotic resistance may present a problem. If antibiotic sensitivity testing cannot be performed, the patient should be carefully observed, and if response to the antibiotic does not occur within 24 to 48 hr., the dosage should be increased or the antibiotic should be changed.

Reaction of the Pulp

The initial reaction of the pulp to bacterial invasion is an inflammatory response. If the number and virulence of the invading organisms are low, the pulp tissue may localize the infection with the formation of a small ulcer. If the number or virulence of the organisms are high, then a series of microabscesses will form which eventually coalesce and destroy a large portion of the pulp tissue. The process usually continues until there is total necrosis of the tissue, since the ability of the pulp tissue for repair is limited. The bacteria are then free to pass into the periapical tissues.

Pathogenesis of Infections of the Periapical Region

If pulpal infection remains untreated, it will spread into the periapical tissue. Initially the periodontal ligament is involved, then the underlying alveolar bone. After spreading through the bone, the infection exits either at the unattached mucosa or further apically into the fascial planes. Infection along the unattached mucosa results in the formation of a *gingival abscess* (parulis). Infection in the fascial planes results in a diffuse cellulitis.

The most common pathway for invasion of the periapical tissues by bacteria is through the apical foramen from an infected pulp and/or pulp canal. The bacteria involved are the same as those causing pulpal infections, and streptococci are the principal invaders. Normally the body defenses can control the infection, but in some instances antibiotic therapy is indicated. Removal of the source of infection by debridement of the pulp canal is essential in order to prevent recurrence of infection. Other potential but relatively rare sources of infection include the blood, periodontal lymphatics, and direct extension through periodontal lesions.

Reaction of the Periapical Tissue

Following the initial invasion of the periapical region, an acute inflammatory response occurs. The severity and outcome of the response depend on the number of organisms present, their virulence, and the resistance of the host. If host resistance is overcome, an acute abscess or cellulitis will develop. If host resistance is strong, infection will persist as a chronic alveolar abscess.

Acute Alveolar Abscess The acute abscess is characterized by a massive growth of the invading bacteria which causes a build-up of periapical pressure, resulting in severe pain. The pressure caused by the bacteria forces the tooth incisally or occlusally and causes it to become loose in its socket. The tooth is extremely sensitive to biting or percussion. The pain can be relieved by releasing the pressure, either by draining through the tooth or by incision and drainage above the apex of the root.

Chronic Alveolar Abscess When a standoff between invading organisms and host defense occurs, a chronic abscess develops and is characterized by the absence of pain, progressive destruction of alveolar bone, the formation of a blood vessel-rich capsule of chronic inflammatory tissue, and a small number of viable organisms. Attempts to isolate organisms from these lesions using cannula type sampling have often been unsuccessful. Organisms must be present in small numbers, as in some skin abscesses, or the lesion would be resolved.

Occasionally, the chronic abscess may develop into an acute suppurative process (phoenix abscess). When this occurs, the pain is moderately severe and the suppuration will drain through a fistula that will form on the gingiva. After drainage, the pain will subside and the fistula will heal, only to recur. The pulp canal remains a continuous source of viable organisms and this nidus of infection must be removed either by endodontic treatment or by extraction of the tooth before the abscess can be resolved.

Dental Granuloma The dental granuloma is a special form of chronic alveolar abscess. The infection is less suppurative. The granulomatous tissue becomes encircled by a fibrous capsule. The size of the lesion is usually more limited than the chronic abscess with less bone destruction. However, the lesion retains the potential of entering an acute suppurative stage. To avoid this possibility, the infected pulp canal must be treated or the tooth extracted whenever a granuloma is present.

Radicular Cyst The shape and initial development of the root of the tooth are determined by Hertwig's epithelial root sheath which is formed from the epithelial dental organ. As the dentin of the root begins to form, the sheath begins to break up and form epithelial remnants (rests of Malassez) which remain in the periodontal ligament space. During formation of the dental granuloma, some of the rests become entrapped in the granulation tissue and begin to proliferate. The proliferations may remain isolated in the granulation tissue or they may coalesce to form a cyst by lining the inner wall of the granulation tissue. The epithelial cells closest to the lumen and away from the nutriment furnished by the granulation tissue will begin to slough and cause osmotic changes in the lumen. The result is an influx of fluid and the enlargement of the cyst.

Dental granulomas and radicular cysts cannot be differentiated clinically. Treatment of patients with periapical pathologic conditions requires an observation period. Cysts which do not respond to conservative endodontic treatment must be removed surgically.

PERIODONTAL DISEASE

Periodontal disease is a general term used to denote disruption of the normal integrity of the investing and supporting tissues of the teeth. Maintenance of these tissues in a state of health is important if the teeth are to remain functional throughout the life span of the individual. Loss of functional support of the tooth accounts for most tooth extractions after the individual reaches early middle age. Destruction of the supporting structures probably has a varied etiology, and the tendency to group these as a single entity may be misleading. In most forms of periodontal disease, there is little doubt that the endogenous flora plays an important role in the progression of the disease. However, different forms of the disease are probably initiated and/or continued by different bacterial species. In order to appreciate the problem of periodontal disease, the ensuing discussion is concerned with the normal flora of the gingival crevice, the result of an overgrowth of the flora, and the possible causes for the overgrowth.

Normal Flora of the Gingival Crevice

The flora of the gingival crevice differs somewhat from that of the saliva, interproximal areas, and pits and fissures of teeth. Study of the flora of the gingival crevice presents the same problems encountered with study of the saliva and the flora of dental surfaces.

A summary of microorganisms found in the gingival crevice is included in Table 17-3. The most obvious conclusion is that the flora of the crevice is predominantly gram-positive (70 percent). The organisms present are almost evenly distributed between cocci and bacilli. Among the cocci, facultative bacteria predominate. The relative numbers and the proportion of bacteria found should be taken as an indicator only, since many bacillary chains are difficult to break up into single cells. Consequently, when a dilution plating technique is used for counting, the method can introduce a sizable margin of error. A similar problem arises when direct cell counts are used, since the individual bacteria in a long chain do not appear in the same plane during counting procedures.

Among gram-negative organisms present in the gingival crevice, anaerobic cocci of the genus *Veillonella* make up a significant portion of the flora. Facultative gram-positive rods are not commonly recovered, but gram-negative anaerobic bacilli are numerous in the flora, especially *Bacteroides melaninogenicus* and *Fusobacterium nucleatum.*

Although spirochetes can be consistently found in the gingival crevice, they make up only a small proportion of the total flora.

Human Periodontal Disease

Acute Gingivitis Acute gingivitis may be localized in a limited area at the gingival crevice or may be diffuse, affecting most areas of the gingival margin on both the upper and lower arches. The lesion is inflammatory in nature, and the free margin of the gingiva usually, but not always, responds with an edematous type of reaction. The lesion frequently responds effectively to local debridement and hot rinses. The microbiology of these lesions has not been elucidated.

Acute necrotizing ulcerative gingivitis is associated with a marked overgrowth of fusobacteria and oral spirochetes *(Borrelia, Treponema).* The disease occurs as either a localized or generalized infection in which the gingival margins become edematous and there is characteristic

Table 17-3 Organisms of the Human Gingival Crevice Region

Group	Approximate percent of cultivatible microbiota
Gram-positive facultative cocci	28.8
Staphylococci	
Enterococci	
S. mutans	
S. sanguis	
S. mitis	
Gram-positive anaerobic cocci	7.4
Peptostreptococcus	
Gram-positive facultative rods	15.3
Corynebacterium	
Lactobacillus	
Nocardia	
Odontomyces viscosus	
B. matruchotii	
Gram-positive anaerobic rods	20.2
A. bifidus	
A. israelii	
A. naeslundii	
A. odontolyticus	
P. acnes	
L. buccalis	
Corynebacterium	
Gram-negative facultative cocci	0.4
Neisseria	
Gram-negative anaerobic cocci	10.7
V. alcalescens	
V. parvula	
Transients	
Gram-negative facultative rods	1.2
Gram-negative anaerobic rods	16.1
B. melaninogenicus	
B. oralis	
V. sputorum	
F. nucleatum	
S. sputigenum	
Spiral organisms	1 to 3
T. denticola	
T. oralis	
T. macrodentium	
B. vincentii	

Source: According to S. S. Socransky, *J. Dent. Res.*, 49:203–222, 1970. (Copyright by the American Dental Association. Reprinted by permission.)

blunting of the interdental papillae. The precise relationship of the fusobacteria and spirochetes to the disease is not well defined. The disease cannot be reproduced in animals or in man, but invasion of the underlying connective tissue by spirochetes during the course of the disease has been demonstrated. It is uncertain, however, whether spirochetal invasion is the cause or effect.

Local irritants and/or systemic disturbances have been implicated as contributing factors in the disease. Thorough debridement with the removal of local irritants does bring about a remarkable recovery of the tissue. The disease also responds well to antibiotic therapy when it is used in severe cases, but removal of local irritants is still indicated.

Chronic Gingivitis Chronic gingivitis results from constant irritation of the free gingiva and is characterized by noticeable edema and a slight bluing of the tissue which results from venal stasis. Overgrowth of the gingival crevice flora may result from improper or total absence of oral hygiene. The only reported alteration in the flora involved a threefold increase in spirochetes.

Periodontitis When infection progresses beyond the gingival crevice and the underlying alveolar bone is involved, the condition is referred to as periodontitis. It is usually initiated by the formation of a periodontal pocket which develops following a break in the epithelial attachment. The flora of the crevice increases in number, and the spread of the lesion seems to occur more as a result of an overgrowth of the endogenous bacteria rather than from invasion of pathogenic forms. The crest of the alveolus is involved initially, and disease may lead to resorption and cupping of the crest. If the disease is permitted to progress in the absence of treatment, it will follow along the periodontal liga-

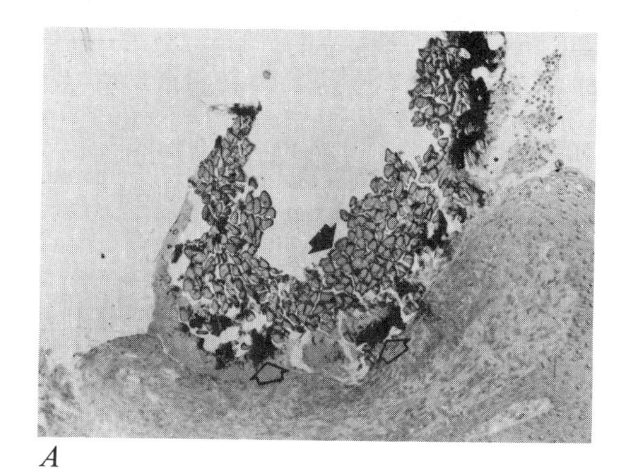

A

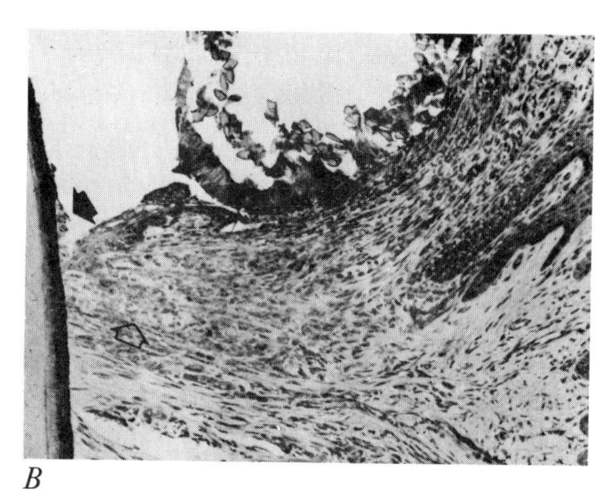

B

Figure 17-5 Serial sections through the gingival sulcus of squirrel monkey tooth 10 weeks after placement of silk ligature. The ligature facilitates accumulation and retention of dental plaque. *A*. Brown and Brenn preparation showing the accumulation of bacteria in contact with underlying gingival tissue (opened arrows). Remnant of the ligature is retained in the preparation (magnification approx. 50 ×). *B*. Hemotoxylin-eosin preparation showing inflammatory infiltration in the gingival connective tissue. The collagen fibers are disoriented (opened arrow), and the crevicular epithelium (closed arrow) is ulcerated (magnification approx. 50 ×). (*Courtesy of M. J. Deasy, College of Medicine and Dentistry of New Jersey, New Jersey Dental School, Newark.*)

ment, destroying the adjacent bone, and will eventuate in crater formation. Progression of the lesion will result in loss of the integrity of the tissue with a resultant decrease in the capacity of the tissue for repair. Surgical intervention is necessary to restore the architecture of the tissue so that removal of plaque and debris is again possible. While it is impossible to indict specific organisms in the etiology of active cases of periodontitis, it may be concluded that bacterial overgrowth accompanies progession of the disease.

Causative Factors

Many factors including dental plaque, occlusal trauma, faulty restorations, calculus formation, areas of food impacting, and improper toothbrushing have been considered as causative factors in periodontal disease. Each of the factors can disturb the integrity of the supporting tissue and permit the endogenous flora to gain an advantage. Whenever present, these factors must be corrected in order to maintain a healthy periodontium.

The mechanism involved in the toxicity of the overgrowing endogenous flora of the gingival crevice has not been elucidated. It may be brought about by an increase in bacterial enzymes (collagenase, hyaluronidase, proteases, and nucleases), but if it is, the mechanism remains obscure. End products of bacterial metabolism may result in chronic inflammation of the tissue cells leading to the release of hydrolytic enzymes from leukocytic lysosomes. The accumulation of bacterial debris may cause sensitivity reactions of the immediate or delayed type with consequent local tissue destruction. The presence of gram-negative organisms may cause local sensitization to endotoxin. Each mechanism suggested has been demonstrated to exist in the gingival sulcus, but what importance it may have in the progression of periodontal disease has not been demonstrated.

INFECTIONS OF THE ORAL MUCOSA

Bacteria

Potentially any microorganism in the endogenous flora can invade the oral mucous membrane if tissue resistance is lowered. Invasion of the connective tissue by spirochetes in acute necrotizing ulcerative gingivitis is a case in point.

In addition to infections caused by the resident bacterial flora, severe infections of the oral mucosa can be caused by group A β-hemolytic streptococci and coagulase-positive staphylococci, especially in debilitated individuals. These stomatitides are characterized by diffuse inflammation of the oral mucosa accompanied by fever and malaise.

Small crater-like ulcerations called *aphthous ulcers* appear on the oral mucosa often in the vestibular space. The exact etiology of such lesions is unknown. L-forms of bacteria and herpes simplex virus have been isolated from the lesions, but there is no evidence directly relating these organisms to the etiology of the lesions. A rare progressive infection of the oral mucous membranes called *noma* may be seen in debilitated children or adults. It is usually secondary to another oral infection and is accompanied by a marked overgrowth of fusobacteria and oral spirochetes.

Actinomycetes

Actinomycetes are a group of organisms with properties intermediate between those of bacteria and fungi but are classified with the bacteria. Anaerobic *Actinomyces israelii,* a member of the normal oral flora, causes cervicofacial actinomycosis in man.

Under appropriate environmental conditions, *A. israelii* produces a penetrating, suppurating infection of the soft tissues and bone. The lesion is usually seen on the mandible and is generally preceded by local trauma. Hypersensitivity to the organism or its products may play a role in pathogenesis in susceptible individuals. Actinomycosis is not a common disease, but anyone who performs manipulations in the oral cavity should be alert to its potential for producing destructive lesions. Sulfur granules are characteristically found in actinomycotic lesions and when examined microscopically under wet mount reveal the presence of the typical central mycelium and peripheral clubs. The mycelial mass adheres to a polysaccharide-protein complex and contains about 50 percent calcium phosphate. The causative agent may be recovered from pus following anaerobic culture at 37°C.

Avoidance of undue trauma in dental operations is suggested as a preventive measure. Treatment involves early diagnosis and thorough surgical debridement along with supportive penicillin or tetracycline chemotherapy. Sulfonamides have also been used effectively in combination with surgical treatment.

Viruses

Herpetic gingivostomatitis is a diffuse infection of the oral tissues that may occur as a result of primary contact with herpes simplex virus. Secondary herpetic infection is commonly seen on the lips. Trauma, the common cold, sunlight, and many other stimulants activate the virus which persists as a latent infection in the epithelial tissues.

Fungi

The fungal infection most commonly seen in the mouth is candidiasis. The causative agent, *Candida albicans,* is a yeast which is part of the normal flora of skin and the oral, intestinal, and vaginal mucosa. In newborn nurseries, candidiasis may become epidemic because of spread by careless handling of contaminated objects by nursery personnel. In debilitated adults, the infection commonly involves the lips, which are cracked and covered by a grayish white membrane. Small, raised white lesions may also be seen on the oral mucous membranes. In the edentulous individual, lesions are often seen under improperly cleansed dentures.

Laboratory diagnosis may be made by culturing on cornmeal and chlamydospore agar and examining the growth microscopically for pseudomycelia and chlamydospores. Direct microscopic examination of wet mounts of portions of the membrane for a mycelial net containing yeast cells is also of diagnostic value. Prevention of the disease in adults involves the maintenance of adequate nutrition and, in the edentulous adult, good oral hygiene. Precautions to prevent the spread of infection should be taken in nurseries. Local applications of nystatin are effective in treatment.

Prolonged administration of antibiotics in adults with a subsequent alteration in the salivary flora can precipitate oral candidiasis. When the therapy is discontinued, the normal flora tends to reestablish itself, and the lesions due to *Candida* overgrowth disappear.

ORAL SIGNS OF SYSTEMIC DISEASE

Bacteria

The major systemic disease producing clinical manifestations in the mouth is syphilis, caused by the species *Treponema pallidum.*

Syphilis may occur as a primary infection of the oral tissues as a result of sexual contact. In this case, the primary lesion (chancre) may be seen at the site of introduction. In untreated patients infected venereally, mucous patches are found during the secondary stage, and gummata, usually located on the palate, are seen during the tertiary stage of the disease. The oral lesions in the primary and secondary stages are literally teeming with organisms, and dentists may contract the disease through small cuts or abrasions on the hands when working on patients with oral lesions.

Granulomatous lesions of tuberculosis are occasionally seen in the mouth and are usually secondary to a pulmonary infection.

Viruses

A number of systemic virus infections, including measles, mumps, varicella, and smallpox, produce oral lesions. The oral signs of measles infection precede the skin lesions and consist of bluish white lesions appearing on the buccal mucosa of the cheek opposite the maxillary molars *(Koplik spots).* In mumps, the orifice of the parotid duct and the parotid gland are inflamed. In varicella and smallpox, lesions similar to those seen on the skin appear on the oral mucosa.

Fungi

Many systemic fungous diseases including histoplasmosis, blastomycosis, paracoccidioidomycosis, and geotrichosis can produce oral granulomatous lesions which are usually secondary to disseminated disease in other tissues (Chap. 23).

THE ORAL FLORA AS THE SOURCE OF ENDOCARDITIS

Many acute oral infections result in systemic manifestations of toxicity such as elevated temperature and malaise. In addition, manipulation of normal and infected oral tissues regularly results in bacteremia (Chap. 14). Bacteremia is of special significance in individuals who have rheumatic carditis or chronic valvular disease, since they may develop bacterial endocarditis. Such individuals should receive protective antibiotic therapy before any dental treatment. Penicillin is the drug of choice, and the recommendations of the American Heart Association for its use are illustrated in Table 17-4.

The relationship of chronic oral foci of infection to systemic disease is less clear. Although direct proof of a cause-and-effect relationship is

Table 17-4 Suggested Prophylaxis for Dental Procedures*

For most patients:

Penicillin administered intramuscularly

600,000 units of procaine penicillin G mixed with 200,000 units of crystalline penicillin G 1 hr. prior to procedure and once daily for the 2 days following the procedure (or longer in the case of delayed healing).

Penicillin administered orally

A. 500 mg of penicillin V or phenethicillin 1 hr. prior to procedure and then 250 mg every 6 hr. for the remainder of that day and for the 2 days following the procedure (or longer in the case of delayed healing).

B. 1,200,000 units of penicillin G 1 hr. prior to procedure and then 600,000 units every 6 hr. for the remainder of that day and for the 2 days following the procedure (or longer in the case of delayed healing).

For patients suspected to be allergic to penicillin or for those on continual oral penicillin for rheumatic fever prophylaxis, who may harbor penicillin-resistant viridans streptococci:

Erythromycin administered orally

For adults—500 mg 1½ to 2 hr. prior to procedure and then 250 mg every 6 hr. for the remainder of that day and for the 2 days following the procedure (or longer in the case of delayed healing).

For children—The dose for small children is 20 mg/kg orally 1½ to 2 hr. prior to the procedure and then 10 mg/kg every 6 hr. for the remainder of that day and for the 2 days following the procedure (or longer in the case of delayed healing).

Erythromycin

Preparations for parenteral use are also available.

* American Heart Association recommendations for prevention of bacterial endocarditis in patients with rheumatic carditis or chronic valvular disease.

Source: J.A.D.A., 85:1378, 1972. (Copyright by the American Dental Association. Reprinted by permission.)

lacking, chronic oral foci (infected teeth or gums) should be treated when diagnosed.

PROSPECTIVE

In the United States much progress has been achieved in providing adequate dental care but only to half of the population. In the developing nations, effective oral hygiene has a low priority in view of their many unresolved, life-threatening confrontations with infectious disease. Greater future emphasis must be placed on preventive dentistry, and the development of sound methods for delivering dental care presents a challenging opportunity to the dental profession, the public, and governmental bodies. In addition to the application of recognized principles of oral hygiene, the prospect of preventing and controlling dental disease will be limited unless a more accurate understanding of the pathogenesis of dental caries and periodontal disease is forthcoming.

BIBLIOGRAPHY

Burnett, G. W., and Scherp, H. W.: *Oral Microbiology and Infectious Disease,* 3d ed., Baltimore, Md.: The Williams & Wilkins Company, 1968.

"Conference on Specific Questions Related to Periodontal Disease," (symposium), *J. Dent. Res.*, vol. 49, no. 2, part I, suppl., 198-275, 1970.

"Current Research Concepts Fundamental to the Improvement of Periodontal Care," (symposium), *J. Dent. Res.*, vol. 50, no. 2, part I, suppl., 184-314, 1971.

Davies, M., and Keddie, N. C.: "Abdominal Actinomycosis," *Br. J. Surg.*, 60:18-22, 1973.

"Evaluation of Agents Used in the Prevention of Oral Disease," *Ann. N.Y. Acad. Sci.*, 153:1-388, 1968.

"Fifth International Conference on Oral Biology," (symposium), *J. Dent. Res.*, vol. 51, no. 2, part I, suppl., 213-442, 1972.

Fitzgerald, R. J.: "Plaque Microbiology and Caries," *Ala. J. Med. Sci.*, 5:239-246, 1968.

Kleinberg, I.: "Formation and Accumulation of Acid on the Tooth Surface," *J. Dent. Res.*, 49:1300-1317, 1970.

Liljemark, W. F., and Gibbons, R. J.: "Proportional Distribution and Relative Adherence of *Streptococcus miteor (mitis)* on Various Surfaces in the Human Oral Cavity," *Infect. Immun.*, 6:852-864, 1972.

"Mechanisms of Dental Caries," *Ann. N.Y. Acad. Sci.*, 131:685-930, 1965.

Mergenhagen, S. E., and Snyderman, R.: "Periodontal Disease: A Model for the Study of Inflammation," *J. Infect. Dis.,* 123:676-677, 1971.

Nolte, W. A. (ed.): *Oral Microbiology,* 2d ed., St. Louis: The C. V. Mosby Company, 1973.

Pindborg, J. J.: *Pathology of the Dental Hard Tissues,* Copenhagen: Munksgaard, 1970.

"Role of Human Foodstuffs in Caries," (symposium), *J. Dent. Res.,* vol. 49, no. 6, part I, suppl., 1194-1352, 1970.

Rushton, M. A., Cooke, B. E., and Duckworth, R.: *Oral Histopathology,* 2d ed., Baltimore, Md.: The Williams & Wilkins Company, 1970.

Scherp, H. W.: "Dental Caries: Prospects for Prevention," *Science,* 173:1199-1205, 1971.

Shovlin, F. E., and Gillis, R. E.: "Biochemical and Antigenic Studies of Lactobacilli Isolated from Deep Dentinal Caries: II. Antigenic Aspects," *J. Dent. Res.,* 51:583-587, 1972.

Sognnaes, R. F. (ed.): *The Chemistry and Prevention of Dental Caries,* Springfield, Ill.: Charles C Thomas, Publisher, 1962.

"The Etiology and Prevention of Dental Caries. Report of a WHO Scientific Group," *W.H.O. Tech. Rep. Ser.,* no. 494, 1972.

vanHoute, J., Gibbons, R. J., and Pulkkinen, A. J.: "Ecology of Human Oral Lactobacilli," *Infect. Immun.,* 6:723-735, 1972.

Volker, J. F.: "Dental Science," *Fed. Proc.,* vol. 31, no. 6, part II, TF71-TF79, 1972.

Chapter 18

Enteric and Urinary Tract Infections

Bernard A. Briody and Zigmund C. Kaminski

PERSPECTIVE

Enteric and urinary tract infections are second only to respiratory diseases as a source of human discomfort. Fortunately, however, most of these infections are either asymptomatic or are limited to the gastrointestinal or urinary tract. On the other hand, both short-term and chronic illnesses may fulminate into a systemic infection which terminates fatally.

The normal intestinal bacterial flora serves as the endogenous source of the great majority of urinary tract infections. Therefore, the normal flora is properly considered in the same context as enteric and urinary infections.

Pathogenic intestinal protozoa and helminths

are identified almost exclusively by direct observation of their typical morphology in material obtained from the patient. In contrast, bacterial pathogens must be isolated, separated, and distinguished from the indigenous flora.

THE NORMAL FLORA OF THE GASTROINTESTINAL TRACT

Commencing shortly after birth and continuing until death the human gastrointestinal tract contains a large population of microbes primarily consisting of bacteria and their viruses and collectively designated as the normal flora. Recently accumulated evidence indicates that the normal flora:

1 Exerts morphogenetic effects that are essential for adequate histological development and healthy function of the gastrointestinal tract
2 Constitutes a major defensive barrier to invasion by pathogenic bacteria
3 Is involved in bacterial overgrowth of the jejunum and malabsorption associated with depressed intestinal motility
4 Serves as the endogenous source of most urinary tract infections as well as many skin and wound infections
5 Is associated with the exchange of genetic markers, including those controlling antibiotic resistance

Population Characteristics

Viable bacteria are normally found in all parts of the gastrointestinal tract. Their number progressively increases from the stomach [10^2 to 10^4 organisms per gram (or per milliliter) of contents] to the jejunum (10^5 to 10^7), to the ileum (10^6 to 10^8), to the large intestine and rectum (10^{11}). At this last concentration, bacteria constitute 10 or 20 percent of the mass of the feces. In the upper part of the gastrointestinal tract the number of bacteria increases in the presence of food and when intestinal motility is depressed.

The numerical distribution of microorganisms comprising the normal enteric flora fluctuates widely with the age of the person, the pH of the intestinal contents, the diet, the use of chemotherapeutic agents, intestinal motility, and many other factors. The stools of normal adults contain about 10^{11} bacteria per gram, mostly obligate anaerobes ($>$ 95 percent). The anaerobic bacteria include the gram-negative *Bacteroides* and the gram-positive *Bifidobacterium*, lactobacilli, *Clostridium perfringens*, and group N streptococci. *Bacteroides*, especially *B. fragilis*, commonly outnumber all other bacteria, and *Bifidobacterium* is the second most prevalent bacterium in the normal fecal flora.

The predominant bacteria, however, vary depending upon the location in the gastrointestinal tract. Gram-positive lactobacilli predominate in the stomach, presumably because of their tolerance to the acid environment. In the jejunum and ileum, lactobacilli and enterococci are the chief organisms and are present in concentrations ranging from 10^5 to 10^8 per gram. Although still found in the large intestine in concentrations of 10^6 to 10^8, lactobacilli and enterococci represent only about 0.1 percent of the flora.

Although comprising only a small fraction of the total bacterial population, the aerobic flora is much more significant in clinical medicine. The bulk of the aerobic flora is composed of the Enterobacteriaceae family of gram-negative enteric bacilli, including *Escherichia*, *Klebsiella*, *Enterobacter* (*Aerobacter*), *Serratia*, *Citrobacter*, and *Proteus*. Other gram-negative enteric bacilli present in the fecal flora include *Pseudomonas aeruginosa* and *Alcaligenes fecalis*, which are not members of the Enterobacteriaceae family. In addition, the flora may contain aerobic species of lactobacilli, enterococci, and staphylococci.

The fecal flora usually includes the aerobic yeast-like fungus *Candida*. Ordinarily, *Candida* organisms are few in number, probably because their growth is restricted by competition from other microorganisms. However, if the bacterial population is depleted by antibiotics, *Candida* can multiply excessively and cause rectal and vaginal irritation.

There are several species of intestinal protozoa that may be present in the normal enteric flora. Included are the intestinal amebas *(Entamoeba coli, Endolimax nana, Iodamoeba bütschlii)* and the intestinal flagellates *[Chilomastix mesnili, Enteromonas hominis, Retortamonas (Embadomonas) intestinalis, Trichomonas hominis]*.

In addition to bacteria, fungi, and protozoa, bacterial viruses (phage, or bacteriophage) are constantly found in intestinal contents. Although not usually considered in this context, unquestionably bacterial viruses are the overwhelmingly predominant microorganisms present in the intestinal tract of man. The fact that most bacteria in the enteric tract carry phage has important implications in terms of phage-mediated transfer of bacterial genes (Chap. 3) and also provides the basis for an exquisitely sensitive procedure for identifying bacteria according to their phage type (Chaps. 14 and 18).

The Enterobacteriaceae

While the Enterobacteriaceae family of bacteria contains many genera that are part of the normal flora, *Escherichia, Klebsiella, Enterobacter, Serratia,* and *Proteus* can produce disease in the urinary tract, the blood (Chap. 14), meninges (Chap. 24), lungs (Chap. 23), and skin and subcutaneous tissues (Chap. 16). In addition, the Enterobacteriaceae include several important enteric pathogens: *Salmonella* species, *Shigella* species, and enteropathogenic and enterotoxin-producing *E. coli*.

The Enterobacteriaceae are short, straight, gram-negative rods (0.5 by 1 to 3 μm) that grow well on artificial media, attack glucose, and produce acid or acid and gas. The bacteria are separated into genera on the basis of several characteristics, including ability to ferment lactose, motility, capsule formation, IMVIC reactions (*i*ndole formation, *m*ethyl red acid determination, *V*oges-Proskauer acetylmethylcarbinol production, *c*itrate utilization), mannitol fermentation, pigment production, H_2S (hydrogen sulfide) production, urease activity, and ornithine and lysine decarboxylase activity (Fig. 18-1). The genera are subdivided into species and types on the basis of additional biochemical reactions, antigenic structure, and phage typing. For practical purposes, *Escherichia coli* will be used as the prototype Enterobacteriaceae. The properties of other members of the family will be taken up in the consideration of enteric bacterial infections *(Salmonella, Shigella)* and urinary tract infections *(Klebsiella, Enterobacter, Serratia, Proteus, Citrobacter)*.

Escherichia coli

Biological Characteristics Probably *E. coli* has been more intensively and exhaustively studied than any other living species. *E. coli* has served as the prototype microorganism for the analysis of growth, nutrition, metabolism, macromolecular synthesis (DNA, RNA, proteins, cell wall components), regulatory mechanisms, microbial genetics, genetic fine structure, radiobiological mechanisms, viral replication, antiseptics, disinfectants, chemotherapeutic agents, and as an index of fecal pollution of water supplies. Much of the basis of molecular biology is the result of studies performed on *E. coli.*

E. coli is a normal inhabitant of the intestinal tract of man and animals, is ubiquitously distributed in nature, and is found in a countless variety of serotypes and phage types. Characteristically, *E. coli* microorganisms are indole and methyl red positive; acetylmethylcarbinol and citrate negative (IMVIC + + − −); and ferment a variety of carbohydrates, including glucose, fructose, galactose, lactose, maltose, arabinose, xylose, rhamnose, and mannitol, producing acid and gas. The bacteria grow well

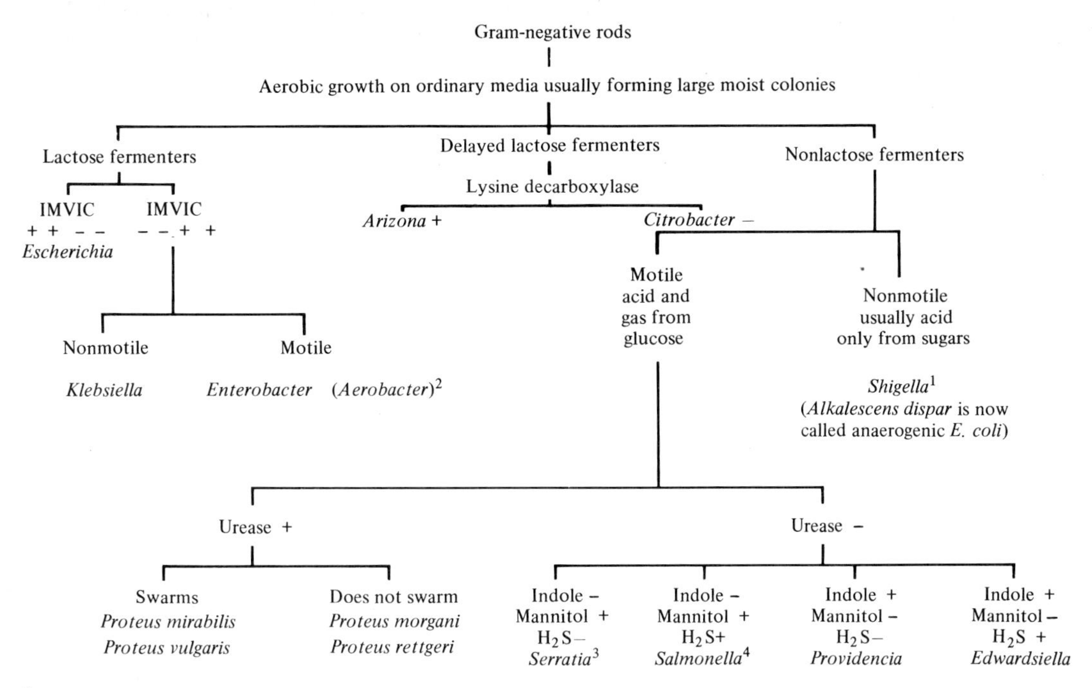

[1] *S. sonnei* is a late lactose fermenter (3 to 9 days).

[2] Includes lactose fermenters (*Enterobacter cloacae*, *E. aerogenes*) and *E. liquefaciens*, *E. aglomerans*, *E. hafniae* (usually nonlactose fermenters).

[3] Usually fails to produce gas in glucose.

[4] *Salmonella typhi* produces acid only in glucose.

Note: The reactions refer to the majority of isolates in the particular genus.

Figure 18-1 Characteristics differentiating Enterobacteriaceae found in man.

aerobically on ordinary laboratory media between 30 and 37°C, with a mean generation time of 20 to 30 min, and are facultatively anaerobic.

Potentially, and apparently practically, one of the most significant properties of *E. coli* is their ability to conjugate with enteric pathogens. As a consequence, multiple resistance to antibiotics can be transferred (Chap. 3).

Pathogenicity and Virulence Clinical isolates of *E. coli* fall into three major categories that might be designated as opportunistic, enteropathogenic, and enterotoxin-producing. The common O serotypes (1, 4, 6, 7, 25, 50, and 75) most frequently isolated from urinary infections, septic infections, bacteremia, meningitis, pulmonary infections, abscesses, and skin and wound infections merely reflect their normal distribution in human stools (Table 18-1). Such microorganisms are designated *opportunistic pathogens* because in their normal habitat they are generally harmless or perhaps even useful, but when they gain access to other sites or tissues they can express their full pathogenic potential. In comparison with other categories, the opportunists have no unique pathogenic potential for man or animals.

Enteropathogenic *E. coli*, as the name implies, are pathogenic within the intestinal tract

Table 18-1 Distribution of O Serotypes among *Escherichia coli*

Source	Pathogenic category	Common O serotypes
Normal flora		1, 4, 6, 7, 25, 50, 75
Extraintestinal disease	Opportunistic	1, 4, 6, 7, 25, 50, 75
Infantile diarrhea	Enteropathogenic	111, 55, 26, 86, 112, 119, 124 to 128
Traveler's disease	Enterotoxin-producing	15, 78, 6

of man, especially in neonates and infants. Most cases of infantile diarrhea have been associated with O serotypes 111 and 55, but O types 28, 86, 112, 119, and 124 to 128 have also been incriminated. Thus, enteropathogenic serotypes are distinctly different from opportunistic serotypes, are naturally virulent for man, and have a characteristic epidemiological pattern. The unique invasive potential of the enteropathogenic serotypes is based on their ability to penetrate the epithelial cells of the intestinal mucosa, but the bacterial component(s) responsible for this property is unknown. The clinical consequences are an acute exudative diarrheal disease with lymphatic involvement and, occasionally, a terminal bacteremia.

Although unable to invade the intestinal mucosa, other *E. coli* release an enterotoxin that adsorbs to epithelial cell membranes and stimulates adenyl cyclase activity; the resultant increase in cyclic adenosine 3′, 5′-monophosphate (cAMP) leads directly to the increased electrolyte secretion of the gut. In this respect, the enterotoxin resembles choleragen but is less potent and acts for a much shorter period of time. Characteristically, enterotoxin-producing bacteria are isolated from cases of traveler's diarrhea, and the O serotypes (15, 78, and 6) involved differ from those commonly encountered in opportunistic and enteropathogenic infections.

Antigenic Structure The complex antigenic structure of the Enterobacteriaceae has been elucidated over a period of many years by Kauffmann, White, Edwards, Ewing, and other investigators and has been successfully applied to the recognition of serological groups and types (serotypes) within the family. In addition to a rough antigen common to all bacteria within the family, Enterobacteriaceae have one or more O somatic antigens; motile members have one or more H flagellar antigens, which may show diphasic variation; and many bacteria have one or more K or Vi capsular, envelope, or sheath antigens.

The O somatic antigens are the endotoxins of the Enterobacteriaceae and are integral components of the cell wall composed of polysaccharide-protein-lipid complexes whose antigenic specificity is determined by the polysaccharide moiety. O antigens are thermostable (100°C) and are resistant to alcohol and dilute acid.

The H flagellar antigens are proteins found only in the flagella of motile bacteria. H antigens are thermolabile (60°C) and are inactivated by alcohol and dilute acid. Some Enterobacteriaceae may mutate from one phase to another (diphasic variation). H antigens included in phase 1 are shared by few other species and are referred to as specific H antigens, whereas phase 2 antigens are shared by a large number of other species and are referred to as group H antigens.

The K antigens are polysaccharides located over the surface of the cell wall as envelopes or as capsules that can mask or inhibit O antigen agglutination. The K antigens are further subdivided into thermolabile (L and B) and thermostable (A) antigens. Heated B antigen can absorb, but will not be agglutinated by B antiserum, whereas heated L antigen will neither absorb nor be agglutinated by L antiserum. The Vi antigen of *Salmonella typhi* is similar to some of the thermolabile K antigens of *Citrobacter* and other *Salmonella* species.

Serological grouping of Enterobacteriaceae is based on the possession of specific O antigens, of which more than 150 have been defined in *E. coli*. Serological typing requires the additional use of K antigens and, in motile bacteria, the H antigens. In *E. coli* there are more than 80 recognized K antigens and more than 50 H antigens. Individual serotypes may possess different sets of antigens (O 111:B 4:—; O 111:B 4:H 2; O 111:B 4:H 12) which frequently facilitate efforts to trace the source of an epidemic or to determine whether a given recurrent infection represents a relapse or a reinfection.

ENTERIC BACTERIAL INFECTIONS

Until the twentieth century the outcome of military expeditions usually was more dependent on the ability of soldiers in opposing armies to survive enteric disorders and to fight while suffering from dysentery than on the effectiveness of their armaments.

Enteric infections commonly follow ingestion of polluted water or food contaminated with excreta from subclinical cases or from asymptomatic carriers (individuals who have recovered from infection or disease but still continue to excrete the pathogens). Subclinical cases or carriers are liable to initiate an epidemic whenever the opportunity arises to contaminate material ingested by others. Such conditions tend to occur in habitations where many people are crowded together with inadequate washing facilities and unsanitary conditions. Thus, mental institutions, orphanages, and camp sites are prone to epidemics of these diseases, and the risk is increased in proportion to the turnover of the occupants. In addition, hospital nurseries are especially liable to outbreaks of enteropathogenic *E. coli* infections, which can be fatal for neonates.

Although enteric bacterial infections are universal, their severity is increased strikingly whenever accompanied by kwashiorkor and other forms of malnutrition. Gastroenteritis, for example, is a major cause of death in infants and young children in some countries in Central and South America, and is also a severe disease in India and other areas of the Orient.

The Causative Agents

Salmonellae Salmonellae are motile, gram-negative rods that fail to attack lactose or produce indole, but can ferment a number of sugars including glucose and mannitol. *Salmonella typhi*, the causative agent of typhoid fever, is an exception in that it produces acid but not gas in glucose, maltose, and mannitol. Although more than 1,300 serotypes of salmonellae have been identified on the basis of O, H, and K (Vi) antigens, the bulk of human infections are caused by a few species limited to five O groups (Table 18-2). *S. typhimurium* is by far the most commonly encountered human pathogen. *S. typhi* and *S. choleraesuis* are recognized as being more pathogenic for man, but the basis of their action has not been determined. All salmonellae can invade the intestinal mucosa, the lymphatics, and the blood, but rarely produce serious disease. Most *Salmonella* infections of man arise from contact with contaminated poultry and meat products.

Shigellae *Shigella* organisms are nonmotile, gram-negative rods that generally fail to attack lactose and produce acid in glucose. Exceptions include *Shigella sonnei*, which can produce acid in lactose in 3 to 9 days, and *S. flexneri* varieties, which can produce acid and gas in glucose. Production of indole, fermentation of mannitol,

Table 18-2 Antigenic Structure of *Salmonella* Commonly Encountered in Human Infections (Kauffmann-White Schema)

			H antigens	
O group	Species	O antigens	Phase 1	Phase 2
A	*S. paratyphi*	1, $\underline{2}$, 12	a	
B	*S. saintpaul*	1, $\underline{4}$, 5, 12	e, h	1, 2
	S. derby	1, $\underline{4}$, 5, 12	f, g	
	S. typhimurium	1, $\underline{4}$, 5, 12	i	1, 2
	S. heidelberg	1, $\underline{4}$, 5, 12	r	1, 2
C	*S. choleraesuis*	$\underline{6}$, 7	c	1, 5
	S. thompson	$\underline{6}$, 7	k	1, 5
	S. infantis	$\underline{6}$, 7	r	1, 5
	S. newport	$\underline{6}$, 8	e, h	1, 2
D	*S. typhi*	$\underline{9}$, 12	d	
	S. enteritidis	1, $\underline{9}$, 12	g, m	
E	*S. anatum*	$\underline{3}$, 10	e, h	1, 6

Note: The underscored O antigen is the major component of the group.

and the presence of major and minor O antigens can be used to separate shigellae into species and serotypes. Shigellae can penetrate the epithelial cells lining the intestinal mucosa and induce acute exudative diarrheal disease, but they rarely, if ever, invade the lymphatics and the blood. Most infections are caused by *S. sonnei* and *S. flexneri* and are usually mild. *S. dysenteriae* characteristically produces a more severe and serious disease, but the basis for its greater pathogenicity for man has not been established. Shigellae are found in the feces of patients and carriers.

Vibrio cholerae The causative agent *V. cholerae* is a motile curved, gram-negative aerobic bacillus that grows well at pH 8.5 to 9.0, reduces nitrates, and forms indole in peptone broth (cholera red positive in the presence of sulfuric acid) and fails to ferment lactose. The bacteria are found in the intestinal contents of cholera patients and carriers. Six antigenic groups have been recognized on the basis of O antigens, with all of the pathogens belonging to group 1. The H and two of the K antigens are common to all cholera vibrios.

All pathogenic cholera vibrios produce an enterotoxin, choleragen, which can account for all the pathophysiological and metabolic alterations observed in cholera. Choleragen is a heat-labile, acid- and pronase-sensitive, highly antigenic protein with a molecular weight of approximately 84,000 which is readily converted to a toxoid by formaldehyde. Choleragen adsorbs to a ganglioside in the intestinal epithelial cell membrane and stimulates adenyl cyclase activity, causing an increase in intracellular cAMP, which induces an active secretion of electrolytes that accounts for the massive abnormal movement of salt and water. In the process, however, the intestinal mucosa remains intact, and the result is an acute nonexudative diarrheal disease.

Vibrio parahemolyticus The most common cause of food poisoning in Japan, *Vibrio parahemolyticus*, has been responsible for numerous summer outbreaks of food poisoning associated with the ingestion of contaminated shellfish and crustaceans (crabs, shrimp) in the Chesapeake Bay, Puget Sound, and Louisiana coastal areas of the United States since 1971. The causative agent is a motile, gram-negative, pleomorphic, facultatively anaerobic rod capable of producing acid but not gas in carbohydrates. The microorganism is unique in its requirement for at least 1 percent NaCl for satisfactory growth, can grow in concentrations of 3 to 7 percent NaCl, and thus is termed a halophil. Thiosulphate citrate bile salts agar (TCBS) is recommended for the primary isolation of *V. parahemolyticus* because the high salt concentration and alkaline pH of the medium suppress the growth of most organisms except halophiles.

Patients infected with *V. parahemolyticus* experience an acute exudative diarrheal disease, presumably the result of the ability of the microorganism to penetrate epithelial cells lining the intestinal mucosa. Severe cases are not unlike those caused by *Shigella* organisms.

Clostridium perfringens Food poisoning associated with type A *C. perfringens* is an infection rather than an intoxication, as indicated by studies on volunteers. The gastroenteritis generally commences 8 to 18 hr. after eating the contaminated food, usually meat. Diarrhea and abdominal cramps are the most prominent clinical features of the illness. Headache and nausea also occur, while fever and vomiting are rarely observed. Recovery is usually uneventful and complete in 12 to 24 hr.

The bacteria involved in *C. perfringens* food poisoning produce an enterotoxin resembling that produced by *E. coli* and thus differ from the typical type A organisms encountered in gas gangrene (Chap. 13). The organism is an anaerobe that is part of the normal flora of the intestinal tract of man and animals. It is also found in soil, water, milk, dust, and sewage.

Readily perishable foods are potentially hazardous and should be thoroughly cooked in order to destroy *C. perfringens*. The food should then be kept hot (140°F or above) or cold (45°F or below) until served. Many outbreaks are known to have occurred when properly cooked meat was allowed to cool slowly for several hours at room temperature before being refrigerated and was subsequently eaten without adequate reheating. Outbreaks of *C. perfringens* food poisoning are receiving increasing attention in the United States but have not been as common as in England, perhaps because of the more extensive commercial and home refrigeration of meats in the United States.

Pathogenesis

Acute Diarrheal Disease The World Health Organization Expert Committee on Enteric Infections has adopted the term *acute diarrheal disease* to identify generically a clinical syndrome characterized by ". . . a disturbance of intestinal motility and absorption which, once and by whatever means initiated, may become self-perpetuating as a disease through the production of dehydration and profound cellular disturbances, which in turn favor the continuing passage of liquid stools." Encompassed within the concept of acute diarrheal disease are clinical entities formerly designated as acute gastroenteritis or food poisoning (Chap. 13), bacillary dysentery, and cholera.

Acute diarrheal disease caused by bacteria is also an epidemiological entity. Man is the primary reservoir of infection in the case of shigellosis, cholera, and enteropathogenic and enterotoxin-producing *E. coli*, whereas poultry, swine, and other animals constitute the major sources of infection in salmonellosis, and shellfish and crustaceans are the reservoir in *Vibrio parahemolyticus* infections.

When it develops, acute diarrheal disease usually occurs 8 to 48 hr. after ingestion of food or water containing millions of bacteria. The severity of the clinical manifestations varies with the virulence of the bacteria and the resistance of the host, and asymptomatic carriers are not uncommon, especially in salmonellosis. As evident from clinical, epidemiological, and experimental observations, depletion of the normal bacterial flora by antibiotics, impaired intestinal motility, malnutrition, and prematurity predispose to infection and are associated with a poorer prognosis. *Shigella dysenteriae* and *Salmonella choleraesuis* may be cited as examples of bacteria associated with severe human infections, in contrast with most other species of *Shigella* and *Salmonella.*

As indicated in Table 18-3, acute diarrheal disease may be characterized as exudative (*Salmonella, Shigella,* enteropathogenic *Escherichia, Vibrio parahemolyticus*) or nonexudative (*Vibrio cholerae, Clostridium perfringens,* enterotoxin-producing *E. coli*) on the basis of the host's tissue response.

The Exudative Form of Acute Diarrheal Disease Primary to an understanding of the sequence which leads to an exudative response is an appreciation of the importance of epithelial cell penetration. Through the use of fluorescein-labeled antibody, the enteropathogen can be identified in epithelial cells and/or the lamina propria of the intestinal mucosa. At the point of bacterial entry the microvilli undergo dissolution, producing a brush border, and the bacteria appear invested by a membrane envelope.

Bacterial multiplication within the epithelial cells and lamina propria incites an inflammatory reaction which secondarily leads to necrosis and sloughing of the mucosa. Not surprisingly, then, microscopic examination of fecal specimens to a greater or lesser extent reveals the presence of erythrocytes, polymorphonuclear leukocytes, mucus, and necrotic mucosa contained in fibrinopurulent exudate. The inflammatory reaction in the human colon may not be distinguishable from idiopathic ulcerative colitis and other inflammatory lesions as observed by electron microscopy.

Salmonella and enteropathogenic *E. coli* are present in and can be isolated from mesenteric lymph nodes, whereas *Shigella, Vibrio cholerae, V. parahemolyticus,* enterotoxin-producing *E. coli,* and *Clostridium perfringens* do not invade lymphatic tissue. Lymphatic involvement may lead to bacteremia in the case of *Salmonella* and *E. coli* but not in *Shigella* infections. However, in severe *Shigella* infections of infants and young children, bacteremia, often due to *E. coli,* is not uncommon.

Despite the fact that bacteremia may be an

Table 18-3 Pathogenesis of Acute Diarrheal Disease

	Exudative				Nonexudative*	
Property	**Enteropathogenic *E. coli***	***Salmonella***	***Shigella***	***Vibrio parahemolyticus***	***Vibrio cholerae***	**Enterotoxin-producing *E. coli***
Mucosa						
Intact	−	−	−	−	+	+
Bacterial penetration	+	+	+	+	−	−
Mesenteric lymph nodes						
Bacteria	+	+	−	−	−	−
Bacteremia	+	+	−	−	−	−
Stool cytology	+	+	+	+	−	−

* *Clostridium perfringens* has recently been shown to produce acute nonexudative diarrheal disease that closely resembles that produced by enterotoxin-producing *E. coli.*

integral component of acute diarrheal disease due to *Salmonella* and enteropathogenic *E. coli,* there are definite advantages for considering the problem of bacteremia separately under the heading of typhoid and other enteric fevers.

The Nonexudative Form of Acute Diarrheal Disease In the nonexudative form of acute diarrheal disease, best exemplified by cholera, the mucosa remains intact throughout the course of infection. The bacteria adhere closely to the mucosal surface but do not penetrate epithelial cells or lamina propria. Microvilli are intact. Epithelial cells and their junctions are undisturbed. However, despite the absence of invasion of the intestinal mucosa by *Vibrio cholerae,* there is a massive loss of fluid and electrolytes. Microscopically, fecal specimens contain a few mononuclear cells, flecks of mucus, and as seen in hanging-drop preparations, actively motile vibrios.

Mechanisms Involved in Production of Acute Diarrheal Disease The invasive potential of the microorganism is critical for the production of the exudative form of acute diarrheal disease (Table 18-3), but the bacterial component(s) responsible for this property is unknown. Ingestion of billions of dead bacteria containing endotoxin produces no effect. Thus, endotoxin, the cell wall component associated with the toxicity of gram-negative bacteria, is not the factor that permits penetration of the intestinal mucosa.

On the other hand, after bacterial multiplication within the epithelial cells and lamina propria, the release of endotoxin on lysis of the bacteria may lead to tissue damage essential to the development of the disease either directly or perhaps by forming biologically active antigen-antibody complexes with cross-reacting antibodies present as a result of previous contact with other gram-negative bacteria.

Infections with *Shigella dysenteriae* characteristically are more severe than those induced by other species of *Shigella.* Attempts have been made to explain this observation on the basis of the fact that *S. dysenteriae,* in contrast with other *Shigella,* contains a heat-labile neurotoxin. When freed by autolysis of the bacteria, the neurotoxin can cause hemorrhage and paralysis in animals. However, involvement of the neurotoxin in human infections has not been demonstrated.

In the nonexudative form of acute diarrheal disease illustrated by cholera, evidence is accumulating that much of the pathophysiology is associated with choleragen, a heat-labile exotoxin of high molecular weight found in the stools of cholera patients and in culture filtrates of *Vibrio cholerae.* Choleragen induces a basic lesion in the jejunal microcirculation, causing striking water and ion fluxes by stimulating a prolonged increase in capillary permeability.

Presumably, choleragen exerts its effect by binding to a ganglioside receptor on epithelial cell membranes, stimulating adenyl cyclase activity and thereby increasing intracellular levels of cyclic adenosine 3′5′-monophosphate (cAMP), which leads directly to the massive electrolyte secretion of the gut. Convalescent cholera serum and secretory IgA (coproantibodies) neutralize choleragen and are probably associated with protection.

Clinical Expression of Acute Diarrheal Disease As indicated by the summary included in Table 18-4, various clinical forms of acute diarrheal disease can be recognized on the basis of frequency, severity, duration, and extent of diarrhea. It must be stressed, however, that the causative agent cannot be identified on the basis of clinical manifestations alone and that the pathophysiology represents a continuum with much overlapping in clinical expression.

Acute Gastroenteritis (Food Poisoning) The most common clinical expression of acute diarrheal disease is characterized by a sudden onset of diarrhea, loss of appetite, and fever with mild to moderate abdominal pain, sometimes accompanied by vomiting. The fever may be caused either by bacterial endotoxin or by endogenous pyrogens released from neutrophils and monocytes following intracellular bacterial multipli-

Table 18-4 Clinical Expression of Acute Diarrheal Disease

	Severity	Duration	Diarrhea	Frequency	Causative agents
			Exudative form		
Acute gastroenteritis	+	+	+	++++	*Salmonella, Shigella,* enteropathogenic *E. coli, Vibrio parahemolyticus*
Dysentery	++	++	+++ (initially) + (later)	++	*Salmonella, Shigella* (especially *S. dysenteriae*), enteropathogenic *E. coli, Vibrio parahemolyticus*
Systemic reaction					
Without bacteremia	++++	++++	±	±	*Shigella dysenteriae* prominently
With bacteremia	++++	++++	±	±	*Salmonella,* enteropathogenic *E. coli*
			Nonexudative form		
Cholera	++++	++	++++	Variable	*Vibrio cholerae*
Traveler's diarrhea	+	+	++	++	Enterotoxin-producing *E. coli*
Clostridium perfringens food poisoning	(Probably similar to traveler's diarrhea)				*Clostridium perfringens*

cation. The stools are watery and light and contain some mucus, leukocytes, and erythrocytes. The duration of illness is short (2 to 5 days) with little debility.

Dysentery (Bad Bowels) A less common but more severe clinical form fits the classic description of bacillary dysentery. Initially, this syndrome is associated with a more intense systemic response with fever, abdominal pain, vomiting, prostration, and the passage of watery stools in large volume. Later, the abdominal pain is more profound; the stool volume decreases and consists largely of mucus tinged with blood, pus, and necrotic intestinal mucosa. The disease persists for 5 to 7 days and is debilitating, requiring 2 weeks or more of convalescence.

Systemic Reaction without Bacteremia An uncommon but much more severe form of dysentery, characteristic of infections with *Shigella dysenteriae,* is dominated by a systemic reaction involving high fever, convulsions, intense abdominal pain, and leukocytosis. Diarrhea is not a prominent feature, and vomiting subsides quickly. The fecal specimens soon consist mainly of mucus, necrotic mucosa, and a fibrinopurulent exudate containing sufficient blood to impart a pink to red color. Dehydration and acidosis progress rapidly, and the abdomen is tender and readily palpated in the colonic area. Convalescence is prolonged, and a fatal outcome may result.

Typhoid and Other Enteric Fevers (Systemic Reactions with Bacteremia) Systemic reactions with bacteremia as a consequence of infection with *Salmonella* and enteropathogenic *E. coli* constitute a spectrum of syndromes involving differences in pathogenesis from the more common clinical manifestations of acute diarrheal diseases as well as from each other. Included as representative of these reactions are such entities as typhoid fever, other enteric fevers, enteropathogenic *E. coli* infections, and septicemia due to *Salmonella choleraesuis.*

Typhoid Fever *Salmonella typhi,* the causative agent of typhoid fever, is unique to man and is transmitted to healthy persons from patients or carriers, i.e., individuals in whom the typhoid bacilli persist indefinitely in the bile passages and in the intestines following recovery from the disease. The pathogenesis of typhoid fever is significantly and characteristically distinct from the common forms of acute diarrheal disease.

Following ingestion of *S. typhi,* and during the course of an incubation period that averages about 10 days, the bacteria do not remain in the intestinal tract but invade the mucosal barrier, pass into the mesenteric lymph nodes, multiply, and enter the blood by way of the thoracic duct. This primary bacteremia is transient, the microorganisms being removed by the phagocytic cells of the reticuloendothelial system including those in the liver. After multiplications in and destruction of reticuloendothelial cells, the bacteria spill over into the blood, producing a more prolonged and extensive secondary bacteremia which spreads the infection to other tissues. The patient has the signs and symptoms of an acute systemic infection, and the bacteria can be isolated from the blood and urine.

Thereafter, the organisms gain access to the intestinal tract following infection of the gallbladder and passage through the bile ducts. Concomitantly, the bacteria multiply in Peyer's patches, killing the lymphoid cells with consequent necrosis and sloughing of the mucosa, hemorrhage, and bloody stools.

Although intravenous infusion of endotoxin in man produces clinical manifestations (fever, chills, headache, nausea, backache, and abdominal pain) which cannot be differentiated from those in typhoid fever, on balance the evidence indicates that circulating endotoxin does not play a major role in the pathogenesis of typhoid fever. Daily intravenous infusions of endotoxin soon lead to the development of tolerance, a finding inconsistent with the sustained febrile course of typhoid fever. Furthermore, induction of tolerance before or during typhoid does not alter the febrile or toxic pattern of the disease.

Clinically, typhoid fever represents a prolonged febrile illness with splenomegaly, lymphadenopathy, leukopenia, abdominal pain, and positive blood, urine, and stool cultures and is occasionally associated with an exanthematous rash on the anterior thorax and abdomen (rose spots), intestinal hemorrhage which may lead to perforation and peritonitis, or focal metastatic infection (cholecystitis, osteomyelitis, chondritis, meningitis, endocarditis, nephritis, bronchitis, pneumonia). The high continued fever (103 to 105°F for 2 to 3 weeks) may result in psychosis, delirium, or mania. As the temperature wanes during the third and fourth weeks, the patients begin the recovery process but may encounter a relapse (5 to 15 percent) which increases to 20 percent of the patients treated with chloramphenicol.

Other Enteric Fevers (Paratyphoid Fever) Certain *Salmonella* species, especially *S. paratyphi* A and *S. paratyphi* B *(S. schottmülleri),* can produce a prolonged febrile illness clinically indistinguishable from typhoid fever. Generally, these infections tend to be milder than typhoid but cannot be differentiated on clinical manifestations in the individual case. Continued fecal excretion of bacteria may occur for several months following recovery, but the long-term carrier state is much less frequent than in typhoid fever.

Bacteremia (Septicemia) A few species of *Salmonella,* most notably *S. choleraesuis* (of swine origin), are highly invasive and cause a clinical syndrome characterized by prolonged fever and intermittent bacteremia, often with evidence of focal metastatic infection in the lungs, heart, kidney, meninges, bones, and joints. Stool cultures are usually negative, but the bacteria can be isolated from blood and urine. Although the sustained high fever, persistent leukopenia, and rose spots of typhoid fever may be absent, infections with *S. choleraesuis* constitute a serious hazard for the patient and may pursue a fulminant course.

Enteropathogenic *E. coli* Infections (Infantile Diarrhea) In neonates, enteropathogenic *E. coli* can cause a serious and life-threatening infection characterized by a short incubation period and large numbers of bacteria, initially in the duodenum but later extending the whole length of the gut and almost completely replacing the aerobic gram-negative organisms in the normal flora. In severe cases the stools are frequent and watery, the temperature rises, and death may occur within a few days accompanied by a sharp loss in weight, acidosis, and dehydration. Macroscopic lesions in the intestines are not prominent. The bacteria do, however, penetrate the intestinal mucosa, resist phagocytosis, multiply extensively, invade the mesenteric lymph nodes, and can cause bacteremia which may lead to severe shock similar to that induced in animals following injection of endotoxin (Chap. 5).

Affected infants excrete enormous numbers of bacteria which rapidly spread to other infants in hospital nurseries. Adults may be carriers and may serve as a source of infection.

Cholera Infections with *Vibrio cholerae* are characterized by a massive loss of fluid and electrolytes. The fluid loss may exceed 10 liters per day. In the absence of treatment, death due to dehydration and electrolyte imbalance may occur within 24 hr. after onset. Fortunately, however, with prompt fluid and electrolyte repletion, recovery is rapid.

Diarrhea Due to Enterotoxin-producing *E. coli* (Traveler's Diarrhea) In recent years evidence has accumulated to show that enterotoxin-producing *E. coli* can cause a nonexudative diarrheal syndrome resembling that of cholera. The bacteria involved synthesize a choleragen-like enterotoxin. The disease can be reproduced in human volunteers or experimentally in ileal loops in rabbits. Unlike the enteropathogenic *E. coli,* the enterotoxin-producing bacteria are unable to invade the epithelial cells of the intestinal mucosa.

The data suggest that enterotoxin-producing strains of *E. coli* are responsible for at least some cases of nonexudative acute diarrheal disease encountered in people who travel from one part of the world to another (traveler's diarrhea). Although the disease may persist in some persons for a few weeks, recovery is usually uneventful and complete.

The Role of Intestinal Bacteria in Malabsorption Syndrome Some enteric diseases (blind-loop syndrome, jejunal diverticulosis, intestinal scleroderma, steatorrhea, strictures, and fistulas) are associated with intestinal hypomotility, bacterial overgrowth in the jejunum, the presence of unconjugated bile salts in jejunal fluid, and malabsorption of vitamin B_{12} and fats (malabsorption syndrome).

Accumulating evidence indicates that intestinal hypomotility facilitates the growth of large numbers of bacteria (bacterial overgrowth) in the jejunum, which usually is sparsely populated with bacteria. The microorganisms involved are members of the normal flora of the large intestine. In the jejunum the bacteria may utilize vitamin B_{12} or block its absorption in some other way, perhaps mechanically. The bacterial overgrowth may include anaerobes *(Bacteroides, Bifidobacterium, Clostridium)* or aerobes (enterococci, staphylococci) that have the capacity to break down conjugated bile salts which are essential for the absorption of fat from the small intestine. Thus, it would appear that when a patient suffers from intestinal hypomotility, bacteria can multiply in large numbers in the small intestine and cause malabsorption by deconjugating bile salts.

Therapy directed against the bacteria can reverse the malabsorption. For example, in carefully evaluated cases, administration of erythromycin led to an improvement in intestinal absorption of fat and vitamin B_{12} and to the disappearance of unconjugated bile salts from jejunal fluid.

Laboratory Diagnosis

Diagnostic and Pathogenic Problems Associated with the Normal Flora Four prominent intestinal pathogens—*Salmonella, Shigella,* and enteropathogenic and enterotoxin-producing *E. coli*—are Enterobacteriaceae closely related to microorganisms of the same family which are part of the normal flora. Consequently, it is of critical importance to utilize selective and differential media when attempting to isolate and identify the common enteric pathogens.

As indicated below, a freshly obtained stool specimen should be immediately streaked on blood, MacConkey and XLD, or Hektoen agar plates and inoculated into gram-negative or selenite-F broth. The blood agar plate is used to detect the possibility of *Candida* or *Staphylococcus aureus* overgrowth. MacConkey's agar inhibits the growth of gram-positive bacteria, permits the growth of aerobic gram-negative enteric bacilli, and provides a basis for differentiating organisms which ferment lactose *(Escherichia, Klebsiella, Enterobacter)* from those which do not (*Salmonella,* most *Shigella*). Lactose fermenters appear as pink to purple colonies as a result of the production of acid which changes the color of the indicator dye (phenol red) incorporated in the medium. Bacteria which do not ferment lactose are present as transparent colorless colonies.

A selective medium is essential for the isolation of *Salmonella* and *Shigella* when they are present in small numbers. *Salmonella-Shigella* (SS) agar, which is still used by many laboratories, is not a satisfactory selective medium because it inhibits the growth of some shigellae. XLD or Hektoen agar is preferable, since *Salmonella* and *Shigella* grow readily, while the lactose fermenters are suppressed.

Inoculation of the stool specimen into an enrichment broth (gram-negative and selenite-F broth) permits *Shigella* and *Salmonella* to initially grow more rapidly than the normal flora. Streak plates on MacConkey and XLD agar prepared from the enrichment broth (after suitable incubation) enhance the probability of isolating *Salmonella* and *Shigella* from the stool specimen.

Suitable biochemical tests are performed on the isolated suspect colonies. If the results indicate a potential pathogen, appropriate antisera are used to confirm the validity of the biochemical data by carrying out slide agglutination tests. Fluorescent antibody techniques are becoming increasingly available and may provide an effective basis for the rapid tentative identification of the organism either directly on the stool specimen or after a period of growth in enrichment broth.

Epidemiology

With the important exception of most salmonellae and *Vibrio parahemolyticus,* man is the reservoir of infection for acute diarrheal disease. In-

Table 18-5 Epidemiological Features of Acute Diarrheal Disease

Reservoir	Human patients, asymptomatic infections, and carriers. In salmonellosis, domestic animals constitute the primary reservoir. Shellfish and crustaceans are the source of most infections from *Vibrio parahemolyticus.*
Geographical distribution	Worldwide except for cholera which, however, in the last 10 years has become pandemic, spreading from India to South Asia, the Western Pacific, the Middle East, and into parts of Europe. The United States has remained free of cholera since 1911.* The distribution of certain *Salmonella* and *Shigella* species, however, varies geographically. For example, *Salmonella hirschfeldii* (paratyphoid C) is a common cause of disease in Eastern Europe and Asia but is extremely rare in the United States. *Shigella dysenteriae* is found in tropical countries, temperate parts of East Asia, and recently has caused extensive epidemics in Central America and Mexico; several cases have been reported in the United States.
Age incidence	All age groups are susceptible to salmonellosis, cholera, and traveler's disease. In shigellosis two-thirds of the cases occur in those under 10 years of age. Infantile diarrhea occurs primarily in neonates and is rarely seen in children over 2 years of age.
Lower socioeconomic factors	Cholera and shigellosis are predominantly encountered in lower socioeconomic groups, especially in areas where poor sanitary facilities, overcrowding, and malnutrition prevail. Salmonellosis is found in every socioeconomic group. Infantile diarrhea and traveler's disease are more common in the affluent because they have access to hospital nurseries or travel more widely.
Severity	The ratio of clinical to subclinical infection is greatest in shigellosis and in nursery epidemics of infantile diarrhea. Clinical severity is greatest in cholera, shigellosis caused by *Shigella dysenteriae,* infantile diarrhea, typhoid, and *Salmonella choleraesuis* infections.
Source of infection	Clinical cases are important in spreading infection, especially in shigellosis, cholera, and nursery epidemics of infantile diarrhea. Long-term carriers are important in typhoid and to a lesser extent in other enteric fevers. Asymptomatic infection is of greatest significance in salmonellosis, traveler's disease, and infantile diarrhea.
Water-borne epidemics	Currently, ingestion of water contaminated with feces is significant in the spread of cholera and, in rural areas, of shigellosis.
Infected food products	Ingestion of infected poultry and meat products (the animal reservoir) is responsible for about 70 percent of cases of salmonellosis, and ingestion of contaminated shellfish or crustaceans is the cause of *Vibrio parahemolyticus* infections. In other forms of acute diarrheal disease, food products must be contaminated from human sources in order to act as a vehicle for transmission.

* A single case of cholera was reported in the United States in 1973.

fections are transmitted by the fecal-oral route. Microorganisms are excreted in feces by patients or carriers, and man acquires infection following the ingestion of food or water contaminated with the pathogen.

Historically, in many countries much has been accomplished in the control of acute diarrheal disease by interrupting the chain of infection through protection, purification, and chlorination of public water supplies; sanitary disposal of human excreta; control of flies; pasteurization of milk and dairy products; sanitary supervision of food processing, distribution, preparation, serving, and storage; and the application of sound principles of personal hygiene. Nonetheless, acute diarrheal disease remains a major cause of illness and mortality in many developing countries because of the lack of adequate sanitary and treatment facilities. Children in most areas of the world face a substantial risk of dying from diarrheal disease.

In more developed countries acute diarrheal disease is second only to respiratory disease as a cause of human discomfort. Although much of this morbidity may result from a break in the application of sanitary procedures, control is inordinately more difficult because of the frequency of unrecognized cases and the persistence of the carrier state in man. In salmonellosis, widespread infection in domestic animals constitutes an ever-present potential hazard for man.

Although the causative agents of acute diarrheal disease induce a spectrum of clinical manifestations with many common epidemiological features, there are recognizable differences in morbidity and mortality according to age, geographical location, socioeconomic factors, and the role of human or animal carriers in the spread of disease. Thus, salmonellosis, shigellosis, cholera, infantile diarrhea, and traveler's diarrhea not only connote etiological entities but also involve concepts that suggest more or less characteristic epidemiological settings, as is illustrated by the data included in Table 18-5.

Prevention and Control

As noted earlier (Chap. 12), the wide application of public health methods and procedures has largely eliminated the scourge of food- and water-borne epidemics of typhoid, cholera, and dysentery in developed countries. Poor sanitary facilities in developing nations, complicated by overcrowding and malnutrition, are chiefly responsible for the continuing threat to life posed by acute diarrheal disease.

Immunization While vaccines in no way diminish or replace the need for adequate sewage disposal and the provision of safe water supplies, limited progress in prevention and control of acute diarrheal disease has been achieved through immunization. For residents and travelers who enter or leave areas where typhoid, other enteric fevers, and cholera are endemic, the use of killed typhoid-paratyphoid A and B (TAB) or cholera vaccines is recommended. Current cholera vaccines afford a three- to fourfold protection for about a year in endemic areas. The efficacy of TAB vaccine is much less convincing but does appear to afford limited protection to those previously unexposed, especially in the case of typhoid fever. It is also recommended that family and other close contacts of typhoid patients be immunized.

An interesting, imaginative, ingenious, and prospectively effective approach to oral immunization against shigellosis may prove to have more widespread application not only to acute diarrheal disease and other infectious agents spread by the fecal-oral route but also to a larger group of microorganisms that attack mucous membranes of the respiratory tract (see section on mucous membrane immunization in

Chap. 12). Currently, two types of living oral vaccines, shown to be effective in preventing shigellosis in monkeys, are being tested in endemic areas. One vaccine includes an avirulent recombinant of *Shigella flexneri* and *E. coli* K 12 (Hfr) which can invade the mucosa but is unable to multiply locally. The other vaccine contains streptomycin-dependent bacteria that grow poorly, if at all, after penetrating the mucosa. Presumably, by penetrating the intestinal mucosa and bringing the shigellae into contact with the appropriate gut-dependent lymphocytes, both vaccines are effective in producing a strong secretory IgA response.

The mild nature of most *Salmonella* infections and the hundreds of antigenic types rule out any attempt at immunization to prevent acute gastroenteritis. Probably a similar situation pertains on a smaller scale in the case of traveler's diarrhea. In the case of infantile diarrhea caused by enteropathogenic *E. coli,* the age incidence of the disease, the number of serotypes involved, and the effectiveness of other control measures preclude any serious effort to develop vaccines.

Chemoprophylaxis Chemoprophylaxis of the family and other close contacts of cholera patients with tetracyclines is effective. In epidemics of diarrhea in newborn nurseries caused by enteropathogenic *E. coli,* some physicians have recommended the prophylactic use of neomycin. Although not routinely employed or currently indicated, clinical trials have established the prophylactic value of neomycin and phthalylsulfathiazole in traveler's diarrhea. In salmonellosis, chemoprophylaxis has not been proposed. However, in persons known to have been exposed to highly virulent organisms such as *S. typhi* or *S. choleraesuis,* it is conceivable that ampicillin might be employed prophylactically.

Among the acute diarrheal diseases chemoprophylaxis has been most extensively and effectively utilized in halting epidemics of shigellosis, especially those occurring in mental institutions, jails, orphanages, and military camps. Formerly, sulfonamides and tetracyclines were the prophylactic drugs of choice. For the past 20 years, however, chemoprophylaxis has become increasingly ineffective and risky because of the widespread transfer of multiple drug resistance by conjugation (Chap. 4) not only among shigellae but also between shigellae, salmonellae, *Escherichia, Klebsiella, Proteus,* and other gram-negative enteric bacteria.

The hazardous and frightening aspect of the transfer of multiple drug resistance through RTF (resistance transfer factor) is indicated by observations recorded since 1968 when epidemics of *Shigella dysenteriae* began to spread widely throughout Central America and Mexico for the first time in 30 years. Four epidemic enteric pathogens—*Shigella dysenteriae* 1, *Salmonella typhi, Shigella flexneri* 2a, and *Shigella flexneri* 6—have since appeared with identical patterns of multiple drug resistance and with enhanced virulence. Each pathogen is resistant to sulfadiazine, tetracycline, chloramphenicol, and streptomycin, and each is sensitive to ampicillin, cephalosporins, gentamicin, polymyxins, kanamycin, nalidixic acid, and nitrofurans. Thus, the collective experience suggests that, in addition to mediating multiple drug resistance, RTF may incorporate and transfer one or more genes that enhance the virulence of enteric pathogens. The demonstration of enhanced virulence accompanying RTF is not entirely unexpected, since naturally occurring isolates of *E. coli* possess RTF's that contain enterotoxin factors associated with ability to produce traveler's disease.

Therapy Most episodes of acute diarrheal disease are of short duration and produce little disability, and chemotherapy is contraindicated in view of the RTF problem. On the other hand, in cholera, infantile diarrhea, the enteric fevers, bacteremias, severe cases of dysentery, and perhaps in protracted cases of diarrhea, chemotherapy is recommended. Currently, with the exception of cholera, antibiotic sensitivity tests are essential because of the frequency of multiple drug resistance associated with RTF.

Despite the fact that replacement of fluid and electrolytes is the first priority, tetracycline therapy of cholera patients is a useful adjunct because it eliminates the causative agent from the feces and shortens the duration and extent of fluid and electrolyte loss. In most cases of infantile diarrhea, therapy must be initiated before the results of antibiotic sensitivity tests become available. The latter are required because epidemics can be caused by *E. coli* resistant to chloramphenicol, neomycin, and other drugs. At present, the most useful drug appears to be neomycin when needed or indicated by the sensitivity pattern of the causative agent. Chloramphenicol, kanamycin, gentamicin, or the polymyxins may also be effective.

In view of the extensive epidemics of typhoid and dysentery associated with bacteria which are multiply resistant to chloramphenicol, tetracycline, streptomycin, and sulfadiazine, chemotherapy of the enteric fevers, bacteremias, and severe cases of diarrhea must be based on the antibiotic sensitivity pattern of the specific causative agent. In typhoid, present use indicates that ampicillin is probably the drug of choice. On the basis of data obtained from sensitivity tests, ampicillin can be continued or switched to a more appropriate drug when indicated. In the past chloramphenicol has proved effective, but current reality dictates that prior to its therapeutic use, it must be established that the causative agent is sensitive. In shigellosis, an increasing incidence of ampicillin-resistant isolates are being reported, and sensitivity tests are critical. In protracted cases of diarrhea without systemic infection, neomycin is a useful drug but should not be employed unless the causative agent has been shown to be sensitive.

Specific Measures in Typhoid Since long-term human carriers play the major role in the perpetuation of typhoid fever, efforts directed at the prevention and elimination of the carrier state are vital to the control of the disease. The specific measures required include (1) detection of the carrier state in patients and contacts, (2) intensive and prolonged chemotherapy of patients and carriers, (3) careful bacteriological monitoring of the effect of chemotherapy in eliminating the carrier state, and (4) cholecystectomy of fecal carriers in whom intensive and prolonged chemotherapy has failed.

Other Methods of Control Under epidemic conditions, emergency measures are undertaken to assure a safe water supply, which often includes boiling or chlorination, and to exclude suspected foods. Other public health measures include case reporting, recognition of the source of the epidemic, and the education of convalescents and carriers in sanitary disposal of feces, in the importance of hand washing after defecation and before eating, and in their exclusion from occupations involving the handling of food. Generally, these procedures are most energetically pursued in the case of cholera, typhoid, institutional epidemics of dysentery, and outbreaks of disease caused by *Shigella dysenteriae.*

Prevention of *Vibrio parahemolyticus* infections can be accomplished in most cases by adequate cooking of shellfish or crustaceans prior to ingestion.

Limiting Factors There are many socioeconomic and biological factors that limit the prospect of preventing and controlling enteric bacterial disease. Included in the category of socioeconomic factors are the provision of safe and abundant public or private supplies of water, sanitary disposal of human excreta, fly control, pasteurization of dairy products, sanitary supervision and refrigeration of food supplies, the elimination of overcrowding and malnutrition, the application of sound principles of personal hygiene, necessary precautions in feeding infants, and public health measures such as case reporting; detection, isolation, surveillance, therapy, and education of patients and carriers; the availability of prompt and adequate rehydration facilities; disinfection of contaminated materials; and when warranted, immunization of contacts, endemic populations, and travelers. Obviously, most developing countries have been unable to provide adequate sanitary and treatment facilities. Consequently, epidemics and endemics of acute diarrheal disease continue to constitute a major social, economic, and health problem whose resolution requires the comprehensive support of the more affluent nations acting in a spirit of willing cooperation.

Prevention and control of acute diarrheal disease are rendered inordinately more difficult, however, by biological factors governing host-parasite interactions. Included in this category are the frequency of mild or unrecognized cases of infections with *Salmonella, Shigella, Escherichia,* and cholera bacteria; the existence of the carrier state in each of the infectious entities; the multiplicity of antigenic types; the transfer of multiple drug resistance through conjugation (Chap. 4); the long-term persistence of human typhoid carriers; and the widespread reservoir of infection and persistence of the carrier state in domestic animals in the case of salmonellosis.

INTESTINAL PROTOZOAL INFECTIONS

Amebiasis

Amebiasis is usually a chronic disease caused by a protozoan parasite of man, *Entamoeba histolytica,* that characteristically affects the colon, occasionally involves the liver, and rarely attacks other tissues. The infection-to-disease ratio is high, especially in countries and population groups where poor sanitary hygiene is practiced. When present, clinical manifestations vary from a mild, intermittent diarrheal disease that may persist for years to an acute amebic dysentery which may terminate fatally.

The Causative Agent The general features of protozoa reviewed in Chapter 2 need no reiteration, but the specific attributes of *Entamoeba histolytica* are worth noting. The parasite has two stages in its life cycle—trophozoite and cyst. Amebic trophozoites are large (20 μm), are actively motile by means of pseudopodia, are uninuclear, divide by binary fission, and have the capacity to invade and lyse tissues, hence, the name histolytica. Amebic cysts are usually smaller in size (5 to 20 μm), are nonmotile, have 1 to 4 nuclei, exhibit nuclear division, lack the capacity to invade tissue, and have a thick, relatively resistant cyst wall. Cysts less than 10 μm in diameter are generally designated as *Entamoeba hartmanni,* a parasite that is held to be of lower pathogenicity.

Pathogenesis Ingested amebic cysts traverse the acid barrier in the stomach and are excysted in the ileocecal region. The released trophozoites multiply rapidly and eventually become established in the cecum where encystation proceeds.

Trophozoites have the capacity to invade the intestinal mucosa, but what triggers the process is unknown. In severe infections, the submucosa is involved, flask-shaped ulcers develop, and the disease may spread widely within the large intestine. Occasionally, the trophozoite may enter the portal circulation, pass by way of the portal vein to the liver, and produce an amebic abscess. The diaphragm and the lungs may become involved as a consequence of extension of the hepatic disease.

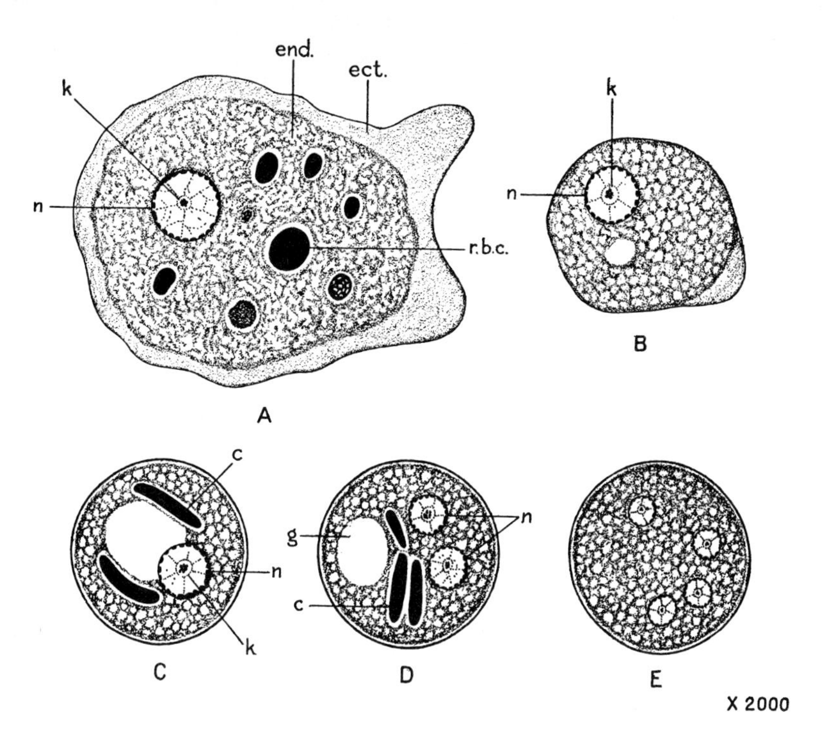

Figure 18-2 Schematic representation of *Entamoeba histolytica. A.* Trophozoite containing red blood cells undergoing digestion. *B.* Precystic ameba devoid of cytoplasmic inclusions. *C.* Young uninucleate cyst. *D.* Binucleate cyst. *E.* Mature quadrinucleate cyst. c, Chromatoid bodies; etc., ectoplasm; end., endoplasm; g, glycogen vacuole; k, karyosome; n, nucleus; r. b. c., red blood cells. (*From H. W. Brown, Basic Clinical Parasitology, 3d ed., New York: Appleton-Century-Crofts, 1969.*)

Laboratory Diagnosis The diagnosis of amebiasis is based on demonstration of the organism in feces or tissues. Formed stools usually reveal the typical cysts, while fluid stools should be examined immediately for the actively motile trophozoites. *Entamoeba histolytica* must be differentiated from nonpathogenic amebas that may be present in the stool, especially *Entamoeba coli.* Trophozoites of *E. histolytica* show progressive motility and may contain ingested red blood cells, in which event the identification is established. *Entamoeba coli* trophozoites are sluggish, their movements are directionless, and they are unable to ingest erythrocytes. *Dientamoeba fragilis* trophozoites (there is no cyst stage) have two nuclei and thus are easily distinguished from *Entamoeba histolytica* and *Entamoeba coli.* If this parasite is pathogenic, as held by some investigators, it produces a mild self-limiting and localized infection.

Some of the important distinguishing features of the cysts of *Entamoeba histolytica* and *Entamoeba coli* are listed in Table 18-6 and illustrated in Figure 18-2. When only cysts are seen and the diagnosis is in doubt, a magnesium sulfate purge should be given on an empty stomach when not contraindicated, as in pregnancy or during abdominal pain. The first passed stool

Table 18-6 Important Diagnostic Characteristics of the Cysts of *Entamoeba histolytica* and *Entamoeba coli*

Characteristic	*E. histolytica*	*E. coli*
Nuclei	1 to 4	1 to 8
Karyosome in nucleus	Central	Off center
Chromatic material on nuclear membrane	Even	Irregular
Chromatoidal bars in cytoplasm	When present, large, thick, rod-shaped bodies	When present, splinter-like bodies

should be examined for cysts, and the subsequent fluid stools should be checked for the motile trophozoites. Supravital stains may be useful in facilitating the identification of trophozoites, and iron hematoxylin stains can be employed to prepare permanent slides for more accurate observation of the structural features of the parasite.

As with all examinations for protozoa and helminths, the stool specimen should be concentrated prior to evaluation. There are a number of suitable techniques including sedimentation, zinc sulfate flotation, and formalin-ether concentration. In examining stools it is important to note that barium and antidiarrheal preparations, antacids, laxatives, and chemotherapeutic agents can interfere with the demonstration of parasites.

A number of serological tests, including gel diffusion precipitin reactions and indirect hemagglutination, are available but do not distinguish between present and past infection. Various culture media are also useful in the hands of specially trained personnel. Other procedures of value in establishing the diagnosis are sigmoidoscopy, x-rays, and liver scans.

Epidemiology Amebiasis is a disease that is worldwide in distribution but is much more prevalent in areas where sanitary conditions are primitive. Epidemics in the United States have resulted largely from direct contamination of the water supply by human feces as a consequence of faulty plumbing connections. The latest large-scale outbreak occurred in 1956 in South Bend, Indiana when the private water system of an industrial plant became contaminated with sewage. Of the 1,500 employees, an estimated 52.4 percent were infected; 31 had amebiasis, and 4 patients died. In accordance with the nature of the disease, amebiasis is more prevalent in developing nations, in rural as opposed to urban areas, in mental institutions, and in individuals returning from endemic areas (missionaries, peace corps volunteers, soldiers). Since 1959 approximately 3,000 cases of amebiasis have been reported annually in the United States with between 54 and 124 deaths.

Prevention and Control Since asymptomatic human carriers are the main source for spreading the disease by way of contaminated feces, prevention must be based on the sanitary disposal of human waste and the protection of water supplies against fecal contamination. Amebic cysts are resistant to chlorination but are removed by diatomaceous earth filters.

Metronidazole is the drug of choice for the treatment of all forms of the disease and is rapidly superseding the older drugs (emetine, chloroquine, and tetracycline) because it is safer and more effective.

Giardiasis

An intestinal pear-shaped flagellate, *Giardia lamblia,* is occasionally associated with acute or chronic diarrhea, especially in children, and less commonly with the malabsorption syndrome. Following ingestion of oval cysts (9 to 12 μm), excystation occurs in the duodenum, and the released binucleate trophozoites (15 μm) multiply by binary fission and adhere by sucking disks to the mucosa of the duodenum and upper jejunum. Intestinal hypomotility facilitates giardial overgrowth, resulting in the malabsorption syndrome. Encystation takes place as the trophozoites pass down the colon. Demonstration of the cysts or trophozoites in the stools establishes the diagnosis. Trophozoites are usually found only when diarrhea is present. When the stools are negative, duodenal aspirates may reveal the presence of the organism in patients with chronic diarrhea and loss of weight. Therapy is based on the use of metronidazole. Prevention and control require the same methods as amebiasis, but the more common involvement of children suggests a more direct fecal-oral route from one child to another.

Balantidiasis

Balantidiasis is a relatively uncommon disease of the colon associated with infection with the largest intestinal protozoa to infect man, the ciliate *Balantidium coli.* After ingestion, the spherical cyst (50 μm) excysts in the small intestine; the released trophozoites (60 by 45 μm) migrate into the cecum where they multiply by binary fission, move down the colon where encystation usually occurs in the lumen, and are passed in the stools. Occasionally, the trophozoites may invade the mucosa of the colon and produce a mild, chronic diarrhea. Less frequently, the submucosa may be invaded, resulting in ulceration and dysentery. Repeated stool examinations may be required to demonstrate the presence of the trophozoites and cysts since the organism is passed intermittently. The use of metronidazole in therapy is superseding diiodohydroxyquin and tetracyclines. Prevention and control are similar to measures recommended for amebiasis and giardiasis. Although porcine strains of *B. coli* have been implicated in human infections, the evidence is unconvincing.

INTESTINAL NEMATODES (ROUNDWORMS)

The general features of the helminths were considered in Chapter 2. In this chapter attention is directed toward the diseases caused by the roundworms in man (ascariasis, trichuriasis or whipworm disease, hookworm disease, strongyloidiasis, enterobiasis or pinworm disease, trichinosis). Except for trichinosis, laboratory diagnosis of disease caused by these parasites is based on the demonstration of eggs and/or larvae in stools or, in the case of enterobiasis, in the folds of the skin in the perianal region. Interestingly, the acute stage of nematode infections or infestations is associated with eosinophilia.

Ascariasis

Ascariasis is usually a chronic disease of children associated with heavy infestation with adult worms *(Ascaris lumbricoides)* and aggravated by concomitant hookworm and whipworm infection. The clinical manifestations can include malnutrition and intestinal obstruction. When irritated, the adult worm migrates and may invade the tissue (bile duct, pancreatic duct, gallbladder, appendix, peritoneum). Rarely, migrating larvae in passing through the lung of a sensitized host may precipitate asthmatic attacks and pulmonary infiltrates. The life cycle of *A. lumbricoides* is indicated diagrammatically below.

Laboratory diagnosis of ascariasis is established by demonstrating the characteristic, large (45 × 65 μm) fertile ova with a mammillated or

Life Cycle of *Ascaris lumbricoides*

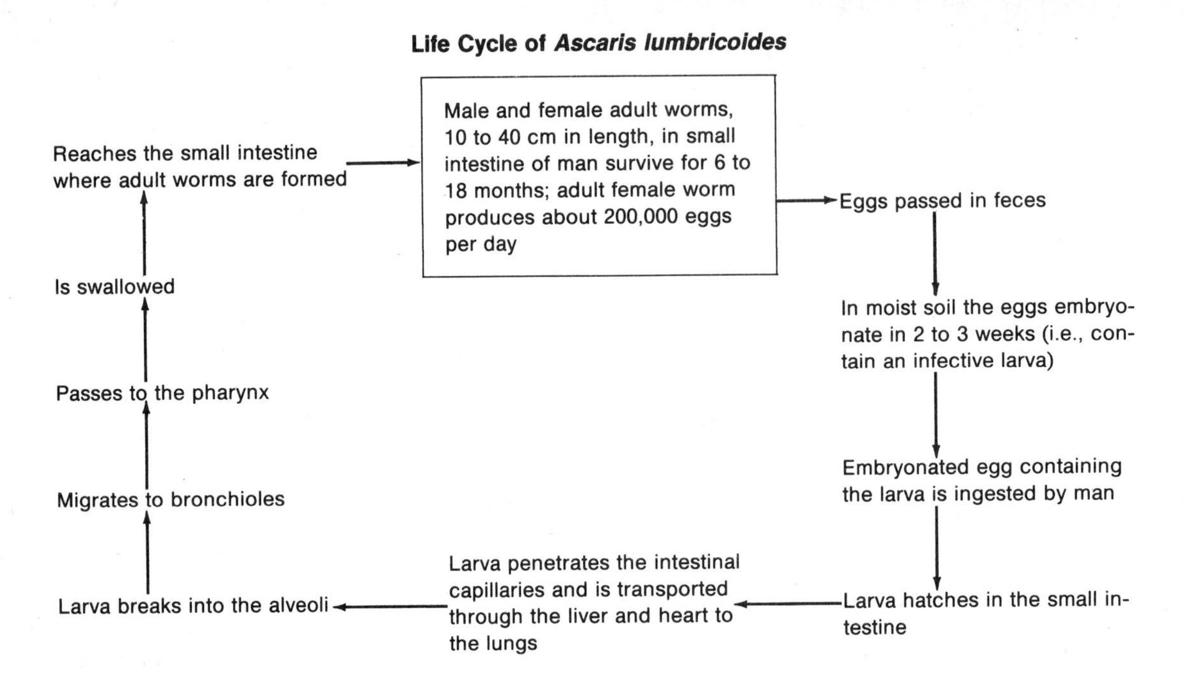

corrugated border or by finding decorticated and infertile ova (Fig. 18-3). After a barium meal, adult worms are readily seen on x-rays. The disease is worldwide in distribution and is especially prevalent in tropical, subtropical, and rural areas with primitive sanitary facilities. An estimated million cases occur annually in the United States, mostly in the rural South. Piperazine and pyrantel pamoate are the drugs of choice in ascariasis, and apparently they act by paralyzing the adult worm, which is then passed in the feces. When other intestinal helminths are also present, ascariasis must be treated first to avoid migration of the adult worms which might be induced by other drugs. Prevention and control are based on personal and environmental hygiene.

Trichuriasis (Whipworm Disease)

Trichuriasis is a disease of the rectum and colon primarily occurring in children heavily infested with adult *Trichuris trichiura* worms. The clinical manifestations may include abdominal pain, diarrhea, and loss of weight, occasionally associated with a bloody diarrhea or rectal prolapse. Laboratory diagnosis is based on the microscopic demonstration of the typical barrel-shaped eggs (50 × 20 μm) with translucent polar plugs (Fig. 18-3). The treatment of choice involves the use of a hexylresorcinol enema preceded by saline purgation. Pyrantel pamoate therapy is being explored and may prove useful. The epidemiology and prevention and control of trichuriasis are generally the same as for ascariasis, although trichuriasis is less prevalent. The life cycle of *T. trichiura* is indicated below.

Hookworm Disease

Hookworm is a chronic disease of man characterized by a variable degree of anemia that is directly proportional to the number of adult *Necator americanus* or *Ancylostoma duodenale* worms that suck blood from the mucosa of the small intestine. In heavy infestations (500 or

Life Cycle of *Trichuris trichiura*

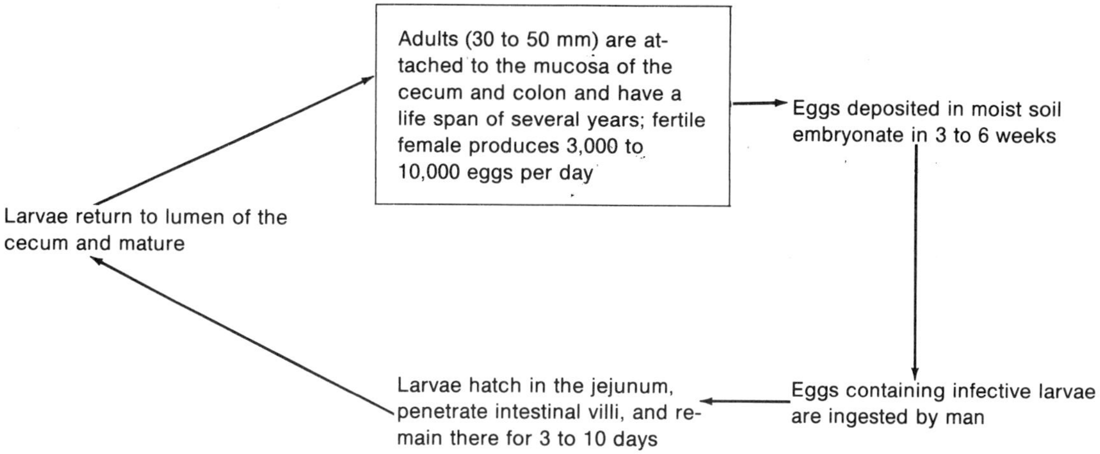

Adults (30 to 50 mm) are attached to the mucosa of the cecum and colon and have a life span of several years; fertile female produces 3,000 to 10,000 eggs per day

→ Eggs deposited in moist soil embryonate in 3 to 6 weeks

→ Eggs containing infective larvae are ingested by man

→ Larvae hatch in the jejunum, penetrate intestinal villi, and remain there for 3 to 10 days

→ Larvae return to lumen of the cecum and mature

more adult worms), a progressive, secondary, hypochromic anemia develops which can be complicated by poor nutrition and, in children, by delayed physical development and mental retardation. As noted by the chart of the life cycle below, the portal of entry is the skin. In addition to the anemia, clinical manifestations may be associated with the migration of the filariform larvae through the skin (ground itch or creeping eruption) or pulmonary infiltrates as the larvae pass through the lungs. Laboratory diagnosis is readily established by detecting oval-shaped eggs (55×40 μm) in routine wet mounts of stool specimens (Fig. 18-3). If the patient is constipated or there is delay in examining the stool, rhabditiform larvae may be seen. In this event, care must be taken to distinguish between hookworm larvae, which have a long buccal capsule, and *Strongyloides* larvae, which have a short buccal capsule. Hookworm disease is often found in the same geographical areas and in the same patient along with ascariasis and trichuriasis. Tetrachlorethylene is the drug of choice in *Necator* infections, and bephenium hydroxynaphthoate is used in *Ancylostoma* infections. Prevention and control are generally similar to that for the other intestinal nematodes with the important exception that the simple expedient of wearing shoes is adequate to prevent infection because the filariform larvae initiate infection by penetrating the skin of the foot.

Strongyloidiasis

Strongyloidiasis is a chronic disease of man caused by *Strongyloides stercoralis,* which is basically similar to the hookworm with the added potential of producing autoinfection which can significantly increase the worm burden in the absence of further external infection. Autoinfection can result when a patient becomes constipated or when rhabditiform larvae are deposited in the perianal skin. Filariform larvae develop under these circumstances and can penetrate the intestinal mucosa or the perianal skin. The life cycle of *Strongyloides* is identical to that of *Necator* and *Ancylostoma,* except that *Strongyloides* has a free-living cycle whereby rhabditiform larvae present in the soil can develop into free-living adults which produce eggs. Man may become infected, as in hookworm, when filariform larvae in the soil penetrate the skin. Fatal, overwhelming strongyloidiasis can occur in patients receiving

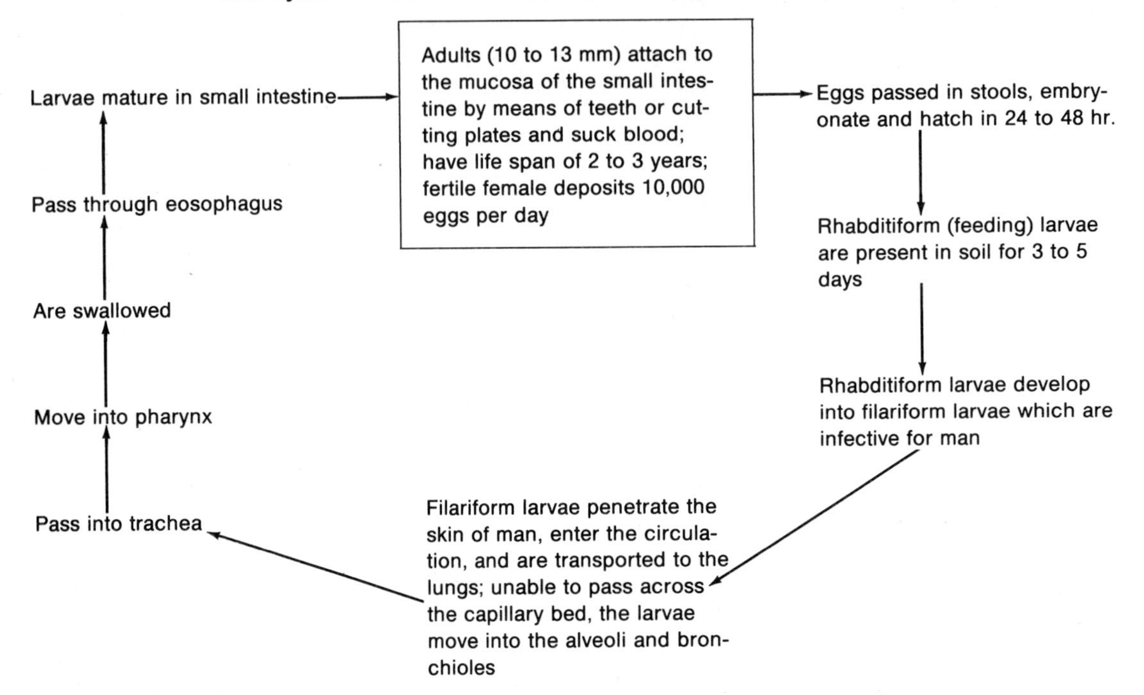

immunosuppressive therapy. For the treatment of strongyloidiasis, thiabendazole is recommended. Prevention and control are the same as for hookworm.

Enterobiasis (Pinworm Disease)

Enterobiasis, or pinworm infection, is usually a mild disease of man, especially children, caused by *Enterobius vermicularis* and characterized primarily by irritation of the perianal area (pruritis ani), restlessness, and disturbed sleep due to nocturnal migration of the gravid female worms. As noted in the chart of the life cycle, autoinfection can occur as a result of the ingestion of eggs deposited in the perianal area or when the eggs hatch in the perianal area and the larvae migrate back into the rectum and mature in the colon (retroinfection). Infection is worldwide in distribution; is transmitted by the fecal-oral route, especially when children sleep together in the same bed; and is particularly prevalent in institutions for retarded children and in orphanages. Stool examination for ova is usually unproductive, but the eggs are easily demonstrated when a scotch tape swab or plastic paddles which are sticky on one side are pressed against the perianal area on rising in the morning. The eggs are oval (55 × 25 μm) and are usually flattened on one side (Fig. 18-3). Treatment involves the use of pyrantel pamoate, but pyrvinium pamoate is also effective. It is recommended that the entire family be treated, thereby lessening the chances of reinfection. Efforts to cut down the spread of infection should be directed toward trimming of the nails to reduce the extent of trauma induced by scratching the perianal area, the use of tight-

Figure 18-3 The eggs of some important enteric and enteric-associated parasites of man as they appear in clinical specimens. (*© Copyright 1962 CIBA Pharmaceutical Company, Division of CIBA-GEIGY Corporation. Reproduced with permission from The CIBA Collection of Medical Illustrations by Frank H. Netter, M.D. All rights reserved.*)

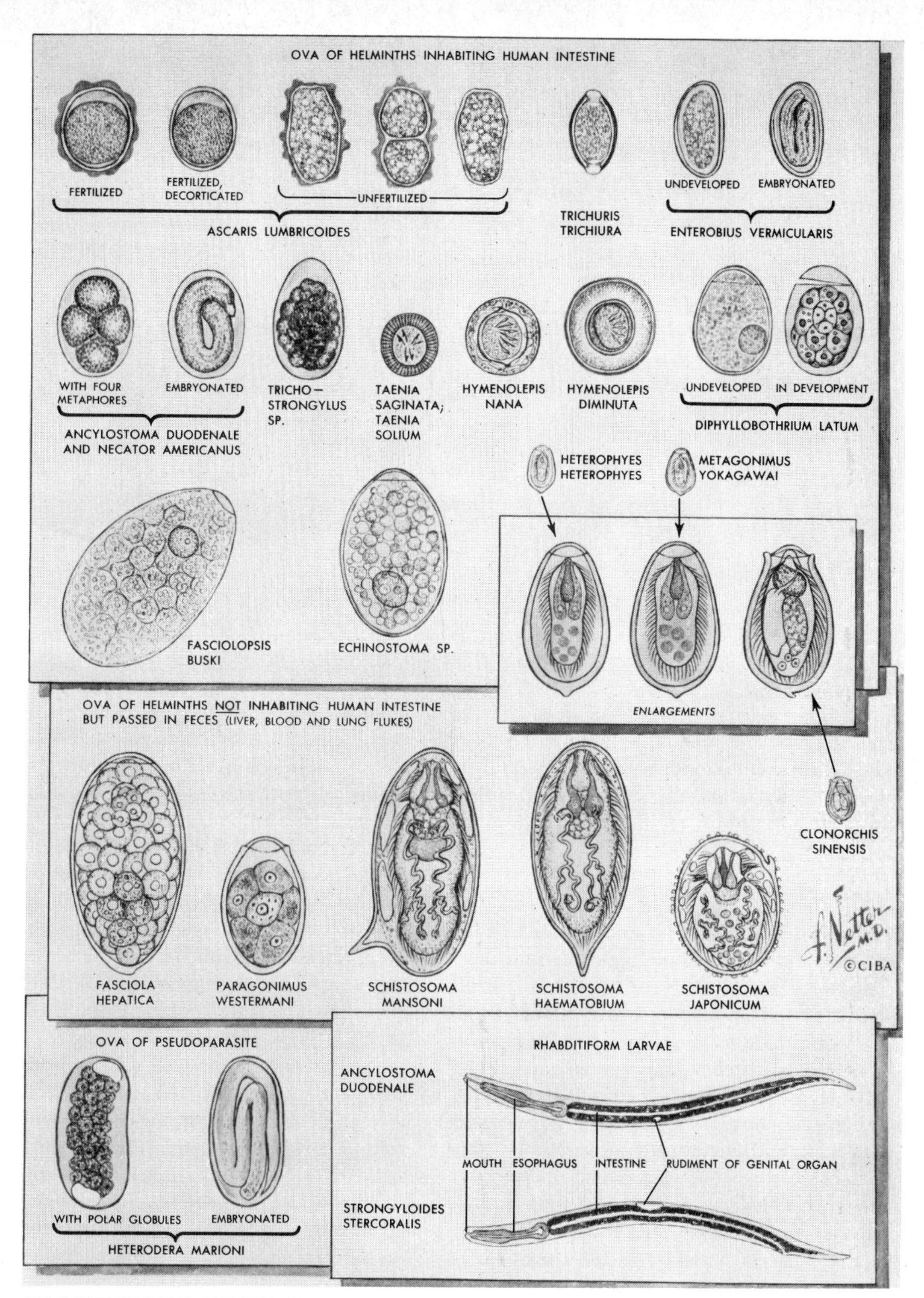

N47-59 DIGESTIVE SYSTEM—PART II PARASITES—OVA AND LARVAE OF HELMINTHS; DIAGNOSIS OF HELMINTHIC INFESTATION BY FECES EXAMINATION

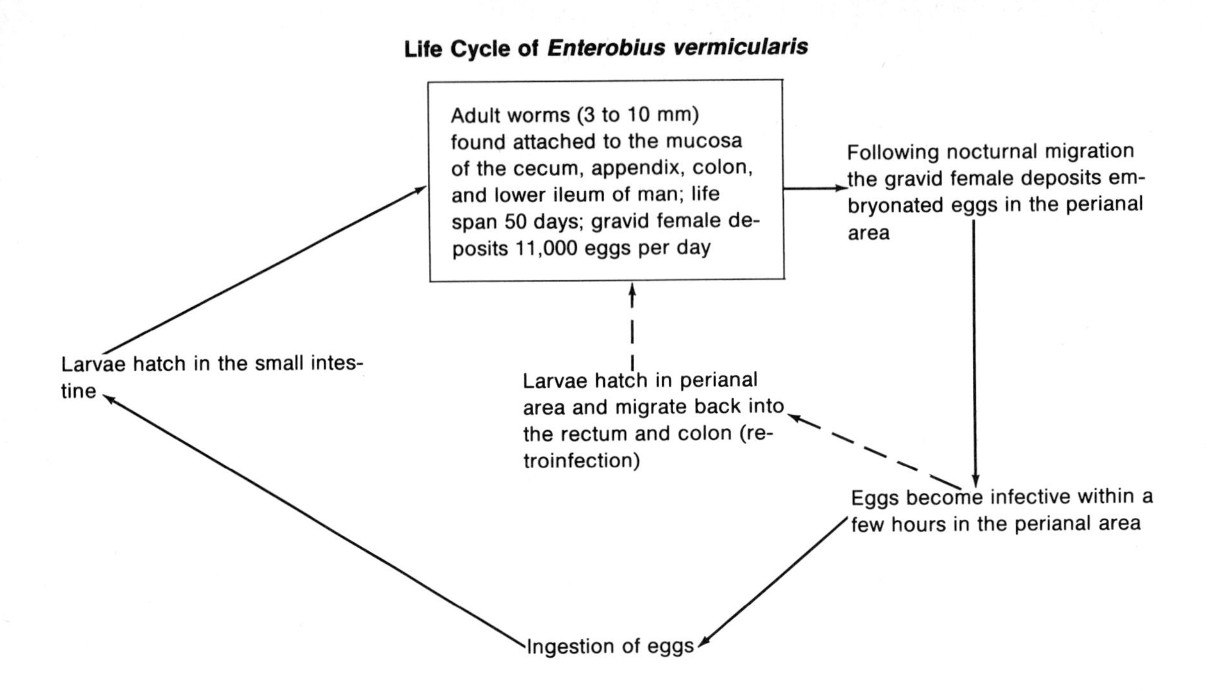

fitting underwear to prevent the spread of the eggs, the taking of frequent showers rather than baths, the use of clean linens, thorough vacuuming of the house and discarding the dust bag, and regular cleaning of toilets with disinfectants.

Trichinosis

Trichinosis is generally a mild disease of man associated with invasion, migration, and especially the encystment of *Trichinella spiralis* larvae. The infection-to-disease ratio is high. Clinical manifestations are dependent upon the number of encysted larvae ingested and may involve fever and abdominal irritation (invasion) and edema, myalgia, and rising eosinophilia (migration and encystment). Respiratory, neurological, cardiac, and rheumatic symptoms are uncommon but may occur 1 to 3 months after ingestion of the larvae. The encysted larvae in striated muscle usually calcify in 6 to 18 months. Trichinosis is worldwide in distribution, but the incidence varies widely with the dietary and cooking habits of individuals and groups and with the use of grain or raw garbage to feed swine. In the United States many factors have combined to sharply reduce the incidence of the disease including the raising of grain-fed swine, laws to prevent the feeding of raw garbage to swine, prolonged salting or smoking of pork which destroys the larvae, the use of frozen foods in which the larvae are killed within 3 days, and adequate cooking of pork products. In 1972 there were only 78 reported cases of trichinosis in the United States. In addition to the domestic life cycle of *T. spiralis* included in the chart below, there is a cycle associated with wild carnivorous animals (bears) which may serve as a source of human infection as in Alaska, and a rat-to-rat cycle has been implicated as a source of infection for swine but is probably a minor factor in transmission of the

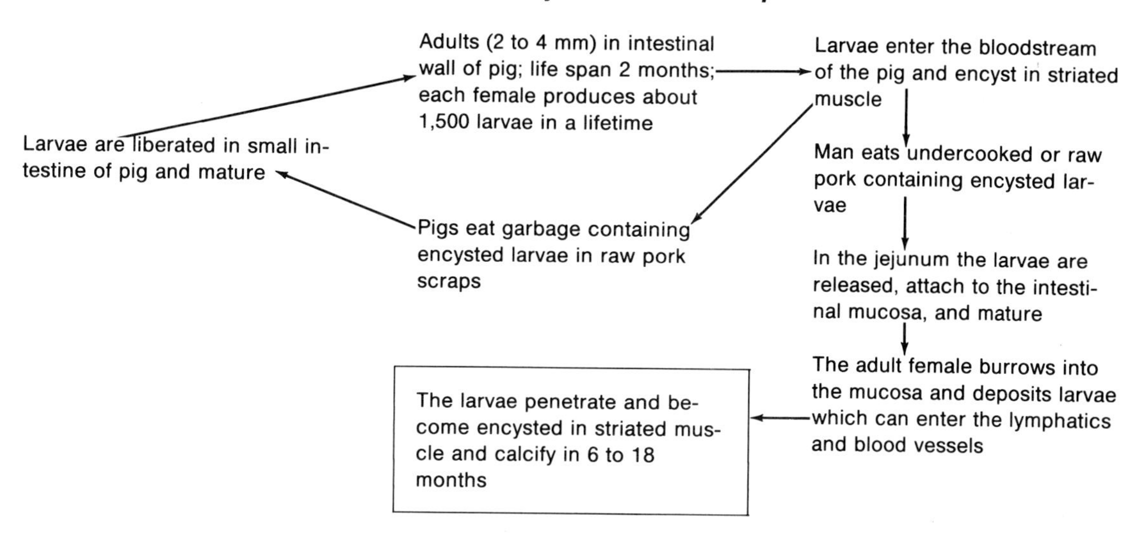

infection to swine. Diagnosis of trichinosis is generally established by a combination of factors including a history of eating pork, muscle biopsy to demonstrate the encysted larvae, a rising eosinophilia, and compatible serological and skin tests. Since there are no eggs and few larvae in the feces, stool examination is worthless. Thiabendazole may prove to be of value in treatment, and the use of corticosteroids usually shortens the course of the disease.

INTESTINAL CESTODES (TAPEWORMS)

The general features of the flatworms, which include the cestodes (tapeworms) and trematodes (flukes), were considered in Chapter 2. In this chapter emphasis will be placed on the beef, pork, fish, and dwarf tapeworms. For convenience, the discussion will also include the tapeworm that causes hydatid cyst disease in the liver and lungs. Morphologically, the tapeworms consist of a scolex (head) used for attachment to the intestinal mucosa, a neck which is the region of growth, and the strobila which includes the individual segments called proglottids. The latter are hermaphroditic and when sexually mature are designated as gravid proglottids.

Taeniasis (Beef Tapeworm Disease)

When caused by the beef tapeworm, *Taenia saginata,* taeniasis is a mild disease occasionally associated with epigastric pain, weight loss, and digestive disturbances. The adult tapeworm may survive in man, the definitive host, for up to 25 years. Disease is caused by only 1 or 2 tapeworms. Human infections occur following ingestion of raw or insufficiently cooked beef containing cysticerci (larvae). In the small intestine the scolex of the cysticercus evaginates, attaches itself to the mucosa, and develops the mature strobila over a period of 2 to 3 months. Ova (35 × 25 μm) are readily demonstrated upon microscopic examination of wet mounts but cannot be differentiated from those of the pork tapeworm (Fig. 18-3). Diagnosis can be

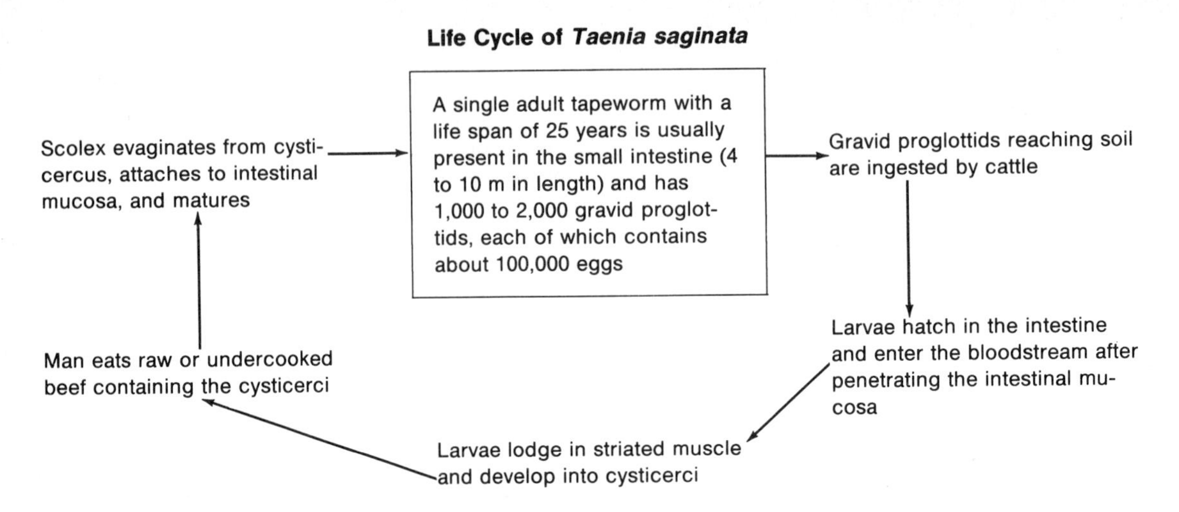

made by examining the proglottid (18 × 6 mm) and counting 15 to 30 lateral uterine branches on each side of the main stem (proglottids of the pork tapeworm usually have fewer than 13 lateral uterine branches). Purgation before and after quinacrine, which is the drug of choice, usually is successful in flushing out the stunned tapeworm. As noted in the chart of the life cycle above, sanitary disposal of human feces would prevent the disease in cattle and man.

Taeniasis (Pork Tapeworm Disease)

When caused by the pork tapeworm, *Taenia solium,* taeniasis can occur as a mild disease similar to that associated with the beef tapeworm or as a more serious disease, cysticercosis. In the latter case, when *T. solium* eggs are ingested by man or enter the small intestine by reverse peristalsis, the eggs hatch, and the larvae penetrate the intestinal mucosa, enter the circulation, and are carried to the tissues (striated muscles, subcutaneous tissues, brain, spinal cord, eye, heart) where they develop into cysticerci and persist for 3 to 5 years. Invasion of the eye, CNS, and heart by cysticerci may present serious complications or death. Epilepsy is a frequent sequel of CNS invasion. The ova are identical with those of *T. saginata* and are regularly present in the stools (Fig. 18-3), but the proglottids usually reveal 7 to 12 lateral uterine branches versus the 15 to 30 seen with *T. saginata.* In addition, the scolex has characteristic hooklets not found on *T. saginata.* Quinacrine is the drug of choice and is usually employed in combination with an antiemetic drug to preclude the possibility of cysticercosis.

Fish Tapeworm Disease

The principal significance of human infections with the fish tapeworm, *Dibothriocephalus latus (Diphyllobothrium latum),* is that in about 1 percent of patients the adult worm attaches to the jejunum, has a tremendous capacity to absorb vitamin B_{12}, and eventually leads to megaloblastic anemia. In nonanemic patients, the adult worm adheres to the ileum, and when present, clinical manifestations are mild, as in beef tapeworm infections. Man acquires infection by ingesting raw or undercooked freshwater fish containing larval forms of the tapeworm. In the small intestine, the larva degenerates and the everted scolex usually attaches to the ileum and develops a strobila. The adult worm is 3 to 10 meters, develops more than 3,000 proglottids, and produces 1 million eggs daily during its life span of 20 years or more. The cycle is perpetuated when human feces containing the ova pollute lakes and streams and are ingested by the copepod *(Diaptomus)* who serves as the first intermediate host, larval development progresses in small fish that eat the copepod and subsequently in larger fish that eat the small fish, and eventually completes development to the infective larval stage in large game fish (pike and walleyed pike), the second intermediate host, who have eaten the larger fish. In addition to man, fish-eating animals including bears may serve as the definitive host. The disease occurs throughout the world and in the United States and Canada is concentrated in the Great Lakes region. Laboratory diagnosis is based on the demonstration of the typical oval-shaped eggs (60×40 μm) which have an operculum or lid at one end that opens to permit the embryo to exit (Fig. 18-3). Quinacrine effects the removal of the tapeworm, and vitamin B_{12} may be used to supplement quinacrine and more rapidly correct the anemia. Sanitary disposal of human feces and adequate cooking of freshwater fish are completely effective in preventing human infection.

Dwarf Tapeworm Disease

Disease in man caused by the dwarf tapeworm *Hymenolepis nana* occurs primarily in children in tropical and subtropical areas and, in heavy infections, may involve abdominal distress, weight loss, and erosion of the villi by cysticercoid larvae. The infection is usually spread by the fecal-oral route among children. After ingestion, the eggs hatch, and the larvae penetrate the intestinal villi and develop to the cysticercoid stage. The cysticercoid adheres to the intestinal mucosa and forms a strobila. Fortunately, the cysticerci do not invade tissues other than the intestinal mucosa. The adult worms are about 20 mm in length, have 200 proglottids, and each proglottid produces 100 ova during its life span of several weeks. Infection may also occur as a result of the ingestion of cysticercoid larvae contained in the body cavity of rat and mouse fleas or grain beetles which had previously eaten the tapeworm eggs. A laboratory diagnosis is readily established following microscopic examination of wet mounts of the stool which reveal embryonated eggs (40×50 μm) containing delicate filaments and an inner and outer shell membrane (Fig. 18-3). *H. nana* has a life cycle in rats and mice as well as man, but this cycle does not appear to be responsible for many human infections. Niclosamide has replaced quinacrine as the drug of choice, but therapy is complicated by the problem of autoinfection following ingestion of the embryonated eggs or constipation, which leads to hatching of the eggs within the intestinal tract.

ECHINOCOCCOSIS (HYDATID CYST DISEASE)

Echinococcosis is a disease of man caused by the larval stage of *Echinococcus granulosus* or, less commonly, *E. multilocularis,* characterized primarily by cystic, enlarging (1 to 7 cm) lesions of the liver and occasionally of the lungs, bone, and CNS. Dogs and other canines are the definitive hosts and man, sheep, and cattle are intermediate hosts. Human infections are acquired following the ingestion of eggs passed in the feces of dogs. The eggs hatch in the small intestine, penetrate the intestinal mucosa, enter the portal circulation, and usually become trapped in the liver. Hydatid cysts form in the liver over a period of many months and years, gradually expanding in size, and consist of a laminated membrane, germinal layer, brood capsule, and hydatid sand (fluid, scolices, hooklets). Clinical manifestations depend primarily on the size and location of the hydatid cyst(s). The chief danger is the accidental rupturing of the cyst, releasing hydatid sand from the walled-off area with the initiation of anaphylactic reactions of varying severity, which occasionally may be fatal. Diagnosis, in most cases, is established on clinical, radiological, and surgical findings (hydatid sand in the cyst). Surgical removal is the only therapy available and must be performed with great care to avoid discharging the contents of the cyst. Prevention and control are based largely on avoiding contact with infected dogs, treating dogs found to be infected, and keeping dogs from feeding on infected tissues of sheep and cattle. Disease caused by *E. multilocularis* is associated with alveolar cysts in the liver which are unencapsulated and progress more rapidly, making surgery more difficult, and may lead to portal hypertension, splenomegaly, and ascites or to metastatic lesions in the bone and brain.

URINARY TRACT INFECTIONS

Except for a few organisms normally found in the lower urethra, the urinary tract is free of bacteria. Urethral contaminants in urine rarely exceed 1,000 per milliliter. In symptomatic or asymptomatic urinary infections, however, bacteria ordinarily are present in concentrations of more than 100,000 per milliliter of urine (bacteriuria). Thus, quantitative studies are of critical importance in distinguishing infection from contamination.

Infections of the urinary tract range from asymptomatic bacteriuria through cystitis and urethritis to pyelonephritis. Asymptomatic bacteriuria is the persistent finding of 100,000 or more bacteria of the same type per milliliter of urine without a history or other evidence of urinary infection. In addition to the presence of bacteria, symptomatic bacteriuria (cystitis and urethritis) is usually associated with frequency of urination, burning pain on urination, and the passage of cloudy, occasionally blood-tinged urine. Acute pyelonephritis is an inflammation of the renal substance accompanied by shaking chills, fever, pain in the costovertebral areas or flanks, symptoms of bladder inflammation, marked pyuria, and the finding of 100,000 or more bacteria per milliliter of urine. Chronic pyelonephritis is used to indicate renal disease resulting from the effects of previous bacterial infection as well as the progressive disease resulting from persisting and recurring bacterial infection. Leukocyte casts in urine sediments are a distinctive finding in chronic pyelonephritis, but generally there are no symptoms of infection.

The Causative Agents

General Characteristics Since the normal flora of the gastrointestinal tract serves as the endogenous source of the great bulk of urinary tract infections, and since urine is a good culture medium for gram-negative enteric bacilli, it is not surprising that the predominant organisms include those of the genera *Escherichia, Proteus, Klebsiella, Enterobacter (Aerobacter), Serratia,* and *Pseudomonas.* Other organisms indigenous to the gastrointestinal tract, such as enterococci, staphylococci, *Candida, Citrobacter,* and *Herellea,* also are involved in urinary infections. Even though lactobacilli, *Bacteroides,* and anaerobic streptococci are present in high concentration in the normal gastrointestinal tract, they are rarely the cause of urinary infections presumably because urine is a poor culture medium for these bacteria.

The frequency with which a particular organism is recovered from urinary tract infections depends largely upon previous history of infection, use of chemotherapy, hospitalization, and instrumentation of the urinary tract. As many as 80 percent or more of initial untreated infections acquired in the community in the absence of instrumentation (uncomplicated cases) are caused by *E. coli.* On the other hand, in patients with a history of treated infection or in those who acquire infection following hospitalization or instrumentation (complicated cases), the

Klebsiella-Enterobacter-Serratia group, enterococci, *Proteus,* and *Pseudomonas* account for the majority of infections (60 to 70 percent), whereas only about 20 percent are due to *E. coli.* Infections associated with enterococci and *Serratia* are almost exclusively acquired in the hospital environment.

Two outstanding characteristics of bacteriuria are persistence and recurrence. The same causative agent is isolated when repeat cultures are obtained over a period of several weeks. Spontaneous cure is rarely documented. Following antimicrobial therapy, recurrent infections are common. A relapse is a recurrence due to the same species and serotype of microorganism present before therapy. A reinfection is a recurrence caused by a microorganism different from the one present before therapy. The balance of evidence suggests that most recurrences are reinfections when bacteriuria is limited to the bladder, whereas most recurrences are relapses when the kidney is also involved.

Escherichia coli The biological properties of *E. coli,* the most frequent cause of urinary tract infections, are the same as those associated with enteropathogenic *E. coli.* The common O serotypes in urinary infections (1, 4, 6, 7, 25, 50, and 75), however, reflect their normal distribution in human stools, and enteropathogenic serotypes are not involved.

***Klebsiella-Enterobacter-Serratia* Group** In respect to their IMVIC reactions, *Klebsiella, Enterobacter (Aerobacter),* and *Serratia* form a natural group. Characteristically, these bacteria are indole- and methyl red-negative and acetylmethylcarbinol- and citrate-positive (IMVIC − − + +).

Klebsiella is nonmotile and ornithine decarboxylase-negative, whereas *Enterobacter* and *Serratia* are motile and ornithine decarboxylase-positive. *Enterobacter* A *(cloacae)* and *Serratia* are highly resistant to cephalothin (250 μg per ml or more in vitro), whereas *Klebsiella* and *Enterobacter* B *(aerogenes)* are highly susceptible. *Serratia* can produce red pigmented, pink, or sectored colonies, but colorless mutants predominate. However, since *Serratia* is inactive in fermenting arabinose, raffinose, and rhamnose, the colorless mutants can be differentiated from *Enterobacter* without difficulty.

When bacteria with aberrant IMVIC reactions (indole or methyl red positive) are isolated, preliminary identification as a member of the *Klebsiella-Enterobacter-Serratia* group should be based on motility and ornithine decarboxylase activity.

The *Klebsiella-Enterobacter-Serratia* group has been classified into a number of serotypes on the basis of their somatic (O), flagellar (H), and capsular (K) antigens. *Klebsiella* has three major O antigens and 72 K antigens. Capsular type 2 and untypable strains have been recovered most frequently from urine. Being nonmotile, *Klebsiella* is devoid of H antigens.

Enterobacter A *(cloacae)* has been separated into 79 serotypes on the basis of 53 somatic O antigens and 56 flagellar H antigens. In *Serratia marcescens* 15 O and 13 H antigens have been recognized.

Hospital isolations of this group of bacteria from urine indicate that about 80 percent are *Klebsiella.* Of the balance, the majority are *Enterobacter* A *(cloacae).*

Proteus The *Proteus* group of bacteria are characteristically motile, lactose negative, and urease positive. They have been separated into *P. vulgaris* and *P. mirabilis* which produce H_2S, liquefy gelatin, and swarm on moist agar and *P. morganii* and *P. rettgeri* which do not. *P. vulgaris* can be differentiated from *P. mirabilis* by its formation of indole and its failure to synthesize ornithine decarboxylase. *P. morganii* can be distinguished from *P. rettgeri* by its production of ornithine decarboxylase and its failure to utilize citrate or to ferment mannitol.

On the basis of somatic and flagellar antigens, the various species of *Proteus* have been separated into more than 100 serotypes. In addition, various cultures of *P. vulgaris* contain somatic antigens designated OX 2, OX 19, and OX K which are agglutinated by the sera of patients convalescing from certain rickettsial diseases, the Weil-Felix reaction (Chap. 22).

Hospital isolations of this group of bacteria from urine reveal that about two-thirds are *P. mirabilis,* 20 percent *P. rettgeri,* and 10 percent *P. morganii.*

Pseudomonas aeruginosa *Pseudomonas aeruginosa* is a motile, lactose-negative, citrate-positive bacillus that produces a soluble bright yellow or blue-green fluorescent pigment and colonies that have an aromatic sour grape odor.

Although *P. aeruginosa* can be separated into antigenic groups on the basis of O and H antigens, phage typing has proved of greater value in classification of the organism.

Other Organisms Involved Among other causative agents, enterococci (Chap. 14) are the most frequently encountered. Staphylococci (Chap. 14) and the yeast *Candida* (Chap. 16) are found occasionally.

Additional gram-negative enteric bacilli, such as *Citrobacter* and *Providencia,* occasionally are involved. *Citrobacter* is motile, usually ferments lactose and other sugars, is indole-negative, methyl red positive, acetylmethylcarbinol-negative, and citrate-positive (IMVIC − + − +). *Providencia* generally resembles *Proteus* in most of its properties, but in contrast with *Proteus* is urease negative (Fig. 18-1). Two major biochemical subdivisions have been recognized on the basis of their action in fermenting adonitol and inositol. Antigenically, it is a diverse group containing more than 150 serotypes based on somatic, flagellar, and capsular antigens. *Citrobacter* also contains more than 150 serotypes involving O and H antigens.

Herellea is sometimes isolated from hospital-acquired cases of urinary infections. Although the source of infection is not known, the finding of *Herellea* on the skin and mucous membranes including the genital area suggests that they may be introduced following catheterization. The organisms are nonmotile, encapsulated, gram-negative diplobacilli or diplococci which oxidize lactose in 10 percent concentration. The IMVIC pattern is − − − +, only citrate being positive. They are closely related in many respects to a variety of other organisms, including *Moraxella (Mima)* (Chap. 19), and *Bacterium anitratum.* Because of their morphology on solid media and the presence of capsules, these bacteria have been confused with *Neisseria* (Chap. 24).

Pathogenesis

Ascending Pathway In the pathogenesis of most urinary tract infections, microorganisms present in the host's own intestinal tract produce surface contamination of the urethra and migrate through the urinary passages from the urethra, bladder, and ureters to the kidneys (ascending pathway). Rarely urinary infections develop as a consequence of systemic disease caused by such pathogens as group A streptococci, typhoid bacilli, and tubercle bacilli (descending pathway).

Progress of the Disease Most infections are asymptomatic, appear to be limited to the urethra and bladder, and are accompanied by persistent bacteriuria. Urethritis and cystitis are usually mild diseases that subside in a week or less, but the bacteriuria continues. Ultimately, a significant but variable proportion of untreated asymptomatic and symptomatic bacteriurias develop renal damage demonstrable by intravenous pyelography or patients experience acute pyelonephritis. Although most episodes of acute pyelonephritis usually terminate in a week to 10 days, the bacteriuria persists, and the disease tends to recur due to relapse or reinfection. Chronic pyelonephritis which results from preexisting infection as well as the progressive disease resulting from persisting or recurring infection is one of the most common and important kinds of chronic renal disease.

Predisposing Factors Foremost among the many unanswered or poorly understood problems dealing with the pathogenesis of urinary tract infections is the question of why certain individuals are prone to infection, to relapse, and to reinfection. Only in about half of the cases is there evidence to indicate that certain predisposing factors facilitate the development and persistence of infection. A few of the more important precipitating factors are considered briefly in the following sections.

Age and Sex Apart from the greater frequency of bacteriuria and pyelonephritis in newborn males which is probably related to their greater frequency of congenital anomalies, spontaneous urinary tract infections are about ten times as frequent in females as in males. Data acquired as a result of long-term study indicate that healthy girls are at about equal risk of acquiring infection from the ages of 1 to 17 and that by the time high school is completed about 5 percent have experienced bacteriuria or overt disease. Among boys the incidence of infection is less than 0.5 percent. The shorter distance between the urethra and the bladder and the closer proximity of the urethra to the causative agents discharged from the rectum are cited as possible reasons for the higher incidence of infection in girls as compared with boys.

During the child-bearing period between 18 and 40, women are more than ten times as likely as men to develop bacteriuria and pyelonephritis. The frequency of bacteriuria among pregnant women generally ranges from 4 to 10 percent. The seriousness of the problem is indicated by the fact that 13 to 40 percent of women found to have asymptomatic bacteriuria early in pregnancy and left untreated develop overt signs of infection, including many episodes of acute pyelonephritis. Among nonbacteriuric pregnant women only about 1 to 1.5 percent experience symptomatic urinary tract infections. These studies provide convincing evidence that bacteriuria can predict future episodes of pyelonephritis.

The prevalence of bacteriuria among women continues to rise with age, reaching 10 to 15 percent in those over 60 years of age. In the absence of prostatism and genitourinary instrumentation, bacteriuria among males rarely exceeds 0.5 percent. In males over the age of 70, the rate is around 3.5 percent. Selected groups, however, such as hospitalized males or those seen in clinic populations, may have rates of bacteriuria of 15 percent or more.

In considering the natural history of urinary tract infections in women, it is difficult to escape the conclusion that pyelonephritis as a troublesome complication of pregnancy and as a common disease of older women has its genesis in childhood. For example, roentgenographic study of 107 bacteriuric children detected in a school survey revealed that 13.1 percent had evidence suggestive of pyelonephritis, 18.7 percent had ureteral vesical reflux (reflux from the bladder into the ureters during micturition), and 6.5 percent had the megacystis syndrome (enlarged bladder). Renal damage, ureteral vesical reflux, and the megacystis syndrome, in turn, predispose to persistent and recurrent urinary tract infections.

Obstruction Any impediment to urine flow significantly increases the opportunity for infection. The obstruction can occur anywhere from the kidney to the urethra and may be associated with an inadequate lumen, intrinsic blockade, extrinsic compression, structural anomaly, disease of the wall, or functional inadequacy. Because it is such a common accompaniment, it has often been said that "infection is the calling card of obstruction." Cystitis and acute pyelonephritis, for example, occur 10 to 20 times more frequently in persons with obstructive lesions than in those without obstruction. Furthermore, the infection is likely to persist, to resist antimicrobial therapy, and to produce progressive renal damage until the obstruction is relieved or removed.

Instrumentation and Hospitalization Catheterization, cystoscopy and other forms of urethral instrumentation, especially the use of an indwelling catheter, are procedures associated with a high risk of inducing urinary tract infections. On an overall basis, instrumentation plays a much greater role in urinary infections in the male than in the female. In both men and women, however, instrumentation and infection increase with age and are clearly related to hospital admissions.

About one-third of infections in hospitalized patients involve the urinary tract. Approximately equal numbers are acquired before and during hospitalization. However, two-thirds of the hospital-acquired infections of the urinary tract are postcatheter, whereas only about 1 to 1.5 percent of the community-acquired infections are postcatheter. As pointed out earlier, the majority of the hospital-acquired infections are caused by microorganisms other than *E. coli.*

Other Observations Urinary tract infections are more prevalent in female diabetics than in paired control subjects (18.8 percent and 7.9 percent) and tend to be more severe in all diabetics, probably because of more frequent instrumentation and lower resistance. *Candida* is more likely to be encountered as the causative agent in diabetics than in nondiabetics but is usually confined to the bladder.

Neuropathies associated with autonomic disturbances of bladder function require catheterization and, consequently, are associated with a high risk of urinary infection.

Persons with the sickle-cell trait are more prone to urinary infection than are comparable persons lacking the trait, possibly because of obstruction associated with sickling and thrombus formation in the blood vessels of the renal medulla.

Complications

Renal Medullary Necrosis Renal medullary necrosis is a severe complication of pyelonephritis seen primarily in patients with diabetes and of urinary tract infection in patients who have habitually consumed large quantities of phenacetin for headache. In some cases, gram-negative bacteremia may supervene.

Gram-negative Bacteremia One of the changing patterns of infectious disease associated with the antibiotic era has been a marked shift in the relative importance of gram-negative organisms in bacteremia, half of all cases being caused by these bacteria. Preceding urinary tract infections are the source of two-thirds of the cases of gram-negative bacteremia. The balance follow surgical disease of the gastrointestinal tract, infected wounds in the skin and subcutaneous tissues, and postpartum or postabortal sepsis.

The clinical manifestations of shaking chills, rising fever, initial leukopenia followed by leukocytosis, and circulatory distress with lowered blood pressure closely resemble the recognized biological effects of gram-negative endotoxins (Chap. 5). When shock and circulatory collapse develop, the fatality rate may be as high as 75 percent.

The causative agents responsible for gram-negative bacteremia are those primarily involved in complicated cases of urinary tract infections.

Pathology Cystitis occurring in the presence of obstruction persists and frequently results in progressive renal damage until the complicating lesion is removed. In the absence of an accompanying pathological process, however, there is little local or systemic damage associated with the disease.

In acute pyelonephritis the lining of the renal pelvis and calyces is inflamed, and infection is usually confined to one or more wedge-shaped areas with apices in the medulla. Upon healing, a linear scar remains. In chronic pyelonephritis there are numerous scars scattered over the renal surfaces and patches of mononuclear infiltration. The scarring process is frequently accompanied by areas of acute pyelonephritis.

Renal medullary necrosis usually involves ischemic necrosis of the renal papilla and adjacent portions of the renal medulla together with lesions of acute and chronic pyelonephritis. The zone of necrosis may be so extensive that chunks of necrotic tissue are sloughed off and are found in the urine sediment.

Although gram-negative bacteremia is associated with endotoxin shock (Chap. 5), the exact mechanism by which shock is induced is not known. One of the intriguing possibilities is that endotoxin triggers the release of lysosomal enzymes, thus initiating the process that culminates in circulatory collapse.

Laboratory Diagnosis

Demonstration of Significant Bacteriuria

Collection of the Specimen In the evaluation of bacteriuria, collecting a proper specimen is of critical importance. The clean-voided, midstream procedure is preferred. This involves careful cleansing of the meatus in the male and collecting the middle portion of the excreted urine. In the female, the vulva is cleansed, the labia spread, and the middle portion of the excreted urine collected. Utilizing this method, surface contaminants are usually reduced to a concentration of 1,000 or less per milliliter of urine. The contaminants most commonly found include diphtheroids, *Staphylcoccus epidermidis,* and microaerophilic streptococci in the male and these bacteria plus Döderlein's bacillus *(Lactobacillus acidophilus)* and enterococci in the female. Because these few contaminants can grow to hundreds of thousands in a few hours at room temperature, the urine specimen must be refrigerated until examined. In the newborn, in infants, and in patients who cannot void spontaneously, suprapubic aspiration is a useful procedure.

Microscopic Examination Microscopic examination of unstained urinary sediment, employing the high dry objective under reduced light, is a rapid procedure which correlates about 80 to 90 percent with quantitative culture when gram-negative bacilli are the causative agents. Another useful method involves the examination of a Gram stain of unspun urine under an oil immersion lens.

Quantitative Determination Whether clinically apparent or not, 95 percent of the specimens obtained from urinary tract infections contain 100,000 or more organisms per milliliter of urine, and the majority (68 to 86 percent) contain 1,000,000 or more. Thus, a criterion of 100,000 or more bacteria per milliliter of urine is employed for the diagnosis of significant bacteriuria. However, in order to insure that no individuals are treated unnecessarily, three consecutive positive cultures should be obtained. This can be accomplished without difficulty since urinary tract infections are characteristically persistent, and spontaneous cure is rarely documented.

The serial dilution pour-plate method is the standard procedure for enumeration of bacteria, but it is too cumbersome for use in clinical laboratories. Consequently, it has been replaced by the calibrated loop surface streak method. In this procedure, streak plate cultures are prepared by direct inoculation of trypticase-soy agar with loops containing 0.01 and 0.001 ml of uncentrifuged urine. The use of calibrated loops provides a simple, reliable method for quantitative urine culture which gives results similar to those obtained by the standard serial dilution pour-plate method.

Isolation and Identification of Gram-negative Enteric Bacilli Since the bulk of urinary infections are caused by gram-negative enteric bacilli, concomitantly with the quantitative urine culture two or three drops of the uncentrifuged urine are streaked on an eosin-methylene blue (EMB) or similar (MacConkey or desoxycholate) agar plate. Such media are used to selectively inhibit the growth of gram-positive bacteria, to indicate whether or not lactose is utilized, on the basis of colonial morphology to distinguish *E. coli* which has a metallic sheen on EMB and the *Klebsiella-Enterobacter-Serratia* group which does not, and to prevent *Proteus* from swarming. Further identification of the bacteria isolated on EMB agar is based on the results of motility, IMVIC, ornithine decarboxylase, cephalothin resistance, sugar, urease, H_2S and gelatin tests, and the production of a soluble bright yellow or blue green fluorescent pigment *(Pseudomonas).*

Definitive identification is rarely performed except when required by the nature of research-oriented investigations. However, the serotype or phage type can be determined and utilized along with other genetic markers (i.e., antibiotic sensitivity pattern) for definitive identification of the causative agent.

Isolation and Identification of Gram-positive Bacteria Although little difficulty is encountered in the isolation of enterococci and staphylococci, which are the principal gram-positive bacteria found in urinary infections, the use of selective plating media does facilitate rapid resolution of specimens containing mixed flora. For this purpose, trypticase-soy agar containing 0.25 percent phenylethyl alcohol by volume is streaked with two or three drops of the specimen. In this medium, gram-positive bacteria grow, but gram-negative bacilli are selectively inhibited. Further identification of enterococci and staphylococci is based on procedures covered in Chapter 14.

Spheroplasts, Protoplasts, and L-forms One of the problems associated with chronic bacteriuria and chronic pyelonephritis in adults is the formation of spheroplasts, protoplasts, and L-forms (Chap. 1) in about 20 percent of patients. During therapy, especially with penicillin, tetracyclines, and chloramphenicol, the causative bacteria may be converted to spheroplasts, protoplasts, or L-forms which manage to survive under conditions of increased tonicity. After discontinuation of antimicrobial therapy, the spheroplasts, protoplasts, or L-forms may revert to the parent bacteria, grow extensively, and cause a relapse.

In efforts to recover spheroplasts, protoplasts, or L-forms, hypertonic early morning urines are cultured in an enriched hypertonic medium containing 10 percent horse serum and 10 percent sucrose. Identification of the species producing the spheroplasts, protoplasts, or L-forms is made by subculturing the colonies and identifying the reverting parent bacteria.

Epidemiology

The important epidemiologic features of urinary tract infections have been considered under pathogenesis (earlier in this chapter) and are graphically and diagrammatically illustrated in Figures 18-4 and 18-5. Briefly summarized, the epidemiologic dynamics of urinary tract infections are complex. Bacteriuria, which is a laboratory diagnosis and not necessarily a disease, is the most common denominator from which emerge cases of urethritis, cystitis, pyelonephritis, renal medullary necrosis, and gram-negative bacteremia. Factors which influence both the prevalence (the number of cases existing in a population at any one point in time) and the incidence (the number of cases arising in a

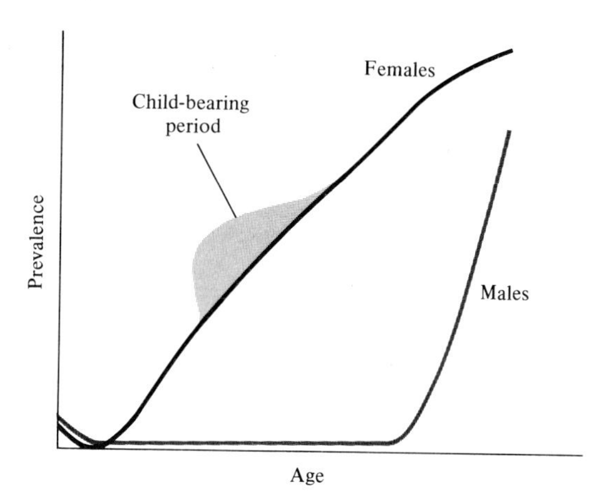

Figure 18-4 Prevalence of urinary tract infections according to age and sex.

population over a specified period of time) are numerous. They include age, sex, obstruction, instrumentation, and predisposing diseases such as diabetes, neuropathies, and sickle-cell trait.

The complexity of the epidemiologic patterns is partly accounted for by the fact that these factors are frequently intertwined. Congenital anomalies, which often obstruct the flow of urine, are more common in males than in females, their effects in terms of urinary tract infections are manifest early in life, and their correction commonly involves instrumentation. Spontaneous asymptomatic infections are common in young females, increase early in pregnancy, and develop into pyelonephritis as a troublesome complication later in pregnancy. Renal damage produced as a result of the pyelonephritis facilitates relapse and reinfection with increasing age. In males, on the other hand, spontaneous infection is uncommon. Urinary tract infections are rare until induced late in life when instrumentation is required for prostatism, bladder hypertrophy, and other reasons.

Prevention and Control

An Important, Complex, and Difficult Problem Prevention and control of urinary tract infections confront the physician with an important, complex, and difficult problem. The high prevalence, in otherwise healthy young girls and pregnant women, in persons in whom the flow of urine is impeded, and in the elderly, together with the tendency to produce progressive renal damage and even bacteremia, testify to the importance of urinary infections. The complexity and difficulty can be illustrated by the diverse number of endogenous microorganisms involved as causative agents and by the tendency of the infections to be asymptomatic, to subside after they become symptomatic, to persist, to recur, to resist therapy, and to develop in those who require urinary instrumentation.

Detection and Bacteriologic Monitoring Since pyelonephritis as a complication of pregnancy and as a common disease of older women undoubtedly has its genesis in the bacteriurias of childhood, the pediatrician is in a unique position to influence the course of urinary tract disease. By early detection, effective treatment, careful bacteriologic monitoring, and when necessary, prompt referral for skilled urological examination, the pediatrician can minimize the

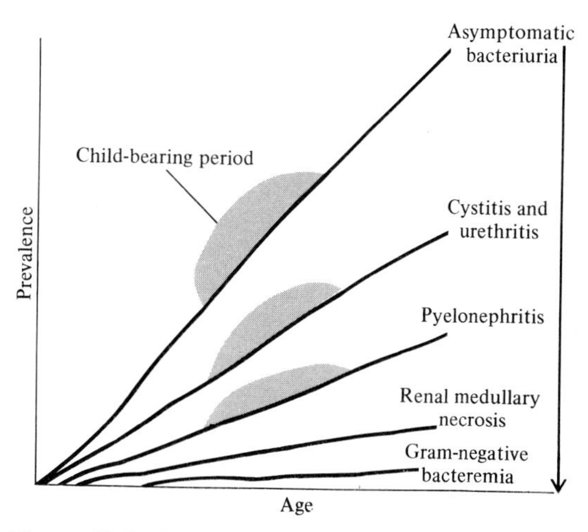

Figure 18-5 Prevalence of urinary tract infections and complications according to age.

extent of renal damage and the prospect of recurrent infection.

The cornerstone of early detection is the quantitative urine culture which will uncover asymptomatic as well as symptomatic bacteriurias. Because persistent asymptomatic infection commonly precedes cystitis and pyelonephritis and because it may be associated with renal damage, quantitative urine cultures may soon become routine health procedures in good pediatric, obstetric, urologic, geriatric, and hospital practice. Previously infected persons, pregnant women, urologic patients, and elderly individuals represent high-risk groups which should have careful bacteriologic monitoring. For example, the high incidence of cystitis and pyelonephritis in pregnant women can be reduced 10- to 40-fold by detection and treatment of asymptomatic bacteriuria which precedes clinical infection. Thus, it is evident that routine quantitative urine cultures are essential to effective obstetric care.

Treatment The diversity of chemotherapeutic agents employed in treatment is a direct reflection both of the great variability in sensitivity of the numerous causative agents and of the magnitude of difficulty encountered in eliminating the microorganism, especially in complicated urinary tract infections. The range of drugs extends from acidifying agents (ammonium chloride, methionine, hippuric acid), to urinary antiseptics (methanamine mandelate, nitrofurantoin, nalidixic acid), to the sulfonamides and includes almost every antibiotic that has become commercially available. The response to the drug of choice varies widely depending on whether infection occurs with or without obstruction, with or without instrumentation, whether acquired in the community or in the hospital, and on the extent of renal damage.

Spontaneous infections acquired in the community in the absence of obstruction or instrumentation respond favorably to antimicrobial therapy. About 80 percent of these infections are caused by *E. coli.* In the presence of obstruction, however, the infections are likely to persist, to resist therapy, and to produce progressive renal damage until the obstruction is removed. Infections induced following instrumentation usually develop in hospitalized patients, are caused by bacteria *(Klebsiella, Enterobacter, Serratia, Pseudomonas, Proteus)* that frequently resist therapy, and are complicated by the underlying disease. The greatest therapeutic problems, however, are presented by patients with chronic recurring urinary infections in whom ultimate control is rarely achieved.

Although a comprehensive consideration of antimicrobial therapy of asymptomatic and symptomatic bacteriuria is beyond the scope of the present discussion, certain general principles must be emphasized, however difficult their successful application may prove to be. The causative agents, even within the same species and serotype, vary widely in their response to chemotherapeutic drugs. Consequently, before initiating therapy, antibiotic sensitivity tests should always be performed, and the results should be used by the physician as a guide in the selection of appropriate antimicrobial therapy.

Since the goal of therapy is elimination rather than suppression of the infection, bactericidal drugs should be employed whenever possible. The response to the drug of choice given in therapeutic dosage should be evaluated by a series of quantitative urine cultures during and following therapy. If the infection is not eliminated, the causative agent should be reidentified, the pattern of antibiotic sensitivity reevaluated, and a search for and relief of an obstructing lesion undertaken promptly.

In patients with chronic recurring urinary infections, the hope for clinical and bacteriological cure is limited by the extent of renal damage, the presence of inoperable obstructions, the necessity for using external urinary drainage appliances, and the resistance to antibiotics of the causative agents commonly involved. Therapeutic failure rates as high as 80 to 90 percent have been reported. At the present time, this gloomy prospect seems to have been substantially improved by the use of gentamicin and kanamycin. Kanamycin is generally effective against *E. coli, Klebsiella, Enterobacter,* and *Proteus* but is ineffective against *Pseudomonas* and *Serratia.* Gentamicin is highly effective against *E. coli, Klebsiella, Enterobacter, Serratia, Pseudomonas, Proteus,* and staphylococci. Only enterococci are resistant. In one recent series of 58 patients with a history of recurring urinary infection, a clinical and bacteriological cure rate of 71 percent has been reported following the use of gentamicin. The failures were encountered in patients with renal calculi, external urinary drainage tubes, intractable vesical neck obstruction, congenital hydronephrosis and ileal loop, and in most cases involved *Pseudomonas* as the causative agent.

In view of the renal and ototoxicity of gentamicin and kanamycin and the probability that resistant mutants will increase with widespread use of these drugs, a healthy skepticism is warranted concerning continuation of the remarkably effective therapeutic responses currently obtainable. For these reasons, and because other drugs produce satisfactory results in the majority of uncomplicated cases, it may be desirable to reserve gentamicin and kanamycin for the treatment of complicated infections that have failed to respond or are unlikely to respond to other antibiotics. Clearly, however, gentamicin is currently the drug of choice in the therapy of most recurrent urinary infections and in most gram-negative bacteremias that occur as complications of these infections.

Instrumentation The high risk of infection associated with urinary instrumentation is most strikingly documented in hospitalized patients and must be avoided whenever possible. For example, a catheter should never be used to collect urine when a clean-voided, midstream specimen is equally satisfactory. When catheterization is required, the administration of a neomycin-polymyxin rinse through a three-way catheter may reduce the incidence of urinary tract infections.

Urinary instrumentation requires careful bacteriological monitoring, since early detection and continued surveillance of infection offer the best chance that subsequent antimicrobial therapy will be effective. Even when the infection cannot be eliminated, it is usually possible to suppress at least temporarily the multiplication of the causative agent and thereby prevent renal damage. In many urological disorders, however, significant bacteriuria frequently recurs and requires appropriate adjustments in the chemotherapeutic regimen.

PROSPECTIVE

The prospect for drastically reducing the incidence and mortality of enteric bacterial, protozoal, and helminthic infections is excellent if the standards of sanitary hygiene in effect in the developed nations could be applied to the rest of the world. Poverty, crowding, and malnutrition are additional problems that must be corrected if adequate progress is to be achieved. Thus, in many respects these illnesses are socioeconomic diseases which can be prevented.

On the other hand, the vastness and pervasiveness of the animal reservoir in salmonellosis present difficulties of much greater magnitude, and there is no solution in sight. Fortunately, however, salmonellosis is generally a relatively mild disease.

With respect to urinary tract infections, the physician is confronted with a more serious, challenging, complex, and difficult problem. In the light of the natural history of the disease, the best prospect for prevention and control is early detection and effective therapy of asymptomatic bacteriuria. To accomplish this goal requires that quantitative urine cultures be utilized as routine health procedures in good pediatric, obstetric, urologic, geriatric, and hospital practice.

BIBLIOGRAPHY

"Amoebiasis. Report of a WHO Expert Committee," *W.H.O. Tech. Rep. Ser.,* no. 421, 1969.

Barrett-Connor, E.: "Travelers' Diarrhea," *Calif. Med.,* 118(1):1-4, 1973.

Berke, R., Wagshol, L. E., and Sullivan, G.: "Incidence of Intestinal Parasites in Vietnam Veterans. Eosinophilia A Guide to Diagnosis," *Am. J. Gastroenterol.,* 57:63-67, 1972.

Biagi, F.: "Unusual Isolates from Clinical Material—*Balantidium coli,*" *Ann. N.Y. Acad. Sci.,* 174:1023-1026, 1970.

Carpenter, C. C. J.: "Cholera and Other Enterotoxin-related Diarrheal Diseases," *J. Infect. Dis.,* 126:551-564, 1972.

Curlin, G. T., Mosley, W. H., and Greenough, W. B., III: "Cholera Antitoxin Titrations: A Comparative Study of Fat-cell, Ileal-loop, and Rabbit-skin Assays," *J. Infect. Dis.,* 127:294-298, 1973.

Formal, S. B., Hornick, R., and DuPont, H.: "Enterotoxic Diarrheal Syndromes," *Annu. Rev. Med.,* 24:103-110, 1973.

Gangarosa, E. J., Bennett, J. V., Wyatt, C., Pierce, P. E., Olarte, J., Hernandes, P. M., Vazquez, V., and Bessudo, D. M.: "An Epidemic-associated Episome?" *J. Infect. Dis.,* 126:212-214, 1972.

Geddes, A. M.: "Enteric Fever, Salmonellosis, and Food Poisoning," *Br. Med. Jr.,* 1:98-100, 1973.

Giannella, R. A., Formal, S. B., Dammin, G. J., and Collins, H.: "Pathogenesis of Salmonellosis. Studies of Fluid Secretion, Mucosal Invasion, and Morphologic Reaction in the Rabbit Ileum," *J. Clin. Invest.,* 52:441-453, 1973.

Hendrickse, R. G.: "Dysentery Including Amebiasis," *Br. Med. J.,* 1:669-672, 1973.

Hsieh, H. C., Stoll, N. R., Reber, E. W., Chen, E. R., Kang, B. T., and Kuo, M.: "Distribution of *Necator americanus* and *Ancylostoma duodenale* in Liberia," *Bull. W.H.O.,* 47:317-324, 1972.

Ironside, A. G.: "Gastroenteritis of Infancy," *Br. Med. J.,* 1:284-286, 1973.

Johns, M. A., Whiteside, R. E., Baker, E. E., and McCabe, W. R.: "Common Enterobacterial Antigen. I. Isolation and Purification from *Salmonella typhosa* 9:901," *J. Immunol.,* 110:781-790, 1973.

Juranek, D. D., and Schultz, M. G.: "Trichinosis in the United States, 1971," *J. Infect. Dis.,* 126:687-689, 1972.

Kelly, J. D.: "Mechanisms of Immunity to Intestinal Helminths," *Aust. Vet. J.,* 49:91-97, 1973.

Klock, L. E., Spruance, S. L., Andersen, F. L., Juranek, D. D., and Kagan, I. G.: "Detection of Asymptomatic Hydatid Disease in a Community Screening Program," *Am. J. Epidemiol.,* 97:16-21, 1973.

Kunin, C. M.: *Detection, Prevention and Management of Urinary Tract Infections,* Philadelphia: Lea & Febiger, 1972.

Leiby, P. D., and Kritsky, D. C.: "*Echinococcus multilocularis:* A Possible Domestic Life Cycle in Central North America and Its Public Health Implications," *J. Parasitol.,* 58:1213-1215, 1972.

Levine, M. M., DuPont, H. L., Formal, S. B., Hornick, R. B., Takeuchi, A., Gangarosa, E. J., Snyder, M. J., and Libonati, J. P.: "Pathogenesis of *Shigella dysenteriae* 1 (Shiga) Dysentery," *J. Infect. Dis.,* 127:261-270, 1973.

Mallory, A., Kern, F., Jr., Smith, J., and Savage, D.: "Patterns of Bile Acids and Microflora in the Human Small Intestine. I. Bile Acids," *Gastroenterology,* 64:26-33, 1973.

———, Savage, D., Kern, F., Jr., and Smith, J. G.: "Patterns of Bile Acids and Microflora in the Human Small Intestine. II. Microflora," *Gastroenterology,* 64:34-42, 1973.

Martin, L. K.: "Hookworm in Georgia. I. Survey of Intestinal Helminth Infections and Anemia in Rural School Children," *Am. J. Trop. Med. Hyg.,* 21:919-929, 1972.

Mathan, V. I., and Baker, S. J.: "Whipworm Disease. Intestinal Structure and Function of Patients with Severe *Trichuris trichiura* Infestation," *Am. J. Dig. Dis.,* 15:913-918, 1970.

Mayers, C. P., and Purvis, R. J.: "Manifestations of Pinworms," *Can. Med. Assoc. J.,* 103:489-493, 1970.

McCabe, W. R., Johns, M., and Digenio, T.: "Common Enterobacterial Antigen. III. Initial Titers and Antibody Response in Bacteremia Caused by

Gram-negative Bacilli," *Infect. Immun.,* 7:393–415, 1973.

"Oral Enteric Bacterial Vaccines. Report of a WHO Scientific Group," *W.H.O. Tech. Rep. Ser.,* no. 500, 1972.

Pawlowski, Z., and Schultz, M. G.: "Taeniasis and Cysticerosis *(Taenia saginata),*" *Adv. Parasitol.,* 10:269–343, 1972.

Powell, S. J.: "Latest Developments in the Treatment of Amebiasis," *Adv. Pharmacol. Chemother.,* 10:91–103, 1972.

Savage, D. C. L., Wilson, M. I., McHardy, M., Dewar, D. A. E., and Fee, W. M.: "Covert Bacteriuria in Childhood. A Clinical and Epidemiological Study," *Arch. Dis. Child.,* 48:8–20, 1973.

Stark, R. L., and Duncan, C. L.: "Purification and Biochemical Properties of *Clostridium perfringens* Type A Enterotoxin," *Infect. Immun.,* 6:662–688, 1972.

Tripathy, K., Duque, E., and Bolanos, O.: "Malabsorption Syndrome in Ascariasis," *Am. J. Clin. Nutr.,* 25:1276–1281, 1972.

Walzer, P. D., Wolfe, M. S., and Schultz, M. G.: "Giardiasis in Travelers," *J. Infect. Dis.,* 124:235–237, 1971.

Zen-Yoji, H., LeClair, R. A., Ohta, K., and Montague, T. S.: "Comparison of *Vibrio parahaemolyticus* Cultures Isolated in the United States with Those Isolated in Japan," *J. Infect. Dis.,* 127:237–241, 1973.

Chapter 19

Infections of the Ear and the Eye

Bernard A. Briody

INFECTIONS OF THE EAR

From the viewpoint of pathogenesis, the ear should be considered as an integral part of the upper respiratory tract when associated with middle ear infections (otitis media) and as a part of the skin in infections of the external auditory canal (otitis externa).

Otitis media is usually an acute condition with earache and an inflamed eardrum or with a sudden onset of discharge from the ear, either following earache or occurring without a previous history of chronic ear disease. In the majority of cases otitis media is preceded within 2 weeks by upper respiratory tract infection and may occasionally be followed by serious complications (mastoiditis, deafness, intracranial infections).

Otitis externa is an acute or chronic infection limited to the external auditory canal and is rarely, if ever, associated with serious complications.

Acute Otitis Media

The Causative Agent The principal bacterial pathogens in acute otitis media are groups A, C, and G streptococci, coagulase-positive staphylococci, *Hemophilus influenzae,* and pneumococci. Mixed cultures may be present in about one-third of the cases. *Pseudomonas, Proteus,* and *Escherichia* may be found in about 10 percent of the cases (Table 19-1), frequently after the use of antibiotics. The biological and other properties of the causative agents are discussed in other chapters (14, 18, and 24).

Pathogenesis The seasonal pattern in the incidence of acute otitis media is almost identical with the incidence of upper respiratory infection. The majority of cases, especially in children (Fig. 19-1), develop within 2 weeks following viral (parainfluenza, measles, influenza, mumps) and bacterial (group A streptococci, *Mycoplasma pneumoniae*) infection of the upper respiratory tract. It is estimated that otitis media will develop in about 3 percent of untreated cases of streptococcal pharyngitis.

Anatomical considerations, preceding respiratory infection, and the fact that the principal causative agents are prominent members of the normal flora of the nasopharynx (pneumococci, coagulase-positive staphylococci, and *H. influenzae*) or are occasionally carried in the nasopharynx (groups A, C, and G streptococci), all suggest that the bacteria reach the middle ear through the eustachian tube.

In acute infections there is hyperemia, edema, and thickening of the cuboidal epithelial mucosa lining the cavity of the middle ear, neutrophils migrate through the mucosa, and the cavity is filled with a purulent fluid. With closure of the lumen of the eustachian tube, the exudate accumulates under pressure and may be discharged through the tympanic membrane (30 percent of cases) with visual perforation of the eardrum occurring in about 12 percent of cases. In about 80 percent of the patients the infection is unilateral.

Following effective destruction of the bacteria by phagocytosis, spontaneous or operative perforation of the tympanic membrane, or chemotherapy, the pressure is relieved, and there is resolution of the inflammatory process.

Complications Prior to the antibiotic era, mastoidectomy was required in about 10 percent of the cases of otitis media and myringotomy in 30 percent. Intracranial complications (meningitis, brain abscess) developed in about 2.2 percent of cases. About 15 percent of all cases of meningitis were preceded by otitis media.

The use of antibiotics has reduced the incidence of acute mastoiditis to 0.4 percent, and mastoidectomy, myringotomy, and intracranial complications occur in less than 0.1 percent. On the other hand, short and ineffective treatment with antibiotics may be responsible for the apparent increase in acute otitis media due to *Pseudomonas, Proteus,* and *Escherichia* and may be associated with the documented increase in cases of nonsuppurative serous otitis media which has become increasingly evident in the last 10 years.

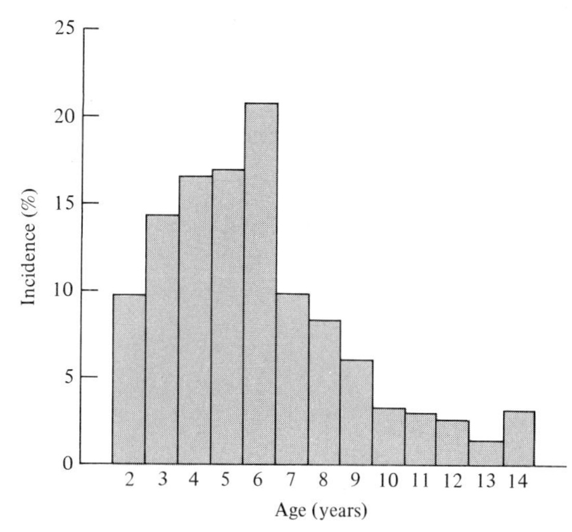

Figure 19-1 Incidence of attacks of otitis media in 10,732 children under 15 years of age in 1955. *(From "Acute Otitis Media in General Practice: Report of a Survey by the Medical Research Council's Working-Party for Research in General Practice," Lancet, 2:510–514, 1957.)*

Deafness The true incidence of persistent loss of hearing following otitis media is not known. In a recent study, in which oral penicillin was routinely utilized in treatment of acute otitis media in children under 11 years of age, 20 percent had deafness of 20 decibels or more when tested 6 months later, and 6.6 percent had not improved when tested 4 years later. Recurrence of otitis media was the only factor that increased the chances of permanent damage to the middle ear and occurred in 75 percent of the patients who subsequently developed impaired hearing.

Table 19-1 The Principal Causative Agents in Acute Otitis Media Compared with the Normal Flora of the Nasopharynx and the Ear Canal

Causative agent	Incidence (percent)	Resistant to penicillin (percent)	Predominant age group	Normal flora—nasopharynx	Normal flora—ear canal
Groups A, C, and G streptococci	34	None	5 to 9 years	Occasionally carried	Not present
Coagulase-positive staphylococci	30	60	Often in older age groups	Prominent feature	Present in 20 percent
Hemophilus influenzae	16	56	Under 5 years	Often present	Not present
Pneumococci	13	None	All age groups	Prominent feature	Not present
Mixed cultures	32	Most	All age groups	Often present	Coagulase-positive staphylococci
Others (*Pseudomonas, Proteus, Escherichia*)	10	All	All age groups	Often present	Occasionally present

Source: Adapted from F. H. Linthicum, *Arch. Otolaryngol.*, 80:489–493, 1964 (Copyright 1964, American Medical Association); J. V. Dadswell, *Lancet*, 1:243–245, 1967; and J. R. Leonard, *Laryngoscope*, 77:663–680, 1967.

Laboratory Diagnosis Laboratory diagnosis of acute otitis media depends upon the recovery of the causative agent from the discharge or from aspirated exudate and its subsequent identification on the basis of its biological, biochemical, and serological properties. Practically all the causative agents will grow on chocolate blood agar plates in the presence of 5 to 10 percent carbon dioxide.

Epidemiology Preceding viral or bacterial infection of the upper respiratory tract paves the way for the more pathogenic members of the normal flora of the nasopharynx to reach the middle ear by way of the eustachian tube. Consequently, the prevalence, age distribution, and seasonal incidence parallel those observed in infections of the upper respiratory tract (Table 19-1 and Figs. 19-1 and 19-2). As indicated in Figure 19-1, the peak incidence of acute otitis media occurs between 3 and 6 years of age. Approximately 68 percent of cases are seen in those under 10 years of age, especially those caused by *H. influenzae* and groups A, C, and G streptococci (Table 19-1).

Prevention and Control Basically, prevention and control of acute otitis media are dependent upon (1) prevention or control of the preceding viral or bacterial infection and (2) appropriate therapy of acute otitis media when it develops. Definite progress in preventing acute otitis media has been achieved by prompt and vigorous penicillin therapy of streptococcal pharyngitis, and progress is being made in the prevention of measles and mumps.

The use of penicillin cannot be considered to represent acceptable treatment of acute otitis media when approximately 40 percent of the causative agents are unlikely to respond to the drug (Table 19-1). Ideally, the causative agent should be isolated and an appropriate drug (or drugs in the case of certain mixed infections) selected on the basis of antibiotic sensitivity tests. Since general practitioners or pediatricians are called upon to treat most patients with acute otitis media, future progress in effective treatment depends largely upon their willingness to take cultures prior to the use of antibiotics and to switch to the antibiotic indicated when cultural and sensitivity data warrant. In addition, the appropriate antibiotic must be used in therapeutic concentration for an adequate period.

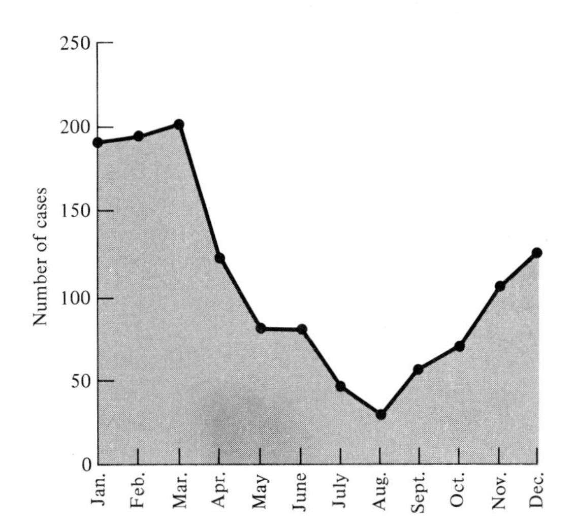

Figure 19-2 Seasonal incidence of attacks of otitis media in 10,732 children under 15 years of age in 1955. (*From "Acute Otitis Media in General Practice: Report of a Survey by the Medical Research Council's Working-Party for Research in General Practice," Lancet, 2:510–514, 1957.*)

Otitis Externa

Acute infections of the external auditory canal are caused primarily by coagulase-positive and coagulase-negative staphylococci in roughly equivalent proportions. Chronic infections are more commonly associated with *Pseudomonas* (especially in tropical countries), fungi (*Aspergillus, Allescheria,* and others), *Proteus,* and a variety of other bacteria. The causative agents and their prevalence largely reflect the prevalence of the microorganism in the normal flora of the external auditory canal. Most infections respond to irrigation and appropriate antibiotics.

Bullous Myringitis

Bullous myringitis is an inflammation of the tympanic membrane characterized by vesicular lesions and frequently associated with mycoplasma infection (Chap. 20). For unknown reasons, bullous myringitis occurs more commonly in experimental human infections with mycoplasma than in natural infections. Mycoplasma, however, have been recovered from the vesicular fluid in naturally infected children. Human infection with mycoplasma primarily involves the upper and lower respiratory tracts, but much remains to be learned concerning the pathogenesis of mycoplasma myringitis.

Other Diseases

A number of systemic infections or infections of nervous tissue may be associated with temporary or permanent deafness including prenatal syphilis (Chap. 21), in utero infection with rubella virus (Chap. 22), meningococcal meningitis (Chap. 24), herpes zoster (Chap. 22), and mumps (Chap. 25). Deafness always means disease of the cochlea or the auditory nerve and its central connections.

INFECTIONS OF THE EYE

The list of microorganisms and parasites that are associated with infections of the eye is impressive (Table 19-2). It includes bacteria, fungi, chlamydiae, viruses, and parasites as significant etiological agents. Destructive infections may be induced by aerobic members of the normal flora (pneumococci, staphylococci, *Pseudomonas, Proteus, Klebsiella, Bacillus subtilis, Candida, Mucor,* and many others), by pathogenic organisms that primarily or frequently attack the eye (trachoma, *Onchocerca*), as a consequence of in utero infection (syphilis, rubella, *Toxoplasma*) or passage through the birth canal (neonatal conjunctivitis due to gonococci, pneumococci, staphylococci), or infection with pathogenic organisms that characteristically produce disease elsewhere in the body (smallpox, vaccinia, leprosy, *Schistosoma,* tubercule bacilli, herpes simplex, varicella-zoster, meningococci, diphtheria bacilli).

Historically, and unfortunately, currently as well, eye infections are a major cause of blindness in many parts of the world. The principal diseases are neonatal gonococcal conjunctivitis, smallpox, prenatal syphilis, trachoma, and in utero infection with rubella virus and *Toxoplasma.* In addition, the inventory would include leprosy, schistosomiasis, onchocerciasis, viral keratoconjunctivitis, and bacterial keratoconjunctivitis.

In the United States there has been a progressive reduction in the proportion of blindness resulting from infection. Of the estimated total cases of blindness recognized in 1940, 1950, 1957, and 1962 the percentage caused by infection was 21, 14, 10, and 5, respectively (Fig. 19-3). In 1962 infections were responsible for 2.2 percent of new cases of blindness, with syphilis accounting for 1.1 percent and trachoma and neonatal gonococcal conjunctivitis for less than 0.1 percent. The successful development and use of rubella vaccine should substantially reduce blindness consequent to in utero infection with rubella virus. Thus, currently the bulk of new cases of blindness in the United States due to infectious disease are probably caused by prenatal syphilis and infections following corneal injury.

In this chapter emphasis will be focused chiefly on bacterial keratoconjunctivitis and trachoma-inclusion conjunctivitis (TRIC) chlamydiae, with brief reference to ophthalmia neonatorum, the specific eye manifestations of in utero infection with rubella virus, epidemic keratoconjunctivitis (adenovirus type 8), onchocerciasis, fungal keratoconjunctivitis and rhino-orbitalcerebral mucormycosis. Further details of other causative agents will be found in Chapter 14 (staphylococci, viridans streptococci, pneumococci), Chapter 15 (leprosy bacilli and tubercle bacilli), Chapter 16 (fungi), Chapter 18 (gram-negative enteric bacteria), Chapter 20 (adenovirus), Chapter 21 (gonococci and syphilitic spirochetes), Chapter 22 (smallpox, vaccinia, rubella, herpes simplex, varicella-zoster), Chapter 23 *(Histoplasma),* Chapter 24 (influenza bacilli and meningococci), and Chapter 25 *(Toxoplasma).*

Bacterial Keratoconjunctivitis

The Causative Agents Since the biological properties of the other causative agents are discussed elsewhere, only *Hemophilus aegyptius* (Koch-Weeks bacillus) and *Moraxella lacunata* (Morax-Axenfeld diplobacilli or *Mima*) will be considered here. *H. aegyptius*, like *H. influenzae* (Chap. 24), is a gram-negative coccobacillus which requires X and V factors for growth, is nonhemolytic, exhibits the "satellite phenomenon" with *Staphylococcus aureus* (Chap. 24), and causes acute conjunctivitis. Unlike pathogenic cultures of *H. influenzae, H. aegyptius* is not encapsulated but does agglutinate human red blood cells. It is generally considered a part of the normal flora of the conjunctiva.

Moraxella lacunata is a gram-negative diplobacillus which does not require X and V factors, grows well on Loeffler's medium, producing colonies that are convex, smooth, glistening and semitransparent. The properties of *Moraxella* are those generally associated with *Herellea* or *Mima* (Chap. 18). The organism is part of the normal conjunctival flora and usually causes a chronic blepharoconjunctivitis and purulent keratitis but may also be responsible for acute conjunctivitis. The chronic form persists for an average of 2 years without corneal change and is often found in children's institutions.

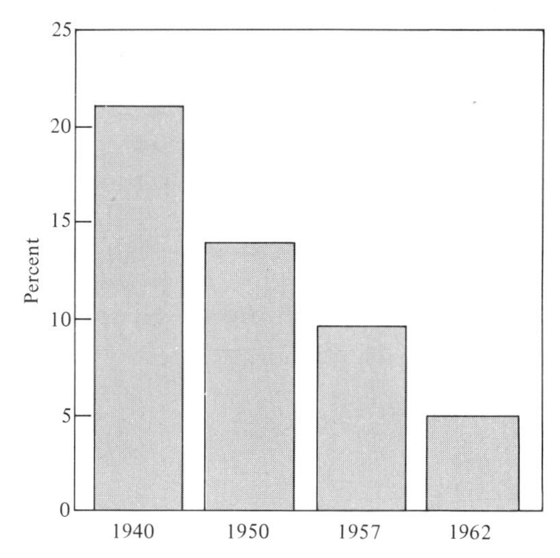

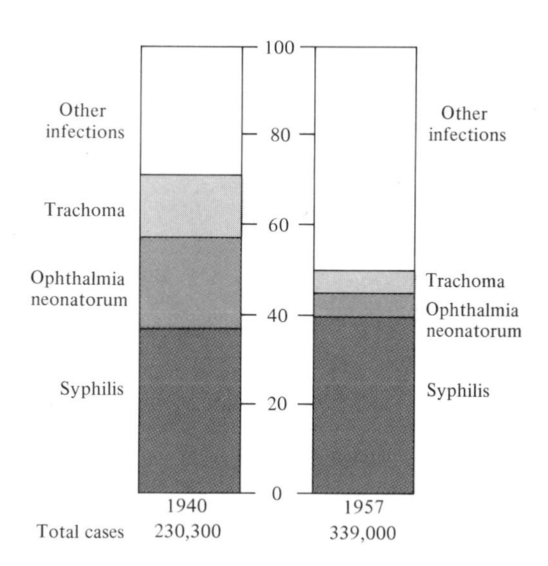

Figure 19-3 Infectious disease as a cause of blindness in the United States, 1940–1962. *(A)* Overall percentage of blindness due to infectious disease in 1940, 1950, 1957, and 1962. *(B)* Major infectious causes of blindness in 1940 and 1957. (*From the NSPB Fact Book: Estimated Statistics on Blindness and Vision Problems, National Society for the Prevention of Blindness, Inc., New York, 1966; and from M. Lerner and O. W. Anderson, Health Progress in the United States, 1900–1960, Chicago: University of Chicago Press, 1963, p. 209.*)

Table 19-2 Eye Infections: Important Characteristics and Causative Agents

Infection	Frequency	Important characteristics	Causative agents
Eyelids			
Hordeolum (sty)	Common	An abscess in the lid glands	Staphylococci
Blepharitis	Common	Chronic bilateral inflammation of the lid margins occasionally complicated by conjunctivitis, superficial keratitis, and chronic hordeolum	Staphylococci
Lacrimal apparatus			
Acute dacryocystitis	Common	An infection of the lacrimal sac almost always secondary to obstruction of the lacrimal duct	Staphylococci, pneumococci
Chronic dacryocystitis	Common	Associated with delayed canalization in infants and with menopausal women, in whom the disease persists until the obstruction is surgically removed	Pneumococci, *Hemophilus influenzae, Candida*
Dacryoadenitis	Uncommon	Inflammation of the lacrimal gland	Mumps virus
Conjunctiva			
Acute purulent bacterial conjunctivitis	Commonest	Bilateral infection of the thin transparent mucous membrane which lines the anterior surface of the eyeball up to the limbus and the posterior surface of the lids. Produces a copious discharge and usually heals spontaneously in 7 to 14 days. Corneal ulceration may complicate gonococcal infection, and viridans streptococcal infection may become chronic.	Pneumococci, staphylococci, meningococci, gonococci, *Hemophilus aegyptius, H. influenzae,* viridans streptococcus, *Proteus, E. coli, Moraxella* (*Mima* ?)
Chronic nonpurulent bacterial conjunctivitis	Occasional	Bilateral infection with scanty discharge and the frequent presence of localized conjunctival lesions. Diphtheritic conjunctivitis often results in conjunctival scarring. Infection with leprosy bacilli is an important cause of blindness in many parts of the world.	Staphylococci, *Moraxella* (*Mima* ?), *N. catarrhalis, Proteus, Corynebacterium diphtheriae, Leptothrix, Actinomyces,* tubercle bacilli, *Francisella tularensis,* leprosy bacilli

Table 19-2 Eye Infections: Important Characteristics and Causative Agents (CONTINUED)

Infection	Frequency	Important characteristics	Causative agents
TRIC chlamydiae conjunctivitis	Extremely common (worldwide)	Bilateral conjunctivitis due to TRIC agents is an important cause of conjunctival and corneal scarring and blindness. Corticosteroids enhance infection. Other chlamydiae (lymphogranuloma venerum, psittacosis) rarely cause conjunctivitis.	Trachoma and inclusion conjunctivitis (TRIC), chlamydiae
Viral conjunctivitis	Common	Unilateral or bilateral conjunctivitis caused by the adeno-, herpes-, pox-, myxo-, and papova- groups of viruses; may be self-limited (adenovirus, Newcastle disease virus), recurrent (herpes simplex and molluscum contagiosum viruses), or severe (smallpox, vaccinia, herpes, varicella-zoster viruses). Often aggravated by corticosteroids.	Adenoviruses (16 of 30 types; types 3, 7, and 8 most common, herpes simplex, varicella-zoster, cytomegalovirus, smallpox, vaccinia, molluscum contagiosum, Newcastle disease, measles, papilloma
Fungal conjunctivitis	Uncommon	May be acute or chronic, often secondary to fungous infections of the skin or mucous membranes. Often aggravated by corticosteroids and initiated after antibiotic therapy.	*Candida, Sporotrichum, Allescheria, Aspergillus, Mucor, Phialophora, Blastomyces*
Parasitic conjunctivitis	Common in Africa and Central America	Infestation with *Onchocerca* is a major cause of blindness; filaria (*Loa loa*) may invade the anterior chamber and vitreous; *Wuchereria* may produce extreme edema resembling elephantiasis in other parts of the body; *Trichinella* may produce muscular pain and edema in extraocular muscles; *Schistosoma haemotobium* may cause a granuloma which requires excision. *Thelazia callipaeda* may cause blindness.	*Onchocera, Loa loa, Wuchereria, Trichinella, Schistosoma haematobium, Cysticercus (T. solium), Echinococcus,* animal parasites (*Thelazia californiensis* and *T. callipaeda*)

Table 19-2 Eye Infections: Important Characteristics and Causative Agents (CONTINUED)

Infection	Frequency	Important characteristics	Causative agents
Cornea			
Keratitis (corneal ulcer)	Common	Frequently develops following injury to cornea. Scarring and perforation is a major cause of blindness. When available, appropriate chemotherapy must be employed within hours after onset if blindness is to be avoided. In some parts of the world smallpox is a major cause of blindness.	Pneumococci, group A streptococcus, *Pseudomonas, Moraxella* (*Mima* ?), syphilitic spirochetes, *Klebsiella,* herpes simplex, smallpox, varicella-zoster, vaccinia, *Candida, Aspergillus, Nocardia, Cephalosporium, Mucor*
Cornea and conjunctiva			
Keratoconjunctivitis	Common	Simultaneous infection of the cornea and the conjunctiva may be caused by many of the agents that infect either one.	Gonococci, *Corynebacterium diphtheriae,* TRIC agents, adenovirus (especially type 8), herpes simplex, smallpox, vaccinia, varicella-zoster, *Candida* and other fungi, *Onchocerca, Wuchereria, Thelazia callipaeda*
Uvea and other tissues			
Uveitis, endophthalmitis	Variable	Inflammation of the vascular coat of the eye involving the iris, ciliary body, and choroid (uveitis) is frequently serious, often the result of in utero infection (syphilis, rubella, *Toxoplasma*), occasionally involves the retina (syphilis, rubella, *Toxoplasma, Histoplasma*) and the lens (rubella). Penicillin and streptomycin chemoprophylaxis preceding cataract surgery decreases the incidence of endophthalmitis but does not eliminate the disease, which is usually found to be due to antibiotic-resistant *Pseudomonas, Proteus,* and staphylococci.	Tubercle bacilli, syphilis, *Brucella,* TRIC agents, rubella virus, infectious mononucleosis?, *Histoplasma, Toxoplasma; Pseudomonas, Proteus,* staphylococci in postoperative endophthalmitis; *Bacillus subtilis* occasionally after severe injury

Pathogenesis

Acute Bacterial Keratoconjunctivitis Acute bacterial keratoconjunctivitis is frequently associated with microorganisms that normally form part of the flora of the conjunctiva (Tables 19-2 and 19-3), the urethra, oral cavity, skin, enteric cavity, and the nasopharynx. It is often preceded by viral infection of the upper respiratory tract, by allergic rhinitis, in the more serious cases, by traumatic injury or ophthalmic surgery (Table 19-2), and by the use of contaminated fluorescent solutions to facilitate ophthalmic diagnosis *(Pseudomonas)*.

Considering the extent and intensity of conjunctival exposure to microorganisms, the variety and persistence of irritating stimuli and the fact that it provides a growth medium that will satisfy the most fastidious bacteria, it is surprising that conjunctivitis with subsequent corneal involvement is not more common. When the lids are closed, the temperature of the conjunctival sac is elevated, and bacterial growth is enhanced. When the lids are open, the absence of a cul-de-sac and the copious production of tears together with the phagocytic activity of leukocytes tend to limit bacterial growth. The lytic effect of lysozyme in tears has often been cited as an important antibacterial phenomenon, but its restricted range of activity on the microorganisms in the normal conjunctival flora suggests that its defensive role has been overemphasized.

Chronic Bacterial Conjunctivitis Chronic bacterial conjunctivitis is much less common than the acute form. It may be associated with members of the normal conjunctival flora or with pathogenic bacteria such as syphilitic spirochetes, leprosy bacilli, tubercle bacilli, diphtheria bacilli, and *Franciscella tularensis* (Table 19-2). When caused by indigenous bacteria, the disease is often associated with improper hygiene, intensive irritation, and eyestrain. When caused by pathogenic bacteria, conjunctival and corneal scarring and blindness may develop (Table 19-2).

Laboratory Diagnosis In most cases, a Gram-stained smear will indicate immediately

Table 19-3 Bacterial and Mycotic Flora of the Conjunctiva*

Bacteria	Present	Fungi	Present
Coagulase-negative staphylococci	Commonly	*Aspergillus*	Commonly
Coagulase-positive staphylococci	Commonly	*Penicillium*	Commonly
Diphtheroids	Commonly	*Candida*	Commonly
Viridans streptococci	Commonly	*Curvalaria*	Commonly
Pseudomonas	Commonly	*Hormodendrum*	Commonly
Klebsiella	Occasionally	*Nocardia*	Commonly
Pneumococcus	Occasionally	*Alternaria*	Commonly
H. influenzae	Occasionally	*Mucor*	Occasionally
Saprophytic *Neisseria*	Occasionally	*Monosporium*	Occasionally
Bacillus subtilis	Occasionally	*Streptomyces*	Occasionally
Bacterium anatratum	Infrequently	*Rodotorula*	Occasionally
Mima (*Moraxella* ?)	Infrequently	*Schizomycetes*	Occasionally
Herellea	Infrequently	*Geotrichum*	Occasionally
Moraxella (*Mima* ?)	Infrequently		

* Listed in the order of relative frequency. Bacteria are recovered in 80 to 100 percent of individuals, fungi from 10 to 24 percent.

Source: Based on data contained in publications by J. C. Hammeke and P. P. Ellis, *Am. J. Ophthalmol.*, 49:1174–1178, 1960; R. Ainley and B. Smith, *Br. J. Ophthalmol.*, 49:505–515, 1965; H. V. Nema, O. P. Ahuja, O. Bal, and L. N. Mohapatra, *Am. J. Ophthalmol.*, 62:968–970, 1966; "Conference on Trachoma and Allied Diseases," *Am. J. Ophthalmol.*, 63:1027–1657, 1967; and S. Sowa, J. Sowa, L. H. Collier, and W. Blyth, "Medical Research Council Special Report 308: Trachoma and Allied Infections in a Gambian Village," Her Majesty's Stationery Office, London, 1965.

whether the causative agent is bacterial, fungal, parasitic, or allergic. The absence of bacteria and fungi and the presence of monocytes suggest a chlamydial or viral etiology.

In the case of corneal injury, stained smears are essential and should be examined while the patient waits (Table 19-2). The smear often provides a presumptive diagnosis which can be used as a guide to antibiotic therapy, but cultures and sensitivity tests must also be performed.

Identification of the causative bacteria depends upon cultural, biochemical, and serological properties. With few exceptions (leprosy bacilli, syphilitic spirochetes, tubercle bacilli, *F. tularensis*), the causative bacteria will grow on chocolate blood agar (Chap. 24) in 5 to 10 percent carbon dioxide.

Epidemiology Keratoconjunctivitis due to indigenous bacteria occurs in all ages at all times of the year, but most commonly in the spring and autumn, perhaps as a result of the precipitating role of allergic rhinitis. The disease is prevalent but characteristically endemic, although the purulent discharge in acute infections may be responsible for multiple household cases.

Keratoconjunctivitis due to pathogenic bacteria follows the pattern observed in the underlying disease (leprosy, diphtheria, tularemia) or is associated with in utero infection (syphilis) or infection during parturition (gonococcal conjunctivitis). When caused by indigenous bacteria, the disease is usually secondary to improper hygiene, irritation, or strain of the eyes.

Prevention and Control In keratoconjunctivitis due to indigenous bacteria, proper hygiene, the avoidance of unnecessary eyestrain and irritation, the use of safety procedures designed to reduce injury (safety eyeglasses in industry), chemoprophylaxis in cataract or other major eye surgery, and prompt and appropriate antibiotic therapy form the basic elements of prevention and control. Chemoprophylaxis with penicillin and streptomycin reduces the incidence of postoperative endophthalmitis approximately 85 percent to a frequency of 1 per 740 operations. When it occurs in those treated prophylactically, postoperative infection is usually associated with antibiotic-resistant gram-negative bacteria (*Proteus, Pseudomonas*). Perhaps preoperative prophylaxis with polymyxin or neomycin should be explored.

Although most cases of acute purulent conjunctivitis are self-limited (7 to 14 days), the use of suitable antibiotics is accompanied by recovery in 1 to 3 days. The application of warm compresses for 15 min., three or four times daily, is a useful adjunct to antibiotic therapy. Injured corneas demand immediate therapy with antibiotics presumed to be effective on the basis of Gram-stained smears.

In addition to more widely used drugs, gentamicin, when employed locally, may prove beneficial in therapy of conjunctivitis caused by *Pseudomonas, Proteus,* and *E. coli.*

Ophthalmia Neonatorum

Neonatal conjunctivitis may be caused not only by gonococci (Chap. 21) but also by pneumococci, coagulase-positive staphylococci, or inclusion conjunctivitis chlamydiae. Appropriate antibiotic therapy is available for the management of all these infections, should they develop, and should be employed without delay. Untreated gonococcal conjunctivitis quickly progresses to corneal ulceration, scarring, and blindness. It is, however, a preventable disease (Chap. 21).

Infections Caused by Trachoma and Inclusion Conjunctivitis (TRIC) Group of Chlamydiae (Bedsoniae)

Formerly, trachoma and inclusion conjunctivitis were regarded as two distinct diseases on pathological, clinical, and epidemiological grounds and were assumed to be caused by two distinct microorganisms. However, in the light of data accumulated in the 15 years since they were first grown in chick embryos, it has become apparent that the TRIC agents comprise an antigenically diverse group of microorganisms of varying virulence, otherwise indistinguishable from each other in the laboratory and capable of causing a continuous spectrum of human diseases of varying severity. The diseases associated with TRIC infections include (1) conjunctivitis without keratitis, (2) punctate keratitis with follicular conjunctivitis, (3) trachoma, (4) urethritis, (5) vulvovaginitis, and (6) cervicitis. Reiter's syndrome of arthritis, urethritis, and conjunctivitis may be caused by TRIC agents, but there is no substantial or conclusive evidence to warrant an etiological relationship at this time.

Characteristically, trachoma is associated with tarsal or limbal follicles, epithelial or subepithelial keratitis, vascular pannus (extension of limbal vessels into the cornea), and conjunctival and corneal scarring which after many years may progress to blindness. Inclusion conjunctivitis is a disease that typically involves follicular conjunctivitis and subepithelial corneal infiltration without pannus and scarring. On the other hand, follicular hypertrophy and pannus have been produced in volunteers with TRIC agents recovered from neonatal conjunctivitis and from the genital tract.

The Causative Agents

Biological Properties The TRIC agents are a subgroup of the chlamydiae (Chap. 2). They are obligate intracellular parasites; 250 to 400 μm in diameter; contain RNA, DNA, and a cell wall; possess limited metabolic activity; are toxic for mice; are inhibited by sulfonamides, tetracyclines, chloramphenicol, and erythromycin; are isolated primarily from the eyes and the genital tract of man; and produce natural infection at these sites. The microorganisms can be propagated serially in the yolk sac of embryonated eggs, growing best at 35°C.

Normally TRIC agents cannot be grown in tissue cultures. However, some isolates have been adapted to growth in human cells (amnion, HeLa, Fraser synovial C HI), and most isolates will produce inclusion bodies in irradiated McCoy cells in 72 hr. even though serial passage cannot be accomplished. TRIC agents that kill mice in 4 to 8 days at dilutions of 10^{-5} to 10^{-7} frequently adapt to tissue culture, while others that are negative in mice do not adapt. TRIC agents that have been passed serially in tissue culture lose pathogenicity for man.

Since typical trachoma is inconsistently induced in the Taiwan monkey *(Macaca cyllopis)*, its most susceptible animal host, volunteer studies in blind individuals are sometimes necessary to prove that a given TRIC agent will induce trachoma.

Antigenic Structure The type-specific protective antigens are proteins or protein-polysaccharide complexes present in the cell wall. The type-specific antigen forms the basis of the mouse toxin protection test (MTPT) in which actively immunized mice are challenged intravenously with toxic doses of the TRIC agent. Nine antigenic types have been identified in testing TRIC agents isolated from man by the MTPT test (Table 19-4). Recent studies show that the fluorescent antibody (FA) test can be employed to determine the antigenic type of TRIC agents and is the most useful tool for studying the natural history and pathogenesis of TRIC infections.

The group-specific antigen is more reactive than the type-specific antigen but does not identify the microorganism as a TRIC agent, only as a chlamydiae.

Preliminary results of gel diffusion tests look promising and may have typing and diagnostic value.

Pathogenesis TRIC agents multiply well in human conjunctival, urethral, and synovial membranes. Clinical manifestations are primarily limited to the eye. Occasionally, disease may

Table 19-4 Association of TRIC Antigenic Types with Trachoma

Source	Number tested	Types A, B, C	Types D, E, F*
Ocular trachoma	64	62	2
Other sources	16	0	16
Total	80	62	18

Source: Adapted from E. R. Alexander, S. P. Wang, and J. T. Grayston, *Am. J. Ophthalmol.*, 63:1469–1478, 1967.

* Three additional types (G, H, I) biologically resembling types D, E, and F have been isolated by S. P. Wang, J. T. Grayston, and J. L. Gale, *J. Immunol.*, 110:873–879, 1973.

involve the genital tract, the joints, the middle ear, and the pharynx. On the other hand, natural infection may in fact be systemic with involvement of lymph nodes, spleen, and other tissues. Live trachoma vaccine multiplies for 3 to 4 weeks in the lymph nodes and spleen of baboons after intravenous or subcutaneous inoculation. Viewed in this context, the recovery of TRIC agents from the joint fluid of patients with arthritis, urethritis, and conjunctivitis (Reiter's syndrome) is not surprising. In addition, TRIC agents have been recovered from the middle ear and pharynx of patients with follicular conjunctivitis and otitis media. In a large number of volunteers inoculated with TRIC agents, otitis media occurred in 14 percent.

TRIC agents are transmitted by direct or indirect, venereal or nonvenereal contact with clinically or subclinically infected persons and carriers. Clinical infections characteristically are acquired during passage through the birth canal (neonatal conjunctivitis) or by direct contact with eye lesions early in life (endemic trachoma). Disease may also be acquired following direct contact with eye lesions later in life (adult conjunctivitis), from the genital tract by way of the fingers to the eye (genitoocular), from the eye by way of the fingers to the genital tract (oculogenital), or by sexual contact.

The recent isolation of TRIC agents from urethritis and vulvovaginitis in young adults with trachoma and from cervicitis in the fiancee of a patient with trachoma is an interesting observation whose precise significance must await further study. The evidence of a direct causal relationship would be greatly strengthened if it were shown that the agents isolated from the eye and the genital tract belonged to the same antigenic type and had other identifying markers.

Although the clinical syndromes of trachoma and inclusion conjunctivitis overlap, trachoma infections appear to produce pannus and conjunctival scarring with greater regularity. On the other hand, many TRIC agents recovered from the genital tract and from neonatal conjunctivitis have the capacity to produce follicular hypertrophy and pannus in volunteers.

It is apparent that much remains to be learned concerning the pathogenesis of TRIC diseases. Among the many factors thought to influence the development of TRIC lesions are the site of localization, the virulence of the particular TRIC agent, the rate of reinfection, the duration of infection, the acquisition of hypersensitivity, and the living conditions of the infected individual. Based largely on extensive studies employing the FA test, trachoma appears to be a disease that waxes and wanes following a single unaggravated infection without any decline in microbiological intensity. Healing may occur without scarring, but relapse is common. Pannus and scarring seem to be a function of the duration of infection. The duration of infection may be determined by the living conditions of the patient that are conducive to a higher reinfection rate with other antigenic types and perhaps by repeated insults to the eye resulting from bacterial infection, adenovirus infection, and physical trauma.

Trachoma In endemic trachoma areas, clinical infections are acquired in early childhood, usually involve the upper lids, and cause a purulent or mucopurulent discharge somewhat less acute than inclusion conjunctivitis. The infection may progress to follicular hypertrophy, epithelial keratitis, extension of the limbal vessels into the cornea (pannus), progression of pannus across the cornea, and may be accompanied by conjunctival and corneal scarring, lid deformities, and blindness over a period of many years. On the other hand, the early lesions may heal without scarring.

In some endemic areas (e.g., Gambia), 80 percent of the population have ocular abnormality, and 2.5 percent have severe visual defects. In other endemic areas (e.g., Jamaica), corneal scars rarely develop.

Inclusion Conjunctivitis Inclusion conjunctivitis characteristically involves the lower lids and causes an acute purulent discharge. After several weeks of intense inflammation during which follicles and subepithelial corneal infiltration may develop, the disease gradually subsides, and the conjunctiva becomes normal. Pannus and scarring, as a rule, do not occur.

Genital Infections Urethritis, vulvovaginitis, and cervicitis may be caused by TRIC agents. Disease in the genital tract, however, is an unusual manifestation of infection. Recent evidence suggests that genital disease may be more common when eye lesions serve as the source for contaminating the genital tract.

Arthritis, Urethritis, and Conjunctivitis (Reiter's Syndrome) The syndrome of arthritis, urethritis, and conjunctivitis has been recognized for a long time. The disease may be the result of infection with a TRIC agent. TRIC agents have been recovered from the joint fluid of 6 of 13 cases of Reiter's syndrome, from 2 of 15 patients thought to have rheumatoid arthritis, and from none of 18 patients with other forms of arthritis. Much further study is required to clarify the role of TRIC agents in the pathogenesis of Reiter's syndrome.

The disease is usually manifest in 3 to 4 weeks (urethritis, conjunctivitis, and arthritis), is found mostly in young male adults, is accompanied by remissions and recurrences (especially in the joints), and in most cases, recovery occurs without sequelae in a few months to a few years. The severity and duration of the disease are primarily associated with the arthritis which commonly involves the knees and the ankles and may occasionally result in residual joint damage.

Laboratory Diagnosis Recognition of infection with TRIC agents depends upon one of the following procedures: (1) demonstration of cytoplasmic inclusions in Giemsa-stained smears of conjunctival scrapings (this is most readily accomplished early in the course of the disease and is an indication of active infection); (2) immunofluorescence with type-specific serum which may provide an indication of probable trachoma (types A, B, or C) or of inclusion conjunctivitis (types D, E, or F) as suggested by Table 19-4; (3) isolation of the agent in the yolk sac of chick embryos or incomplete growth of the agent in irradiated McCoy cells together with the finding of cytoplasmic inclusions or specific immunofluorescence.

The demonstration of cytoplasmic inclusions in smears prepared directly from suspected lesions is the least sensitive method and is frequently negative in mild infections with TRIC agents. Immunofluorescence is the most useful tool available for studying the behavior of TRIC agents and is many times more sensitive than the detection of inclusion bodies. Isolation of the agent in eggs is highly sensitive but often requires several passages before the agent can be demonstrated and even when positive on first passage usually requires 9 to 13 days before inclusion bodies can be recognized. Using irradiated McCoy cells inclusion bodies can be demonstrated with greater facility in less time (3 days), but the tissue culture system cannot support continuous growth of the agent, and isolation must be carried out in eggs.

The FA test is positive prior to the appearance of inclusion bodies, during the active phase of the disease, after clinical signs have abated, when reinfection or relapse occurs, in infections which never become clinically manifest, and for a prolonged period following treatment. The speed, convenience, and specificity of the FA test are superior to the other procedures available. It does appear, however, to be less sensitive than isolation of the agent in eggs.

Epidemiology

Source The human eye and genital tract are the natural habitat of TRIC agents. In these sites the microorganisms may induce clinical or subclinical infections or may be present without producing a serological response (carrier state). Clinical infection is common in the eye but rare in the genital tract. In addition, TRIC agents can cause otitis media and arthritis and have been recovered from the pharynx.

Infection may be acquired from infected persons or carriers. Asymptomatic infections are the rule in the genital tract and are common in contacts of patients with trachoma as demonstrated by FA tests and isolation of the agent in eggs. Infection is almost always the result of implantation of the agent in the eye or the genital tract of a susceptible person. The arthritis that occurs in association with urethritis and conjunctivitis (Reiter's syndrome) probably is an offshoot of a basic oculogenital or genitoocular infection and suggests that TRIC infections may be systemic and involve the reticuloendothelial system as do other chlamydiae infections (Chaps. 21 and 23).

Incidence in Endemic Trachoma Areas It is estimated that 400 million persons in endemic areas throughout the world (especially Africa and Asia) have trachoma and that 20 million are blind as a result of the disease. The severely debilitating effects of trachoma are tragically illustrated in recent careful studies in a Gambian village. The incidence of active trachoma increases to a maximum of 91 percent in the 5- to 9-year age group and then declines steadily with advancing age. Inclusion bodies were demonstrated in 42 percent of the active cases, and TRIC agents were isolated from 70 percent of the cases. Ocular abnormality was present in 80 percent of the population, and 2.5 percent had severe visual defects. The conjunctivae of only 3 percent of the population were free from potentially pathogenic bacteria, but bacterial conjunctivitis was unusual and did not appear to affect the course of trachoma. In a study of the flora of trachomatous and nontrachomatous children on American Indian reservations in the United States, only *Moraxella* bacteria occurred significantly more often in trachomatous children.

The natural history of trachoma in the Gambian village unfortunately prevails in many parts of the world. On the other hand, sometimes even in neighboring areas of the same country, trachoma is a much milder disease. In Jamaica, for example, where mild trachoma is endemic, corneal scarring is rarely seen. In an Indian school in the United States at a time when no active cases of trachoma were present, 25 percent of the children had positive FA tests.

Traditionally, trachoma has been associated with poor hygienic conditions and the scarcity of water and is complicated by bacterial conjunctivitis. However, the one factor that correlates best with progressive pannus is the duration of infection. The duration of infection, in turn, is dependent upon the prevalence of trachoma and the frequency of reinfection, probably with an antigenically distinct TRIC type. The roles of bacterial conjunctivitis, adenovirus conjunctivitis, and physical trauma in progressive trachoma, although assumed, have not been established by recent microbiological and serological studies.

Incidence of Inclusion Conjunctivitis (Neonatal Conjunctivitis) Most clinical infections are sporadic cases acquired by newborn infants during passage through infected birth canals. TRIC agents have been isolated from the cervix of the mother and from the conjunctiva in the infant. Secondary cases in contacts of patients with neonatal or adult conjunctivitis are extremely rare.

Adult eye infections can often be traced to swimming in unchlorinated pools or ponds, presumably contaminated by genital secretions. Swimming pool conjunctivitis, a name formerly used synonymously with inclusion conjunctivitis, is not particularly appropriate because (1) TRIC agents are inactivated by chlorine and most swimming pools are chlorinated, and (2) most eye infections acquired by swimming in chlorinated pools are caused by adenoviruses which are resistant to chlorine.

Incidence of Other TRIC Diseases The incidence of urethritis, vulvovaginitis, cervicitis, and arthritis due to TRIC agents is apparently low, but precise knowledge must await further study. Otitis media due to TRIC agents usually occurs concomitantly with eye involvement.

The recovery of TRIC agents from human abortion specimens (4 to 22 samples examined) may only be a reflection of the carrier state in the mother and contamination of the embryo. On the other hand, it is conceivable that there may be a causal relation between the abortion and the presence of the TRIC agent. The problem obviously merits further study.

Prevention and Control

Early Treatment Early treatment is currently the most effective method to prevent the spread and to control diseases caused by TRIC agents. The sporadic nature of inclusion conjunctivitis and its rapid response to chemotherapy with tetracyclines or sulfonamides present no difficulty. On the other hand, many factors combine to interfere with effective prevention and control of trachoma. These include the prevalence of subclinical infections, the frequency of relapse and reinfection, and the persistence of the agent during and after treatment with the most effective drugs (tetracyclines and sulfonamides).

There is no doubt that intensive chemotherapy can eradicate TRIC agents early in the course of trachoma. The effectiveness of the response is inversely proportional to the duration of infection. In most endemic areas this means that preschool age children are the ones most likely to be cured of their infections. This group is also the most difficult group to reach with effective treatment.

Topical tetracyclines (1 percent ointment applied four times daily for 6 weeks) or oral sulfonamides (0.5 Gm daily for 3 weeks) produce a clinical and microbiological cure if given early in the course of the disease. A recent study employing topical tetracyclines (1 percent ointment three times daily for 2 weeks) or sulfisoxazole (a total of 1 Gm per day in three doses continued for 2 weeks) provides an indication of the persistence of TRIC agents during chemotherapy. In the majority of the treated patients, the FA test was positive for 2 to 10 weeks and then became negative. In patients remaining positive for 10 weeks, a second course of therapy was given with results that paralleled the first course of therapy; i.e., the majority became FA negative in 2 to 10 weeks, but in other patients the FA remained positive, and in some cases relapse occurred.

Mass Treatment In endemic trachoma areas where universal infection early in life is the rule, mass treatment campaigns with topical tetracyclines (1 percent ointment applied daily for 3 to 6 days each month for 6 months) would seem to be more desirable than intensive therapy of individual cases. The latter can be cured, but would probably be reinfected. Although eradication cannot be obtained by mass campaigns, clinical improvement and the prevention of sequelae may be dramatic. In a large proportion of treated cases, complications are avoided. An effect on the chain of infection might also result but has not been achieved by the mass campaigns used to date.

Vaccines A variety of attenuated and killed vaccines have been employed experimentally and under field conditions in endemic areas. Type-specific protection can be induced in monkeys and man. Under field conditions the vaccines have given limited protection. For example, in an endemic area of high prevalence two injections of sucrose KCl gradient or genetron (fluorocarbon) purified vaccines at 3-month intervals gave 70 and 50 percent protection for 1 year and a decrease in the FA conversion rate from 37 percent in the unvaccinated to 10 percent in the vaccinated. However, the protection afforded by the vaccines declined progressively at 2, 8, and 12 months following vaccination.

Perhaps the protection afforded by trachoma vaccines can be enhanced by using attenuated TRIC agents, including each of the six recognized antigenic types in the vaccine, and employing improved vaccines in combination with early treatment and mass treatment campaigns.

Corticosteroids The topical use of corticosteroids may reactivate trachoma and has no role in treatment. However, corticosteroids have been employed as a test to determine if treatment has successfully eradicated TRIC agents.

Other Control Measures Theoretically, the availability of proper hygienic measures and instruction in their use should reduce the prevalence of trachoma, but these have rarely been effective in endemic areas and often are beyond the economic resources of the area.

Ocular Manifestations of In Utero Infection with Rubella Virus

Although in utero infection with rubella virus has been recognized since 1941 as a major cause of blindness, it is only in the past few years that the availability of virological and serological methods has permitted an accurate assessment of the problem. It is estimated that approximately 6,000 infants are blind as a result of the major rubella epidemic (Chap. 22) which occurred in the United States in 1964.

Table 19-5 Ocular Manifestations of Rubella Infection in Utero

Ocular manifestation*		Number of eyes involved
Cataracts		30
Monocular	8	
Binocular	11	
Retinopathy		18
Nystagmus		18
Iris hypoplasia		16
Microcornea		12

* The total number of patients was 49, 24 of whom had ocular manifestations.

Source: Adapted from A. I. Geltzer, D. Guber, and M. L. Sears, *Am. J. Ophthalmol.*, 63:221–229, 1967.

The data included in Table 19-5, based on a study of 49 patients with virologically or serologically confirmed in utero infections with rubella virus, indicate the range and frequency of ocular manifestations. Most of the patients with eye involvement showed multiple abnormalities. Five of 13 infants with ocular lesions were positive for conjunctival virus when culture was attempted, but none of five without ocular lesions were positive for virus. The pathogenesis of the ocular lesions is the result of viral invasion (Chap. 22), and the frequent damage to the lens and the retina is in accord with their rapid maturation at the time of viral infection.

Epidemic Adenovirus Type 8 Keratoconjunctivitis

Epidemic keratoconjunctivitis (shipyard eye) is an acute conjunctivitis accompanied by enlarged, tender preauricular nodes which develop 5 to 7 days after infection with adenovirus type 8 and followed by keratitis. The disease usually persists for about 2 to 4 weeks before complete recovery occurs. However, subepithelial opacities in the cornea (with reduced vision) may be present for up to 2 years before resolution. Other manifestations of adenovirus infection (Chap. 20) are rarely present in epidemic keratoconjunctivitis.

Onchocerciasis

Onchocerciasis is a disease caused by a tissue nematode, *Onchocerca volvulus*. Adult worms and microfilariae are found in fibrous subcutaneous nodules (1 to 4 cm). Transmission is accomplished by the small black fly *(Simulium)* which ingests the microfilariae when it bites the skin of an infected person and transfers the microfilariae when it feeds on the skin of a susceptible individual.

Ocular involvement is the most serious complication of the disease and occurs in 10 to 85 percent of those infected. As many as 5 percent of those infected may be blinded. Numerous microfilariae are found throughout the eye and may be associated with photophobia, irritation, conjunctivitis, punctate keratitis, pannus, hypertrophy of the iris followed by atrophy, and destruction of the optic nerve. The pathogenesis of the destructive eye lesions is unknown but may be a combination of toxicity and hypersensitivity.

In endemic areas (Africa and focal areas of infection in Guatemala, Mexico, Venezuela, and South Arabia) the finding of subcutaneous nodules, visual manifestations, and ocular lesions suggests onchocerciasis. Diagnosis is established by demonstrating the microfilariae under the low power of the microscope in a thin section of skin.

Early detection and treatment consisting of surgical removal of the subcutaneous nodules and the use of diethylcarbamazine for the microfilariae and suramin for the adult worms over a period of 2 months are effective in preventing serious eye involvement. Since the black fly is a daytime biter, repellents should be used by outdoor workers in endemic areas. Larvacides are of value in reducing the population of flies by destroying their breeding places.

Fungal Keratoconjunctivitis

Fungal infections of the eye are usually encountered following (1) the use of antibiotics to which the fungi are resistant, (2) the use of corticosteroids which enhance fungal growth, (3) corneal injury, or (4) uncontrolled diabetes. In most cases, the causative agents are members of the normal conjunctival flora (Tables 19-2 and 19-3).

Fungal infection should be suspected in any purulent discharge or corneal ulcer from which bacteria are not isolated. Smears and cultures which are negative may become positive after 2 weeks. In pathogenicity tests, the organisms may be recovered only from animals receiving betamethasone-neomycin drops equivalent to those used in therapy of the patient. Either nystatin or amphotericin B is of value in treatment of infections associated with some of the causative agents.

Rhinoorbitalcerebral phycomycosis, due to *Mucor* and other saprophytic genera occasionally present in the normal conjunctiva, occurs as a well-defined clinical syndrome in adults with uncontrolled diabetes, usually patients in acidosis. Infected persons develop facial pain and headache, rhinitis with epistaxis, lid edema, internal and external ophthalmoplegia, ptosis, chemosis, proptosis, and severe visual loss, all unilateral. Rapid deterioration follows with coma and death in 2 weeks.

The pathogenesis appears to initially involve nasal tissue with progression to the paranasal sinuses and the orbit, a predilection for intravascular invasion, thrombosis of internal carotid or ophthalmic arteries, sudden and complete loss of vision, and spread to the meninges and the brain. A similar picture develops in rats with alloxan diabetes.

Diagnosis is based on the demonstration of the fungus with its pathognomonic, nonseptate, broad branching hyphae up to 50 μm in diameter in the tissue involved. Since the eye involvement appears early in the course of the disease, prompt recognition and effective treatment with amphotericin B can prevent an otherwise fatal infection.

BIBLIOGRAPHY

Beiram, M. M. O.: "Blindness in the Sudan: Prevalence and Causes in the Blue Nile Province," *Bull. W.H.O.,* 45:511-515, 1971.

Dawson, C. R., Hanna, L., and Togni, B.: "Adenovirus Type 8 Infections in the United States. IV. Observations on the Pathogenesis of Lesions in Severe Eye Disease," *Arch. Ophthalmol.,* 87:258-268, 1972.

———, Ostler, H. B., Hanna, L., Hoshiwara, I., and Jawetz, E.: "Tetracyclines in the Treatment of Chronic Trachoma in American Indians," *J. Infect. Dis.,* 124:255-263, 1971.

Goscienski, P. J., and Sexton, R. R.: "Follow-up Studies in Neonatal Inclusion Conjunctivitis," *Am. J. Dis. Child.,* 124:180-182, 1972.

Kuo, C. C., Wang, S. P., Wentworth, B. B., and Grayston, J. T.: "Primary Isolation of TRIC Organisms in HeLa 229 Cells Treated with DEAE-Dextran," *J. Infect. Dis.,* 125:665-668, 1972.

Lindsay, J. R.: "Profound Childhood Deafness. Inner Ear Pathology," *Ann. Otol. Rhinol. Laryngol.,* 82(suppl. 5):4-121, 1973.

McMaster, P. R., Aranson, S. B., and Moore, T. E., Jr.: "The Role of Indigenous Bacteria in Producing Anterior Ocular Inflammation," *Arch. Ophthalmol.,* 86:443-445, 1971.

Paul, E. V., and Zimmerman, L. E.: "Some Observations on the Ocular Pathology of Onchocerciasis," *Hum. Pathol.,* 1:581-594, 1970.

Snowe, R. J., and Wilfert, C. M.: "Epidemic Reappearance of Gonococcal Ophthalmia Neonatorum," *Pediatrics,* 51:110-114, 1973.

Stephan, T., Busis, S. N., Arena, S., Khurana, R. C., and Danowski, T. S.: "Rhinocerebral Phycomycosis (Mucormycosis)," *Laryngoscope,* 83:173-178, 1973.

Thelmo, W., Csordas, J., Davis, P., and Marshall, K. G.: "The Cytology of Acute Bacterial and Follicular Conjunctivitis," *Acta Cytol. (Baltimore),* 16:172-177, 1972.

Chapter 20

Localized Infections of the Respiratory Tract

Bernard A. Briody

PERSPECTIVE

Numerous surveys and carefully controlled studies utilizing clinical, epidemiological, microbiological, and serological data have amply documented that localized respiratory infections account both for the majority of all human illness and the bulk of human infections (Table 20-1). Viruses are the causative agents in more than 90 percent of localized respiratory infections, while bacteria are responsible for the balance.

In terms of the etiology of localized respiratory infections, there are significant differences apparent when the upper respiratory tract, as opposed to the lower respiratory tract, is involved and when children are contrasted with adults (Table 20-2). In addition, when reinfection occurs with the same antigenic type of the causative agent [respiratory syncytial (RS) and parainfluenza viruses, mycoplasma], disease is almost always limited to the upper respiratory tract. As noted in Tables 20-2 and 20-3, rhinoviruses and adenoviruses are the major causes of upper respiratory tract infection in man, whereas infections of the lower respiratory tract are induced primarily by RS virus, parainfluenza viruses, influenza viruses, adenoviruses, and *Mycoplasma*.

Table 20-1 Localized Respiratory Infections As a Proportion of All Infections and Illnesses in the United States

Site of infection	All infections, %	All illnesses, %
Upper respiratory tract	48	39
Lower respiratory tract	30	24
Totals	78	63

Source: Adapted from the United States National Health Survey, *Acute Conditions: Incidence and Associated Disability, United States, July, 1958–June, 1959,* series B-18, Government Printing Office, 1960.

In this chapter emphasis will be given to a consideration of the rhinoviruses, adenoviruses, influenza viruses, parainfluenza viruses, RS virus, coronaviruses, *Mycoplasma pneumoniae,* and *Bordetella pertussis.* The other causative agents involved in localized respiratory infections are discussed elsewhere in the text (diphtheria bacilli in Chap. 13, streptococci in Chap. 14, herpesvirus in Chap. 22, and influenza bacilli, Coxsackie viruses, and echoviruses in Chap. 24).

Table 20-2 Causative Agents in Localized Respiratory Infections According to the Clinical Syndrome

Clinical syndrome	Causative agents
Upper respiratory tract	
Common cold	Rhinoviruses,* influenza viruses, parainfluenza viruses, respiratory syncytial (RS) virus, coronaviruses, adenoviruses, Coxsackie A and B viruses, echoviruses; *Mycoplasma*
Sinusitis	Pneumococci, staphylococci, streptococci secondary to acute upper respiratory tract viral* and bacterial infections
Acute respiratory disease and febrile pharyngitis	Adenoviruses;* streptococci;* influenza viruses, parainfluenza viruses, RS virus, coronaviruses, Coxsackie A virus, herpesviruses; *Mycoplasma*
Lower respiratory tract	
Bronchitis	
Infants and children	RS virus,* parainfluenza viruses;* *Mycoplasma;** rhinoviruses; influenza bacilli
Adults	Influenza virus
Chronic bronchitis, emphysema, and bronchiectasis	
Adults	Aggravated by acute bronchitis associated with influenza bacilli,* and pneumococci* following viral infections of the upper respiratory tract
Bronchiolitis	
Infants and children	RS virus,* parainfluenza viruses;* *Mycoplasma;** adenoviruses, and rhinoviruses
Adults	Influenza virus
Epiglottitis, laryngitis, laryngotracheobronchitis (croup)	
Infants and children	RS virus,* parainfluenza viruses,* influenza viruses;* *Mycoplasma,* influenza bacilli
Tracheobronchitis	
Children	Influenza;* pertussis
Adults	Influenza*
Bronchopneumonia	
Infants	RS virus,* parainfluenza viruses*
Children	*Mycoplasma**
Adults	Influenza viruses,* adenoviruses;* *Mycoplasma**

* These causative agents are most commonly involved in the indicated syndrome.

THE CAUSATIVE AGENTS

As is evident from the data included in Tables 20-2, 20-3, and 20-4, localized respiratory infections are caused by numerous viruses and a few bacteria. For convenience and in order to avoid needless repetition, some of the more important properties of viruses isolated from respiratory infections are summarized in Table 20-4, and the various clinical syndromes are briefly described in Table 20-5.

Table 20-3 Frequency of Virus Isolations from Respiratory Specimens*

Virus group	Number of isolates
Rhinoviruses	378
Adenoviruses	170
Myxoviruses	126
Echoviruses	91
Herpes simplex	75
Coxsackie viruses	25
Cytomegaloviruses	17
Ungrouped	4

* Excluding 142 poliovirus isolations which reflect the use of the attenuated Sabin vaccine.

Source: Modified from M. K. Cooney, C. E. Hall, and J. P. Fox, *Am. J. Epidemiol.*, 96:286–305, 1972.

As noted in Table 20-4, attempts to isolate viruses from respiratory secretions are based on the use of appropriate tissue cultures incubated on roller drums at 33°C for 14 days and periodic examination of the cultures for cytopathogenicity (CPE) and hemadsorption (HAD).

Rhinoviruses

In terms of morbidity, rhinoviruses are the most common cause of human illness and account for an estimated 40 percent of respiratory infections. In infants and young children, clinical disease is divided approximately equally between the common cold on the one hand and bronchitis, bronchiolitis, bronchopneumonia, and croup on the other hand, with no disease occurring in about 12 percent of patients infected with the virus. In adults, about 95 percent of infections are clinically characterized as a common cold with no disease occurring in 3 percent and bronchitis in 2 percent. At any

Table 20-4 Properties of Viruses Causing Localized Respiratory Infections

Virus	Nucleic acid	Number of antigenic types	Essential lipid	Symmetry	Stability at pH 3.0	Hemagglutinin	Isolation of virus*
Adenoviruses	DNA	31	−	Icosahedral	+	+ Types 12, 18 −	HEK
Myxoviruses							
Influenza virus	RNA	Numerous	+	Helical	−	+	HEK
Parainfluenza virus	RNA	4	+	Helical	−	+	HEK
RS virus	RNA	1	+	Helical	−	−	HEE
Coronaviruses	RNA	Probably numerous	+	Helical	−	−	HEK and WI-38**
Picornaviruses							
Rhinovirus	RNA	>90	−	Icosahedral	−	−	WI-38
Coxsackie virus	RNA	30	−	Icosahedral	+	+	HEK
Echovirus	RNA	33	−	Icosahedral	+	+	WI-38

* All tissue cultures should be incubated on roller drums at 33°C for 14 days and periodically examined for cytopathogenicity (CPE) and hemadsorption. For other viruses, efficient recovery of poliovirus requires both HEK and WI-38 cells; herpes simplex can be isolated in WI-38; cytomegalovirus is best recovered in human fetal tonsil tissue culture.

** Some isolates of coronavirus can be recovered only in human embryonic tracheal organ cultures.

Key to abbreviations in table: RS = respiratory syncytial virus; HEK = human embryonic kidney tissue culture; HEE = human heteroploid esophageal epithelium tissue culture; WI-38 = Wistar Institute human diploid tissue culture.

Table 20-5 Clinical Syndromes Encountered in Localized Respiratory Infections

Syndrome	Brief description
Common cold	An acute afebrile inflammation of the nasal mucous membranes accompanied by excessive secretions (catarrh), nasal stuffiness, sneezing, and a sore or dry throat.
Acute respiratory disease	An acute febrile illness characterized by pharyngitis, often with laryngitis, and accompanied by cough, hoarseness, and a sore throat with little or no faucial exudate.
Pharyngoconjunctival fever	An acute febrile illness, usually of children, characterized by nonexudative pharyngitis, submandibular lymphadenopathy, and unilateral, nonpurulent follicular conjunctivitis.
Febrile pharyngitis	An acute febrile illness, usually of children, characterized by nonexudative pharyngitis and submandibular lymphadenopathy.
Sinusitis	An acute afebrile illness that usually follows viral infections of the upper respiratory tract and is associated with the accumulation of mucous secretions in the paranasal sinuses, pain, and secondary bacterial infection.
Epiglottitis, laryngitis and laryngotracheobronchitis (croup)	Acute febrile illnesses of mild to fulminating character often associated with a sore throat, hoarseness, and a barking cough and in severe or fulminating cases by the rapid development of toxicity, prostration, difficulty in breathing, cyanosis, and death.
Acute bronchitis	An acute febrile illness characterized primarily by an initial nonproductive cough which soon becomes mucopurulent and is usually preceded by inflammation of the nasal mucous membranes and a sore throat.
Chronic bronchitis, emphysema, and bronchiectasis	Chronic bronchitis is arbitrarily defined as cough with the production of sputum occurring on most days for at least 3 months in the year during at least 2 years. The disease predisposes to recurrent respiratory infection and emphysema, i.e., dilatation and destruction of the walls of the air passages distal to the terminal bronchioles. Bronchiectasis is dilatation of the bronchial tree characterized by cough, mucopurulent sputum, hemoptysis (bloody mucus), and recurrent pneumonitis.
Bronchiolitis	An acute febrile illness characterized by exudation in the bronchioles which leads to obstruction, difficulty in breathing, prostration, and anoxia and is usually preceded by inflammation of the nasal mucosa and cough.
Tracheobronchitis	When caused by influenza virus, an acute febrile illness characterized by headache, myalgia, and prostration with destruction of the ciliated epithelial cells and their replacement by squamous epithelium. When caused by pertussis bacteria, an acute febrile illness associated initially with catarrh and characteristically with paroxysmal cough which terminates in a deep, forced inspiration (whoop).
Bronchopneumonia	The bronchopneumonia that occurs in localized respiratory infections may be primary (RS, influenza, or parainfluenza viruses; adenoviruses; *Mycoplasma*) or secondary to influenza and pertussis and caused by bacteria. Clinical manifestations partly reflect the preceding illness. Evidence of bronchopneumonia is best obtained by roentgenograms that often reveal a patchy or diffuse consolidation radiating from the hilar region. The outcome in most cases is recovery, but primary influenza virus pneumonia can lead to vascular collapse and death in a few days.

given time, multiple antigenic types are circulating in the community.

Adenoviruses

With the exception of croup, adenoviruses, especially types 3, 4, and 7, can produce the full spectrum of clinical syndromes listed in Table 20-5. In children, adenovirus infection is frequently associated with pharyngitis, conjunctivitis, cervical lymphadenopathy, and fever (pharyngoconjunctival fever). Adenovirus pneumonia in infants and in military recruits is an infrequent but serious disease. Adenovirus type 8 is responsible for epidemic keratoconjunctivitis (Chap. 19), which attacks all age groups. In addition, adenovirus may occasionally be involved in viral meningitis, in producing a generalized exanthem, or in causing acute hemorrhagic cystitis.

Adenoviruses are interesting from a structural and biological point of view. The capsid of the virus consists of 252 capsomeres composed of several different macromolecular entities: (1) *Hexons* are polygonal hollow structures distributed on the faces and edges of the triangular surfaces of the icosahedron, and each hexon has six neighbors, is a multimeric protein present in all adenoviruses, and can be detected by complement fixation; (2) *pentons* are similar structures found on the 12 vertex units of the icosahedron, and each penton has five neighbors and is associated with a penton fiber of variable length; (3) penton fibers are string-like structures with a terminal knob, appear to be composed of two immunologically distinct proteins, and are associated with hemagglutinating activity for rhesus or rat cells.

Adenoviruses are isolated from persons with respiratory illness (Tables 20-2 and 20-3); from the respiratory secretions, adenoids, and tonsils of healthy persons; and most commonly from the stools of persons with respiratory illness or healthy persons. Adenoviruses do not produce disease in the enteric tract, but somewhat surprisingly are recovered three times more frequently from fecal specimens than either Coxsackie viruses or echoviruses. Two percent of specimens from ill patients are positive for adenovirus, while only 0.5 percent of specimens from well persons are positive, a ratio of 4 to 1. By comparison, the ratio between ill and well persons is 5.3 to 1 for rhinoviruses, 15 to 1 for myxoviruses, but only 1.5 to 1 for enteroviruses (Coxsackie viruses and echoviruses). In addition, as noted in Chapter 2, adenovirus types 12, 18, and 31 (and to a lesser extent, types 3, 7, 14, 16, and 21) can transform cells in vitro and can induce tumors when injected into newborn hamsters. The highly oncogenic adenoviruses (types 12, 18, and 31) have a guanine-cytosine content of 48 percent in their DNA which closely approximates that of human DNA, whereas nononcogenic adenoviruses have a guanine-cytosine content of 58 percent. There is, however, no evidence that adenoviruses are involved as causative agents in human cancer (Chap. 2).

Influenza Viruses

Historically, influenza viruses have caused the greatest *pandemics* (worldwide epidemics) known to man. It is estimated that the influenza pandemic of 1918–1919 caused 20 to 40 million deaths and that the influenza pandemic of 1957–1958 was responsible for even more cases, although fewer deaths. Consequently, it is not surprising that influenza virus has been more intensively studied than any other animal virus.

Influenza viruses can be grown conveniently in the laboratory both in chick embryos and in tissue cultures. Despite the fact that the viruses induce little CPE, their presence can be detected by hemagglutination and HAD. The structure of the virus is characterized by protein spikes that project through the envelope of the virus. The hemagglutinin (HA) spikes and the neuraminidase spikes comprise the principal antigenic sites of the virus and are involved in the attachment of the virus to cells. After growth in susceptible cells, the virus is slowly released from the surface of the plasma membrane. Addition of red blood cells to the virus preparation leads to HAD with the projecting spikes of the virus combining with glycoprotein receptors on the surface of the erythrocytes.

Ferrets have been the animals of choice for experimentally reproducing the human disease. Most of the major features of human influenza, including the destruction of ciliated tracheobronchial cells and their replacement by squamous epithelial cells, are present in the ferret.

Probably, the outstanding and unique feature of influenza viruses is their propensity for antigenic variation. Genetically determined changes occur in both the HA and the neuraminidase antigens. Over a period of time the antigenic variants that survive are those that are less and less susceptible to the antibodies present in the population. Consequently, in time there are a sufficient number of susceptible individuals in the population to permit the virus to initiate an epidemic.

Antigenic variation is most marked within influenza viruses classified as type A, is less marked in type B, and apparently is of no consequence in type C. The designation of types A, B, and C is based on an S (soluble) antigen specific for the type which is present in the nucleocapsid of the virus but is also produced in excess in infected cells and thus occurs as a soluble antigen in crude virus preparations. The S antigen can easily be separated from the virus by centrifugation and can be conveniently detected by complement fixation.

Parainfluenza Viruses

As noted in Tables 20-2 and 20-4, parainfluenza viruses are members of the myxovirus group that have many properties in common with influenza viruses, are capable of producing a wide spectrum of clinical manifestations, and are second only to RS virus in causing serious disease of the lower respiratory tract in infants and young children. Antigenic variation, however, is not a problem with the parainfluenza viruses. On the contrary, heterotypic antibody responses are common in the parainfluenza viruses; i.e., an infant or child infected with one type (type 1) will develop antibodies to types 1, 2, and 3. In addition, parainfluenza viruses share common antigens with Newcastle disease and mumps viruses. Parainfluenza types 1 and 3 cause more severe infections in children than do types 2 and 4. On the other hand, reinfections in both children and adults are limited to common colds. In tissue cultures, parainfluenza viruses often induce the formation of *syncytia* (giant cells).

Respiratory Syncytial (RS) Virus

RS virus is the most important respiratory pathogen of infants and young children, especially in infants less than 6 months of age. An estimated 30 percent of infections of the lower respiratory tract in infants and young children are caused by RS virus. Bronchiolitis and bronchopneumonia are particularly common in those under 6 months of age. Children between 1 and 3 years of age are more likely to develop upper respiratory tract infection or tracheobronchitis and croup. There is a single antigenic type of the virus, and as the name implies, the virus can induce syncytial (giant cell) formation in tissue cultures. RS virus is a member of the myxovirus group but fails to produce hemagglutination.

Coronaviruses

Coronaviruses share some properties with the myxoviruses (Table 20-4) but differ in other respects. Coronaviruses are similar in size to influenza virus (100 nm) and have surface projections. However, the pleomorphic envelope has widely spaced club-shaped surface projections which do not possess hemagglutinating or neuraminidase activity. The viruses are rarely found in infants and young children with lower respiratory tract infections but are encountered in upper respiratory tract infections (Table 20-2). Some estimates of the role of coronaviruses in upper respiratory infection in adults suggest that they may account for 10 to 25 percent of disease. Recovery of virus from clinical specimens is complicated by the necessity for using human embryonic tracheal organ cultures.

Mycoplasma pneumoniae (Eaton Agent)

Mycoplasma pneumoniae, the only recognized human pathogen in the mycoplasma or pleuropneumonia-like group, are spherical microorganisms (about 0.5 μm) that lack a cell wall, divide by binary fission (budding), require cholesterol, grow on media containing serum and yeast extract, and produce small, smooth colonies (about 500 μm) in contrast to the fried-egg colonies produced by the other classic mycoplasmas and the tiny rough colonies of the T mycoplasmas. On primary isolation from respiratory specimens, colony formation may require 2 to 3 weeks. Thallium acetate and penicillin are usually added to the medium to inhibit the growth of other bacteria. After the organisms are passed a few times in the laboratory, colonies develop in 3 to 6 days. *Mycoplasma pneumoniae* can produce β-hemolysis of guinea pig or sheep erythrocytes, can be inhibited by tetracyclines and erythromycin, belong to a single antigenic type, and can be inhibited by specific antibody. As noted in Table 20-2, the organism can produce disease in both the upper and lower respiratory tract of children and adults.

Bordetella pertussis

Bordetella pertussis, when isolated from patients with pertussis (whooping cough), are small gram-negative encapsulated coccobacilli (1.2 × 0.4 μm) that produce small, smooth colonies on potato-blood-glycerol agar containing penicillin. Such bacteria have a full complement of antigens including an agglutinogen, hemagglutinin, heat-stable toxin, and protective antigen and are designated as phase I. Disease caused by the organism is a tracheobronchitis primarily occurring in infants and young children. Growth of the bacteria is inhibited by erythromycin, tetracyclines, and chloramphenicol. Similar but antigenically distinct bacteria *(B. parapertussis* and *B. bronchiseptica)* may produce a comparable but usually milder syndrome.

PATHOGENESIS

Viruses

Man is the reservoir for agents that cause localized infections of the respiratory tract. Infection is spread from man to man following inhalation of infected droplets which deposit the microorganisms on the respiratory epithelial mucosa. The viruses presumably adsorb to receptors on the surface of the plasma membrane, are taken up by the cells lining the respiratory tract by pinocytosis, intracellular replication ensues, progeny virus is released, additional cells are infected, and the cycle repeated. Within 1 to 2 days (rhinoviruses, influenza viruses, RS virus, coronaviruses) or in 5 to 6 days (parainfluenza viruses, adenoviruses), the mucosal epithelial cells are damaged to the extent that clinical manifestations (Table 20-5) become apparent.

Infection usually commences in the upper respiratory tract and may extend to involve the lower respiratory tract, especially in primary infections of infants and young children with RS and parainfluenza viruses and in primary or subsequent infections caused by influenza viruses in all age groups. In influenza, the destruction of the ciliated tracheobronchial cells is virtually complete in many patients. Repair of the mucosal damage involves the formation of a squamous cell epithelium which is gradually replaced over a period of a month or more by a new layer of ciliated epithelial cells. While the squamous epithelium persists, the individual is resistant to infection with the same or different types of influenza virus, since the virus cannot adsorb to or replicate in the squamous cells.

Although most of these viruses can produce serious disease in the lower respiratory tract (Table 20-2), the most important consequence of respiratory viral infection is secondary bacterial pneumonia which follows influenza. The principal bacteria involved are pneumococci and staphylococci. The pneumonia consistently takes a heavy toll in every influenza epidemic. Fatal cases are concentrated in patients over 55 years old who have underlying cardiovascular, cardiorenal, or cardiopulmonary disease. To a lesser extent, parainfluenza virus infection is associated with bacterial invasion. In addition to pneumonia, respiratory viral infection is the major predisposing factor in otitis media (Chap. 19) and in sinusitis (Table 20-2).

With the exception of influenza viruses and adenoviruses, recurrent infections with the same or a different antigenic type are usually limited to the upper respiratory tract and are much less frequently followed by secondary bacterial infection. Regardless of the causative agent the clinical manifestations are those associated with the common cold.

Adenoviruses can enter by way of the conjunctiva, especially when traumatized or irritated by foreign material. When this occurs, however, the respiratory tract is invariably involved except in epidemic keratoconjunctivitis caused by type 8. Probably in most cases, however, the infection is spread by infected droplets.

To what extent the pathogenesis of localized respiratory infections can be accounted for by the formation of immune complexes between the causative agent and IgG antibody remains to be delineated. However, as discussed more fully elsewhere (Chap. 12), the available data strongly suggest that infection with RS virus in those under 1 year of age is in fact an immune complex disease. Theoretically, the same mechanism could apply to infections of the lower respiratory tract caused by rhinoviruses and parainfluenza viruses in those under 1 year of age and for older children and adults when mycoplasmas, influenza viruses, and adenoviruses are involved.

Bacteria

Following inhalation of *Mycoplasma pneumoniae* or *Bordetella pertussis* in infected droplets, the microorganisms adhere to and cannot be expelled by the ciliated epithelial cells. Electron microscopy utilizing ferritin-labeled antibody and fluorescent antibody studies have clearly demonstrated extracellularly replicating mycoplasmas buried deep in invaginations of the plasma membrane and masses of pertussis bacteria entangled in the ciliated epithelium and enmeshed in a mucopurulent exudate. The mechanism by which mycoplasmas and pertussis bacteria damage the host are not understood. As judged by the ability of the normal bacterial flora to induce secondary bacterial pneumonia, impairment of the integrity of the mucous membrane is much more extensive in pertussis than in mycoplasma infection. In fact, most deaths in pertussis are caused by secondary bacterial pneumonia, especially in those under 1 year of age.

LABORATORY DIAGNOSIS

Without doubt, the best and most rapid method of establishing a laboratory diagnosis of localized respiratory infection would be to demonstrate positive fluorescent antibody reactions on exfoliated epithelial cells. In the hands of experts, this procedure is practical in certain limited situations (influenza, RS, and parainfluenza viruses; mycoplasma; pertussis). However, the multiplicity of the antigenic types of the other causative agents, the expertise required, and the expense entailed generally preclude the adoption of this method as a routine procedure.

As with most infections, a laboratory diagnosis of the microorganism causing localized respiratory infection depends on the isolation and identification of the agent or the demonstration of a fourfold rise in antibody titer with paired acute and convalescent serum samples. When attempts are made to recover virus, appropriate tissue cultures are inoculated as indicated in Table 20-4. If hemadsorption can be demonstrated, the virus may be either an influenza or parainfluenza virus. If syncytia are present, RS or parainfluenza virus may be the causative agent. However, the virus must be identified by any one of a battery of tests, including HA-inhibition, complement fixation (CF), neutralization, or fluorescent antibody staining. Generally, complement fixation and HA-inhibition are used whenever feasible, but in some cases neutralization tests are essential in order to identify the antigenic type of the virus. Similarly, when attempts are made to establish a serological diagnosis, the CF and HA-inhibition tests are preferred. Obviously, however, as indicated in Table 20-4, the HA-inhibition test cannot be employed in the case of rhinoviruses, RS virus, and coronaviruses.

EPIDEMIOLOGY

Even though complicated by diverse etiology and variable and overlapping clinical syndromes caused by the same or different microorganisms, considerable progress has been achieved in the past 20 years in elucidating the epidemiology of localized respiratory infections. The general epidemiological features include the following observations:

1. There is a high attack rate in susceptible persons, as illustrated by pertussis and RS, parainfluenza, and influenza viruses.
2. With the exception of adenoviruses, there is a high correlation between ability to recover the agent and the presence of clinical manifestations.
3. Children form the main cohort of infection and are usually responsible for introducing the infection into the family unit.
4. The causative agents are spread from man to man by droplet infection during the respiratory season (late fall, winter, early spring).
5. With the important exception of influenza, the severity of the disease is inversely related to age. Pneumonia in young adults caused by *Mycoplasma* and by adenovirus is a rare occurrence in individuals who escaped infection earlier in life and has a favorable prognosis. In addition, *Mycoplasma* infections spread more slowly than the other causative agents and show a peak incidence in persons between the ages of 5 and 20.
6. Recurrent infections with the same antigenic type of the microorganism usually are limited to the upper respiratory tract.
7. With the exception of influenza virus, the causative agents appear to be constantly present and circulating within the community.

Epidemic peaks and frequencies vary with the causative agent, the number of antigenic types, and the immune status of the population. For example, multiple rhinovirus serotypes are usually circulating in the community at any given time. Adenovirus types 1, 2, and 5 infections are acquired early in life and are characterized clinically by a febrile pharyngitis; types 3, 4, and 7 are more commonly associated with acute respiratory disease, pharyngoconjunctival fever, and pneumonia and cover a wider age spectrum. Pneumonia in infants caused by adenovirus types 3 and 7 is a highly fatal illness and may occur sporadically or in epidemics.

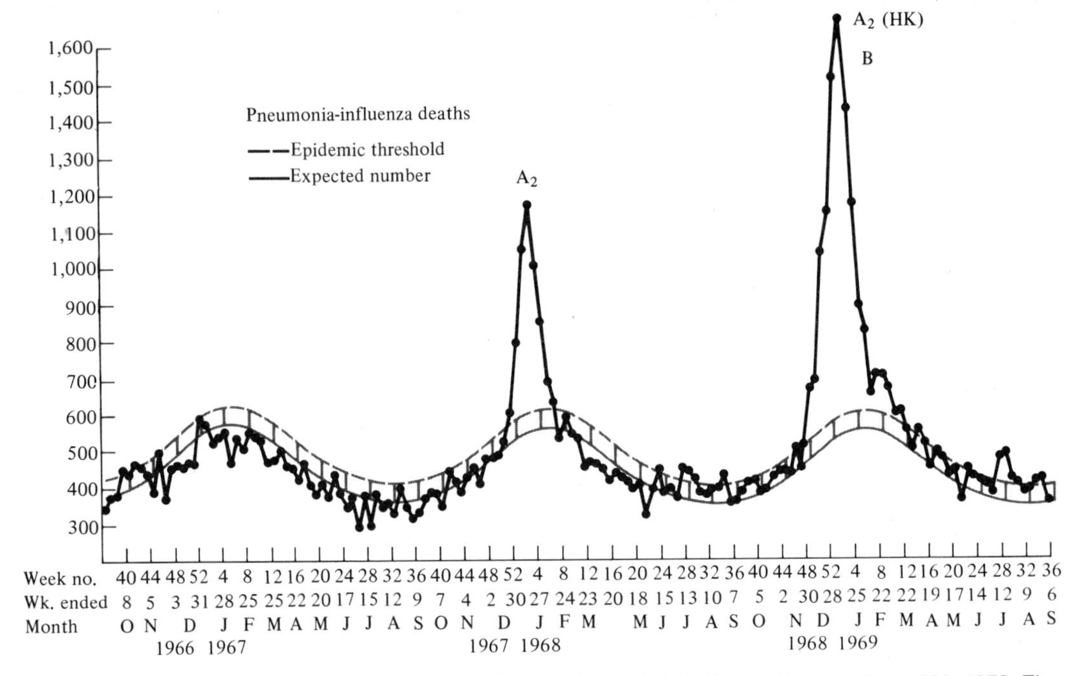

Figure 20-1 Pneumonia-influenza deaths in 122 United States cities, 1966–1973. The peaks of deaths correspond closely with epidemics of influenza caused by A_2 (Hong-

Influenza virus can spread explosively under epidemic conditions but virtually disappears from the community during interepidemic periods. School children between 5 and 14 years of age experience the highest attack rates. Within a few weeks more than 40 percent can become infected. The virus is subsequently widely disseminated in the community and can involve 50 percent or more of a country in a few months. The rate of spread is facilitated by the short incubation period of the disease (18 to 36 hr.), by the high concentrations of virus present in respiratory secretions, and by the susceptibility of the population, but much remains to be explained concerning the genetic markers that condition the virulence of the virus.

At best, the antigenic classification of influenza viruses is a historical accident. At worst, it has created a confusing and chaotic situation. According to orthodoxy, there are three antigenic types—A, B, and C. The types are recognized on the basis of their soluble S or ribonucleoprotein antigen which does not cross-react between types and which can be conveniently assayed by complement fixation. Type C influenza viruses do belong to a single antigenic type, are responsible for mild disease, and rarely, if ever, cause epidemics. Type A influenza viruses include a diverse group of viruses which confer little, if any, cross-protection and are characteristically associated with epidemics that recur at intervals of 2 to 3 years and with pandemics that occur at intervals of 30 to 40 years (1889–1890, 1918–1919, 1957–1958). Within type A influenza viruses, antigenic variation is recognized to be one of the central problems if prevention of the epidemic disease is to become a reality. Type B influenza viruses also include diverse viruses that confer minimal cross-protection and are associated with epidemics that recur at 3- to 6-year intervals but have not yet been incriminated in pandemic influenza, possibly because they are less labile antigenically.

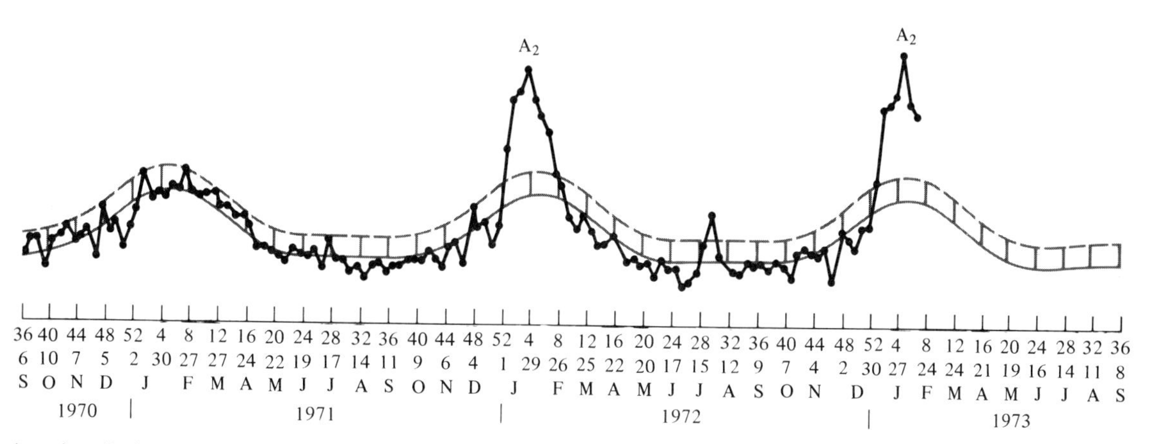

kong) or B viruses. (*From Morbidity Mortality Weekly Report, 17(53):1, 1969; and from Morbidity Mortality Weekly Report, 22(7):61, 1973.*)

Among the parainfluenza viruses, type 2 spreads more rapidly than types 1 and 3. Most children have neutralizing antibody to type 2 by 2 years of age and to types 1 and 3 by 6 years of age. In accordance with these findings, parainfluenza viruses are constantly present in the community and are major causes of lower respiratory tract infection in infants and young children, especially types 1 and 3.

RS virus is responsible for yearly outbreaks among susceptible persons with attack rates as high as 60 percent or more. The virus is constantly present in the community and is the most important respiratory pathogen in those under 1 year of age. Disease caused by RS virus is more common in clinic patients, both in urban and rural areas, than in patients who have access to private physicians. Above the age of 1 year, RS virus infections increasingly involve the upper respiratory tract and spare the lower respiratory tract.

Disease caused by *Mycoplasma* covers a broad spectrum (Table 20-2), spreads slowly (incubation period of 12 to 14 days), and is characteristically endemic rather than epidemic. The most serious consequence of *Mycoplasma* infection is bronchopneumonia which, however, has a favorable prognosis. Mycoplasmal pneumonia exhibits wide fluctuations in frequency, depending upon a number of variables, but generally may involve 3 to 10 percent of those infected.

In unimmunized populations, the attack rate in pertussis approaches that observed in measles and varicella. The incidence and mortality are greatest in those under 1 year of age, with death usually being caused by secondary bacterial pneumonia. Among immunized populations, the incidence and mortality decline sharply. There is a trend toward a higher incidence in older children and adults whose immunity has declined, but the disease is generally less severe. Only about 3,000 cases are reported annually in the United States, with a mortality of about 1 percent.

PREVENTION AND CONTROL

The major problems associated with the development of effective immunizing agents were documented in Chapter 12 and are especially applicable to localized respiratory infections. The difficulties relate to the (1) incubation period, (2) localization of infection to mucous membranes, (3) necessity for administering the antigen(s) in a physical state and by a route that will ensure an effective secretory IgA response, and (4) multiplicity of antigenic types.

The two outstanding successes in prevention of localized respiratory infections involve the use of killed phase I pertussis vaccine and live enteric-coated adenovirus type 4 (Chap. 12). There has, however, been a disastrous failure associated with the use of killed RS virus vaccine (Chap. 12) and less evident disease-enhancing effects associated with the use of killed parainfluenza virus and mycoplasma vaccines.

At best, the efficacy of currently recommended influenza virus vaccines is marginal. This is particularly tragic because whenever there is an epidemic of influenza A or B or a pandemic of influenza A, there will be an excess number of cases of pneumonia and pneumonia-influenza deaths (Fig. 20-1). In the United States in the past 20 years, influenza epidemics have been associated with from 10,000 to more than 100,000 excess deaths due to pneumonia, many of which are caused by pneumococci and staphylococci.

In influenza, in addition to the short incubation period (18 to 36 hr.), the localization of the infection to mucous membranes, the failure to administer the vaccine in a physical state or by a route calculated to ensure an effective secretory IgA response, and the multiplicity of antigenic types (far greater than that suggested by the designation of types A, B, and C or the latest proposed notation which includes strain designation and a description of the hemagglutinin and neuraminidase antigens), there is the unique problem of antigenic variation. Needless to state, the problem of immunization against influenza is being totally reevaluated.

Encompassed within the framework of current and projected investigations are the following approaches.

1 The development of vaccines (attenuated, attenuated temperature-sensitive mutant, attenuated recombined, killed recombinant, subviral) that can be administered in a physical state and by a route that will produce an effective secretory IgA response and protection against exposure to the natural disease
2 The successive and predictable reproduction of past antigenic variations in the virus under controlled laboratory conditions in order to formulate a mechanism for predicting and developing the antigenic variants that will occur in nature in the future
3 Further study and evaluation of the significance of the six distinct and separable pieces of viral RNA within the nucleocapsid of the virus in terms of antigenic variation and genetic recombination among different influenza viruses
4 The more accurate assessment of antigenic variation in the avian, swine, and equine influenza A viruses and an evaluation of their role, if any, in antigenic variation in human influenza A viruses and in human infection

PROSPECTIVE

The prospects for preventing and controlling localized respiratory infections could scarcely be considered encouraging. Only in pertussis, which can be controlled by immunization, and in *Mycoplasma* pneumonia, in which the course of the disease can be shortened by therapy with tetracyclines or erythromycin, has demonstrated progress been achieved. Perhaps extension of the concept of mucous membrane immunization which has been employed successfully with adenovirus type 4 (Chap. 12) may lead to further successes with other viruses. On the other hand, in view of the nature of the problem and in the light of the available data, it is appropriate to maintain a healthy skepticism concerning potential developments that might improve the situation.

BIBLIOGRAPHY

Bradburne, A. F., and Tyrrell, D. A. J.: "Coronaviruses of Man," *Progr. Med. Virol.,* 13:373-403, 1971.

Brown, R. S., Nogrady, M. B., Spence, L., and Wiglesworth, F. W.: "An Outbreak of Adenovirus Type 7 Infection in Children in Montreal," *Can. Med. Assoc. J.,* 108:434-439, 1973.

Eckert, E. A.: "Properties of an Antigenic Glycoprotein Isolated from Influenza Virus Hemagglutinin," *J. Virol.,* 11:183-192, 1973.

Foy, H. M., Cooney, M. K., Maletzky, A. J., and Grayston, J. T.: "Incidence and Etiology of Pneumonia, Croup and Bronchiolitis in Preschool Children Belonging to a Prepaid Medical Care Group over a Four-year Period," *Am. J. Epidemiol.,* 97:80-92, 1973.

———, Cooney, M. K., McMahan, R., and Grayston, J. T.: "Viral and Mycoplasmal Pneumonia in a Prepaid Medical Care Group during an Eight-year Period," *Am. J. Epidemiol.,* 97:93-102, 1973.

Ginsberg, H. S.: "Adenoviruses," *Am. J. Clin. Pathol.,* 57:771-776, 1972.

Glezen, W. P., and Denny, F. W.: "Epidemiology of Acute Lower Respiratory Disease in Children," *N. Engl. J. Med.,* 288:498-505, 1973.

Jackson, G. G., and Muldoon, R. L.: "Viruses Causing Common Respiratory Infections in Man," *J. Infect. Dis.,* 127:328-355, 1973.

Jamieson, W. M.: "Whooping Cough," *Br. Med. J.,* 1:223-225, 1973.

Kapikian, A. Z., Almeida, J. D., and Stott, E. J.: "Immune Electron Microscopy of Rhinoviruses," *J. Virol.,* 10:142-146, 1972.

———, James, H. D., Jr., Kelly, S. J., and Vaughn, A. L.: "Detection of Coronavirus Strain 692 by Immune Electron Microscopy," *Infect. Immun.,* 7:111-116, 1973.

Kilbourne, E. D., Butler, W. T., and Rosen, R. D.: "Specific Immunity in Influenza—Summary of Influenza Workshop III," *J. Infect. Dis.,* 127:220-236, 1973.

Knight, V. (ed.): *Viral and Mycoplasmal Diseases of the Respiratory Tract,* Philadelphia: Lea & Febiger, 1973.

Lamy, M. E., Pouthier-Simon, F., and Debacker-Willame, E.: "Respiratory Viral Infections in Hospital Patients with Chronic Bronchitis. Observations during Periods of Exacerbation and Quiescence," *Chest,* 63:336-341, 1973.

Laver, W. G., and Webster, R. G.: "Studies on the Origin of Pandemic Influenza. III. Evidence Implicating Duck and Equine Influenza Viruses As Possible Progenitors of the Hong Kong Strain of Human Influenza," *Virology,* 51:383-391, 1973.

Shore, S. L., Potter, C. W., and McLaren, C.: "Immunity to Influenza in Ferrets. IV. Antibody in Nasal Secretions," *J. Infect. Dis.,* 126:394-400, 1972.

Stuart-Harris, C. H.: "Immunity to Influenza," *J. Infect. Dis.,* 126:466-468, 1972.

"Symposium on Mycoplasmas," *J. Infect. Dis.,* 127(suppl.):1-92, 1973.

Ward, T. G.: "Viruses of the Respiratory Tract," *Progr. Med. Virol.,* 15:126-158, 1973.

Chapter 21

Venereal Infections

Bernard A. Briody

Syphilis
Gonorrhea
Other Venereal Infections

SYPHILIS

For every case of syphilis identified, treated, and reported by physicians, there are nine cases identified, treated, and not reported. With more than 75 percent of all cases identified and treated by physicians, it is obvious from the above that the number of actual cases of syphilis is much greater than reported. A remedy for this dangerous situation must be sought.

By exploring those facts essential to an understanding of the disease, the ensuing discussion attempts to provide a stimulus for effective cooperative action between physicians and public health authorities. The problem of syphilis cannot be solved by either group acting independently of the other.

Perspective

Although the controversy will probably never be resolved, the most plausible evidence indicates that syphilis was introduced into Barcelona in 1493 when Columbus' first expedition returned from America. In 1494 many Spaniards infected with the disease accompanied the army of the French King Charles on his invasion of Italy. Within 5 years the disease appeared in France, Germany, Switzerland, Holland, Greece, England, Scotland, Hungary, and Russia. The "syphilization" of the Western world proceeded rapidly after 1500.

At the peak of the Industrial Revolution in the nineteenth century, at least 15 percent of the population in urban areas was syphilitic. In the latter half of the nineteenth century, a period of great social change and rapid rise in the standard of living, there was a decline in the incidence of syphilis which cannot be attributed to treatment or control measures.

With the discovery of the causative agent by Schaudinn and Hoffmann, the introduction of the complement-fixation test by Wassermann, and the advent of arsphenamine therapy by Ehrlich between 1905 and 1910, effective public treatment and control programs were applied, and the attack rate was reduced. The introduction of sulfonamides (1938) and, more important, of penicillin (1943) revolutionized the treatment of the disease and led to a further sharp decline, with a low reached in 1957. But from 1957 to date there has been a persistent, significant increased incidence, most marked in Europe and North America.

The Causative Agent

Biologic Properties *Treponema pallidum,* the causative agent of syphilis, is a strict and fragile parasite found naturally only in the tissues of infected man. The organism is a slender, motile spiral (0.2 μm diameter and 5 to 15 μm in length) with pointed ends and coils spaced at intervals of 1 μm. Staining is difficult, but the organism may be seen in tissues stained with silver by Levaditi's method. The spirochetes are best visualized using the dark-field microscope. Efforts to grow the organism on artificial media, in chick embryos, and in tissue culture have failed. However, *T. pallidum* grows readily in the testes of the experimentally inoculated rabbit.

Viability outside the animal body is short. The organism is rapidly killed by oxygen, soap, common bactericidal agents, and drying. The observation that the organism is destroyed in infected tissues at temperatures between 39 and 42°C formed a rational basis for the treatment of late syphilis by fever, often purposely induced by malaria. In whole blood or plasma stored at 4°C the organism is killed in a few days and is, therefore, unlikely to be transmitted by properly stored blood. Preservation of the organism is best accomplished by lyophilization.

Antigenic Structure Little is known concerning the antigenic structure of *T. pallidum* because of the impossibility of culturing the organism and the difficulty of separating the organism from animal tissue.

Serologic Tests

A battery of serologic tests has been developed and has proved to be of great value in the diagnosis of syphilis. Basically, the tests may be classified as those which measure Wassermann antibody, or reagin, and those which measure antibody reactive with suspensions of *T. pallidum.* In the following sections only a few of the more practical or promising tests are noted.

Reagin Tests Wassermann discovered that extracts of human fetal liver tissue swarming with *T. pallidum* reacted with antibody in the serum of patients with syphilis and that the mixture had the power to fix complement. It was soon found that the antibody could be demonstrated when normal liver or other tissues were used as the antigen. The antigen used at present is a purified lipid extracted by alcohol from beef heart (cardiolipin) to which lecithin and cholesterol have been added. Thus, the Wassermann test is an empirical complement-fixation (CF) reaction between a nonspecific antigen and a substance found in syphilitic serum called reagin. It is important to recognize that reagin is produced in a number of acute and chronic diseases which, therefore, can produce biological false positive tests for syphilis. In fact, about 50 percent of those with positive tests have some other disease.

Reagin can also be detected by the direct mixture of syphilitic sera with cardiolipin antigen, which leads to the formation of visible aggregates, particularly when shaken. This is the flocculation reaction which in various modifications is the basis of the Hinton, Kahn, Kline, Mazzini, Meinicke, Venereal Disease Research Laboratory (VDRL), rapid plasma reagin (RPR), and other tests. It permits the rapid and economical screening of large numbers of sera.

Results of the flocculation test closely parallel those of the CF reaction. In general, it is technically more simple and somewhat more sensitive than the CF test. On the other hand, it is more likely to become positive in diseases other than syphilis; i.e., the more sensitive the test, the less specific it is.

Treponemal Tests Although there are a number of procedures, including agglutination, immune adherence, complement-fixation, and methylene blue tests, in which the antigens used are derived from *T. pallidum,* the *Treponema pallidum* immobilization (TPI) test was the first one to unravel many diagnostic problems that could not be solved by other serological techniques. In the TPI test, virulent, motile *T. pallidum* obtained by needle puncture of a syphiloma maintained in rabbit testes are mixed with the serum and complement and are allowed to incubate. The test is read by comparing the number of immobile treponemes to that in an untreated control using the dark-field microscope. While the test is complicated and expensive, it is of great practical value in distinguishing between biological false positive and true positive reagin tests. Although its chemical nature is unknown, the reactive material participating in the TPI test is located on the surface of the organism.

An indirect fluorescent treponemal antibody test (FTA) has largely replaced the TPI test in the diagnosis of syphilis. After prior absorption with nonpathogenic Reiter treponemes to remove cross-reacting antibodies, syphilitic antibodies in the patient's serum will combine specifically with the Nichols strain of *T. pallidum* and can be demonstrated following the addition of fluorescein-labeled antibody to human immunoglobulins.

Pathogenesis

Pathology The two basic pathologic lesions in syphilis are endarteritis and chronic inflammation of the hypersensitive type. There are few clinicopathologic manifestations of syphilis which are unrelated to one or the other phenomenon. Primary and secondary syphilis proceeds as an endarteritis about the small vessels; cardiovascular syphilis is a consequence of recurrent inflammation and healing in the wall of the aorta; and inflammation of the cerebral vessels is prominently involved in diffuse meningovascular syphilis as well as in general paresis. Chronic inflammation of the hypersensitive type is most conspicuous in the development of the gummata.

Portal of Entry The disease is practically always acquired by sexual contact. Although a surface lesion is almost always involved in the sexual transfer of infection, it is often painless, inconspicuous, or hidden. Since more than half of the recently reported cases in males in urban areas of France, the United Kingdom, and the United States have been in homosexuals, the oral cavity and the anorectal area not uncommonly serve as the portal of entry. In prenatal (congenital) syphilis the infection may be transmitted to the fetus in utero by placental transfer from the mother.

Incubation Period The organism first penetrates the mucous membrane or, in rare instances, a break in the skin. It multiplies locally, spreads to the regional lymph nodes in a matter of hours, and without further delay enters the bloodstream. For about 3 weeks extensive local and systemic multiplication of the organism proceeds in the absence of signs or symptoms of infection. At this time the incubation period comes to an end with the appearance of a primary lesion (hard chancre) at the site of infection.

Primary Syphilis The typical hard chancre, usually located on the penis or the vulva, has an indurated base and an eroded surface with se-

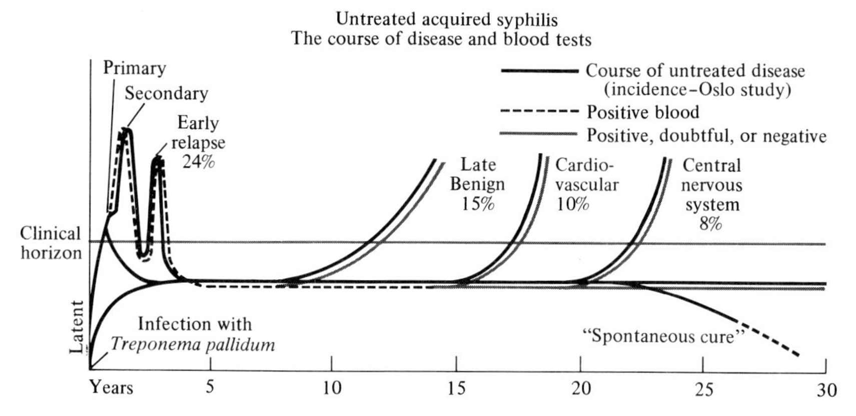

Figure 21-1 The natural history of untreated acquired syphilis. (*E. G. Clark and N. Danbolt, Med. Clin. North Am., 48:613–623, 1964; R. H. Kampmeier, Med. Clin. North Am., 48:667–697, 1964; and H. J. Morgan, South. Med. J., 26:18–22, 1933.*)

rous discharge, is painless, and red in color. Lesions commonly appear as areas of simple induration. In other cases the primary lesion may be so inapparent that it escapes the notice of the infected individual, especially when it is located on the cervix. Extragenital primary lesions of the fingers, lips, and tongue tend to be painful and prominent, whereas those in other parts of the oral cavity and the perianal region are inconspicuous and not painful.

The appearance of the chancre is usually accompanied by enlargement of the regional lymph nodes without suppuration.

Healing of the primary lesion begins in 3 to 8 weeks, and new epithelium eventually grows over the surface. The degree of scarring is variable, and none may be evident. The regional lymphadenopathy subsides gradually and may persist to some extent for several months.

Secondary Syphilis The secondary stage, which frequently but not invariably develops 1 to 3 months after spontaneous healing of the primary lesion, is characterized by the appearance of widespread mucocutaneous lesions. The typical rash is maculopapular, symmetrical, and diffuse, involving the entire skin, including the palms of the hands and the soles of the feet. In the oral cavity, the lesions are usually eroded (mucous patches), and around the genitalia lesions may become condylomatous. The genital lesions are large, flat, elevated plaques which may be as large as 2 to 3 cm in diameter.

The secondary stage is the most highly contagious because the lesions are literally teeming with spirochetes and because there are many lesions from which the infection may spread instead of the usual single lesion of primary syphilis. Secondary lesions on glabrous skin are not infectious because they are covered with a protective epithelial coat. In the genital area, the lesions become eroded because of the constant moisture, and the disease retains its essential venereal character.

As noted in Figure 21-1, evidence of secondary relapse occurs in 24 percent of cases and may involve multiple episodes. Clinically and epidemiologically it is important to observe that in 85 percent of relapses the lesions appeared in the mouth, throat, or anogenital areas. The majority of relapses (69 percent) occur within 6 months, 88 percent within 1 year, and 95 percent within 2 years. In general, they occur somewhat earlier in males than in females. Thereafter, 65 percent of untreated syphilitics are "cured," i.e., do not experience clinical manifestations.

Latent Stage The latent, or quiescent, phase commences with the spontaneous resolution of secondary syphilis and may persist for 2 to 20 years or longer. Since there are no clinical signs or symptoms during this stage, the diagnosis is based on a high titer of reagin in the serum confirmed as syphilitic by a treponemal test.

Latent Benign (Tertiary) Syphilis In the past, the late manifestations of the disease commonly appeared as granulomatous lesions (gummata) about 10 to 20 years or longer after infection. The gummata had a predilection for the skin, the bones, and the mucous membranes of the upper respiratory tract and the oral cavity. Today, gummata are rarely seen.

Late Cardiovascular (Tertiary) Syphilis The basic pathological lesion of cardiovascular syphilis is aortitis which develops 10 to 20 years after infection except in persons infected before the age of 15. Its clinical complications are aortic insufficiency, saccular aneurysm of the aorta, or stenosis of the coronary arteries. The incidence is almost twice as high in males as in females, with the highest rates occurring between the ages of 35 and 55. Although not the most frequent cause of death in syphilis, the most common lesion at necropsy is found in the cardiovascular system. Aneurysms of the thoracic aorta are more prevalent than those in the abdominal aorta, and the prognosis is gloomy.

Late (Tertiary) Neurosyphilis Aortitis and neurosyphilis frequently occur together. In contrast to cardiovascular syphilis, neurosyphilis develops in 6.1 percent, but cardiovascular syphilis appears in none of those infected before 15 years of age. When initial infection occurs in patients over 40 years of age, the nervous system is rarely involved. In neurosyphilis the male-to-female ratio is 4 to 1 or greater.

The earliest clinical manifestations involve the meninges and the cerebral vessels. The meningitis which results may be acute or chronic. The leptomeninges show opacity, patches of fibrous thickening, and small discrete focal lesions or gummata. The large and medium-sized vessels show endarteritis with necrosis and fibrosis of the media, leading to secondary thrombosis and rupture. Similar changes occur in the veins, and the lumina of the smaller arteries are reduced. The end result is a reduction in the blood supply to the brain. Hemiplegia is not uncommon.

The hallmarks of late neurosyphilis are general paresis and tabes dorsalis, which in the majority of instances appear 10 to 30 years following infection. General paresis, formerly one of the commonest causes of admission to mental hospitals, is an inflammatory destructive disease of the entire brain. The disease progresses over a period of 1 to 5 years with steady intellectual and physical deterioration, ultimately terminating in death.

Tabes dorsalis is manifest as a chronic degenerative disease involving sensory roots, afferent fibers, dorsal columns of the spinal cord, and occasionally the cranial nerves. Although the disease may become quiescent, in the majority of cases it is marked by intense spasmodic pains in the legs, ataxia, diplopia, hypesthesia, and hyperesthesia. Over a period of many years there is evidence of increasing disability and invalidism, and ultimately death may result. About 10 to 15 percent of all tabetics develop optic atrophy which frequently progresses to total blindness in 2 to 10 years.

Prenatal (Congenital) Syphilis Prenatal syphilis occurs when a pregnant woman with primary, secondary, or latent syphilis transmits the infection across the placenta to the fetus after the fourth month of gestation. The conse-

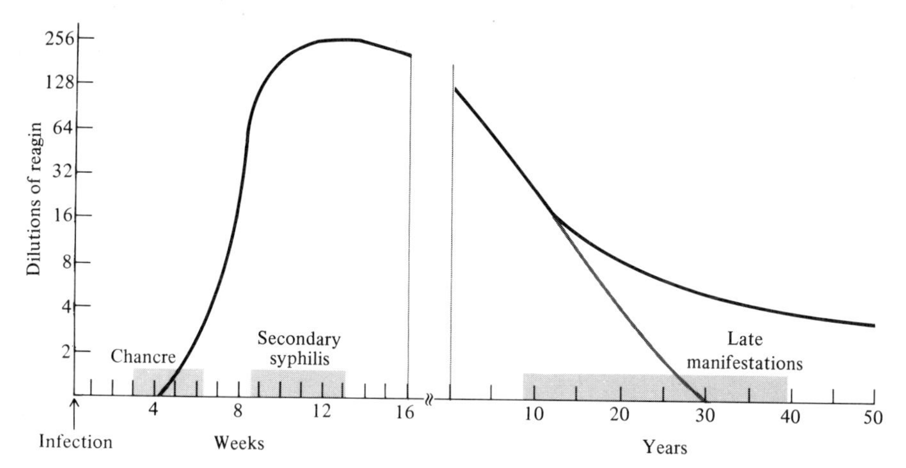

Figure 21-2 Time course of reagin antibody in untreated syphilis. Thirty years after infection about 50 percent of reagin tests are nonreactive. (*Public Health Service Publication, no. 743, July 1961.*)

quences for the fetus are devastating. About 25 percent of prenatal infections produce death before birth, while 25 to 30 percent of newborn infants die shortly after birth, and 40 percent develop late syphilis. Early postnatal manifestations include lesions of the mucous membranes and mucocutaneous areas. Rhinitis is an early finding and may be accompanied by a hemorrhagic nasal discharge. Fissures which heal by scarring may occur about the lips and perianally. Cutaneous lesions resemble those of secondary syphilis and are most common around the lips, on the palms and soles, and in the anogenital area. The most common lesion is osteochondritis of the nose and lower legs, which is associated with intense pain and tenderness. Hepatosplenomegaly occurs in almost two-thirds of the cases, and meningitis may be found in half.

Spirochetes may be demonstrated in umbilical blood by dark-field examination in more than half the cases. Cutaneous and mucocutaneous lesions are regularly positive, and the spirochetes are particularly abundant in the nasal discharge. Spirochetes are so abundant in fetal syphilitic liver that this tissue was used as the original source of the antigen for complement fixation. Placental transfer of both reagin and treponemal antibodies occurs and complicates but does not preclude a serological diagnosis.

The late lesions of prenatally acquired syphilis may develop after 2 years of age and seldom occur after the age of 30. In decreasing frequency the lesions involve interstitial keratitis, neurosyphilis, bilateral synovitis affecting the knees, arthritis, and neural deafness. Cardiovascular involvement is extremely rare. Some of the lesions of prenatal syphilis produce scars which persist as stigmata. The most common condition, and pathognomonic of the disease, is the presence of Hutchinson's upper central incisors which are barrel-shaped or show a convergence of both lateral margins toward the cutting edge. Syphilitic involvement of the first molar also occurs. Another manifestation, saddlenose, results from destructive osseous changes. Previous tibial osteitis persists as saber shin.

Laboratory Diagnosis

Dark-field Examination Properly prepared and quickly executed dark-field examination will reveal the organism in most open or abraded primary and secondary syphilitic lesions and permits an immediate diagnosis of the disease. An experienced observer will encounter no difficulty in demonstrating the organism in the base of penile chancres. In contrast, darkfield identification of *T. pallidum* in lesions in the female genital tract, the oral cavity, and the anorectal area is difficult because of the presence of other spirochetes as part of the normal flora. Differentiation of these spirochetes from *T. pallidum* is based on size, type of coil, and motility and is best done by experts.

Serologic Tests Tests for reagin usually become positive 4 to 5 weeks after infection or about 1 to 2 weeks after the appearance of the primary lesion. In secondary syphilis reagin tests are almost always positive. Reagin usually persists in the serum of untreated syphilitics for 10 years or more. Thereafter, the reagin test may spontaneously revert to negative in untreated "cures." Thirty years after infection, about 50 percent of reagin tests in untreated syphilitics are negative (Fig. 21-2).

The two greatest limitations of reagin tests are the frequency of biologic false positive reactions and the lack of reactivity (false negative), especially in tabes dorsalis but occasionally in cardiovascular syphilis and neurosyphilis. Biologic false positive reactions are most common in malaria and leprosy and occur with a frequency of 10 percent or more in a number of diseases including typhus, vaccinia, *Mycoplasma* pneumonia, lymphogranuloma venereum, infectious mononucleosis, lupus erythematosus, and infectious hepatitis.

Quantitative reagin titers are especially useful in assessing the adequacy of treatment in adults and in following infants suspected of having prenatal syphilis. Despite their limitations, qualitative reagin tests are invaluable as screening procedures when correlated with clinical observation and when employed in conjunction with epidemiologic investigations.

Table 21-1 The Long-Term Fate of Untreated Syphilis

"Spontaneous cure"		65%
Primary cause of death		11%
Excess mortality (all ages)		58%
Secondary relapses		24%
Multiple episodes	23%	
Location in mouth, throat, anogenital area	85%	
In 6 months	69%	
In 1 year	88%	
In 2 years	95%	
In 5 years	100%	
Late cardiovascular syphilis		10%
Aortic insufficiency	60%	
Saccular aneurysm	30%	
Stenosis of coronary arteries	6%	
Uncomplicated aortitis	4%	
Late neurosyphilis		8%
Diffuse meningovascular	37%	
General paresis	33%	
Tabes dorsalis	27%	
Gummata of the brain	3%	

Source: Adapted from E. G. Clark and N. Danbolt, *Med. Clin. North Am.*, 48:613–623, 1964; and R. H. Kampmeier, *Med. Clin. North Am.*, 48:667–697, 1964.

The chief value of the FTA test is that it can be used to distinguish the true positives from the biologic false positive reagin group. The FTA test is positive in one-third of patients with primary syphilis, two-thirds of patients with secondary syphilis, and almost all patients in other stages of syphilis. Treponemal antibody, once present, persists for life. However, the appearance of this antibody can be prevented by chemotherapy early in the course of syphilis.

Epidemiology

Incidence

Morbidity and Mortality The essential venereal nature and the characteristic early clinical manifestations of syphilis were recognized and recorded at the close of the fifteenth century.

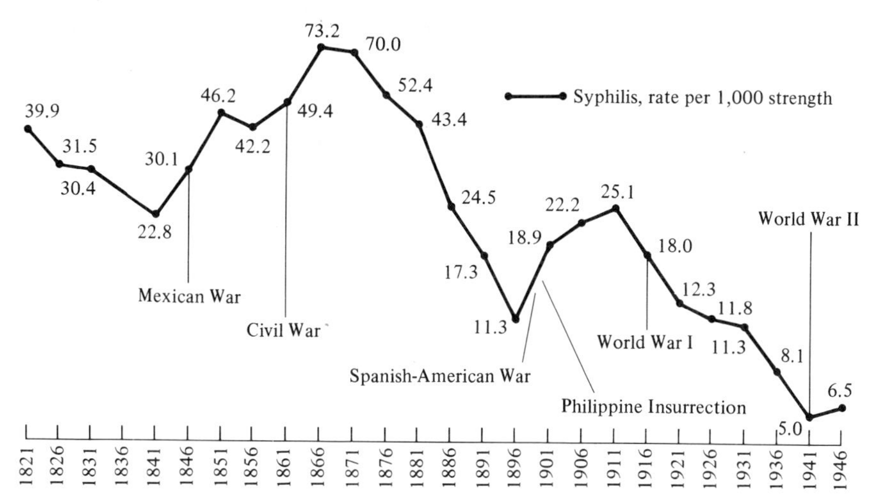

Figure 21-3 Syphilis in the United States Army. (*W. L. Fleming, Med. Clin. North Am., 48:587–612, 1964; and J. E. Moore, Am. J. Syph. Gon. Vener. Dis., 35:101–134, 1951.*)

Since that time syphilis has been one of the world's major health problems, especially among armies and seafaring populations. The data included in Figure 21-3 show the increased incidence which followed the Mexican, Civil, and Spanish-American Wars. The expected upsurge after World Wars I and II was prevented by the application of effective treatment and control programs. The introduction of serological tests and dark-field microscopy in the first decade of the twentieth century provided the tools needed to develop an understanding of the natural history of the disease. The Oslo study accurately assessed the long-term risks for untreated syphilitics in an outstanding example of the epidemiological method (Fig. 21-1 and Table 21-1).

Among World War II draftees in the United States serological tests were positive in 1.8 percent of whites and 24.5 percent of nonwhites. The data do not indicate the actual prevalence of syphilis because the actual number of biological false positives is not known, but they do provide a rough indication of the relative frequency of syphilis in the two groups. Rates for both whites and nonwhites were highest in the South.

The Changing Scene Historically, and in many countries today, the prostitute is important in the spread of syphilis. In Western countries, however, spread of the disease is most effectively accomplished by the promiscuous amateur, the teen-ager, and the homosexual. Half of the cases of infectious syphilis are in persons under 25 years of age, and 15 percent or more are in those under 20. Recent investigations in urban areas of the United States, the United Kingdom, and France have shown that between 44.5 and 70 percent of all cases of syphilis occur in male homosexuals because of their greater promiscuity. Ordinarily the homosexual experiences three times the number of contacts as does the heterosexual. One recently reported homosexual with syphilis had 86 different contacts including 11 women in the 4 weeks preceding the recognition of his infection.

The various clinical forms of the disease have shown conflicting trends between 1958 and 1973 (Fig. 21-4). The most striking and alarming

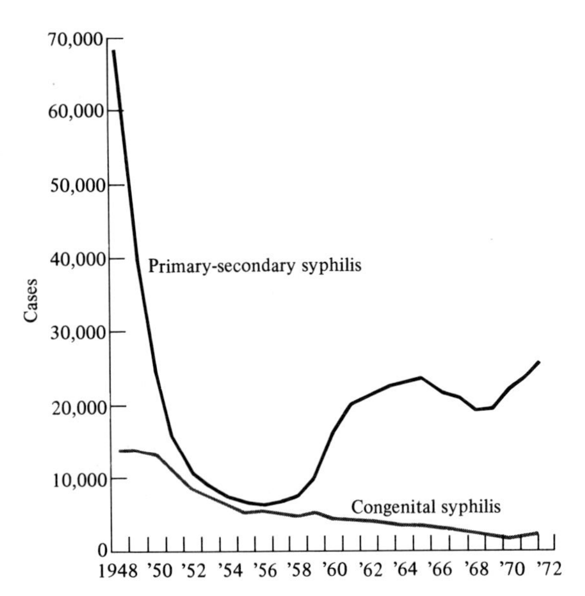

Figure 21-4 Primary, secondary, and congenital syphilis—reported civilian cases in the United States from 1948 to 1972. [*Morbidity Mortality Weekly Report, 20(53):66, 1972; and Morbidity Mortality Weekly Report, 21(52):445, 1972.*]

change during this period has been the threefold increase in primary and secondary syphilis in the United States. The rate of late syphilis has continued to decline.

Prevention and Control

The Central Problem The central problem in the prevention and control of syphilis is associated with the failure to detect the majority of cases. Effective methods are available to establish a definitive diagnosis early in the course of the disease, to eliminate the infection with adequate doses of penicillin, and to uncover hidden cases by contact and cluster interviewing. Nonetheless, accomplishment falls far short of possible attainment, primarily because only 1 of 10 cases seen by the physician is reported. Thus, the contacts, suspected contacts, and associates of 9 of every 10 cases treated by the physician represent a vast reservoir of infection that is free

Table 21-2 Major Findings of the Oslo Study of Untreated Syphilitics

About 65 percent of untreated syphilitics recover spontaneously after passing through the primary and secondary stages of the disease.
There is no way to predict the outcome in the individual case.
Secondary relapse or the appearance of late benign syphilis has no prognostic significance.
Secondary relapses prolong the period during which the infection may be transmitted.
Serious late manifestations including cardiovascular syphilis, neurosyphilis, and death occur twice as frequently in males as in females.
Syphilitics show a greater mortality from other conditions than do nonsyphilitics. Excess deaths are greatest between the ages of 30 and 50.

Source: Adapted from E. G. Clark and N. Danbolt, *Med. Clin. North Am.*, 48:613–623, 1964; and R. H. Kampmeier, *Med. Clin. North Am.*, 48:667–697, 1964.

to be furtively and extensively spread through the community.

Figure 21-5 indicates the recommended procedures and the typical results of contact and cluster interviewing which should be immediately and thoroughly applied in each newly diagnosed case. The first essential step in this process is for the physician to report every identified case promptly to public health authorities skilled in interviewing and in avoiding embarrassment to the patient.

Secondary factors interfering with case finding are related to the inherent nature of the disease, including those factors listed in Table 21-2.

Mechanical prophylaxis through the use of condoms offers the best method of personal protection, but these are rarely employed by those having the greatest exposure.

Treatment The target of an effective control program in syphilis is the adequate treatment of every early case. For this purpose, penicillin

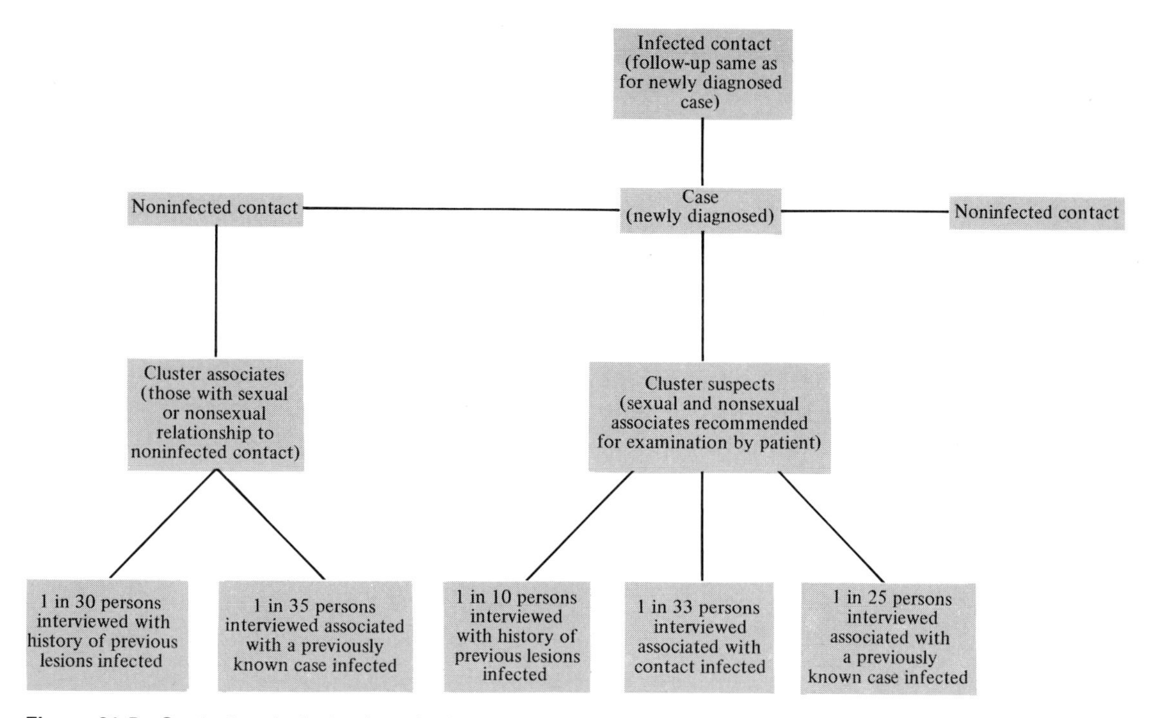

Figure 21-5 Contact and cluster interviewing in syphilis and the detection of cases based on serological findings.

produces a dramatic result as measured by the rapid healing of primary and secondary lesions followed by a loss of serologic reactivity and continued freedom from clinical disease. As indicated in Table 21-3, penicillin is the drug of choice for all stages of the disease.

Clinical inspection and quantitative reagin tests are important parts of the follow-up program for every treated patient. In patients with primary, secondary, or early latent syphilis, reagin tests on serum are performed monthly for 6 months, then at 3-month intervals for 1 year. The spinal fluid is examined for reagin 1 year after completion of chemotherapy. In latent syphilis, late benign, and cardiovascular syphilis, the patient's serum should be tested for reagin at 6-month intervals for 2 years, and a negative spinal fluid examination should be obtained either at diagnosis or before discharge. In patients with neurosyphilis, quantitative reagin tests on serum and spinal fluid are performed at 3-month intervals for the first year and at 6-month intervals for the second year. When the cell count and total protein in the spinal fluid return to normal, the disease is no longer active.

In cardiovascular syphilis, damaged or scarred vessels and valves do not return to normal function. In neurosyphilis, the destructive progression of the lesions will be halted. With healing, some recovery of impaired activities may occur; but obviously, where neuronal necrosis has occurred, recovery of function is not possible. While the detection and management of cardiovascular syphilis and neurosyphilis present a special and enduring problem for the physician, he can largely prevent their future occurrence by reporting to public health authorities every case of primary, secondary, and early latent syphilis he treats. Prenatal (congenital) syphilis, on the other hand, is an entirely preventable disease when the pregnant mother is treated with penicillin prior to the fourth month of her pregnancy.

Prognosis of Treated Syphilis Arsphenamine, fever therapy, sulfonamides, and penicillin have exerted profound influences on the long-term fate of infection with *T. pallidum*, and mortality has dropped sharply. A reversal in the proportion of deaths from neurosyphilis and cardiovascular syphilis was in large part a consequence of the introduction of fever therapy for the treatment of paresis. In the Oslo study and in the United States in 1900, the ratio of deaths from neurosyphilis to those from cardiovascular syphilis was approximately 3 to 1, whereas in 1958 the ratio was 1 to 3.5.

With the use of penicillin in the treatment of syphilis and, of incidental but perhaps equal importance, its use for other infections, the decline in late clinical manifestations of syphilis has been greatly accelerated. Gummata have virtually disappeared, syphilitic aortic aneurysms have become extremely rare, and there has been a sharp decline in neurosyphilis.

The course of syphilis has been confused by the apparent widespread use of penicillin, often in inadequate dosage, by exposed or infected individuals in attempts at personal prophylaxis or treatment. Self-treatment makes recognition of primary and secondary lesions more difficult. In addition, it creates a potentially dangerous situation for the patient which may eventually result in neurosyphilis or cardiovascular syphilis.

Immunity There can be no doubt that a relative state of specific immunity develops 2 years or more after infection with *T. pallidum*. In the untreated disease literally billions of organisms are killed as the primary and secondary lesions heal, and the spirochetes are later effectively removed from the blood. Thereafter, and in the absence of treatment, 65 percent of previously infected individuals never exhibit any further clinical manifestations of syphilis. Experiments with previously uninfected volunteers have

Table 21-3 The Result of Effective Treatment of Syphilis with Penicillin*

Stage of disease	Recommended dose of penicillin (units in millions)	Reagin titer	Prognosis
Primary	2.4 to 4.8	Quickly becomes nonreactive	Excellent
Secondary	4.8	Reverts steadily and becomes nonreactive, but not as rapidly as in primary stage	Excellent
Early latent	4.8 to 9.6	Remains stable or declines gradually	Excellent
Late latent			
CSF negative	9.6	Remains stable or declines gradually	Excellent
CSF positive	14.4	Remains stable or declines gradually	Good
Late	14.4	Remains stable or declines gradually	Unsatisfactory unless treatment is begun early

* The indicated chemotherapy with penicillin would also prove adequate for the treatment of gonorrhea, which is often simultaneously present in syphilitic patients.

shown that 57 spirochetes sufficed to induce syphilis in half of those challenged, whereas 100,000 spirochetes were necessary to cause reinfection in 10 of 26 volunteers who had been treated for primary, secondary, or early latent syphilis of less than 2 years' duration. More significantly, none of five volunteers with untreated latent syphilis of more than 2 years' duration were reinfected when challenged with 100,000 organisms. There is abundant evidence that reagin is totally unrelated to specific immunity, and no direct relationship of treponemal antibody has been established.

Prospective

The physician occupies a pivotal position in efforts to control syphilis. Unless he reports every case he identifies and treats to public health authorities, syphilis will continue its recent increase. Public health authorities must be prepared to pursue a vigorous program of contact and cluster interviewing to search out and bring to treatment every early case of syphilis. But the battle must not end with this accomplished. Syphilis has proved to be an unrelenting foe. The program must not only be continued, it must be expanded. It ultimately must encompass every member of society, but initially must concentrate on an education and social action program concerned with those at greatest risk. In this category are to be found the poor and uneducated, the promiscuous amateur, the teenager, and the homosexual. Those especially concerned with these groups include parents, teachers, clergymen, lawyers, judges, sociologists, psychiatrists, and public health officials. Tomorrow others will replace those at greatest current risk. The problem of syphilis is the problem of society itself.

GONORRHEA

Gonorrhea has existed throughout the centuries and in spite of the efficacy of modern treatment continues to prevail. Incidence has increased in each year since 1957. For cogent reasons which will be developed in the succeeding pages, gonorrhea is proving to be more difficult to control effectively than syphilis or, indeed, most other diseases.

Perspective

Although the disease is unquestionably more ancient, the name *gonorrhea,* or *flow of seed,* was first applied to it by Galen in A.D. 130. A means of clinical recognition and a description of gonorrhea were recorded in 1376 by John of Arderne, surgeon to Richard II and Henry IV of England. It was not until 1879 that the causative agent was identified by Neisser and named the gonococcus. Bumm grew the organism in pure culture in 1885.

Early efforts at treatment were time-consuming, painful, prolonged, and not particularly effective. The sulfonamides were introduced into treatment in the late 1930s and following a brief interval of declining effectiveness were succeeded in 1943 by penicillin, which remains the drug of choice.

The Causative Agent

Biological Properties Man is the only known host. The causative organism, *Neisseria gonorrhoeae,* is found most commonly in urethral or vaginal discharges of infected persons and in other areas of the genital tract in asymptomatic carriers—primarily the female. Occasionally, it may be found in synovial fluid and more rarely in blood, skin lesions, and spinal fluid. In acute cases of gonorrhea the microorganism is characteristically located in the cytoplasm of polymorphonuclear leukocytes, and in smears of urethral exudate it is observed to be a gram-negative diplococcus, oval or kidney-shaped, with an overall size somewhat less than 1 μm.

Antigenic Structure The fluorescent antibody (FA) test, following appropriate preliminary absorption with other *Neisseria,* is of value in the specific identification of the organism. The antibody appears to be produced in response to a species-specific surface antigen with characteristics similar to Vi and K antigens of the gram-negative enteric bacteria (Chap. 18). The antigen may, in fact, be associated with the virulence of the gonococcus. The virulent clonal type (type 1) is stimulated by ferric ion in a modified chocolate agar medium.

Pathogenesis and Natural History of the Disease

Infection with the gonococcus occurs following sexual intercourse or, on occasion, following pederasty. The person transmitting the organism may be symptomatic (a male or less frequently a female with urethral discharge) or an asymptomatic female carrier. During the incubation period of 3 to 5 days the gonococcus invades the anterior urethra in males and quickly produces a purulent discharge. This rarely occurs in females. The infection may spread posteriorly to other areas of the genital tract containing columnar epithelium. The prostate, epididymis, seminal vesicles, and testes may become involved in the male. In females, infection may traverse the cervix and involve the fallopian tubes. If this occurs, sterility frequently results because of adhesions, stricture, and pyosalpinx secondary to salpingitis. Portions of the genital tract containing stratified squamous epithelium are spared. Spontaneous cure is common but is often delayed for several months in females (Fig. 21-6). In 1.5 to 2.5 percent of untreated cases, arthritis (usually monoarticular) may occur 1 to 4 weeks after infection, commonly involving the knee, wrist, and ankle. In rare instances, gonococcemia, endocarditis, or meningitis results.

Ophthalmia Neonatorum Gonococci present in the birth canal may infect the conjunctiva of the newborn during parturition. Subsequent involvement of the cornea is followed by ulceration, vascularization, healing, formation of scar tissue, and blindness. Instillation of a 1 percent solution of silver nitrate into the conjunctival sacs of every newborn infant, introduced by Credé in 1881, has proved to be an excellent method of chemoprophylaxis and has virtually eliminated gonococcal ophthalmia neonatorum. This disease accounted for 28 percent of new cases of blindness in 1907, but less than 0.1 percent in 1957.

Vulvovaginitis In prepubescent females gonococci may produce vulvovaginitis. The infection is transmitted by sexual contact. In most cases of vulvovaginitis, the gonococcus is not the causative agent.

Laboratory Diagnosis

Stained Smears The presence of gram-negative diplococci in the cytoplasm of polymorphonuclear leukocytes seen on smears prepared from acute clinical cases with purulent discharge is strong presumptive evidence of gonococcal infection. The diagnosis should be confirmed by culture and sugar fermentation reactions or by FA technique.

Culture The organism is fastidious in its growth requirements. Primary isolation of pathogenic *Neisseria (N. gonorrhoeae* and *N. meningitidis)* is best achieved on chocolate agar containing 3 units of vancomycin, 7.5 μg colistimethate, and 12.5 units of nystatin per ml of medium when incubated in an atmosphere containing 2 to 10 percent carbon dioxide. After heating, blood agar becomes a chocolate brown color as a result of lysis of the erythrocytes and denaturation and coagulation of the proteins and is less toxic to the gonococci. The antibiotics added to the medium almost completely pre-

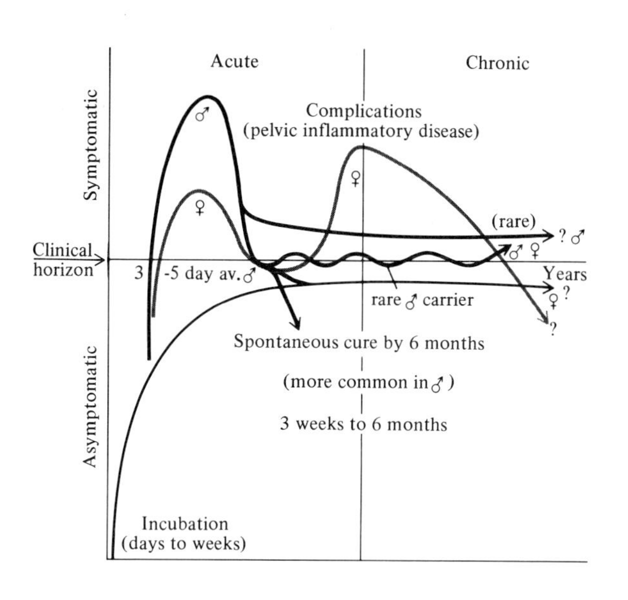

Portal of entry:
- Mucous membranes of the genital tract possessing columnar epithelial cells

Mechanism of transmission:
- Sexual intercourse

Source of infection in:
- Male contact
  - Urethral discharge (greater than 90 percent)
- Female contact
  - Asymptomatic carrier (greater than 90 percent)

Incubation period:
- 85 percent in 3–5 days

Spontaneous cure:
- Common in males
- Common but delayed in females

Posterior spread:
- Male
  - Prostatitis (15 percent)
  - Epididymitis (17 percent)(possible cause of sterility)
  - Urethral stricture (percentage unknown)
- Female
  - Salpingitis (14 percent)

Complications:
- Arthritis (1.5 to 2.5 percent)
- Gonococcemia (occasional)
- Endocarditis (rare)
- Meningitis (rare)

Figure 21-6 The pathogenesis and long-term fate of untreated infections with *Neisseria gonorrhoeae*. (*W.H.O. Tech. Rep. Ser., no. 262, 1963.*)

vent the growth of the normal bacterial flora—many of which are also gram-negative and oxidase-positive. These include *Mima* species and the saprophytic *N. sicca* and *N. catarrhalis*. However, it is important to note that *N. lactamica*, an organism with limited pathogenic potential, will grow in the presence of the antibiotics. *N. lactamica* is usually cultured from the pharynx, but can be isolated from genital specimens.

This selective medium has been particularly valuable in isolating *N. gonorrhoeae* from cervical, vaginal, and rectal specimens. As a consequence, the finding of oxidase-positive colonies of gram-negative diplococci on this medium represents a convenient, presumptive diagnostic procedure. In the absence of the antibiotics, oxidase-positive colonies resembling *N. gonorrhoeae* are recovered from approximately 16 percent of specimens from the genital tract of normal uninfected women.

Oxidase Test *Neisseria* colonies rapidly oxidize dimethyl-*p*-phenylenediamine HCl due to the presence of the enzyme indophenol oxidase. The oxidation is accompanied by the gradual development of a black color on the colonies.

Fluorescent Antibody As indicated by the data included in Table 21-4, the use of the delayed immunofluorescent technique for the detection and identification of gonococci in specimens from the genital tract of asymptomatic females represents a distinct improvement over the culture method. In the delayed FA procedure, the specimen is cultured for 16 to 20 hr. to accumulate gonococci in sufficient numbers for detection by fluorescent microscopy. In the direct FA method, the labeled antibody is immediately added to a smear prepared from the specimen and examined for fluorescence. A definitive identification by the direct FA tech-

Table 21-4 Identification of *N. gonorrhoeae* in 85,000 Specimens from the Urethra, Cervix, and Vagina of Asymptomatic Females

Method of identification	Composite group (% positive)	Gonorrheal contacts (% positive)
Oxidase-positive colonies on chocolate agar	22	59
Direct FA on smears	15	43
Delayed FA on culture of exudate	37	79

Source: Adapted from J. D. Thayer and M. B. Moore, Jr., *Med. Clin. North Am.*, 48:755–765, 1964.

nique requires less than 1 hr. Unfortunately, however, this technique is less sensitive than the delayed FA procedure and also exhibits nonspecific fluorescence.

Latex Agglutination Test The presence of gonorrheal antibody in serum can be demonstrated by the rapid agglutination of latex particles coated with antigen extracted from *N. gonorrhoeae.* Before testing, the patient's serum is reacted with antigen prepared from guinea pig and beef tissue in order to remove interfering substances which may be found in some serum samples. The latex test may be negative in patients from whom positive cultures are obtained, cannot distinguish between active gonorrhea and past infection, and is frequently positive in meningococcal infections and carriers. Nonetheless, the test is a useful adjunct to diagnosis, similar to reagin flocculation tests in syphilis, especially in asymptomatic females. A positive latex test in females is an indication for a complete culture work-up utilizing specimens obtained from the cervix, rectum, and pharynx. Suspect cultures are then confirmed by sugar fermentation reactions or by FA tests.

Epidemiology

Prevalence Gonorrhea is the most prevalent of the venereal diseases. In the United States an estimated 3.75 million new cases, of which 750,000 are reported, occur annually (Fig. 21-7). Gonorrhea ranks third to measles and streptococcal infections among reported cases of notifiable diseases in the United States; but in actual fact, its incidence is believed to be greatest, although this is unconfirmed because of the widespread failure to report cases. Studies have shown that the actual incidence of gonorrhea exceeds that reported by a factor of 5 or even 100. Annual incidence on a worldwide basis is estimated at 60 to 65 million infections, with an estimated 7.6 million occurring annually in India alone.

Among reported cases, the male-to-female ratio varies between 2 to 1 and 4 to 1. This ratio is highly unreliable, however, as is demonstrated whenever investigation is made. In Denmark, the United States, and England, the true male-to-female ratios for all ages are 1 to 1.6, 1 to 1.7, and 1 to 1.9, respectively. Partially because of earlier sexual maturity in women, gonorrhea is much more common in teen-age females than in teen-age males. In England, for example, in the 15- to 19-year-old group the ratio is 1 to 4, while in the 20- to 24-year-old group the ratio is 1 to 1.4. In females in the Scandinavian countries, the greatest number of cases occur in the 15- to 19-year-old group, and the rate per 100,000 is highest in this age group. Not only are the rates higher among teen-agers but in almost all countries they have steadily increased since 1957. Figures vary somewhat, depending on the completeness of the study and the particular country

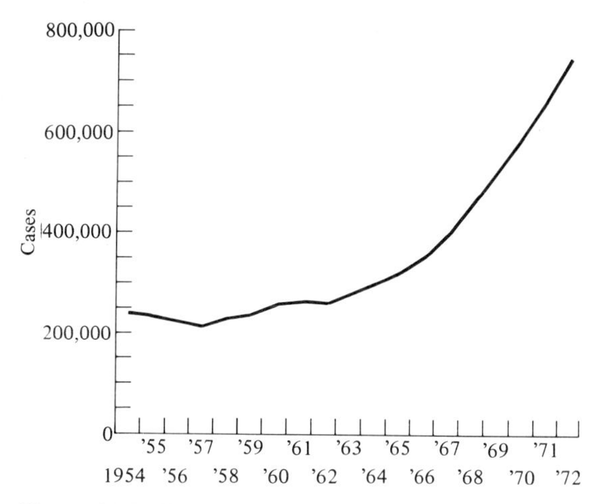

Figure 21-7 Reported civilian cases of gonorrhea in the United States from 1954 to 1972. [*Morbidity Mortality Weekly Report, 20(53):67, 1972; and Morbidity Mortality Weekly Report, 21(52):445, 1972.*]

or area involved, but it is estimated at present that 1 to 2 percent of the world's population between 15 and 24 years of age is infected with gonococci.

The problem groups include prostitutes, promiscuous amateurs, teen-agers, homosexuals, servicemen, and migrants. The role that each plays varies geographically. Between 30 and 50 percent of prostitutes have asymptomatic gonorrhea. In Africa and Asia, the proportion of infections originating from prostitutes is estimated to be between 80 and 97 percent; in Europe the prostitute serves as the source of infection in 16 to 34 percent of cases. In the United States and Canada, the promiscuous amateur, the teen-ager, and the homosexual have taken over from the prostitute as the main sources of infection. Gonorrhea is much more common in military as contrasted with civilian populations. For example, the military-to-civilian ratio in Japan was 7.5 to 1 and 5.2 to 1 in 1951 and 1956, respectively. In England and Wales in 1961 migrant workers from other countries constituted 1.4 percent of the population but 27.3 percent of the cases of gonorrhea. A survey conducted on Swedish ships between 1957 and 1960 revealed that 7 percent of the crew members were infected with gonococci. An important finding in this study was that 90 percent of those infected had a urethral discharge. This is almost the exact reverse of the situation which obtains in females proved to be sources of infection, 90 percent of whom are asymptomatic.

Two particularly difficult groups are repeaters and defaulters. *Repeaters* are those who have been successfully treated and quickly become reinfected. Approximately 20 to 30 percent of cases seen annually represent second infections within the same year. *Defaulters* are those who do not return for clinical evaluation and cultures and who are lost to effective epidemiological control. In one study less than 10 percent of those treated were observed for the recommended period of 3 months.

The Reservoir The reservoir of gonococcal infection is much more extensive than that in syphilis. More than half of all gonococcal infections (90 percent in females) are both asymptomatic and chronic, thus favoring the spread of the infection through the community. The latex agglutination test may prove useful in the detection of the asymptomatic carrier state in the female, but must be substantiated by positive cultures. No effective immunity develops in gonorrhea. Consequently, a person who recovers from gonorrhea or who is successfully treated can be readily reinfected.

Because of the short incubation period of 3 to 5 days and the efficiency of the method of transmission, the potential for spreading gonorrhea is great. It has been calculated that starting with 1 infected patient, and assuming only 1 contact per infected person, 64 persons could acquire gonorrhea in 21 days (the incubation period of syphilis) and in a period of 63 days, 1,048,576 cases of gonorrhea could result, as compared to 10 in syphilis.

The short incubation period is responsible for

another major problem: the difficulty of finding and treating contacts before they have spread the infection. In addition, there are many accessory factors which contribute to the expansion of the reservoir. These include the attitude of infected persons toward the disease, their educational and economic status, the recognition that gonorrhea is a less serious disease than syphilis, and the development of strains of *N. gonorrhoeae* that are increasingly resistant to penicillin. In addition, the public health effort has been diverted to syphilis and away from gonorrhea. Inadequate numbers of experienced investigators and insufficient public health budgets have hampered wide-scale contact and cluster interviewing within 6 days after recognition of a case of gonorrhea *(speed zone epidemiology)*. On the other hand, the latex agglutination test may facilitate epidemiological evaluation because great numbers of patients can be screened rapidly.

Prevention and Control

The Central Problems Prevention and control of gonorrhea are largely impeded by the nature of the disease. In the male, the detection of gonorrhea is relatively simple because most infections present external clinical manifestations, primarily urethral discharge. On the other hand, the female diagnosis is difficult because 90 percent of infections are asymptomatic. The most sensitive methods permit laboratory detection of only 80 percent of asymptomatic females, but this situation might be improved by the development of a more specific latex agglutination test.

No practical immunity develops upon natural recovery or following adequate chemotherapy. This is most unfortunate because studies reveal that 54 percent of infections among teen-agers occur in problem groups (repeaters and defaulters). Despite intense educational efforts, 26 percent of these young people become reinfected in 6 months.

Personal protection against reinfection is best achieved through the use of condoms, but these are rarely employed by individuals having the greatest exposure.

Treatment Since its introduction in 1943, penicillin has been the drug of choice in the treatment of gonorrhea. Although there has been a gradual change in the sensitivity to penicillin of cultures of gonococci, most gonorrheal infections can be successfully treated with 4,800,000 or more units of penicillin. This dosage of penicillin will also effectively suppress syphilitic infections prior to onset of the primary lesion.

Penicillin resistance of gonococci is less of a problem in the United States than in some other countries largely as a result of the practice in this country of using high concentrations of penicillin for the treatment of gonorrhea. In addition to inadequate chemotherapy, so-called treatment "failures" may occasionally be due to reinfection with the gonococcus or to nongonococcal urethritis. The majority of patients harboring strains of gonococci most resistant to penicillin have been exposed to prostitutes outside the United States who have received low doses of penicillin at semimonthly intervals as a prophylactic measure against syphilis. While syphilis is thus prevented, these concentrations of the drug readily permit the selection of penicillin-resistant strains of gonococci.

Since the introduction of penicillin, the incidence of gonococcal epididymitis has been reduced from 17 to 0.7 percent; however, the incidence of gonococcal salpingitis has declined only slightly from 14 to 9 percent, mainly because of the large number of asymptomatic female cases which remain undetected until salpingitis develops.

Prospective

In working toward the prevention and control of gonorrhea one of the key questions is where to start. Since the disease may be readily diagnosed in the male, this is a reasonable place to begin. An attainable goal would be to bring every infected male to examination and treatment. This will accomplish little, however, unless there is a rapid and extensive program of contact and cluster interviewing. Every female contact, cluster suspect, and cluster associate must be singled out for special attention and examined repeatedly for the presence of gonococci by the culture and delayed FA methods. When any male becomes infected following sexual contact with a female member of this group, that female should be considered to have gonorrhea and should be placed under treatment. To have any impact on the incidence of gonorrhea in a community, the program must be continuous and comprehensive.

At this point, it is pertinent to pose a few questions. Are the public health authorities prepared to institute such a program which can at best keep the lid on gonorrhea? Apparently not. The response to this approach in pilot studies of problem groups has been discouraging. On the national level, less than 15 percent of all cases of gonorrhea are subjected to any epidemiological control at all. Where are the trained investigators and the necessary funds to be found to pursue an effective program of epidemiological control? Will this situation change if a more specific latex agglutination test can be developed?

It has become obvious that other methods must be considered and evaluated. What would happen if public health authorities mobilized their resources to mount a long-range nationwide educational campaign directed at the level of those 13 to 14 years of age in cooperation with the parents, the schools, the churches, and the press on a community-wide basis? Is the nation prepared to accept such a campaign? The only acceptable answer is that it must be prepared. It is recognized that in slum areas the campaign must begin at an earlier age. Without a concomitant frontal attack on social problems in general, the hope for success is negligible. It is easy to be pessimistic and difficult to be optimistic about the prospects for preventing and controlling gonorrhea, but the problem can no longer be ignored.

OTHER VENEREAL INFECTIONS

Compared to syphilis and gonorrhea, other infections which are transmitted venereally are of secondary importance. Included in this group are those infections which are regularly transmitted by sexual contact (chancroid, granuloma inguinale, lymphogranuloma venereum, and trichomonas vulvovaginitis). These are briefly considered in this chapter. In addition, there are a number of infections which may be transmitted venereally, such as inclusion conjunctivitis (Chap. 19) and herpes (Chap. 22).

Chancroid (Soft Chancre)

Hemophilus ducreyi, the etiological agent of chancroid, is a short, gram-negative bacillus, 1 to 2 μm in length and 0.5 μm in width. The organism is a strict parasite of man. It grows well in 24 hr. in fresh rabbit blood containing hemin (X factor). The disease is transmitted by sexual contact. Its initial sign is a small papule or vesicle which appears after an incubation period of 4 to 10 days. A pustule marked by redness, edema, and induration rapidly forms, becomes necrotic, and ulcerates. Lymph node swellings in the groin (buboes) frequently occur, a few of which may progress and produce large suppurative lesions. Ordinarily, however, the ulcer heals in from 1 week to several months. The organism rarely invades the body beyond the regional lymph nodes. Although *H. ducreyi* seems to belong to a single antigenic type, no significant level of immunity accompanies recovery from the infection.

A laboratory diagnosis depends on (1) demonstration of the organisms in smears from the ulcerating lesions or buboes, preferably from material obtained by biopsy; (2) culture of the organism on blood agar plates; (3) a positive skin test of the delayed hypersensitivity type with the reaction appearing 24 to 48 hr. after the intradermal injection of a phenol-killed preparation of the organisms; (4) production of a local ulcerating lesion following autoinoculation of a pure culture of the organism into the skin of the forearm of the suspected patient; and (5) exclusion of other venereal infections by specific laboratory tests. Smears which are positive in 60 to 90 percent of cases usually suffice to establish the diagnosis. The skin test is positive in about two-thirds of patients.

The infection is found more commonly in the southern part of the United States and in warmer climates. Since 1954 reported cases of chancroid have declined steadily from 3,000 to 1,250 in 1964. When used, condoms provide the best method of prophylaxis. Sulfonamides are effective in chemotherapy, and when necessary streptomycin or the tetracyclines may be employed. Control is based on adequate treatment of the infected individual, and in appropriate situations, by case-finding techniques.

Granuloma Inguinale

Calymmatobacterium granulomatis (Klebsiella granulomatis) is a gram-negative bacillus with a well-defined capsule which is characteristically located in clusters (Donovan bodies) within the cytoplasm of monocytes present in the granulomatous or ulcerating lesions. Morphologically and antigenically the organism is closely related to numerous species of *Klebsiella* (Chap. 18). It grows best at a low redox (OR) potential on a modified chocolate agar. Capsular material obtained from the organism reacts with antibody from patients with the disease in precipitin and CF tests. A heat-killed suspension of the microorganisms produces a delayed type of hypersensitivity following intradermal inoculation in patients with current or past infection.

The incubation period is long (45 days in experimental human infections). The resulting disease primarily involves the skin and the mucous membranes. It occurs as a chronic, slowly progressive, granulomatous and ulcerative disease, usually localized in the genital and perianal area but occasionally involving the mouth, nose, and pharynx. The lesions spread by direct extension, often accompanied by thickening and fibrosis of the skin and subcutaneous tissues. Hyperplasias and active areas of regeneration often accompany inflammation of skin and mucous membranes. Some are so florid that they have been referred to as pseudocarcinomatous hyperplasias, yet few are associated with subsequent carcinomas. Spontaneous cure is uncommon.

A laboratory diagnosis usually depends upon the demonstration of the Donovan bodies in stained smears from the lesions or recovery of the organism on culture. Occasionally the diagnosis must be established by exclusion or by noting the therapeutic response to streptomycin or the tetracyclines. The disease occurs more frequently in the southern part of the United States and in tropical and subtropical areas of the world. Less than 150 cases are reported annually in the United States. Control may be partly provided by the use of condoms and by thorough washing with soap and water immediately after coitus. Treatment with streptomycin or the tetracyclines usually results in a cure.

Lymphogranuloma Venereum

The causative agent of lymphogranuloma venereum is an obligate intracellular parasite of man which for numerous reasons (cited in Chap. 2) is best regarded as a member of a group of agents known as chlamydiae (bedsoniae). The organism is most conveniently cultured in the yolk sac of the chick embryo. As a member of the chlamydiae group, the agent shares group-specific antigens with and has biological properties similar to psittacosis and trachoma and inclusion conjunctivitis organisms. The agent possesses specific antigens which react in CF and neutralization tests as well as a toxin which can be neutralized by specific antibody (Chap. 2). There is only one antigenic type.

The infection is transmitted during coitus. After an incubation period of 7 to 12 days, the disease begins as a small transient ulceration, often inconspicuous and unnoticed, at the site of contact on the penis or the vulva. In men, but only rarely in women, this is followed in a few days by enlargement and suppuration of the regional lymph nodes (buboes). At this time, systemic dissemination of the organism may occur, evidenced by constitutional signs and symptoms which in rare instances may eventuate in arthritis, conjunctivitis, or meningoencephalitis. Although the majority of infections, especially in the male, heal spontaneously, the inguinal lymphadenitis may persist for weeks or months.

In an unknown but significant number of females, the disease may progress, influenced by the proximity of the vagina to the rectum and by the lymphatic distribution in the perianal region. The vulvar lesions may result in urethral stricture, puffy swelling of the labia, and vaginal stenosis. The infection may spread in the vaginal tissue planes to invade the rectum where the fascia is thinnest and where rectum and vagina are closest together. The initial proctocolitis may be followed by rectal stricture in a few months to several years. Rectovaginal fistulas develop in about one-third of the patients with proctocolitis. During most of this time the women remain infectious.

A laboratory diagnosis may be established by isolation of the agent in the yolk sac of the chick embryo, followed by identification on the basis of morphology, staining reactions, and serological tests. Stained smears of pus, buboes, or biopsy material may be examined for the agent but are not of great value. CF tests are useful when the specific lymphogranuloma venereum antigen is used but are definitely diagnostic only when a rise in antibody titer is demonstrated in paired sera. A delayed hypersensitivity skin test (Frei test) is based on the intradermal injection of the heat-inactivated agent (commercially available as Lygranum). A positive test is manifest by the appearance of an inflammatory reaction which reaches a maximum in 2 to 4 days and means only that infection has occurred. If, however, the test is initially negative and then becomes positive, a definite diagnosis may be established.

Lymphogranuloma venereum exists throughout the world but is most common in the tropics. In 1964 less than 750 cases were reported in the United States, and most of these occurred in the southern part of the country. Immunity following recovery from the disease is somewhat obscured by the frequent persistence of the organism in spite of the presence of antibody, a property shared with other members of the chlamydiae group. Whatever its nature, immunity persists for life following recovery from a clinical attack. Treatment should be initiated early with sulfonamides, tetracyclines, or chloramphenicol. When treatment is delayed, stricture of genitoanorectal tissues may result. If the disease is far advanced at the time of diagnosis surgical intervention is almost always indicated. Control of the disease is difficult in the female because inguinal buboes are uncommon and the disease is often unrecognized for months or years after onset. During most of this interval, the women remain infectious and can transmit the disease to susceptible males. In areas and groups where lymphogranuloma venereum is prevalent, skin tests should be performed periodically, and positive reactors should be carefully evaluated clinically for evidence of disease.

Trichomonas Vulvovaginitis

Vulvovaginitis is the most common gynecological disorder. In addition to *Candida albicans*

(Chap. 16), the disease is frequently caused by large (15 to 18 μm), actively motile flagellates *(Trichomonas vaginalis).* The flagellate is found only in the trophozoite stage, moves by means of anterior flagella and an undulating membrane, and multiplies by binary fission.

The incidence of the disease is the reverse of that for gonorrhea in that females experience a high incidence of clinical infection, whereas males are generally asymptomatic and serve as a reservoir of infection. Infection is usually transmitted venereally but may be acquired by neonatal females born of infected mothers or indirectly when there is a breakdown in personal or communal hygiene (contaminated towels, for example). The disease is uncommon in young girls and postmenopausal women but may involve approximately 25 percent of the female population, especially those who practice poor personal hygiene or those who are concurrently affected with other venereal diseases. Other predisposing factors include pregnancy, estrogen deficiency, diabetes, carcinoma, and the use of antibiotics. Clinically, the vaginal mucosa is markedly hyperemic and painful, and there is a copious discharge of yellowish purulent material. Microscopic examination of freshly prepared wet mounts of cervical smears or vaginal discharge reveal the presence of large, motile trophozoites. In males, the flagellate can be demonstrated microscopically in the centrifuged specimen of first morning urine (15 ml).

Prevention and control are based on good personal hygiene, prompt treatment of the patient with metronidazole administered orally for about 10 days, and the detection and treatment of carriers among the sexual contacts of the patient.

BIBLIOGRAPHY

Fam, A., McGillivray, D., Stein, J., and Little, H.: "Gonococcal Arthritis: A Report of Six Cases," *Can. Med. Assoc. J.,* 108:319–325, 1973.

Gardner, H. L., and Kaufman, R. H. (eds.): "Viral Infections in Gynecology and Obstetrics," *Clin. Obstet. Gynecol.,* 15:856–1030, 1972.

"Gonorrhea," (symposium), *Br. J. Vener. Dis.,* 48: 496–521, 1972.

Jeerapaet, P., and Ackerman, A. B.: "Histologic Patterns in Secondary Syphilis," *Arch. Dermatol.,* 107:373–377, 1973.

Monif, G. R. G. (ed.): *Infectious Diseases in Obstetrics and Gynecology,* New York: Harper & Row, Publishers, Incorporated, 1973.

Nelson, M.: "Uncomplicated Male Gonorrhea," *Calif. Med.,* 118(1):10–13, 1973.

"Present Status of Gonorrhoea Control," (symposium), *Postgrad. Med. J.,* 48(suppl. 1):5–80, 1972.

Ris, H. W., and Dodge, R. W.: "Trichomonas and Yeast Vaginitis in Institutionalized Adolescent Girls," *Am. J. Dis. Child.,* 125:206–209, 1973.

"Serological and Immunological Tests in Treponemal Disease," (symposium), *Br. J. Vener. Dis.,* 48:460–495, 1972.

"Trichomoniasis," (symposium), *Br. J. Vener. Dis.,* 48:522–533, 1972.

"Venereal Disease," (symposium), *Practitioner,* 209:601–653, 1972.

Webster, B. (ed.): "Venereal Diseases," *Med. Clin. North Am.,* 56:1055–1220, 1972.

Chapter 22

Systemic Infections with Skin Lesions in Which Man Is the Reservoir

Bernard A. Briody

PERSPECTIVE

Skin lesions (exanthemata or rashes) are of diverse appearance and etiology. An understanding of their pathogenesis requires a comprehensive knowledge of medicine. In appearance the lesions may be vesicular, pustular, macular, papular, petechial, purpuric, urticarial, nodular, granulomatous, or may occur in various combinations. In etiology they may be due to allergic reactions to organic chemicals, proteins, and infectious agents; to bacterial products (erythrogenic toxin of group A beta-hemolytic streptococci); or to a considerable number of viruses, rickettsiae, bacteria, fungi, protozoa, and metazoa (Tables 22-1, 22-2 and 22-3). The causative agents may have a human or an animal reservoir and may produce localized or systemic, acute or chronic, subclinical or clinical, mild or fatal infections.

In this chapter, emphasis will be given to viruses of the pox-, herpes-, myxo-, and arbogroups which produce systemic infections with skin lesions and in which man is the reservoir. The diseases include smallpox, varicella, zoster, herpes, rubella, dengue, and epidemic typhus (a

Table 22-1 Systemic Infections with Skin Lesions in Which Man Is the Reservoir

- Viruses
  - Poxviruses
    - Smallpox (variola)
    - Vaccinia
  - Herpesviruses
    - Herpes
    - Varicella-Zoster
    - Cytomegalovirus disease
  - Myxoviruses
    - Measles
    - Rubella
  - Arboviruses
    - Dengue
  - Picornaviruses
    - Coxsackie virus infections (Chap. 24)
    - Echovirus infections (Chap. 24)
  - Miscellaneous Viruses
    - Roseola (exanthem subitum)
    - Erythema infectiosum (fifth disease)
- Rickettsiae
  - Epidemic typhus
- Bacteria
  - Syphilis (Chap. 21)
  - Meningococcal infections (Chap. 24)
  - Typhoid (Chap. 18)
  - Tuberculosis (Chap. 15)
  - Bartonellosis (Chap. 25)
  - Bejel (Chap. 16)
  - Actinomycosis (Chap. 17)
- Protozoa
  - Trypanosomiasis (*T. gambiense*) (Chap. 25)
- Roundworms
  - Hookworm disease (Chap. 18)
  - Strongyloidiasis (Chap. 18)

Table 22-2 Systemic Human Infections with Skin Lesions in Which Animals Are the Reservoir

- Viruses
  - Poxviruses
    - Cowpox
    - Milkers' nodules (pseudocowpox)
    - Orf (contagious pustular dermatitis of sheep)
  - Herpesviruses
    - B virus (monkeys)
  - Arboviruses
    - Chikungunya
    - O' Nyong-Nyong
    - West Nile (birds)
    - Crimean-Central Asian hemorrhagic fever
  - Picornaviruses
    - Foot and mouth disease (cattle)
- Rickettsiae
  - Endemic typhus (rats)
  - Scrub typhus (rodents)
  - Rocky Mountain spotted fever (rodents, rabbits)
  - Rickettsialpox (mice)
- Bacteria
  - Anthrax (sheep)
  - Glanders (horses)
  - Plague (rodents)
  - Leptospirosis (rodents, dogs, swine, cattle)
  - Rat-bite fever
  - Erysipelothrix* (fish, poultry, swine, sheep, cattle, horses)
  - Relapsing fever (rodents)
- Protozoa
  - Trypanosomiasis (cattle, opossums, armadillos)

* May also occur as a localized infection.

Table 22-3 Systemic Human Infections: Skin Lesions Infrequently Present

Viruses
Arboviruses: Sindbis, Omsk hemorrhagic fever, Bunyamwera, Colorado tick fever
Reoviruses
Infectious mononucleosis
Cat-scratch fever
Fungi
Aspergillosis*
Blastomycosis*
Candidiasis*
Chromomycosis*
Cryptococcosis
Sporotrichosis*
Rhinosporidiosis*
Roundworms
Trichinosis

* May also occur as a localized infection.

rickettsial infection). Systemic exanthematous diseases which are transmitted from animals to man are considered in Chapter 26, and localized infections with skin lesions are discussed in Chapter 16.

SMALLPOX

The term *pock*—or its plural, *pox*—refers to the pustular eruption of skin associated with smallpox in man. Smallpox (variola) virus is a natural human parasite. Initial contact with the virus frequently results in a clinical infection. Classic smallpox (variola major) is a severe disease with a high case fatality rate (about 50 percent). Alastrim (variola minor) is a mild form of the disease with a low case fatality rate, usually less than 1 percent.

An antigenically closely related virus, vaccinia, is used for immunization of man against smallpox. On extremely rare occasions (2 per 100,000), immunization with vaccinia virus may be followed by generalized vaccinia, a disease which resembles smallpox and has a mortality of about 5 percent.

The Causative Agent

Biologic Properties of Smallpox Virus Poxviruses are large, complex, brick-shaped particles ($300 \times 200 \times 100$ nm) with rounded ends and central bulges in the narrow aspect. They contain DNA, have essential lipid in the envelope, are sensitive to pH 3.0, multiply in the cytoplasm of susceptible cells, and share a common internal nucleoprotein antigen.

Man is the natural host for smallpox virus (used here to include the causative agents of classic smallpox and alastrim). The virus is widely disseminated throughout the tissues, and the environment is contaminated largely by the respiratory secretions and skin lesions of infected individuals.

Because the virus is resistant to drying, it may persist in the environment for more than a year at ambient temperatures of 20 to 25°C. The virus is also resistant to glycerol, phenol, and many of the common disinfectants. However, it is readily inactivated when heated at 56°C for 30 min.

Typical small pocks are produced by the virus on the chorioallantois of the chick embryo in 48 to 72 hr. The lesions show little tendency to necrosis and fail to develop at temperatures of 39°C or higher. The virus is not highly virulent for laboratory animals but may produce keratitis following corneal inoculation in rabbits, usually multiplies in suckling mice, and may cause systemic disease in monkeys. A wide variety of mammalian tissue cultures support the growth of the virus and show cytopathic changes with the formation of eosinophilic cytoplasmic inclusions.

Vaccinia Virus Vaccinia virus appears to be a laboratory variant of cowpox virus, the causative agent of a natural disease of cattle which may occasionally be transmitted to man. Vaccinia virus differs from smallpox virus primarily in the basis of its lesser virulence for man and its greater virulence for the chick embryo and the rabbit. The pox produced by vaccinia virus on the chorioallantois of the chick embryo are larger, more necrotic, more hemorrhagic, and more umbilicated than those induced by smallpox virus. In addition, vaccinial lesions regularly develop at temperatures (40°C) which inhibit the growth of smallpox virus. Vaccinia virus regularly produces lesions in rabbit skin which can be passed serially, whereas the lesions induced by smallpox virus cannot be passed serially.

Antigenic Structure Smallpox virus is closely related to vaccinia, cowpox, monkeypox, rabbitpox, and ectromelia (mousepox) viruses. Collectively, these viruses are known as the vaccinia subgroup of the poxviruses.

Although the definitive antigenic structure of the vaccinia subgroup of poxviruses has not been established, the viruses are known to contain several important antigens (Table 22-4). These include the protein (LS) antigen, nucleoprotein (NP) antigens, and a soluble lipoprotein hemagglutinin (HA) antigen.

LS Antigen Although the soluble LS antigen is readily separable from the virus by filtration or centrifugation, it also constitutes part of the surface of the virus. LS antigen combines with antibody in precipitin, CF, and FA tests.

NP Antigens The NP antigens contain two reactive components or two distinct antigens which are extracted by the same procedure. The group-specific NP component common to all poxviruses is located in the core of the virus and is demonstrable by precipitin, CF, and FA tests. The subgroup-specific NP component is located on the surface of the virus, induces the formation of *neutralizing* antibody, and reacts with antibody in precipitin, CF, and FA tests. The precise relationship of the subgroup-specific NP component to a soluble protective antigen with a molecular weight of 100,000 to 200,000 remains to be determined.

HA Antigen HA antigen is a by-product of viral multiplication. It is demonstrable by agglutination of the red blood cells of certain chickens, by inhibition of this agglutination with antibody, and by FA tests. Although HA precipitates with antibody, it does not give the typical quantitative precipitin curve seen when the LS and NP antigens react with their antibodies. HA fails to elute from agglutinated cells, is inactivated by lecithinase, remains stable on heating, is devoid of ability to incite the formation of neutralizing antibody, and is associated with particles having a diameter of 65 nm and a density of 1.1. The ratio of plaque-forming units to HA units in the usual viral preparation is 1 million to 1.

Table 22-4 Antigens of the Vaccinia Subgroup of the Poxviruses

Characteristic	LS antigen	NP antigens	HA antigen
Chemical nature	Protein	Nucleoprotein	Lipoprotein
Antigenic specificity	Subgroup	Group Subgroup	Subgroup
Location of virus	Surface	Core Surface	Not part of virus
Time of synthesis (hours after infection)	4 hr.	5–6 hr.	10 hr.
Physical features	Molecular weight of 240,000	Makes up 50 percent or more of virus	65 nm in diameter

Pathogenesis

The more virulent members of the vaccinia subgroup of the poxviruses show a more or less uniform pattern in their pathogenesis. In essence the virus multiples at the portal of entry and quickly progresses to the regional lymph nodes, from which, by way of the blood, it travels to the liver, spleen, and other tissues; after extensive multiplication, it passes by way of the blood to the skin and mucous membranes.

In smallpox, the typical course of events appears to be as follows. After local multiplication at the site of entry in the respiratory tract, the virus quickly progresses to the regional lymph nodes where replication also occurs. The few virus particles entering the blood (primary viremia) via the efferent lymphatics are rapidly removed by macrophages lining the sinusoids of the liver, the sinuses of the spleen, the lymph nodes, and the capillaries of the lungs, kidneys, adrenals, and other organs. After multiplication in the macrophages, the virus is released and replicates extensively in the parenchymal cells of these organs. Consequently, the virus literally overflows into the blood (secondary viremia) in increasing concentration and is distributed to the skin and mucous membranes. The virus multiplies rapidly in the epithelial cells of the skin, pharynx, uvula, tongue, other portions of the oropharynx, larynx, esophagus, and trachea. The usual incubation period of 12 to 13 days ends with the appearance of a macular rash on the face and upper extremities which then spreads to the trunk and the lower limbs. Thereafter, the rash becomes papular, vesicular, and then pustular. Early in the disease the characteristic cytoplasmic inclusions are found in the epithelium of the skin and mucous membranes. The skin lesions heal gradually over a period of a few weeks.

Aberrant patterns may occur, depending largely on the severity of the disease. For example, in fulminating cases (purpuric smallpox) the patient may die before the appearance of the rash with hemorrhages in the skin, mouth, nose, intestine, and other epithelial surfaces. In the eruptive form of the disease the severity parallels the extent of the skin lesions. For example, when hemorrhage occurs between the skin lesions (hemorrhagic smallpox), the mortality may be about 80 percent. In patients with confluent skin lesions, the mortality may be about 40 to 50 percent. On the other hand, in patients with discrete skin lesions, the mortality is low, averaging about 5 percent, finally, in the mildest form of the disease, usually seen in partially immune individuals, the lesions may fail to develop (smallpox sine eruptione).

Laboratory Diagnosis

Because of the minimum time required (2 to 12 hr.), the most useful method of establishing a laboratory diagnosis of smallpox is the demonstration of antigen in the skin lesions. In this procedure the antigen in the form of fluid or crusts from a number of lesions is reacted with antivaccinial rabbit serum in a CF, gel diffusion, or FA test. Since the lesions may not contain sufficient antigen, additional procedures are indicated.

Microscopic examination of a stained smear (Giemsa, Gutstein, Herzberg, Morosow) from the skin lesion is suggestive of smallpox when it reveals numerous virus particles (elementary bodies) in the absence of giant cells. In all cases, however, the suspect material should be inoculated onto the chorioallantois of the chick embryo or onto tissue culture monolayers. The pocks or plaques produced can be identified by their antigenic reactivity in neutralization, hemadsorption, FA or CF tests. In addition to the skin lesions, virus may be regularly recovered from the saliva and, in severe cases of smallpox, from the blood.

Demonstration of a rise in antibody (CF, HA-inhibition) between the acute and convalescent phases of the disease will serve to establish a diagnosis of smallpox but is of little practical value.

In the rare situation in which it becomes necessary to distinguish the lesions of smallpox from those due to generalized vaccinia, this can be most readily accomplished by showing that vaccinia virus produces pocks on the chorioallantois of the chick embryo at 40°C, whereas smallpox virus fails to grow at this temperature.

Epidemiology

Source Man is the reservoir of infection in smallpox. The source of infection is the patient with the disease. Most patients become infectious with the appearance of the rash. At this time, as a consequence of viral multiplication in the mucous membranes lining the oral cavity and the nasopharynx, virus is present in the oral and nasal discharges. Thereafter, the skin lesions serve as an important additional source for contaminating the environment for a period of 2 to 3 weeks.

The virus is transmitted by the airborne route as a result of direct contact with infected droplets or indirectly through articles and materials (bedclothes, etc.) contaminated with the virus.

A particularly dangerous source of infection is the partially immune person who experiences a mild illness which is not recognized as smallpox.

Occurrence Today, as in the past, classic smallpox (variola major) is endemic in the countries of southeastern Asia and in Africa. From these areas, it was introduced into Europe and America where it was a devastating disease for centuries, declining only with the widespread use of vaccination. The persistence of the endemic disease in Asia and Africa represents a continuing threat to all countries, since it may be introduced by international travelers into countries free of the disease.

Unvaccinated persons of all countries, races, and ages are susceptible. In highly endemic areas, smallpox is primarily a disease of children. On the other hand, in countries where universal vaccination of infants is carried out, cases of smallpox are found primarily in adults whose immunity has waned.

Alastrim (variola minor) is endemic in Africa and in South America, particularly in the countries of Venezuela, Colombia, Brazil, Bolivia, Peru, and Paraguay. Because of failure to employ universal vaccination, the milder nature of the disease, and the resulting failure to report infectious cases, alastrim remained endemic in the United States and in Great Britain until 1930.

Prevention and Control

Variolation Smallpox was the first disease in which active immunization was employed. The earliest attempts to prevent smallpox were made by the Chinese who placed the dried crusts of skin lesions in the noses of susceptible persons in the hope of producing a mild form of the disease. Although success was achieved in some instances, in other cases fatal smallpox ensued. In addition, the inoculated persons served as sources of infection for those who had previously escaped the disease.

During the eighteenth century the practice of inoculating material from smallpox lesions by incision or puncture of the skin (variolation) became popular. The usual result of variolation was the production of smallpox which had a short incubation period (7 to 8 days) and a milder course than the naturally acquired disease. Although variolation was a distinct improvement over the Chinese method, the procedure was not without risk to the inoculated and to the community. At best, the mortality in the inoculated was 0.2 percent. Since the practice of inoculating whole communities at one time and isolating the susceptible individuals from the inoculated was not widely employed, spread of smallpox from the inoculated to the susceptible population was an almost constant threat.

Vaccination In 1798 Jenner's finding that the inoculation of cowpox (vaccination) in the skin of man protected against subsequent exposure to smallpox led to the abandonment of variolation and established the foundation for the modern method of preventing the disease. Cowpox is a mild endemic disease in cattle which occasionally causes a mild infection in farm workers (Chap. 26). When the causative cowpox virus is passed repeatedly in different animals and tissues, it is referred to as vaccinia virus.

Smallpox Vaccine The standard smallpox vaccine is prepared from vaccinial lesions of the skin of inoculated calves or sheep and contains infective virus to which glycerol has been added (glycerinated calf lymph or glycerinated sheep lymph). Lyophilized vaccines are more stable at higher temperatures than glycerinated lymph and are particularly useful in the tropics where continuous refrigeration is rarely available. Other vaccines have been prepared from vaccinia virus grown on the chorioallantois of chick embryos and from infected tissue cultures of chick embryos or bovine embryo skin.

Multiple Pressure Method of Vaccination Smallpox vaccine is introduced into the superficial layers of the skin by the multiple pressure method. In this procedure a drop of vaccine is placed on the dry, previously cleansed skin over the deltoid area of the arm. With the side of a needle, 10 rapid pressures are made through the vaccine drop for a primary vaccination (30 for revaccination). Firm pressure is applied while holding the needle parallel to the skin in order to avoid the vascular layer. The multiple pressure technique is preferred to the scratch and scarification methods because it is the least traumatic and gives the smallest reactions.

Reactions to Smallpox Vaccine The time when the maximum diameter of erythema appears around the inoculated site forms the basis for determining the response to smallpox vaccine. In a fully susceptible person the reaction reaches its maximum extent usually in 8 to 10 days (primary vaccinia or primary reaction). In a person with some residual immunity erythema is maximal in 3 to 7 days (vaccinoid or accelerated reaction). If the reaction is most intense in 2 or 3 days, the person is sensitive to the virus or other materials in the vaccine (early or immediate reaction).

In primary vaccinia a small papule appears in 4 days and quickly becomes a vesicle which enlarges in size and is accompanied by erythema. In 8 or 9 days the center of the vesicle becomes depressed and the contents become turbid. At this time axillary adenitis and fever may be noted. Thereafter, the pustule dries up and a scab is formed which separates in a week. In vaccinoid reactions vesiculation always occurs, and in early reactions the local lesion is usually papular but may vesiculate.

Duration of Immunity Following Vaccination Primary vaccinia is followed by a high level of immunity to smallpox which usually persists for several years. It is estimated that the increased resistance to smallpox is 1,000-fold for 1 year, 200-fold for 3 years, 8-fold for 10 years, and 2-fold for 20 years. Comparable estimates for persons showing vaccinoid reactions are not available, but the level of immunity would presumably be higher and more durable than that induced by primary vaccinia. Persons showing early reactions should be revaccinated with vaccine known to be potent.

Complications Following Vaccination Vaccination is a relatively safe and effective immunizing procedure, but serious complications may occur. In a recent survey of 6 million vaccinated children in the United States, three deaths and a number of complications were recorded (Table 22-5). The risk of serious complications following primary vaccination is greatest in those under 1 year of age and is much lower in those between 1 and 4 years of age. Following revaccination, complications are negligible.

Because of the risk of eczema vaccinatum, persons with chronic dermatitis should not be vaccinated and should avoid contact with vaccinated persons. Because of the risk of developing generalized vaccinia or progressive vaccinia, pregnant women, patients with leukemia, lymphoma, blood dyscrasias, and dysgammaglobulinemia; and patients who have had recent therapy with steroids, antimetabolites, alkylating agents, or ionizing radiation should not be given smallpox vaccine. Pyoderma may be largely avoided by vaccinating during the cool seasons of the year.

If there is imminent danger of smallpox and vaccination must be performed in pregnant women or in patients with the diseases listed above, human vaccinal immune gamma globulin should be injected concurrently.

Recommendations Ideally, primary vaccination should be performed between 1 and 2 years of age in order to minimize the risk of postvaccinal encephalitis, vaccinia necrosum, and eczema vaccinatum. To maintain a high level of immunity against smallpox, revaccination of the general population at intervals of 5 years is recommended. For those at greater risk, revaccination should be performed every 3 years. In endemic areas, yearly revaccination is indicated.

In 1971, however, the U.S.P.H.S. recommended that routine smallpox vaccination be discontinued, indicating that the risk of smallpox in the United States was insufficient to warrant universal primary vaccination of infants and children. In other words, the mortality associated with smallpox vaccination in the United States in the past 25 years was greater than the actual mortality experience of smallpox importations into unvaccinated European populations during the same period. At the same time, the U.S.P.H.S. strongly emphasized the (1) need for adequate immunization of health service personnel and travelers to endemic areas and (2) the necessity of an effective national surveillance system to identify suspect cases and to prevent outbreaks should importations occur. Within 6 months of the issuance of 1971 recommendations, the distribution of smallpox vaccine declined by more than 90 percent, and requests for vaccinia immune globulin for prophylaxis or treatment of the complications of smallpox vaccination were reduced by 75 percent. Only four states still have both a mandatory smallpox vaccination for school entrance and a state health department policy supporting routine vaccination.

Prophylaxis after Contact Several measures are available to reduce the risk that smallpox will develop in close contacts. These include vaccination, human vaccinial immune gamma globulin, and the antiviral drug, N-methylisatin

Table 22-5 The Incidence of Complications Following Primary Vaccination of 6 Million Children

	Rate per 1,000,000 vaccinated children		
Complication	**All ages**	**Under 1 year of age**	**1 to 4 years of age**
Death	0.5		
Postvaccinal encephalitis	1.8	1.5	0.7
Progressive vaccinia	1.1	1.5	0.3
Eczema vaccinatum	8.7	24.5	7.4
Generalized vaccinia	20.8		
Accidental vaccination	13.6		

Source: Adapted from J. M. Neff, J. M. Lane, J. H. Pert, R. Moore, J. D. Millar, and D. A. Henderson, *N. Engl. J. Med.*, 276:125–132, 1967.

β-thiosemicarbazone. Vaccination within 3 days after exposure confers a significant level of protection on previously unvaccinated contacts. Further delay in the vaccination of smallpox contacts greatly reduces the ability to prevent or modify the disease. When vaccinated contacts are also given immune gamma globulin, protection is enhanced (8 cases in 400 close family contacts versus 29 cases in 400 close family contacts who were vaccinated only). However, preliminary trials indicated that N-methylisatin β-thiosemicarbazone is the most effective agent for preventing smallpox in close contacts.

Treatment There are no specific measures for the treatment of smallpox. However, massive doses of human vaccinial immune gamma globulin have proved to be effective in the treatment of eczema vaccinatum and progressive vaccinia. The apparent success of N-methylisatin β-thiosemicarbazone in the treatment of a few cases of progressive vaccinia awaits further confirmation.

Other Control Measures Although universal vaccination and revaccination at appropriate intervals form the basis for the control of smallpox, a number of accessory measures are helpful. These include prompt and accurate reporting and isolation of cases, disinfection of contaminated discharges and materials by reliable methods (incineration, autoclaving, boiling), finding the immediate prior case, surveillance of contacts for 16 days, and insisting upon recent vaccination or revaccination as a condition for entry to or departure from a country.

HERPES

Infections caused by herpesvirus are associated with tissues derived from the embryonic ectoderm (skin, mucous membranes, CNS). The protean clinical manifestations of the disease may be primary or recurrent.

Primary Herpes On initial contact with herpesvirus type 1, more than 90 percent of persons develop a subclinical infection. Acute gingivostomatitis is the commonest clinical manifestation of primary infection. Other syndromes observed include meningoencephalitis, aseptic meningitis, generalized vesicular eruption, eczema herpeticum, and neonatal herpes with involvement of the liver, adrenals, lungs, and CNS.

Recurrent Herpes Persons who recover from infection with primary herpesvirus type 1 develop neutralizing antibodies, carry the virus in a latent form, and maintain a high level of neutralizing antibodies for the balance of their lives. Periodically the virus may be reactivated following disturbance in the external or internal environment. Recurrent herpes is characterized by the repeated formation of superficial vesicles in the same mucocutaneous area of the body. Herpes simplex (herpes labialis, cold sores, fever blisters), the commonest manifestation of recurrent disease, involves the mucocutaneous junction of the lip.

Primary or Recurrent Herpes Other clinical manifestations may be characteristic of either primary or recurrent herpes. These include keratitis, keratoconjunctivitis, vulvovaginitis, herpes progenitalis, traumatic herpes, and herpetic whitlow.

Genital Herpes (Primary and Recurrent) In recent years herpesvirus type 2 has been recognized as the causative agent of primary and recurrent disease involving the genital tract. The primary disease is most commonly transmitted venereally. In females, infection is associated with lesions in the cervix, vulva, vagina, and urethra and in males with the penis and urethra. The clinical manifestations may include fever, dysuria, inguinal adenopathy, and genital soreness. Certain sex practices can be associated with lesions in the anus or the mouth. In addition, genital infection with herpesvirus type 2 in pregnant women may result in serious neonatal disease with dissemination of the virus to the skin, eyes, CNS, and visceral organs.

Recurrent genital herpes is frequent. In women, the cervix is usually involved, and the infection is subclinical. In men, herpetic vesicles are commonly present on the penis as in the primary disease, but constitutional signs of infection are generally absent.

The Causative Agent

Biologic Properties Infectivity in the herpes group of viruses is primarily associated with medium-sized particles with a core containing DNA (78 nm in diameter) enclosed in an icosahedral protein capsid (105 nm in diameter) and surrounded by an envelope containing essential lipid (180 nm in diameter). Naked particles (those without envelopes but containing the core enclosed in the capsid) are also infectious, but they are much less efficiently adsorbed to susceptible cells than are the enveloped particles. In addition, noninfectious viral particles without cores (empty particles), with and without envelopes, are produced. In some infected cells 90 to 95 percent of the viral particles formed may be empty.

The herpes group of viruses are labile. Infectivity of the viruses is rapidly inactivated at pH 3.0, at temperatures of 37°C, and by organic solvents, detergents, and enzymes.

Preservation of the virus is best accomplished by storage at −70°C in the presence of material rich in protein. Less effectively, the virus may be preserved in 40 percent glycerol at −20°C.

Man is the natural host for herpesvirus. The virus is widely disseminated throughout the world as evidenced by the finding of neutralizing antibodies in as much as 90 percent of the population. Furthermore, the majority of the population carry the virus in a latent form and are potential periodic excretors of the virus. The environment is contaminated largely by the saliva of asymptomatic adults, approximately 2.5 percent of whom excrete the virus at any given time.

In contrast with varicella-zoster virus which has a narrow host range, herpesvirus grows and produces intranuclear inclusions in chick embryos, mice, rabbits, guinea pigs, hamsters, cotton rats, and many types of tissue culture cells (rabbit kidney, HeLa, WI-38, and Hep-2). Isolation and experimental study of herpesvirus are most effectively carried out in tissue cultures, chick embryos, and mice. Assay of the virus is based on plaque formation in tissue cultures and pock formation on the chorioallantoic membrane of chick embryos.

In tissue cultures the virus characteristically produces large syncytial giant cells, although some strains of the virus cause rounding of cells which may or may not pile up. In chick embryos the formation of small raised pox (1 to 2 mm in diameter) in 24 to 48 hr. is preceded by the development of Feulgen-positive intranuclear inclusions in the infected cells. Encephalitis and death occur in suckling mice following intracerebral or intraperitoneal inoculation with the virus and in adult mice injected intracerebrally.

Replication of herpesvirus in tissue cultures is associated with the formation of viral CF antigens in 2 hr., the synthesis of viral DNA in 5 hr., and the formation of infectious particles in 6 hr. Viral DNA synthesis levels off at 7 hr., and the synthesis of virus at 9 hr.

Antigenic Structure Two types of herpesvirus were originally distinguished on the basis of the kinetics of virus neutralization by antiserum in a microquantal test performed in rabbit kidney tissue cultures. Subsequently, it was demonstrated that the two types differed in respect to the source of the virus and biological, biochemical, and biophysical properties. Type 1 is primarily responsible for early childhood infection (asymptomatic and gingivostomatitis), herpes labialis, keratitis, and keratoconjunctivitis, and dermatitis above the waist. Type 2 is the principal cause of genital infections and dermatitis below the waist. Both types can cause severe and fatal infections in the neonatal period.

Types 1 and 2 also differ in terms of virulence for rabbits, mice, and guinea pigs; in the size of pocks produced on the chorioallantois of chick embryos or plaques on human, rabbit, and monkey cells; in ability to induce plaques in chick embryo cells; and in inactivation by heat and ultraviolet light. Both show only 40 to 47 percent homology in viral DNA.

On the basis of serological epidemiology, type 2 herpesvirus has been associated with human cervical carcinoma and has been isolated from degenerated cervical tumor cells grown in vitro; type 2 antigens have been detected in exfoliated but not in biopsied tumor cells, and ultraviolet irradiated virus can transform hamster embryo fibroblasts in vitro which can then induce fibrosarcomas in newborn hamsters. From 1 to 5 percent of the transformed cells contained type 2 antigens in the cytoplasm, and the tumor-bearing hamsters developed neutralizing antibody. The suggestion has been made that both the human cervical carcinoma and the hamster fibrosarcoma cells harbor the viral genome in a repressed state. On the other hand, whether or not herpesvirus type 2 is the causative agent of human cervical carcinoma remains to be determined.

Herpes virus is antigenically related to B virus of monkeys and pseudorabies virus of pigs.

Pathogenesis

Primary Herpes (Generalized Infection)

Acute Gingivostomatitis Although the predominant features of acute gingivostomatitis are usually localized to the oral cavity, the disease is basically a generalized infection accompanied by viremia, by hepatic involvement in the more severe cases, and by necrosis of the liver, adrenals, lungs, and CNS in neonates. The chief local manifestations of acute gingivostomatitis are pain, red swollen gums, a vesicular eruption on the oral mucous membranes, and submaxillary lymphadenopathy. Type 1 herpesvirus is the causative agent.

Acute gingivostomatitis most commonly develops in young children (1 to 3 years of age) 6 to 7 days following contact with an asymptomatic carrier. The lesions are characterized by the presence of giant cells and intranuclear inclusions. Although the vesicles may ulcerate before healing, scarring is rarely seen. Virus may be excreted in the saliva for as long as 7 weeks, may be found in the stool, and may be present in the blood for a few days. Uneventful recovery usually occurs in 1 to 2 weeks.

Neonatal Herpes Most herpes infections acquired just before or after birth terminate fatally. The onset of the illness occurs 4 to 7 days after birth, without stomatitis or vesicles. The disease progresses rapidly with dyspnea, jaundice, convulsions, mucocutaneous hemorrhages, and death in less than a week. Virus is widely disseminated throughout the tissues including the liver, adrenals, lungs, and CNS. Both types 1 and 2 herpesviruses can cause the syndrome, but type 2 infections are more common.

For unknown reasons, in a few virologically and serologically proved cases the neonatal disease is mild with the lesions apparently limited to the skin and the mucous membranes of the nose.

CNS Infection As indicated above, neonatal infection often results in CNS involvement with necrosis of the temporal cortex, the basal ganglia, and the brain stem. In rare instances, meningoencephalitis may accompany primary mucocutaneous herpes in older children and adults. In addition, CNS infection may occur in the absence of other herpetic manifestations. Except for neonatal disease, meningoencephalitis is caused by type 1 herpesvirus.

The severity of the disease varies from meningitis with uneventful recovery to an acute encephalitis with paresis, sensory changes, convulsions, coma, and death in 1 to 2 weeks. Although the mechanism by which the virus invades the CNS is not known, clinical and experimental evidence suggests that the virus may spread centripetally along the nerves.

Recurrent Herpes (Localized Infection)

Herpes Simplex (Herpes Labialis, Fever Blisters, Cold Sores) Persons who have had primary infection with herpesvirus type 1 are candidates to develop recurrent herpes at periodic intervals throughout their lives. Most commonly the recurrent disease occurs at the mucocutaneous junction of the lips and face (herpes simplex). The lesions appear as red papules which quickly vesiculate. The fully developed lesions consist of a crop of superficial clear vesicles on an erythematous base. Healing without scarring is usually complete in 2 to 7 days. Virus may be isolated from the vesicles for 24 to 48 hr.

There is great individual variation in the frequency with which recurrent herpes occurs and in the nature of the provocative stimulus which triggers the localized disease. Some persons regularly develop the disease following brief exposure to sunlight or heat. Other individuals consistently show the fever blisters following fever, minor respiratory or gastrointestinal infection, trauma, trigeminal neuralgia or operative section of the trigeminal nerve, or physical exertion. Attacks may also be precipitated by menstruation, pregnancy, or emotional strain. The most resistant persons develop herpes simplex following severe pneumococcal pneumonia or bacterial meningitis. If there is a common mechanism which reactivates the latent infection and leads to herpes simplex, it probably involves disturbance in the local tissue blood supply.

Herpetic Keratitis and Keratoconjunctivitis A more chronic and potentially more severe form of the recurrent type 1 disease is associated with involvement of the conjunctiva and the cornea. The disease may be superficial and limited to the conjunctiva, or it may lead to the formation of dendritic ulcers, corneal erosion, necrosis, rupture, and scarring or to iridocyclitis (severe pain, circumcorneal flush, and multiple keratitic precipitates).

Genital Herpes As noted earlier, genital herpes may occur either as a primary or recurrent disease after venereal transmission of type 2 herpesvirus. When primary infection occurs in patients who have type 1 antibody, the disease is usually more mild than in those without antibody.

Laboratory Diagnosis

A variety of methods may be employed to suggest or establish a laboratory diagnosis of herpes infection. These include the demonstration of giant cells and intranuclear inclusions in smears taken from the base of fresh vesicles; the use of the FA test on smears or sections of infected tissues; the isolation of the virus from the local vesicles, the saliva, the blood, or the viscera or CNS at autopsy; and in the case of the primary disease, by demonstrating a rise in specific antibody. Isolation of virus on the chorioallantoic membrane of chick embryos or in appropriate tissue cultures (rabbit kidney, WI-38, Hep-2, and HeLa cells) and its identification by neutralization or CF tests comprise the procedure of choice. If a rise in specific antibody is to be demonstrated in the primary disease, the initial serum specimen must be taken before the fifth day of the disease, and the second serum specimen must be obtained 2 to 3 weeks after onset. Identification of the herpesvirus as type 1 or 2 is usually determined on the microquantal neutralization test in rabbit kidney tissue culture. Similarly, identification of the infection on the basis of the production of neutralizing antibody must be made on a greater increase in homotypic versus heterotypic antibody.

Epidemiology

Source Man is the reservoir of infection in both primary and recurrent herpes. The main cohort of infection is the large number of subclinically infected carriers, 2.5 percent of whom have the virus in the saliva at any given time. The patient with the primary or recurrent disease can also transmit the infection but appears to play a minor role.

Spread of the virus to susceptible persons (those without antibody) most commonly occurs as a result of close contact. The virus enters by way of the oral route, the conjunctiva, the respiratory tract, the genitalia, the traumatized skin, or during passage through the birth canal and may be transferred across the placenta. In susceptible adults the infection is usually transmitted by kissing or by sexual intercourse. In the latter case, type 2 herpesvirus is involved, whereas oral transmission (kissing) involves type 1 herpesvirus.

As noted earlier, the recurrent disease is the result of an endogenous infection following alteration of the external or internal environment by a variety of stimuli.

Age Incidence The incidence of primary herpes caused by type 1 herpesvirus reaches a peak in young children between 1 and 3 years of age. Approximately 90 percent of infants are born of immune mothers and are highly protected for about 6 months. Infants born of nonimmune mothers are susceptible from birth and provide the candidates for the severe neonatal form of the disease.

The incidence of infection is considerably greater among persons living in a lower socioeconomic environment then those at a higher level. The explanation is related at least in part to overcrowding and to the level of hygiene practiced. The recurrent disease, on the other hand, chiefly involves adults.

Type 2 infections, both primary and secondary, are spread venereally. Consequently, except for rare neonatal infections, antibodies do not appear until puberty and then rise steadily, reaching a peak of about 50 percent in the adult population.

Occurrence Primary and recurrent infection is found throughout the world. Characteristically, primary disease appears sporadically, a finding that is not surprising in view of the fact that the ratio of infections to disease is at least 10 to 1. However, under unusual circumstances, as in orphanages, hospital wards, or susceptible families, epidemics of the disease may occur.

Prevention and Control

No specific measures have been developed as yet to prevent or control the disease. The practice of using smallpox vaccine in an effort to prevent recurrent herpes simplex is no more effective than placebos, has no rational basis, and may be dangerous in patients with malignancy who are concurrently being treated with immunosuppressive drugs.

Treatment Properly utilized in cases without chronic tissue damage, 5-iodo-2′-deoxyuridine (IDUR) has proved valuable in the treatment of herpetic keratitis. IDUR is a thymidine analogue which presumably acts by making fraudulent noninfectious viral DNA, but which may function by inhibiting enzymes involved in the utilization of thymidine in DNA synthesis. IDUR-resistant mutants of herpesvirus have developed. For these mutants, cytosine arabinoside and other purine and pyrimidine analogues have been employed in treatment.

VARICELLA-ZOSTER

Varicella and zoster are two clinical entities caused by a single virus—varicella-zoster, or V-Z. Virus isolations from typical cases of varicella and zoster are identical in morphology, antigenic structure, host range, ability to form intranuclear inclusion bodies and multinucleate giant cells, type of response induced in tissue cultures, and ability to serve as a reciprocal source of infection.

It is increasingly attractive to look upon the clinical and epidemiological differences between varicella and zoster which are itemized below as no more striking than those encountered between primary and recurrent herpes. According to this concept, varicella is the disease acquired as a result of initial contact with V-Z virus. Zoster, on the other hand, represents the reactivation of V-Z virus in a person who already has antibody as a result of previous contact.

Characteristic	Varicella	Zoster
Type of cases	Epidemic	Sporadic
Skin lesions	Widespread	Along peripheral sensory nerves
Predominant age incidence	Children under 10 years old	Adults
Seasonal prevalence	In winter and spring	None
Antibody at onset of illness	Absent	Present

The Causative Agent

Biologic Properties V-Z virus is a member of the herpes group of viruses. It differs from herpesvirus primarily in host range, in the fact that in tissue cultures infectious virus remains within the cell (i.e., is cell-associated), and in antigenic structure.

Replication of V-Z virus occurs in a variety of primary cultures and cell lines of human and monkey origin. Virus spreads contiguously from cell to cell and is rarely found in the extracellular fluid. Neighboring cells are infected in 8 to 16 hr., indicating that no more than 8 hr. are required for the synthesis of virus. As the plaque develops the cells become rounded, multinucleate giant cells appear, and intranuclear inclusion bodies are seen in stained preparations.

Man is the natural host for the virus. Experimentally, the virus has been transmitted only to man.

Antigenic Structure Analysis of the antigenic structure of V-Z virus is hampered by the cell-associated property of the virus and the inability to produce antiserum in animals. The antigens of the virus can be detected in plaque neutralization tests in tissue culture and in FA, CF, and gel diffusion precipitation tests. There are probably at least four antigenic components associated with the virus; three have been observed in gel diffusion tests, and another antigen reacts in the CF test.

Pathogenesis

Varicella Varicella is usually acquired by droplet infection from a patient with the disease, although a patient with zoster may also be the source of varicella. During the incubation period of 14 to 17 days it is thought that the virus multiplies at the portal of entry and quickly passes by way of the lymphatic system and the blood (primary viremia) to the lungs, liver, spleen, and other organs. From the viscera it is returned to the blood (secondary viremia) and is filtered out by the endothelial cells of the vessels in the corium. The formation of the vesicles is preceded by ballooning degeneration of cells in the corium, involvement of the overlying epidermis, the formation of intranuclear inclusion bodies and multinucleate giant cells, exudation, and the accumulation of clear fluid. Successive crops of vesicles showing a centripetal concentration appear over a period of 2 to 5 days. In contrast with extracellular fluids of tissue cultures, virus is present in high concentration in the clear fluid of young vesicles.

Although the vesicles may cause pain, pruritis, and may be secondarily infected, varicella is usually a benign disease with healing of the lesions without scarring in 7 to 10 days. Occasionally, however, primary varicella pneumonia may develop, more commonly in adults than in children. In children with leukemia or some other malignant disease or in patients receiving cortisone therapy, varicella is a severe and often fatal disease. The other potentially serious consequence of varicella is postinfectious encephalitis (Chap. 24).

Zoster The pathogenesis of the segmental lesion in the involved dorsal root ganglion that is pathognomonic of zoster is unknown. Presumably, the disease represents the reactivation of virus which has silently persisted since the childhood attack of varicella. In many patients the disease is precipitated by malignancy, cortisone therapy, trauma, or concurrent infection, including tuberculosis.

The vesicular eruption is usually unilaterial, showing an irregular, bandlike distribution corresponding to the involved dorsal root or the sensory division of a cranial nerve. The eruption is most commonly located on the trunk, is frequently accompanied by pain and regional lymphadenopathy, and generally heals within 2 weeks. Occasionally, however, complications may ensue. These include pain which persists for several months, corneal scarring resulting from ophthalmic zoster, or paralysis and motor damage.

Laboratory Diagnosis

A laboratory diagnosis in varicella and zoster is best accomplished by isolation of the virus from the fluid of early vesicles in primary cultures or cell lines of human or monkey origin and its subsequent identification on the basis of its immunological reactivity. For varicella the diagnosis may also be made by demonstrating a rise in antibody titer between the acute and convalescent phase of the disease by the use of neutralization or CF tests.

Epidemiology

Varicella The patient with varicella is the usual source of infection of susceptible individuals who subsequently develop varicella, but patients with zoster may initiate outbreaks of varicella. Varicella is a highly contagious disease, ranking second only to measles. More than 70 percent of susceptible persons are infected on exposure to a patient with varicella, but only 15 percent of susceptible persons exposed to a patient with zoster will develop varicella.

The disease is found throughout the world and characteristically occurs in epidemics at intervals of a few years during the winter and spring in temperate climates. Approximately 29 percent of cases develop in those under 4 years of age, and 62 percent occur in those between 5 and 9 years of age.

Zoster In contrast with varicella, zoster presumably represents an endogenous infection which occurs sporadically without a particular seasonal prevalence. The disease predominantly affects adults, appearing with increasing frequency and severity in those over 45 years old.

The incidence of zoster is higher than generally acknowledged. In selected adult groups rates of 13 to 200 per 100,000 per year have been reported.

Prevention and Control

Apart from the use of zoster immune globulin (ZIG) there are no specific measures for the prevention and control of varicella. ZIG is a gamma globulin fraction of plasma with a high titer of antibody from patients convalescing from zoster. ZIG can prevent clinical and laboratory evidence of varicella in susceptible children when given within 72 hr. of household exposure. The use of ZIG is indicated for children at high risk of severe varicella, including those with immunodeficiency diseases, leukemia, or lymphoma or those receiving immunosuppressive agents. In such children varicella poses the threat of pneumonia, encephalitis, purpura, or death. In the United States ZIG is available for authorized use in high-risk children through the Center for Disease Control, Atlanta, Georgia and seven ZIG regional consultants.

Effective vaccines have not yet been developed but may become available in the future. In the event an attenuated vaccine were used, a key problem would revolve around its efficacy in reducing the incidence of zoster.

RUBELLA (GERMAN MEASLES)

Until the classic observations of Gregg in 1941, associating congenital cataract, congenital heart disease, and other abnormalities with maternal rubella, the disease was recognized as a mild exanthematous illness of short duration. Today, however, the overwhelming personal tragedy, the extent of fetal wastage, and the expense involved indict rubella as a major medical and social problem.

Detailed virologic and serologic studies have established the fact that the teratogenic effects of rubella virus are devastating and may involve virtually every tissue. In utero infection with rubella virus may be associated with an overall mortality within 1 year of birth of more than 10 percent (more than 35 percent in those with purpura). Affected newborns have a low birth weight (4.5 to 5.5 lb) and frequently develop congenital heart disease, deafness, eye defects (cataracts, microphthalmia, retinopathy, glaucoma, corneal clouding), thrombocytopenic purpura, psychomotor retardation, myocardial necrosis, hepatomegaly, splenomegaly, hepatitis, jaundice, metaphyseal rarefaction of long bones, large anterior fontanel, microcephaly, generalized adenopathy, hemolytic anemia, pneumonitis, and dermatoglyphic abnormalities. Less common findings include hypoplastic anemia, CSF pleocytosis, and spastic quadripareses.

The Causative Agent

Biological Properties The classification of rubella virus is uncertain, but it generally resembles the arboviruses. The virus is spherical in shape, approximately 60 nm in diameter, has an RNA nucleocapsid with a double membrane, an envelope containing essential lipid, and characteristic projecting spicule surface subunits. The virus is sensitive to pH 3.0 and is readily inactivated by treatment with ether, chloroform, sodium desoxycholate, and Formalin. Preservation of the virus is best accomplished by storage at −70°C in media with a high protein content.

Intracellular infectivity titers are consistently higher than extracellular titers at 24 and 48 hr. but are nearly equal at 72 hr. The peak titer for intracellular virus ($10^{7.8}$ per milliliter) is reached at 48 hr. and that for extracellular virus ($10^{6.8}$ per milliliter) is reached at 72 hr. CF antigen is first detected at 48 hr. and reaches a maximum titer at 72 hr., followed by a sharp decrease due in part to thermal inactivation.

Man is the only natural host for rubella virus.

Experimentally infected rhesus and grivet monkeys may develop a mild illness or a subclinical infection.

In tissue cultures the virus has been grown in a variety of primary cells and cell lines of human, simian, rabbit, and bovine origin. Perhaps the most useful data have been derived from studies with continuous monkey and rabbit kidney cell lines and primary grivet monkey kidney and rabbit embryo cultures. Cytopathogenetic effects (CPE) and high virus titers are produced in monkey and rabbit kidney cells. Earlier assay techniques were indirect and based on the ability of rubella virus to multiply in cells without accompanying cytopathology and to prevent typical CPE produced by echovirus 11, Coxsackie virus A9, Sindbis virus, and other viruses (interference). A recent adaptation of this technique, which involves interference with hemadsorption with Newcastle disease virus, permits the recognition of rubella plaques which stand out as hemadsorption-negative areas. Rubella hemagglutinin (HA) is active on erythrocytes of 1-day-old chicks and adult geese and pigeon cells but not on human or guinea pig cells which can be agglutinated by Newcastle disease virus.

Antigenic Structure Analysis of numerous isolations of rubella virus indicates that they are antigenically homogeneous on the basis of neutralization, HA-inhibition, and CF tests. The CF antigen is produced in parallel with extracellular virus in rabbit kidney cultures. It is not yet known, however, whether the neutralization, CF, and HA-inhibition tests are measuring the same antigen or antigens. The CF antigen and the virus show a similar rate of thermal inactivation, but the CF antigen retains reactivity after prolonged irradiation with ultraviolet light, whereas infectivity is rapidly inactivated.

Specific antisera may be prepared in rabbits following repeated inoculation of virus and used for identification of the virus.

Pathogenesis

Postnatal Infection Children and young adults usually acquire rubella by droplet infection from a patient with the clinical disease and, in some cases, from persons with inapparent infection. The result is an acute, mild exanthematous disease of short duration (3 to 5 days). During the incubation period of 16 to 21 days, it is thought that the virus multiplies in the pharynx and quickly passes by way of the lymphatic system and the blood (primary viremia) to the visceral organs. From the viscera, and perhaps the lymphatic system as well, it overflows into the blood (secondary viremia) and invades the skin where it produces a maculopapular eruption suggestive of scarlet fever. The rash persists for 3 days or less, and recovery quickly ensues.

Posterior cervical lymphadenopathy characteristically develops prior to the rash (often a week before), and enlargement of the preauricular, postauricular, and suboccipital nodes is commonly observed. Rubella without rash may occur in one-third of the cases, and in certain groups (military recruits) the ratio of subclinical infection to overt rubella may be 6.5 to 1.

Virus is found in highest concentration in the pharynx and has been isolated 7 days prior to and 21 days after the rash. Viremia is present 7 days prior to the rash and drops precipitously with the appearance of the rash. The stool may contain virus for a few days after the rash develops, possibly as an overflow from the pharynx or perhaps as a consequence of viral multiplication in the lymphatic tissue of the small intestine. Antibody develops 1 to 2 days after the rash, reaches a peak within 1 month, and persists at a high level for 6 to 12 months.

Arthritis with swelling, erythema, and pain of the finger, wrist, knee, or ankle joints is a relatively common complication of rubella, especially in young females beyond the age of puberty and in adults.

Experimental rubella pursues a generally

similar but somewhat accelerated course. The rash usually appears in 13 to 16 days. The disease may be transmitted by intramuscular injection, by spraying the nasopharynx, or by prolonged contact. Persons with an antibody titer of 1 to 4 are uniformly resistant (no cases in 37 of those inoculated), whereas individuals who do not have neutralizing antibody in a titer of 1 to 4 are highly susceptible (46 cases in 54 of those inoculated).

In Utero Infection

The Basis For the pregnant woman rubella is a mild disease of short duration. For the fetus infected during the first 4 months of pregnancy rubella frequently has grave and disastrous consequences. The placenta and the fetus are infected as a result of the secondary viremia which is an integral feature of the pathogenesis of subclinical as well as clinical rubella.

In the fetus the virus is widely disseminated. For example, in a study involving a 12-week fetus, 3 logs of virus per gram of tissue were found in the eye, and 2 logs per gram of tissue were found in the cord, gut, kidney, liver, and spleen; virus was also isolated from the lung. In other studies virus has been isolated from the following tissues: adrenal gland, aqueous fluid, long bones, petrous bones, bone marrow, brain, CSF, ductus arteriosus, eye, intestine, kidney, liver, lung, lymph nodes, muscle, myocardium, pancreas, peritoneal fluid, skin, spleen, testes, and thymus.

The Timing Fetal infection with rubella virus is a major hazard during the second through the sixth week of gestation when the embryonic organs are being formed (heart, eyes,,etc.). The risk, however, continues until the fourth month. At this time, the immunocompetency of the fetus (Chap. 7) is developed to the extent that it can manage the challenge of rubella infection with an efficiency approximating that of the mother.

Congenital heart lesions are associated with infection in the first 8 weeks of pregnancy, eye lesions with infection in the first 10 weeks, and deafness with infections between the eighth and twelfth weeks. On the other hand, there is a general lack of correlation between the precise timing of infection and the particular stage of embryonic development. This is probably related to the fact that the virus persists throughout pregnancy.

The Consequences When fetal infection occurs in the first 3 months of pregnancy, the most vulnerable targets are the heart, ears, eyes, brain, and platelets. The most striking aspect of congenital rubella is the chronic nature of the infection. This is in sharp contrast to the acute, mild exanthematous illness of short duration in postnatal rubella.

Despite the presence of neutralizing antibody which may be formed by the fetus as early as the third month, virus frequently persists throughout fetal development and for several months of postnatal life. In one study of infants with congenital rubella, virus was isolated from 63 percent in the first month, from 31 percent from the fifth to seventh months, and from 7 percent from the tenth to thirteenth months. No virus was isolated from children 3 to 15 years of age with a history of congenital rubella. The data indicated that infants who carry the virus for the longest period are likely to have the most serious involvement.

Affected infants excrete the virus in their nasopharyngeal secretions, urine, and stools and can spread the infection to susceptible physicians, nurses, and members of the family after close and prolonged contact.

A history of maternal rubella in the first 3 months of pregnancy does not inevitably lead to serious consequences for the fetus, as is indicated by the results included in Table 22-6. It is evident that there are three syndromes associated with proved rubella infection during the first trimester. The classic rubella syndrome is associated with defects involving the heart, ears,

Table 22-6 The Consequences of First Trimester Maternal Rubella for the Fetus and the Developing Infant

Consequence	Classic syndrome	Expanded syndrome	Hepatosplenomegaly syndrome
Number of patients	37	34	10
Mortality (%)	8	32	0
Virus isolation (% positive)	25	66	50
Mean birth weight	2,533 Gm	2,178 Gm	3,327 Gm
Thrombocytopenia (%)	0	100	0
Purpura (%)	0	78	0
Cardiac defects (%)	86	78	0
Hepatomegaly (%)	86	85	20
Splenomegaly (%)	62	76	10
Eye defects (%)	54	41	0
Full fontanel (%)	43	69	0
Long bone changes* (%)	21	45	0
Large anterior fontanel (%)	17	56	0

* There is a defect in bone formation primarily involving the deposit and calcification of osteoid. The changes are probably secondary to metabolic or nutritional disturbance.

Source: Adapted from A. J. Rudolph, E. B. Singleton, H. S. Rosenberg, D. B. Singer, and C. A. Phillips, *Am. J. Dis. Child.*, 110:428–433, 1965 (Copyright 1965, American Medical Association).

eyes, brain, bones, liver, and spleen, a low birth weight, and a mortality of 8 percent. The expanded rubella syndrome, in addition to the findings occurring in the classic disease, is marked by thrombocytopenic purpura, a mortality of 32 percent, and a lower birth weight. The hepatosplenomegaly rubella syndrome is evident initially by hepatic and splenic involvement but may, as the study continues, prove to be associated with other defects (i.e., deafness). These infants have a normal weight at birth and are known to excrete virus.

The Mechanism Although the clinical manifestations of congenital rubella are caused by the virus, the precise mechanism by which the changes are brought about are unknown. Embryonic material obtained by therapeutic abortion from rubella-infected mothers, and used to initiate fibroblast cell strains in vitro, shows an increased frequency of chromosome breakage. The findings, however, do not indicate that chromosome damage or transmitted mitotic errors play a significant role in the teratogenic effects of the virus. A more likely possibility is that rubella virus inhibits the multiplication of certain kinds of human cells. The finding that many of the organs of infants who die with congenital rubella are undergrown and have fewer than the normal number of cells is compatible with this suggestion.

Laboratory Diagnosis

Indirect Method A number of procedures have been developed to permit the isolation and identification of rubella virus. The indirect method based on interference of rubella with the CPE of other viruses (echovirus II, Coxsackie virus A9, and Sindbis virus) has been most often used for diagnostic work because of the difficulty in detecting CPE on initial isolation of rubella in primary human amnion and monkey kidney cells as well as in the rabbit kidney cell line. Identification of the virus as rubella is based on the specific reversal of this interference by rubella antiserum. An improved modification of the interference method (inhibition of hemadsorption with Newcastle disease virus) permits the recognition of rubella plaques which appear as hemadsorption-negative areas. Reversal of the hemadsorption-negative areas by rubella antiserum identified the plaques as being caused by rubella virus.

Direct Method More direct and satisfactory methods for the isolation and identification of rubella virus have been devised recently. These include the production of distinct CPE on primary cultures of rabbit embryo cells (perhaps also on an established line of rabbit cornea cells) within 6 to 8 days after inoculation of clinical materials. Neutralization of the CPE by rubella antiserum indicates the presence of rubella virus. Identification of the virus as rubella, however, is more commonly based on its ability to fix complement or to inhibit HA in the presence of specific antiserum.

Serologic Procedures A serological diagnosis may be established by demonstrating a rise in neutralizing, CF, or HA-inhibiting antibodies, provided that the acute phase serum is collected in the first few days of the disease. Because of speed and economy, the micro-CF or HA-inhibition tests are the preferred methods for a serological diagnosis of rubella. The CF and HA antigens are best prepared from virus grown in the rabbit kidney cell line.

An indirect FA technique, using a chronically infected continuous line of monkey kidney cells as the antigen, has also been developed to assay the antibody content of human serum.

A more sophisticated procedure, useful in establishing the diagnosis in infants congenitally infected with rubella but who do not excrete virus, involves the fractionation of the serum into 7S and 19S components. If a normal infant has rubella antibody as a result of placental transfer from the mother, it is located in the 7S fraction, since 19S antibody cannot pass the placenta. A congenitally infected infant, on the other hand, has rubella antibody in both the 7S and the 19S fractions. The 19S antibody is predominant, is formed in utero by the fetus, and reaches a maximal level in the infant between 4 and 7 months. Some affected infants may also contain antibody in the IgA fraction.

Epidemiology

The 1963–1965 Epidemic in the United States

The major rubella epidemic which developed in the United States in the winter and spring of 1963 and 1964 and which did not involve the Far West until the winter and spring of 1964 and 1965 was the largest since 1935 (Fig. 22-1). The magnitude of the epidemic can be gauged from several parameters. It is estimated that 1,800,000 cases occurred in 1964 alone, producing congenital defects in 20,000 infants. It has been calculated that 1 in every 200 infants born in Philadelphia during the 1964 epidemic had congenital rubella, excluding over 100 therapeutic abortions performed because of maternal rubella in the first trimester of pregnancy.

Source Man is the reservoir of infection in both congenital and postnatal infections. The main cohort of infection is the clinical case of rubella (with or without rash), but inapparent infections with the virus can also serve as the source. Postnatal infection as a rule requires prolonged and close contact with the infected patient. For example, 16 of 17 susceptible persons exposed to prolonged contact with rubella patients acquired the infection, 12 having clinical and 4 subclinical illness. On the other hand, only 1 to 5 susceptible persons having a single brief contact with rubella patients acquired the infection. Infants with congenital rubella also provide a potent source of infection, as indicated by one study which showed that 5 of 7 exposed student nurses developed the disease. Data indicate that under conditions of natural exposure approximately half of the susceptible contacts will acquire the disease, but there is

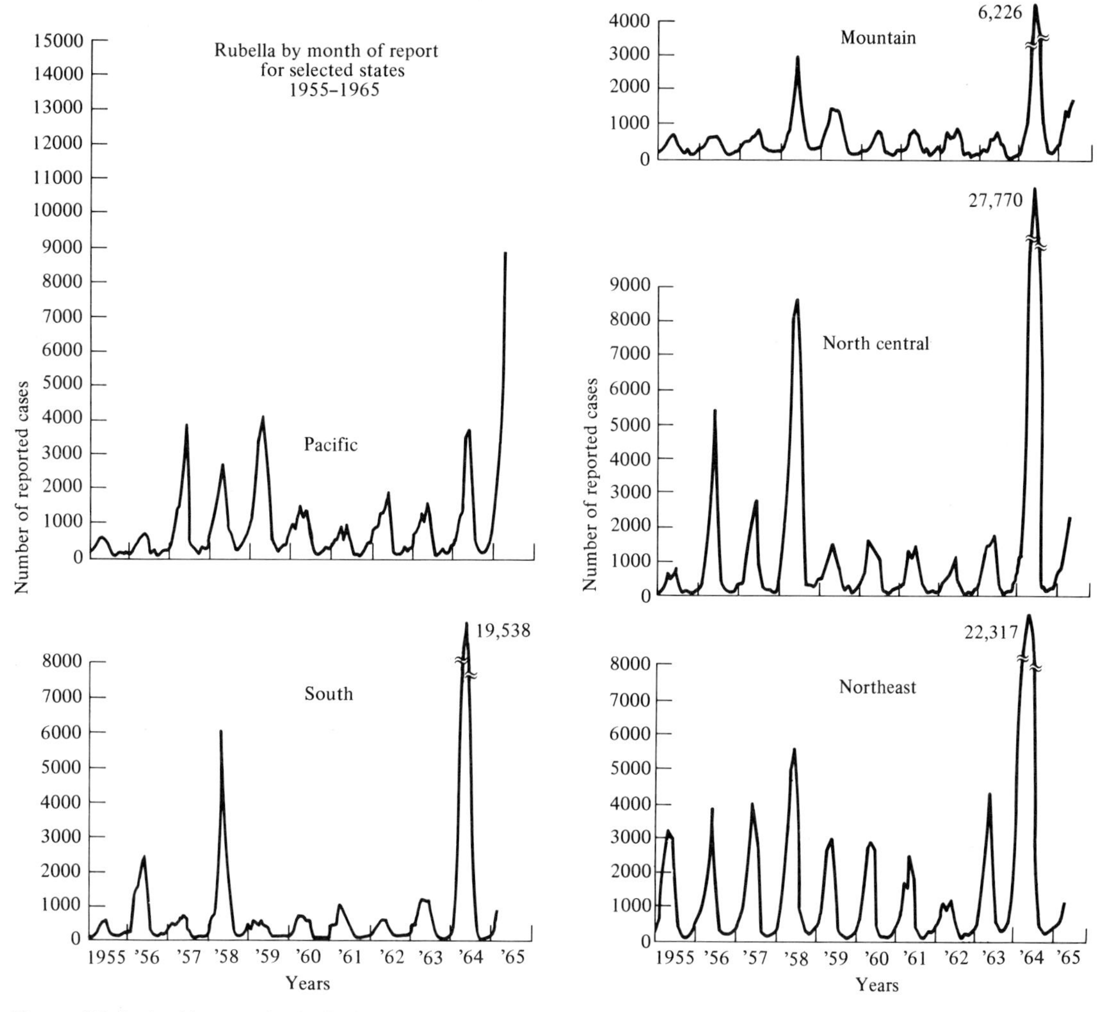

Figure 22-1 Incidence of rubella in the United States from 1955 to 1965. [*Morbidity Mortality Weekly Report, 14(16):139, 1965.*]

wide variation within particular groups, as indicated below.

Age Incidence Rubella is primarily a disease of children and young adults. Approximately 15 percent of women attending prenatal clinics and 15 percent of young military recruits do not have antibody and, consequently, are susceptible to infection with rubella virus. The infection-to-disease ratio is close to 1 to 1 for the fetus of a woman who develops rubella in the first trimester of pregnancy. In young children who are susceptible the ratio is probably close to 2 to 1, whereas in young recruits the ratio may be as high as 6.5 to 1.

Occurrence Rubella occurs throughout the world and, in temperate climates, shows the seasonal prevalence in the winter and spring that is characteristic of infections spread by the respiratory route. When maternal rubella develops in the first trimester of pregnancy, 15 to 20 percent of the infants can be expected to have major congenital malformations. The risk is highest in the first month (about 47 percent), less in the second month (about 22 percent), and least in the third month (about 7 percent).

Evaluation of the 1963–1965 epidemic, the first one in which effective virological and serological procedures could be employed, provided a more accurate assessment of the risks associated with maternal rubella and clearly indicated that the risk of fetal damage was greater than previously estimated. The reasons for the greater extent of fetal damage are based on the following observations: (1) virus isolation and neutralizing antibody studies show that congenital infection can occur in infants who appear to be normal during the early months of life; (2) approximately one-third of cases of rubella occur without rash, and consequently, congenital infection may not be suspected, and there may be no history of maternal rubella; (3) clinically inapparent infection in pregnant women occurs with high frequency. In one study, for example, 15 of 245 women with a history of first trimester exposure, but no clinical rubella, showed seroconversion. When the fact that 85 percent of the women were probably immune at the time of exposure is taken into account, the true rate of seroconversion without clinical rubella is 15 of the 37 susceptible women.

Prevention and Control

Vaccination Attenuated rubella virus vaccines were licensed for use in the United States in 1969. Attenuation of the viruses was achieved following extensive serial passage in tissue cultures of duck embryo, rabbit kidney, or dog kidney. Since 1971 combined attenuated vaccines have become available, and currently several products are licensed. These include measles-rubella, rubella-mumps, and measles-mumps-rubella vaccines. The latter vaccine has been given simultaneously with the third dose of trivalent oral poliomyelitis vaccine. In addition, measles and rubella vaccines have been administered at the same time at separate sites. Surprisingly, currently available data indicate that each of the many combinations and regimens produce antibody responses that are comparable to those which follow administration of the vaccines at different times.

With respect to the use of rubella vaccine, current recommendations suggest that the vaccine be administered between the ages of 1 year and puberty, either singly or in combination. However, in view of the demonstrated efficacy of measles-mumps-rubella combined vaccine when given simultaneously with the third dose of trivalent oral poliomyelitis vaccine, it is probable that this regimen will become adopted as standard procedure in the future.

If rubella vaccine is employed in postpubertal females, its use should be limited to patients who are negative for HA-inhibiting antibody before vaccination, and pregnancy precautions should be observed. The vaccine should not be given to pregnant women. Although the data are limited, in pregnant women who have received rubella vaccine, the vaccine virus has been demonstrated to persist in placental tissue for as long as 69 days after vaccination, and some degree of histopathological changes in decidua and/or placenta occur which are similar to changes seen with gestational rubella. The findings reemphasize the necessity of caution and selectivity in administering rubella vaccine to females of childbearing age and strongly reinforce the desirability of early immunization, preferably during the second year of life. In addition, although there is little likelihood that the vaccine virus can spread from the vaccinated to the unvaccinated, precautions should be taken to avoid contact between pregnant women and vaccinated individuals.

Accurate evaluation of the long-term efficacy of rubella vaccine in the prevention of rubella must await further study, but current results are highly encouraging. The principal untoward effect of the vaccine has been associated with self-limited arthralgia and arthritis in postpubertal females.

Prophylaxis with Human Gamma Globulin The value of human gamma globulin is controversial, and in any event, it does not represent an adequate solution to the problem of preventing congenital rubella for the following reasons:

1 There is little evidence to indicate that globulin (titers of 1:32 to 1:128) protects against experimental rubella.
2 Only 45 percent of pregnant women with first trimester rubella (proved by virological and serological procedures) provide a history of exposure to rubella in the 12 to 21 days prior to illness. Thus, 55 percent of those at risk would not receive gamma globulin.
3 A number of infants have been born with congenital rubella in spite of the administration of gamma globulin to their mothers.

In the most favorable report on the protective effect of human globulin, 15 to 20 ml per patient were given within 5 days of exposure. Apparent protection against clinical rubella persisted for 1 month, but not for 2 months. At 1 month there were two cases of rubella among 145 naturally exposed to the disease who received gamma (γ) globulin (an incidence of 1.4 percent) and 58 cases among 524 women who did not receive γ-globulin (an incidence of 11.1 percent). In the absence of serological evaluation of both groups and follow-up virological and serological studies on the infants delivered of these women, on the basis of the natural history of rubella and the evaluation of γ-globulin in measles, infectious hepatitis, serum hepatitis, poliomyelitis, and other diseases, the most logical deduction is not that γ-globulin exerted an eightfold protection against congenital rubella but that it increased the incidence of inapparent maternal infection without necessarily altering the incidence of congenital rubella.

Other Control Measures

Isolation Isolation procedures are unlikely to be highly effective in view of the many inapparent cases in children and young adults and the fact that congenitally infected infants may be normal in appearance for several months when virus is excreted in high concentration. Nonetheless, it is important to isolate all those known to have rubella from pregnant women.

Abortion Like the administration of gamma globulin, therapeutic termination of pregnancy because of maternal rubella represents a controversial and ineffective solution to the problem. If there are no legal or moral obstacles, therapeutic abortion may be indicated providing:

1 The risk of developing congenital defects is taken into account (estimated to be seven times higher in the first month than in the third month).
2 A definitive diagnosis of rubella in the mother has been established by isolation and identification of the virus or by demonstrating a rising titer of CF or HA-inhibiting antibodies in the mother.

There is no excuse for failing to perform, at least, the necessary CF or HA-inhibition tests. As indicated by the data included in Tables 22-1, 22-2, and 22-3, skin lesions resembling rubella are caused by allergens, by bacterial products, and by a large number of viruses, rickettsia, bacteria, fungi, protozoa, and metazoa.

Treatment

Chemotherapy There is little prospect that effective chemotherapeutic agents will be developed, although amantadine hydrochloride does inhibit an early phase of rubella virus replication in tissue cultures.

Surgical Repair Surgery is one of the few useful methods available for the treatment of infants with congenital defects. The outlook, however, varies with the specific lesion. A patent ductus arteriosus can be readily repaired, septal defects require more complicated open-heart surgery, and cataracts are difficult to repair and affected children may have little vision.

Other Methods In deafness caused by rubella, nerve damage is usually not complete. Consequently, hearing aids and auditory training can be helpful.

Infants who carry and excrete virus for long periods tend to have the most serious involvement. They fail to gain weight and show increasing evidence of mental and physical retardation which, however, may not be apparent for several months. The outlook for these infants is grim since there is no available method for halting the progression of the disease.

By comparison, infants who survive the acute neonatal episode of thrombocytopenic purpura frequently clear up spontaneously along with some of the accompanying lesions, such as hepatitis, anemia, and bone defects.

MEASLES

Measles has been recognized as a clinical entity for about 2,000 years. The major epidemiological features of the disease (an attack rate of almost 100 percent in susceptible contacts, spread by droplet infection prior to the appearance of the rash, an incubation period of 14 days, and prolonged immunity following recovery from a single attack) were initially reported by Panum in 1846.

In the past 20 years reliable techniques for the isolation, cultivation, and identification of the virus have become available and have made possible the development of an effective vaccine, which, if used widely, should bring the disease under control.

In the ensuing discussion emphasis will be placed on the pathogenesis of measles because it is a prerequisite for a basic understanding of the disease and because it illustrates in a unique way the close interrelationships between replication and distribution of virus and the developing pathology, clinical features, and complications associated with the disease. In no other disease of man, with the possible exception of yellow fever, is it possible to show such a precise correlation between the behavior of the causative agent and clinical pathology.

The Causative Agent

Biologic Properties Measles is one of the larger myxoviruses, spherical in shape, 120 to 250 nm in diameter, with a core containing RNA surrounded by an envelope containing essential lipid. The core is composed primarily of a ribonucleoprotein with a coiled herringbone appearance and a protein spacing of 45 to 55 Å. The ribonucleoprotein is about 4,000 nm in length, consists of about 10,000 nucleotides, and has an RNA content of 3×10^6 molecular weight units.

The virus is sensitive to pH 3.0, to heat at 37°C, and is readily inactivated by ether, acetone, formalin, and ultraviolet light. Storage of the virus is improved by protein materials, and the virus may survive for several months at 4°C, for several years at 4°C in the lyophilized state, and indefinitely at −70°C.

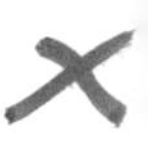

Synthesis of viral components occurs in both the nucleus and the cytoplasm. Peak viral titers (10^6 to 10^8 per milliliter) are found 2 to 4 days after inoculation of stable cell lines with higher concentrations present within the cells as compared with the fluid phase.

Man is the primary and essential host for the virus. Monkeys may acquire a subclinical infection after human contact but apparently do not transmit the infection to other monkeys or to man. In addition, the virus has been adapted to multiply in suckling mice and hamsters.

In tissue cultures the virus has been grown in a variety of primary cells and cell lines of human, simian, canine, and chicken origin. Primary cultures of monkey kidney are the cells of choice for the isolation of the virus from clinical materials. Attenuated vaccine strains are propagated in chick embryo cell cultures. CPE produced by measles includes (1) the formation of syncytia or giant cells containing nuclear and cytoplasmic inclusions and (2) the conversion of epithelial cells to a spindle cell form with nuclear inclusions. Syncytia predominate on primary isolation, and the spindle cell changes increase with serial passage of the virus.

Virus assays are based on end-point titration of CPE in tube cultures, plaque production under agar overlay, and focal areas of immunofluorescence or hemadsorption.

Antigenic Structure There is only one antigenic type of measles virus, and a single attack of the disease confers prolonged immunity.

The envelope is the source of antigens capable of inducing the formation of neutralizing, hemagglutinin-inhibiting (HAI), hemolysis-inhibiting, and CF antibodies.

Hemolysis The hemolytic activity for primate cells is lost on treatment with ether and appears to be associated with a lipoprotein. This antigen causes early, nontransmissible CPE and may be related to the formation of syncytia.

HA Antigen The HA antigen is present on the surface of the virus and at the surface membranes of infected cells where the virus acquires its envelope. The latter location of the antigen is responsible for hemadsorption and for mixed agglutination of infected cells with primate red blood cells (RBC).

The HA does not elute from RBC, cannot be removed from RBC by neuraminidase, causes best agglutination at 37°C, and is associated primarily with noninfective particles. As indicated by the data included in Table 22-7, the HA exists in a variety of forms under natural or native conditions. The antigen may be separated from the envelope by a mixture of ether and Tween 80. Purified ether–Tween 80 HA is highly antigenic, inducing the formation of neutralizing and HAI antibodies in titers comparable to those produced by a formalinized, alum-adsorbed, whole virus vaccine.

Ribonucleoprotein (NP) Antigen NP antigen, located in the core of the virus, may be released from the virus by treatment with ether–Tween 80 and separated by density gradient centrifugation in cesium chloride. The NP antigen fixes complement in the presence of specific antibody but does not induce the formation of neutralizing or HAI antibodies.

Antigenic Relationships to Other Viruses Measles virus shares neutralizing and CF antigens, located in the envelope and the core respectively, with bovine rinderpest and canine distemper viruses. Cross-reactivity is reciprocal between measles and rinderpest but only occurs in one direction between measles and distemper; i.e., antibodies reacting with distemper virus develop in measles infection in man, but the reverse does not occur.

Table 22-7 Naturally Occurring Forms of Measles Hemagglutinin

Size	Density	Infectivity	Hemolytic activity	CF activity	Probable structure
Large	High	+	+	+	Intact virus
Large	High	–	+	+	Partially intact virus
Small	Low	– (early CPE)	+	(–)	Intact envelopes without NP
Small	Low	–	–	(–)	Damaged envelopes
Small	High	–	–	+	35 to 50 nm rosettes
Purified ether–Tween 80 HA	High	–	–	+	35 to 50 nm rosettes

Source: Adapted from A. P. Waterson, *Arch. Gesamte Virusforsch.*, 16:57–80, 1965.
Note: (–), probably negative.

Days	Developments	Associated pathology
0–2	Virus excreted from the pharynx and urine of patients with measles enters susceptible contacts by way of the respiratory tract, or possibly the conjunctiva, and multiplies in lymphatic tissue.	
2–3	Primary viremia occurs with resulting seeding of the entire RES.	
3–5	Viral multiplication ensues within the RES.	Leukopenia develops.
5–15	A massive and prolonged secondary viremia, primarily cell-associated (virus found in washed leukocyte fraction of blood).	
7–11	Visceral spread of virus is accomplished.	
9–14 Incubation period ends	Prodromal manifestations are associated with the following concomitant developments: Virus is found in increasing concentration in the blood, respiratory tract, conjunctiva, oropharynx, urine, feces, lymphatic tissue (lymph nodes, adenoids, tonsils, spleen, thymus, Peyer's patches, appendix), and lungs.	Coryza; epithelial giant cells (some with cytoplasmic and nuclear inclusions) in trachea, bronchi, and some bronchioles; Koplik spots on buccal mucosa with similar lesions on the conjunctiva and the large intestine; conjunctivitis often present; large, multinucleate RES giant cells (some with cytoplasmic inclusions) and hyperplasia in lymph nodes, tonsils, spleen, thymus, Peyer's patches, and appendix; in some cases, appendicitis develops, and surgery is undertaken prior to the appearance of the rash. RES also shows hemorrhage and necrosis.
	Rash appears and virus may be isolated from the rash. The skin lesions may be due wholly or partly to a direct effect of the virus or may be due to an indirect response to a virus-antibody complex.	Skin lesions are associated with focal epidermal necrosis, destruction of hair follicles and papillae, perivascular exudation of serum and infiltration of lymphocytes, proliferation of endothelial cells. Koplik spots show focal necrosis of the buccal mucosal epithelium with formation of tiny white papules or vesicles.
	Viremia ceases. Antibody appears. Virus disappears from the pharynx, conjunctiva, urine, and feces.	Epithelial giant cells are sloughed off from the respiratory epithelium and appear in the bronchial lumen.
	Antibody titer increases. Rash evolves. Patient recovers.	Squamous metaplasia of the bronchial mucosa develops. Chromosomal breakage occurs in 30 to 70 percent of peripheral leukocytes versus 0 to 5 percent of controls, but the significance of the damage is uncertain.
	Complications preceding or following rash	1 Respiratory complications include croup, bronchinolitis, and interstitial pneumonia. 2 Postinfectious encephalitis, occurs with a frequency of 1:1,000 to 1:10,000, but measles is the leading cause (Chap. 24).

Figure 22-2 The natural history and pathogenesis of measles. *[Adapted from (A) M. V. Milovanovic, J. F. Enders, and A. Mitus, Proc. Soc. Exp. Biol. Med., 95:120–127, 1957;*

Diagrammatic representation

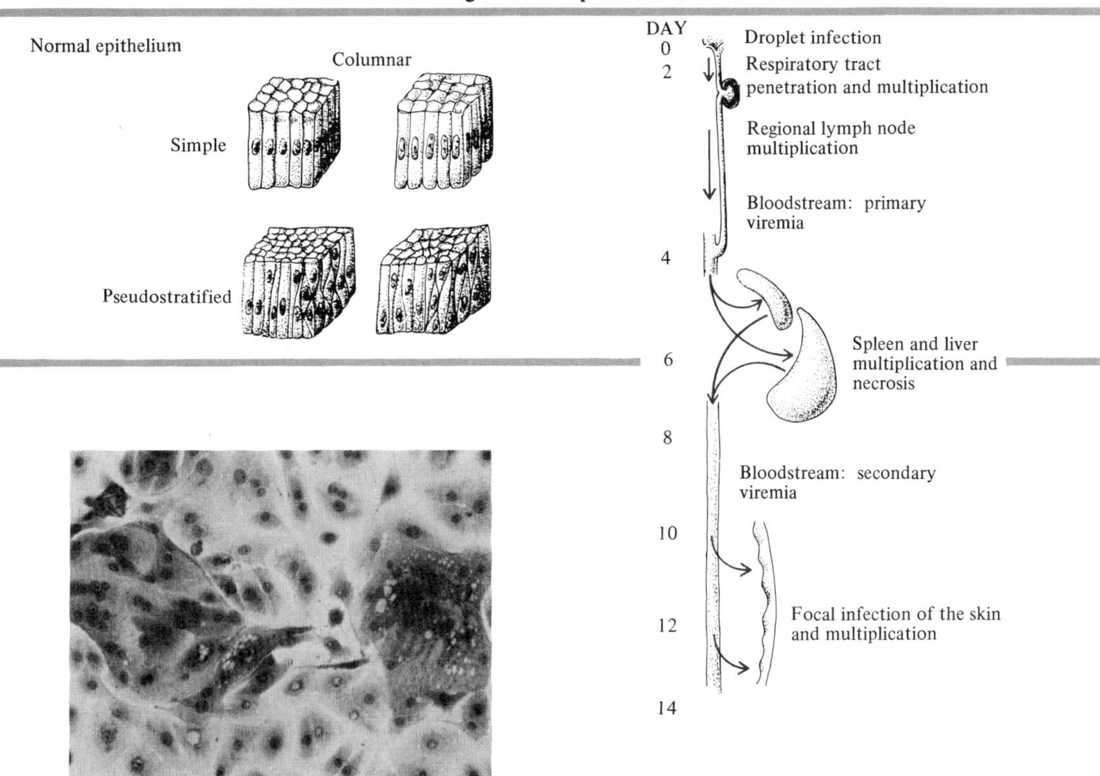

A Multinuclear giant cells *B*

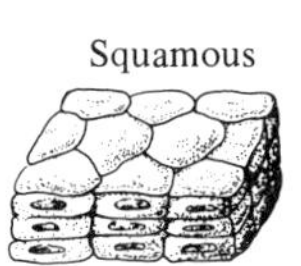

Pseudostratified

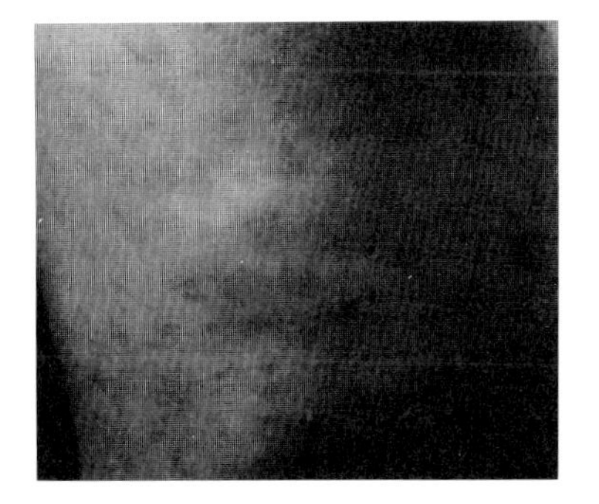

C Early measles skin lesions

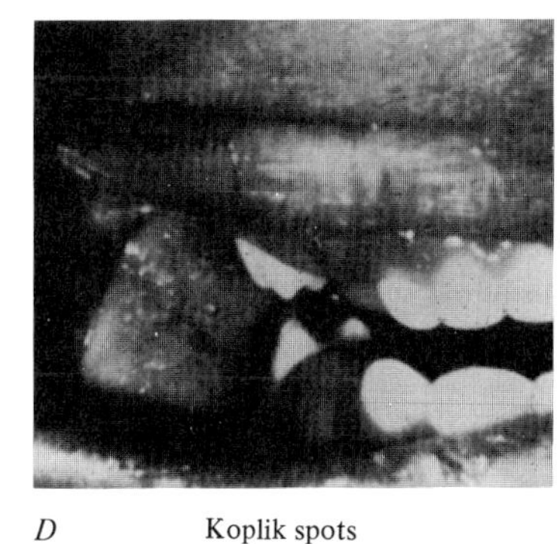

D Koplik spots

3 Secondary bacterial infection, frequently involving otitis media or bronchopneumonia, is one of the major hazards associated with measles.

4 In leukemic children, measles usually results in an overwhelming and fatal pneumonia with giant cells containing intranuclear and intracytoplasmic inclusions.

5 Measles in pregnancy may cause a high rate of spontaneous abortions and premature deliveries without inducing the congenital anomalies characteristic of rubella.

6 Other complications include thrombocytopenic purpura and exacerbation of tuberculosis or kwashiorkor.

(B) F. Fenner, J. Pathol. Bacteriol., 60:529–552, 1948; (C and D) D. W. R. Suringa, L. J. Bank, and A. B. Ackerman, N. Engl. J. Med., 283:1139–1142, 1970.]

Pathogenesis

As evident from a detailed summary of the natural history and pathogenesis of measles (Fig. 22-2), the virus multiplies widely throughout the body of the infected patient with a marked predilection for epithelial and lymphatic tissues. It is doubtful if there is an epithelial surface or lymphatic organ that escapes infection with the virus. Furthermore, most of the clinical pathology associated with the disease is the direct result of virus action on these tissues.

Apart from definitive infectivity assays the movements of the virus through the tissues of the body can be followed by microscopic examination. Infected epithelial and lymphatic tissue cells coalesce to form giant cells, many of which contain cytoplasmic and nuclear inclusions.

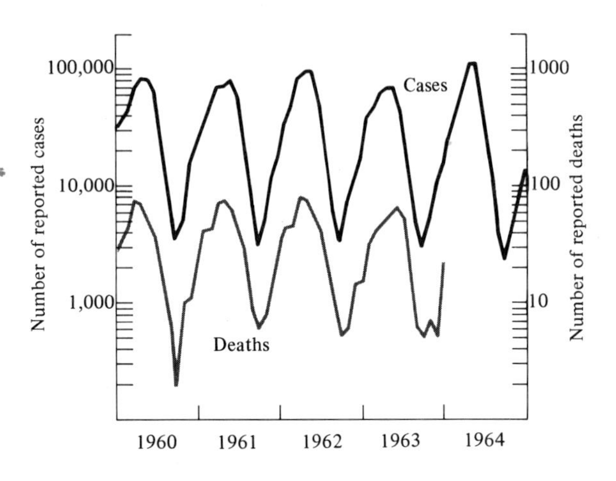

Figure 22-3 Reported cases and deaths due to measles in the United States prior to vaccination from 1960 to 1964. [*Morbidity Mortality Weekly Report, 13(54):38, 1965.*]

Laboratory Diagnosis

Strong presumptive evidence of measles is furnished by the finding of Koplik spots (80 to 95 percent of cases) on combination with the generalized maculopapular rash and the presence of giant cells containing cytoplasmic and nuclear inclusions.

Laboratory confirmation may be obtained by isolating the virus from the patient, preferably from the pharynx, and by inoculating primary monkey kidney tissue cultures prepared from monkeys known not to be infected. The virus may be identified by appropriate immunological reactions, of which the most widely used is the HAI reaction because it is the most sensitive and economical. Neutralization tests, based on inhibition of CPE, hemadsorption, or plaque formation, are rarely employed. CF tests are much less sensitive than HAI tests, and FA tests have not yet been applied to routine diagnosis.

In the absence of virological studies, a laboratory diagnosis may be established by demonstrating a rise in HAI antibodies between the acute and convalescent phases of the disease. Because of the early appearance of antibody, it is essential that the acute phase serum be obtained within 48 hr. after onset. Maximum antibody titers develop 1 to 3 weeks after the appearance of the rash, decline slowly over a period of 6 months, and with the exception of CF antibodies, persist for years.

Epidemiology

Except for isolated areas, usually having a total population of less than 200,000, measles is endemic throughout the world. Epidemic peaks tend to occur at regular intervals of 1 to 3 years, depending on climate, season, and population growth. In temperate countries, the epidemics occur predominantly in the winter and spring, as do other infectious diseases spread by droplet infection. In endemic areas infants are protected for 6 to 9 months as a result of passive transfer of antibody across the placenta. A number of epidemiological parameters, illustrative of the situation in the United States prior to the development of effective vaccines, are indicated in Figure 22-3.

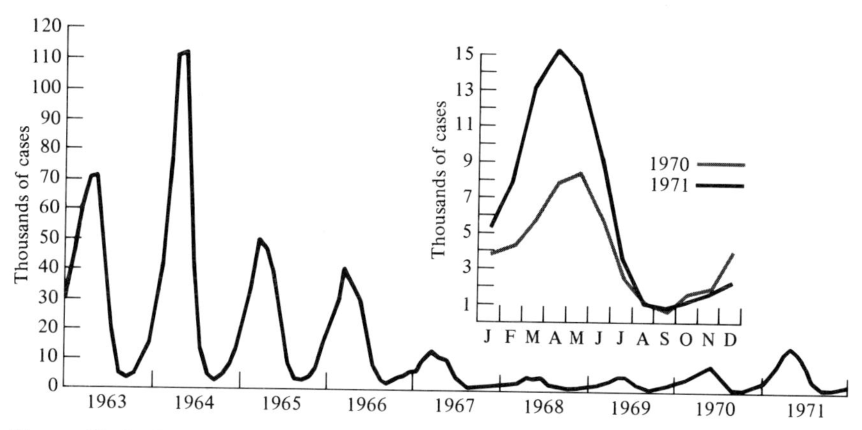

Figure 22-4 Reported cases of measles in the United States before and after the use of vaccine. [*Morbidity Mortality Weekly Report, 20(53):48, 1972.*]

Prevention and Control

Vaccination

Current Status Highly effective, safe vaccines are available for eliminating measles throughout the world. All susceptible children should be immunized with attenuated measles vaccine, except for those who have leukemia, lymphoma, or other generalized malignancy; those whose resistance is altered as a result of therapy with steroids, alkylating drugs, antimetabolites, or x-irradiation; those who have severe febrile illnesses or tuberculosis; and those who are sensitive to egg protein. Preference should be given to susceptible individuals at greatest risk (those with heart disease, cystic fibrosis, or chronic pulmonary disease; those 1 year of age; those in nursery, kindergarten, and elementary school).

Attenuated vaccines are useful in preventing the natural disease in exposed contacts if given on the day of exposure. Several studies have established that, like the Sabin poliovirus, yellow fever, and smallpox vaccines, attenuated measles vaccines can quickly halt epidemics of the disease, especially those that are concentrated in nursery, kindergarten, and elementary schools and hospital pediatric wards. Programs directed toward the continuing vaccination of those attaining their first birthday should be supplemented by community-wide immunization campaigns when the proportion of individuals so protected is known to be low. Even though attenuated vaccines have not been used as extensively as they could be, they have already produced a dramatic effect on the nationwide incidence of measles (Fig. 22-4). Further progress will depend upon a definite improvement in the proportion of the 1- to 4-year-old age group that are vaccinated (61 percent in 1971).

Attenuated Vaccines Through the use of attenuated measles vaccines, optimal immunization can be achieved with one dose in the absence of significant clinical reactions. The protection afforded is quickly induced and is equivalent to that which develops following the natural disease. The vaccinated person cannot spread the infection to susceptible contacts.

Pilot studies have shown that attenuated measles vaccine can be combined with smallpox and yellow fever vaccines. Jet inoculation of the triple vaccine resulted in seroconversion rates (98, 100, and 85 percent) that compare favorably with those achieved for the separate vaccines (97, 100, and 97 percent). In addition, combined measles-mumps-rubella vaccines are effective.

Despite the potential drawbacks associated with attenuated measles vaccines (postinfectious encephalitis, chronic latent infection, contamination with oncogenic avian viruses, and ability to produced chromosome breakage), experience with more than 60 million doses administered in the United States indicates that the vaccine is one of the safest immunizing agents in use. Postinfectious encephalitis has not proved to be a problem. Even though avian leukemia resistance-inducing factor was present in the vaccine, no leukemia antibodies were produced when large amounts were administered to six adults. The amount of chromosomal damage induced in the peripheral leukocytes of patients receiving the vaccine was much less than that encountered in patients who develop the natural disease.

Inactivated Vaccines In view of the great efficacy of the attenuated vaccines, there appears to be only a limited value associated with the projected use of inactivated vaccines. The major disadvantages of inactivated vaccines are related to the four doses that are required, the time required, the delay in achieving a protective effect, and the fact that satisfactory protection is afforded for only a few months and declines rapidly thereafter.

Prophylaxis with Gamma Globulin As indicated by the data included in Figure 22-2, gamma globulin may be used to attenuate or to prevent measles, providing it is administered in adequate concentration within 6 days of exposure. It is especially recommended for exposed children under 3 years of age and for children who are chronically ill. Gamma globulin to attenuate measles is accompanied by a marked reduction in the incidence of postinfectious encephalitis and secondary bacterial pneumonia.

Another form of prophylaxis with gamma globulin is to halt an epidemic of measles in nursery, kindergarten, and elementary schools and in hospital pediatric wards.

DENGUE

Dengue is an acute, mosquito-transmitted (primarily *Aëdes aegypti*) disease of man caused by several distinct antigenic types of a group B arbovirus. The worldwide distribution of the disease between 30 and 40° latitude north and south of the equator closely parallels the distribution of the principal insect vector.

Dengue viruses produce two main clinical syndromes: (1) a mild febrile illness characterized by a maculopapular rash, muscle and joint pain, and generalized lymphadenopathy; and (2) a severe hemorrhagic disease, primarily in children, associated with epistaxis, hematemesis, hepatomegaly, intestinal bleeding, cutaneous petechiae and ecchymoses, thrombocytopenia, prolonged bleeding time, and hemoconcentration which may progress to shock and death.

The assessment of the role that dengue viruses exert in the production of disease is hampered by (1) the fact that the clinical syndromes caused by dengue viruses have also been shown to be due to several different group A and B arboviruses and (2) the long interval required for identification of dengue viruses after their isolation (a year is not unusual). In the latter case, however, the use of the indirect interference test in tissue culture and a FA-CF method in suckling mouse brain have greatly facilitated the identification of dengue viruses.

The Causative Agents

Biological Properties On primary isolation from man dengue viruses multiply without producing cytopathology in suckling mice and hamsters, in continuous lines of grivet and rhesus monkey kidney cells, in hamster kidney cells, and in human cell lines (HeLa and KB). Recent reports, however, suggest that dengue virus can be successfully recovered on primary isolation in *Aëdes albopictus* cell cultures.

After adaptation and continued passage, especially in suckling mice, dengue viruses acquire the capacity to produce lethal infections in newborn and adult mice, plaques in primary cultures of rhesus kidney cells and in KB cells, paralytic disease in monkeys following intracerebral inoculation, and to grow in the chick embryo.

6 types

Antigenic Structure Based on appropriate neutralization tests, there appear to be at least six distinct antigenic types of dengue virus. The dengue viruses, however, share cross-reactive CF and HA antigens with each other and to a lesser extent with other group B arboviruses.

Pathogenesis

Virus is injected through the skin by the mosquito and may enter the blood directly or after passing through the lymphatic channels, nodes, and the thoracic duct. Subsequently, the virus multiplies in virtually every tissue in the body and spills over into the blood, from which the skin is infected. The CNS seems to be spared for the most part, but the skin, muscles, joints, spleen, lymph nodes, intestines, and heart are frequently involved.

The basic lesions are vascular and associated primarily with increased capillary permeability which leads to hemorrhages and effusions of varying intensity. There is no apparent explanation for the mildness of most cases of dengue and the severe hemorrhagic disease associated with other infections with the same virus.

Failure of dengue viruses to produce cytopathology in animals or tissue cultures on primary isolation has led to the development and use of two indirect methods for the identification of the virus. These procedures utilize the techniques of viral interference and fluorescent antibody. However, if the *Aëdes albopictus* cell cultures prove effective for primary isolation, the former methods will probably be replaced.

Laboratory Diagnosis

Indirect Interference Test Continuous cultures of grivet monkey kidney cells are readily infected by dengue viruses of several types on primary isolation from human blood. In this tissue culture system the data show that dengue virus replicates in 2 days and reaches a maximal titer in 4 days which is maintained for 6 more days. Although CPE is not produced by dengue virus, the infected cells develop complete resistance to the cytopathic effect of type 2 poliovirus on the sixth day which is retained for 4 more days. The induction of resistance to poliovirus CPE is associated with and presumably is due to the production of interferon which is initiated by dengue virus.

The indirect interference test is useful in the performance of virus neutralization tests and thus may be employed to identify the agents isolated as dengue viruses.

Fluorescent Antibody, Complement-Fixation Method (FA-CF) In this procedure impression smears of infected suckling mouse brains are reacted with known dengue antiserum and guinea pig complement. Fluorescent-labeled rabbit anti-guinea pig complement is then added. Immunofluorescent staining of the infected cells in the impression indicates the presence of a group B arbovirus rather than the specific presence of dengue virus because of reciprocal cross-reactions among group B arboviruses. On the other hand, the performance of quantitative titers in the FA-CF test provides strong presumptive evidence of the presence of dengue virus. Any one of the type-specific dengue antisera can be used to detect all the antigenic types of the virus because of the intensity of the cross-reactions.

Epidemiology

As with other arboviruses (Chap. 24), the geographical and seasonal distribution and the epidemic pattern of the disease are primarily determined by the efficiency and population density of the vectors.

Prevention and Control

Vaccination Attenuated vaccines for several of the antigenic types of dengue virus have been prepared. They are capable of inducing the formation of protective antibody without producing clinical illness, and vaccinated persons cannot serve as a source of infection for mosquitoes. Extensive field trials, however, have not been completed and commercial vaccines are not available.

The large-scale epidemics which in the past 10 years have spread widely throughout the East and the Far East, Australia, and the Caribbean region (Puerto Rico and Jamaica) together with the severity of the hemorrhagic form of the disease should provide an added stimulus for the development and use of effective attenuated vaccines in endemic areas.

Vector Control The elimination of dengue from many parts of the Western Hemisphere has been accomplished by the systematic eradication of the vector (*Aëdes aegypti*) which is exclusively domestic in its habits and has been man's companion for centuries. The antimosquito methods were used to control urban yellow fever (Chap. 25) but also brought about the control of dengue.

The situation in the Far East, on the other hand, is complicated. An important vector, *Aëdes albopictus,* although it readily adapts to a domestic environment (and thus is efficient in spreading dengue), breeds well in jungle areas. Antimosquito measures attempting to eliminate *Aëdes albopictus* from jungle areas are virtually doomed to fail. In such endemic regions, therefore, attenuated vaccines represent the only logical method of preventing and controlling dengue.

TYPHUS FEVER

Although caused by the same rickettsial organism, the two forms of typhus fever seen in man represent distinct clinical and epidemiological entities and show characteristic serological differences as well. Epidemic typhus is a severe primary disease spread from man to man by the human body louse *(Pediculus humanus).* Recrudescent typhus (Brill-Zinsser disease) is a relatively mild disease occurring in the absence of lice and represents a recrudescence in a person who has undergone a primary attack many years earlier.

Significantly, when lice feed on patients with recrudescent typhus, they become infected with the organism, they can spread the disease to susceptible persons, and consequently, epidemics of louse-borne typhus may ensue.

The Causative Agent

Rickettsia prowazekii, the causative agent of epidemic and recrudescent typhus, is an obligate intracellular parasite that multiplies in the cytoplasm of susceptible cells of man and louse. Like bacteria, rickettsiae reproduce by binary fission, contain both DNA and RNA, possess cell walls, are sensitive to the tetracyclines and chloramphenicol, and appear as minute cocci or rod-shaped organisms occurring singly, in pairs, or chains and having a diameter of 0.3 μm and a length of 1 to 2 μm.

Although rickettsiae have retained most of the major enzyme systems, they have lost many mechanisms for buffering themselves against unfavorable environments. The basis of their obligate intracellular parasitism is probably related to their dependence on the host cell for glutamate (chief energy source), other substrates and cofactors, and a complex environment in which cellular integrity and function are maintained (Chap. 2).

The organisms are labile even at refrigerator temperatures. Viability may be retained somewhat longer when the rickettsiae are suspended in skimmed milk, sucrose, or louse feces. Long-term preservation can be accomplished by storage at −70°C provided that the organisms are placed in sealed glass ampules, quickly frozen, and quickly thawed.

Growth of the organism is best obtained in 6- or 7-day-old chick embryos inoculated via the yolk sac and incubated at 34 to 36°C for several days. The yolk-sac membranes of infected embryos contain high concentrations of viable rickettsiae (10^9 per milliliter). Cultivation is possible in various types of tissue culture, but the rickettsial yields are much lower than in chick embryos.

Lice are readily infected by taking a blood meal containing rickettsiae or by injecting the organism into the insect's rectum. The rickettsiae multiply in the intestinal lining cells and appear in the feces in 3 to 5 days, and the louse usually dies of the infection in 7 to 10 days.

Experimental infection of monkeys, guinea pigs, cotton rats, and mice usually results in an inapparent infection or one marked chiefly by a febrile response.

Antigenic Structure There is a single antigenic type of *R. prowazekii* which contains a number of different antigens. Specific antibodies can be demonstrated by a battery of tests including CF, agglutination of rickettsiae, precipitin reactions, opsonic tests, neutralization tests, protection tests, FA reactions, agglutination of erythrocytes coated with erythrocyte-sensitizing substance (ESS), and agglutination of *Proteus* OX 19 bacteria (Weil-Felix test). The antigens involved in agglutination of *Proteus* OX 19, ESS, and CF are known to be distinct from each other and probably also from the antigen (s) responsible for the induction of protective antibodies.

R. prowazekii is antigenically closely related to *R. mooseri*, the causative agent of murine typhus (Chap. 26). Reciprocal cross-protection occurs in infections caused by *R. prowazekii* and *R. mooseri*, and reciprocal cross-reactions are also evident in ESS *Proteus* OX 19 agglutination tests. In the latter case, *R. prowazekii, R. mooseri*, and *Proteus* OX 19 share a common carbohydrate antigen which forms the basis of the cross-reactions observed.

Pathogenesis

Patients with epidemic and recrudescent typhus have *rickettsemia* during the febrile period. Lice ingest the rickettsiae while taking a blood meal. The organisms multiply in the intestinal cells of the louse, destroy the cells, appear in the feces in quantities infective for man in 3 to 5 days, and usually cause the death of the louse in 7 to 10 days.

When an infected louse bites while taking a blood meal from a susceptible person, it makes a small puncture in the skin and defecates at the same time. The bite is irritating, the person scratches, and rubs the feces containing the rickettsiae into the injured skin.

During the ensuing incubation period of 10 to 14 days, the rickettsiae multiply extensively in the endothelial cells lining the small blood vessels leading to the appearance of vascular lesions which are most numerous in the skin, CNS, myocardium, and kidneys. The accumulation of neutrophils, macrophages, and lymphoid cells around the vascular lesions results in the formation of microscopic nodules.

The louse-borne disease is usually marked by headache which increases in severity, by fever (39 to 41°C) which is present after the third day and persists for about 2 weeks, by a generalized maculopapular rash which appears in 4 to 7 days and which may become petechial in the

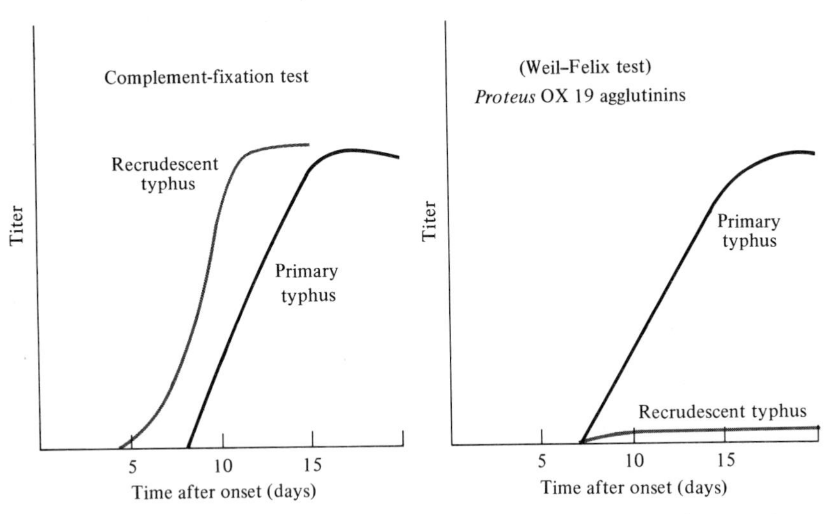

Figure 22-5 Complement fixation and *Proteus* OX 19 agglutinins in primary and recrudescent forms of epidemic typhus. (*Adapted from E. S. Murray, J. A. Gaon, J. M. O'Connor, and M. Mulahasanović, J. Immunol., 94:723–733, 1965; and E. S. Murray, J. M. O'Connor, and J. A. Gaon, J. Immunol., 94:734–740, 1965.*)

second week, by "typhus" (smoky or hazy), a confused mental state with a tendency toward stupor, which develops in the second week, and by renal insufficiency terminating in the third week either in the death or recovery of the patient. Despite the severe involvement of several vital tissues, serious sequelae are usually absent, and recovery is usually complete in 2 to 3 months.

In recrudescent typhus the disease is shorter in duration, the fever curve more irregular, the rash is frequently absent, and the severity is greatly reduced.

Laboratory Diagnosis

Because of the time, expense, and difficulty involved in attempting to isolate and identify *R. prowazekii* from the blood or skin lesions of patients with epidemic and recrudescent typhus, serological procedures are the methods of choice in establishing the laboratory diagnosis. The most useful techniques include the demonstration of antibodies that agglutinate *Proteus* OX 19 (Weil-Felix test), agglutination of erythrocytes coated with ESS, and complement fixation. The interpretation of the results obtained depends on the presence or absence of antibody, the time when they are detected, and their relative titer (Fig. 22-5 and Table 22-8).

***Proteus* OX 19 Agglutinins (Weil-Felix Test)** Since *R. prowazekii* and *R. mooseri* (Chap. 26) share a common carbohydrate antigen with *Proteus* OX 19, it is not surprising that patients with epidemic and murine typhus develop agglutinins for *Proteus* OX 19. On the other hand, failure to detect *Proteus* OX 19 agglutinins in most cases of recrudescent typhus is unexplained but is, nevertheless, a useful diagnostic finding.

In epidemic typhus, agglutinins for *Proteus* OX 19 appear during the second week after onset, reach peak titers of 1:160 to 1:5,000 in the third to fifth week, and fall rapidly in a few more weeks to levels below 1:160. Demonstration of a rise in titer above 1:160 has diagnostic significance but does not distinguish between epidemic and murine typhus. Either tube or slide agglutination tests may be performed with

Table 22-8 Serologic Findings in Epidemic and Recrudescent Typhus (Brill-Zinsser Disease)

Test	Epidemic typhus	Recrudescent typhus
Units of antigen required to obtain maximum CF antibody titers	4 to 8	1
Effect of 60°C for 30 min. on CF antibody titers	Markedly lower	Unaffected
Proteus OX 19 (Weil-Felix) antibody titers (10 to 20 days)	Usually greater than 1:160	Usually negative or less than 1:80
Cross-reacting antibodies to specific murine typhus antigens	Not present	Present*
Species of antibody	19S	7S

* The antibody titers with the murine typhus antigen are two to eight times lower than with epidemic typhus antigen.

Source: Adapted from the data of E. S. Murray, J. A. Gaon, J. M. O'Connor, and M. Mulahasanović, *J. Immunol.*, 94:723–733, 1965; and E. S. Murray, J. M. O'Connor, and J. A. Gaon, *J. Immunol.*, 94:734–740, 1965.

living or killed *Proteus* OX 19 organisms, provided that the cultures are in the O form.

Erythrocyte-Sensitizing Substance Test The test is based on the observation that a serologically active fraction (ESS), isolated from *R. prowazekii* by treatment with ether, heat, and alkali, can coat sheep or human group O erythrocytes. The sensitized erythrocytes are specifically agglutinated by the sera of patients with epidemic typhus.

The agglutinins for the sensitized erythrocytes appear during the second week after onset and persist for long periods after recovery. As with *Proteus* OX 19 agglutinins, a rise in ESS titer has diagnostic significance but does not distinguish between epidemic and murine typhus.

Complement Fixation Specific antigens suitable for distinguishing antibodies of epidemic typhus from those of murine typhus can be prepared by repeated washing of suspensions of *R. prowazekii* grown in yolk-sac membranes.

Complement-fixing antibodies appear early in the course of the disease and reach peak titers in about 2 weeks. Thereafter, the titer falls slowly over a period of months to low levels which may persist for years.

As illustrated in Figure 22-5, CF antibodies appear earlier in recrudescent typhus than in epidemic typhus, reaching peak titers in about 8 to 10 days. Furthermore, as noted in Table 22-8, cross-reacting antibodies to murine typhus antigens are present in the sera of patients with recrudescent typhus but are absent in epidemic typhus. On the other hand, it may not be possible to distinguish epidemic typhus from murine typhus by CF tests on the sera of patients who have been vaccinated with rickettsial vaccines.

Epidemiology

Epidemic Typhus The chief epidemiological features of epidemic typhus are associated with those conditions which favor infestation with lice. For more than 2,000 years typhus fever has been a regular accompaniment of wars, famines, and human misery, especially in colder climates where people are overcrowded, fuel is short, water for bathing is scarce, and the same clothes are worn continuously for months.

In contrast with other rickettsiae (Chap. 26), only infected man and his lice are necessary for perpetuation of typhus fever. *R. prowazekii* has been isolated from goats, but there is no evidence that these animals serve as a natural reservoir of epidemic typhus.

Although persons of all ages are susceptible, the disease is mild in children and severe in adults. The case fatality rate rises sharply with age, the mortality being as low as 1 percent in young children to more than 50 percent in older adults.

Recovery from epidemic typhus is usually followed by prolonged immunity to both epidemic and murine typhus.

Recrudescent Typhus (Brill-Zinsser Disease) Of those who recover from epidemic typhus about 20 to 30 percent retain CF antibodies against *R. prowazekii* for 25 years or more. Some or all of these persons harbor *R. prowazekii.* In one study, fully virulent *R. prowazekii* were recovered from the inguinal nodes of 2 of 31 healthy patients who had CF antibodies in their sera.

The factors that precipitate an attack of recrudescent typhus in these persons with CF antibodies are unknown. The consequences, however, may prove to be disastrous. Lice feeding on such patients acquire the rickettsiae and can spread the infection to susceptible persons, thus initiating new epidemics of typhus.

Prevention and Control

Prevention of Louse Infestation Epidemic typhus has been eliminated from large geographical areas throughout the world by the simple device of preventing infestation with lice. This is accomplished largely by providing an adequate supply of water to suitably heated homes, thereby permitting frequent bathing and frequent change of clothes during the winter months.

Vaccination In highly endemic environments or under conditions where persons are likely to be exposed to the danger of louse-borne typhus, vaccination is recommended. Killed vaccines prepared from yolk-sac membranes were widely used in American troops in World War II with excellent results. Only 64 cases of typhus were recorded, all of whom recovered.

Another vaccine containing the attenuated E variant of *R. prowazekii* has been inoculated into several thousand persons without serious reactions. The E variant can induce immunity to direct challenge with a virulent epidemic strain of *R. prowazekii.* The immunity induced by the E variant persists for at least 5 years.

Controlling Epidemics Delousing can be achieved by heating the clothes of infected persons while they bathe and has been shown to be effective in controlling epidemics of typhus.

The most satisfactory method of delousing, however, involves the use of DDT (dichlorodiphenyltrichloroethane). DDT can be used to treat large numbers of people without removing their garments and retains its lethal effect on lice for more than 2 weeks. Although DDT-resistant lice occur, DDT appears to have retained its effectiveness in controlling epidemics. In the event that resistance becomes a problem, other residual insecticides are available.

Treatment A patient with epidemic typhus should be deloused by bathing and his clothes disinfected by heat. Thereafter, the patient and his garments should be dusted with DDT.

Both tetracyclines and chloramphenicol are highly effective in the treatment of epidemic typhus. The antibiotic employed should be given for 3 days after the temperature returns to normal.

Delirious or stuporous patients require skillful nursing care.

PROSPECTIVE

Man is his own reservoir for the major exanthematous diseases that have been or still are widely endemic throughout the world. For most of these diseases vaccination represents the most rewarding approach to effective control.

Wherever smallpox vaccine has been suitably utilized, the disease has vanished. The use of measles vaccine in the United States in the past few years has resulted in an encouraging reduction in incidence. Further widespread use of this vaccine in the 1- to 4-year-old age group may cause the disease to disappear. Attenuated vaccines for the prevention of rubella and dengue should exert a similar effect.

Elimination of herpes and varicella-zoster by vaccination may prove to be more difficult because of the long-term persistence of the causative agents in large segments of the population. In any event, vaccines have not yet been developed against these diseases.

Although typhus vaccines are available and are useful under highly endemic or epidemic situations, the disease can be more effectively contained by preventing infestation with human body lice by providing homes with an adequate water supply for regular bathing and for the frequent washing of clothes. Another complicating factor in any attempt to control typhus by vaccination is the long-term persistence of *R. prowazekii* in many patients who have recovered from epidemic typhus. Relapse in these patients (recrudescent typhus) may be followed by an epidemic of louse-borne typhus.

BIBLIOGRAPHY

Blattner, R. J., Williamson, A. P., and Heys, F. M.: "Role of Virus in the Etiology of Congenital Malformations," *Progr. Med. Virol.,* 15:41, 1973.

Boese, J. L., Wisseman, C. L., Jr., and Fabrikant, I. B.: "Simple Field Method for Disinfesting Lice-infected Clothing with Dichlorvos Strips," *Trans. R. Soc. Trop. Med. Hyg.,* 66:950–953, 1972.

Boniuk, M. (ed.): "Rubella and Other Intraocular Viral Diseases in Infancy," *Int. Ophthalmol. Clin.,* 12:3–223, 1972.

Breitfeld, V., Hashida, Y., Sherman, F. E., Odagari, K., and Yunis, E. J.: "Fatal Measles Infection in Children with Leukemia," *Lab. Invest.,* 28:279–291, 1973.

Brunell, P. A., and Gershon, A. A.: "Passive Immunization against Varicella-Zoster Infections and Other Modes of Therapy," *J. Infect. Dis.,* 127:415–423, 1973.

Carne, S., Dewhurst, C. J., and Hurley, R.: "Rubella Epidemic in a Maternity Unit," *Br. Med. J.,* 1:444–446, 1973.

Fuccillo, D. A., and Sever, J. L.: "Viral Teratology," *Bacteriol. Rev.,* 37:19–31, 1973.

Hammon, W. M.: "Dengue Hemorrhagic Fever—Do We Know Its Cause?" *Am. J. Trop. Med.,* 22:82–91, 1973.

Hutton, R. D., Ewert, D. L., and French, G. R.: "Differentiation of Types 1 and 2 Herpes Simplex Virus by Plaque Inhibition with Sulfated Polyanions," *Proc. Soc. Exp. Biol. Med.,* 142:27–29, 1973.

Judelsohn, R. G., and Wyll, S. A.: "Rubella in Bermuda. Termination of an Epidemic by Mass Vaccination," *J.A.M.A.,* 223:401–406, 1973.

Juel-Jensen, B. E.: "Herpes Simplex and Zoster," *Br. Med. J.,* 1:406–410, 1973.

Landrigan, P. J., Murphy, K. B., Meyer, H. M. Jr., Parkman, P. D., Eddins, D. L., and Witte, J. J.: "Combined Measles-Rubella Vaccines. Virus Dose and Serologic Response," *Am. J. Dis. Child.,* 125: 65–67, 1973.

Mack, T. M.: "Smallpox in Europe, 1950–1971," *J. Infect. Dis.,* 125:161–169, 1972.

"Rubella and Its Control," *Postgrad. Med. J.,* 48(suppl. 3):5–59, 1972.

Sharp, J. C. M., and Fletcher, W. B.: "Experience of Anti-vaccinia Immunoglobulin in the United Kingdom," *Lancet,* 1:656–659, 1973.

Tauraso, N. M., Myers, M. G., Nau, E. V. O'Brien, T. C., Spindel, S. S., and Trimmer, R. W.: "Effect of Interval between Inoculation of Live Smallpox and Yellow-fever Vaccines on Antigenicity in Man," *J. Infect. Dis.,* 126:362–371, 1972.

Taylor-Robinson, D., and Caunt, A. E.: "Varicella Virus," *Virology Monogr.,* 12:1-88, 1972.

Weibel, R. E., Buynak, E. B., Stokes, J., Jr., and Hilleman, M. R.: "Persistence of Immunity Following Monovalent and Combined Live Measles, Mumps, and Rubella Virus Vaccines," *Pediatrics,* 51:467-475, 1973.

Wenner, H. A.: "The Enteroviruses," *Am. J. Clin. Pathol.,* 57:751-761, 1972.

"WHO Expert Committee on Smallpox Eradication. Second Report," *W.H.O. Tech. Rep. Ser.,* no. 493, 1972.

Wyll, S. A., and Herrmann, K. L.: "Inadvertent Rubella Vaccination of Pregnant Women: Fetal Risk in 215 Cases," *J.A.M.A.,* 225:1472-1476, 1973.

Chapter 23

Systemic Infections Involving the Respiratory Tract

Bernard A. Briody and Zigmund C. Kaminski

PERSPECTIVE

Among infectious diseases pneumonia is the leading cause of mortality, and it ranks fifth among all causes of death. In the United States an estimated 3 million cases occur annually. The average pneumonia is associated with 11 days of bed disability and 17 days of restricted activity. Roughly 10 percent of hospital admissions for acute medical service are due to pneumonia. Such data provide a graphic illustration of the role that pneumonia occupies in the professional activities of the physician.

Pneumonia may be caused by bacteria, fungi, viruses, rickettsiae, chlamydiae, and protozoa. The disease may be localized to the respiratory tract (Chap. 20) or may spread to involve other tissues (Chaps. 14, 15, and 22 to 26). The causative agents of greatest significance are the bacterial members of the endogenous flora, but pneumonia can be produced by bacteria and other microorganisms that are transmitted from exogenous sources. When indigenous bacteria cause pneumonia, the patients invariably have serious underlying disease and/or impaired resistance which most commonly occurs as a consequence of a preceding infection with influenza virus.

Although the widespread use of antibiotics, corticosteroids, and immunosuppressive agents has led to an increased incidence and awareness of pneumonia due to gram-negative enteric bacilli, anaerobic bacteria, fungi, and *Pneumocystis* and to the disappearance of group A streptococcal pneumonia, the pneumococcus (Chap. 14) still accounts for about 90 percent of bacterial pneumonia. In addition, tubercle bacilli continue to be importantly involved in pulmonary pathology even though the morbidity and mortality are progressively declining (Chap. 15).

In this chapter, brief consideration will be assigned to pneumonia caused by bacteria other than the pneumococcus and the tubercle bacillus, to fungi which often are associated with pulmonary pathology but also produce disseminated disease (histoplasmosis, coccidioidomycosis, blastomycosis, paracoccidioidomycosis, aspergillosis), to Q fever, to psittacosis, to *Pneumocystis,* and to a few viruses that induce systemic disease but are occasionally associated with pneumonia.

BACTERIAL PNEUMONIA

Causative Agents

Apart from pneumococci and tubercle bacilli, a large number of bacteria may cause pneumonia. Included are aerobic bacteria, such as staphylococci, gram-negative enteric bacilli (*Klebsiella, Pseudomonas, Escherichia, Proteus, Serratia*), *Nocardia,* and anaerobic bacteria (peptococci, peptostreptococci, *Bacteroides, Fusobacterium, Clostridium, Actinomyces*). Of the aerobes and anaerobes listed, only *Nocardia* is not a member of the normal flora. Because the other organisms are considered elsewhere in the text, the description of the causative agents will be limited to *Nocardia.*

Nocardia asteroides *Nocardia asteroides* is an aerobic, gram-positive, partially acid-fast, branching filamentous bacillus (1 μm in diameter) found in the soil. The organism grows well in 48 to 72 hr. at 37°C on blood agar, media used for mycobacteria, and Sabouraud's glucose agar, producing wrinkled, dry, white or pigmented colonies that penetrate the agar and have a powdery aerial mycelium. Growth is inhibited by sulfonamides. *Nocardia* cell walls contain peptidoglycans, *meso*-diaminopimelic acid, arabinose, and galactose. Following inhalation the organism can produce pulmonary lesions and may spread by direct extension or via the lymph and the blood in about 20 percent of patients. The disseminated disease is almost always accompanied by brain abscesses.

Pathogenesis

Predisposing Factors An essential component of the pathogenesis of bacterial pneumonia is the debilitated or injured host who cannot prevent the organisms from reaching the lower respiratory tract or cannot expel the bacteria before disease results. With the exception of *Nocardia,* the bacteria are members of the normal flora of the oral cavity (Chap. 17), upper respiratory tract (Chap. 14), or the intestinal tract (Chap. 18). For convenience, some of the more commonly recognized predisposing factors are listed in Table 23-1 together with the bacteria encountered.

Endogenous Bacteria As noted above, the members of the indigenous flora of the oral cavity and the upper respiratory tract enter the lower respiratory tract when the resistance of the host is compromised (Table 23-1). The ensuing inflammatory response leads to an alveolar exudate which displaces air, resulting in faulty gaseous exchange, hypoxemia, and spread by spillage into bronchioles and thence by aspiration into other alveoli. A number of the bacteria can also spread as a consequence of necrosis of the alveolar walls, bronchioles, bronchi, and invasion of blood vessels. Necrotizing bacteria include staphylococci, *Klebsiella, Pseudomonas,* anaerobic cocci, *Bacteroides,* and fusobacteria. Empyema is a major complication associated

Table 23-1 Some Predisposing Factors in Bacterial Pneumonia

Predisposing factor	Bacteria involved
Influenza viral destruction of ciliated epithelial cells	Pneumococci, staphylococci, *Hemophilus influenzae*
Extremes of age	Pneumococci, aerobic gram-negative enteric bacilli
Aspiration, regurgitation	Aerobic gram-negative enteric bacilli, anaerobic cocci, *Bacteroides,* fusobacteria
Altered consciousness	
Alcoholism	*Klebsiella*
Oral surgery	Anaerobic cocci, *Bacteroides,* fusobacteria, *Actinomyces,* aerobic gram-negative enteric bacilli
Gastrointestinal and genitourinary surgery	Aerobic gram-negative enteric bacilli, *Bacteroides, Clostridium perfringens*
Postpartum and postabortal states	Anaerobic cocci, *Clostridium perfringens*
Tracheostomy, tracheal intubation, inhalation therapy	Aerobic gram-negative enteric bacilli, staphylococci
Cardiac and neurosurgery	Pneumococci, staphylococci, aerobic gram-negative bacilli
Diabetic acidosis	*Klebsiella*
Noxious gases (ozone, nitrogen dioxide)	Pneumococci
Neoplastic bronchial stenosis	Pneumococci, aerobic gram-negative enteric bacilli, anaerobic cocci, *Bacteroides,* fusobacteria
Chronic obstructive pulmonary disease and cystic fibrosis	Pneumococci, *Hemophilus influenzae,* aerobic gram-negative enteric bacilli
Congestive heart failure	Pneumococci, aerobic gram-negative enteric bacilli
Antibiotics, corticosteroids, immunosuppressive agents, lymphoreticular malignancy	Staphylococci, aerobic gram-negative enteric bacilli, and *Nocardia*

with necrosis, and generalized infection may occasionally occur.

Other Pathogenetic Mechanisms Deposition of *Nocardia asteroides* in the pulmonary alveoli following inhalation from the soil is facilitated when the host is compromised (Table 23-1). Since the organism can cause necrosis of pulmonary tissue, the disease process can progress by direct extension and may penetrate the chest wall or spread hematogenously. Unless the pulmonary disease is promptly recognized and treated, systemic spread occurs in about 20 percent of the patients and is invariably accompanied by brain abscesses with a high mortality (about 80 percent).

Bacterial pneumonia may also occur as a primary disease following inhalation (anthrax, plague, tularemia, Chap. 26), as a result of bacteremia from another focus of infection (abscess, endocarditis, pyelonephritis), by direct intravenous injection along with heroin in addicts, and during the course of inhalation therapy in contaminated aerosol solutions. The latter situation has presented a serious problem because the most common bacteria involved are *Klebsiella* and *Pseudomonas,* which possess necrotizing capacity and are difficult infections to eradicate with antimicrobial drugs.

Laboratory Diagnosis

Because of the numerous causative agents involved in pneumonia (bacteria, fungi, viruses, rickettsiae, chlamydiae, protozoa), the physician is generally confronted with a difficult diagnostic problem. While the clinical manifestations and the acuteness of their onset; the physical and radiologic findings; the extent, consistency, and odor of the sputum; and the presence or absence of leukocytosis often provide clues to the diagnosis, the physician must be guided initially by microscopic examination of a Gram stain and acid-fast stain of sputum or a tracheal aspirate and ultimately by the results of appropriate cultures.

Cultures should be performed to provide for the recovery of aerobic and anaerobic bacteria, tubercle bacilli, and fungi. Consequently, the clinical specimens must be inoculated on blood agar plates and on Sabouraud's glucose agar which are incubated both aerobically and anaerobically and, in addition, on mycobacterial media to permit the isolation of tubercle bacilli. The sources of the clinical specimen should include sputum, bronchial washings, transtracheal aspirates, and blood.

Epidemiology

While bacterial pneumonia is caused predominantly by parasites that are almost exclusively human in origin, the disease does not spread from man to man. In many respects, the epidemiology of bacterial pneumonia follows a pattern that varies little except when influenza epidemics occur (Fig. 20-1). The only other significant epidemiological trends are a higher incidence at the extremes of age and a higher incidence in males as opposed to females.

Prevention and Control

Since the pneumococcus is responsible for about 90 percent of the morbidity associated with bacterial pneumonia, efforts directed at prevention and control must be directed at this problem. As indicated in Chapter 14, the two major approaches involve (1) immunization against the prevalent types of pneumococci and (2) prevention of viral and bacterial infections that predispose to pneumococcal infection. Immunization has not been fully exploited, but much progress has been achieved in the prevention of smallpox, measles, and pertussis. The major unresolved problem is associated with influenza (Chap. 20). On the other hand, even if influenza could be prevented, the many other predisposing factors would remain unresolved. Probably the greatest progress has been accomplished in the therapy of pneumococcal pneumonia which is now associated with a mortality of 5 percent versus 30 percent prior to the use of antibiotics.

The necrotizing action of bacteria may involve a mortality of about 15 percent in pneumonia caused by anaerobic bacteria but is much higher (25 to 60 percent) in the case of disease caused by staphylococci, *Klebsiella*, and *Pseudomonas* even with the most effective antimicrobial therapy. The drugs of choice generally include penicillin G for pneumococci and actinomycetes; clindamycin for *Bacteroides*; penicillinase-resistant penicillins for staphylococci; sulfonamides for *Nocardia*; gentamicin for *Klebsiella*; gentamicin and carbenicillin for *Pseudomonas*; ampicillin for *Hemophilus influenzae*, and chloramphenicol for patients who are critically ill. However, the therapy must be adjusted on the basis of clinical response and sensitivity as determined by antibiotic disk tests and often must be administered for 4 to 6 weeks. Prompt diagnosis and antimicrobial therapy are prerequisites for the prevention of nocardial brain abscesses.

In prevention and control of bacterial pneumonia it is also important to avoid whenever possible any situation, such as administration of a general anesthesic, that facilitates aspiration of material into the tracheobronchial tree; if aspiration does occur, prompt removal is indicated.

FUNGAL PNEUMONIAS

Histoplasmosis

Respiratory infection with the dimorphic fungus *Histoplasma capsulatum* is one of the most commonly encountered in man. Fortunately, pulmonary disease probably occurs with a frequency of less than 1 in 1,000 infections, and disseminated disease is a rare event which is generally limited to patients with impaired resistance (lymphoreticular and bronchogenic malignancy, diabetes, prolonged therapy with corticosteroids and immunosuppressive agents).

In tissues, *H. capsulatum* is a yeast (3 μm) found within reticuloendothelial cells. The organism does not have a capsule as the name implies, but during tissue fixation the cytoplasm retracts from the wall and gives the appearance of a capsule. When cultured on blood agar plates at 37°C, moist white colonies appear which contain small, oval budding yeasts similar to those found in tissues. On Sabouraud's glucose agar at 24°C, however, the organism grows as a mold, producing a cottony aerial mycelium which later becomes buff or brown in color. Microscopically, the hyphal filaments bear spherical microconidia or spores (3 μm) and the characteristic, diagnostic larger tuberculate macroconidia (8 to 15 μm) that are covered with short, stubby, finger-like projections.

In nature, the organism grows as a mold in soil throughout the world but is unevenly distributed. The fungus is concentrated in the great river valleys of the world (Mississippi, Missouri, Ohio, Amazon, Orinoco, La Plata, Congo, and Niger Rivers) that provide an environment, ambient temperature, and humidity conducive for growth. The organism is especially abundant in soil that contains an accumulation of chicken, starling, blackbird, and bat droppings.

Man acquires infection following inhalation of airborne microconidia which are deposited in the alveoli. The fungal spores are phagocytized by alveolar macrophages and replicate in the yeast phase. Thereafter, the organism is widely disseminated in the reticuloendothelial cells and can be recovered from the sputum, blood, and urine. Clinically, there is either no detectable illness or a mild respiratory disease. Thus, most infected patients never are aware of the existence of infection, but upon recovery calcified lesions in the lung, spleen, liver, or adrenals can be detected radiologically, and the patient develops delayed hypersensitivity to histoplasmin (a filtrate of the organism), antibodies to both yeast and mycelial antigens, and a solid immunity to reinfection.

If the intensity of exposure is massive, as in chicken coops, in play areas contaminated with droppings from starling or blackbird nests, or in bat caves, epidemics of clinical disease may occur within 14 days, including acute or chronic pulmonary histoplasmosis and acute or chronic disseminated histoplasmosis. Patients with acute pulmonary histoplasmosis invariably recover completely after an illness of several weeks. Chronic pulmonary histoplasmosis closely mimics tuberculosis and is associated with a mortality of 50 percent within 5 years. The acute and chronic disseminated disease is almost invariably fatal within weeks or months. Cultures of sputum, blood, bone marrow, lymph nodes, and biopsy material are frequently positive. In contrast with the subclinical, benign, or acute pulmonary disease in which CF antibodies appear and quickly disappear, in the chronic pulmonary or disseminated disease high titers of CF antibodies persist and are associated with a poor prognosis.

Diagnosis must be based on isolation of the organism and demonstration of the typical tuberculate macroconidia on Sabouraud's glucose agar containing chloramphenicol at 24°C. A positive histoplasmin skin test simply indicates past exposure and is often negative during the acute disease. Rising CF titers can be used to confirm the data obtained from cultures and to indicate the prognosis.

Therapy with amphotericin B has greatly improved the prognosis of chronic pulmonary histoplasmosis and the disseminated disease but leaves much to be desired because of its toxicity and the necessity for intravenous administration. The mortality in chronic pulmonary histoplasmosis can be reduced from 50 to 25 percent with amphotericin B. If disseminated histoplasmosis is detected early and treated energetically with amphotericin, the mortality can be reduced from more than 90 percent to as low as 10 percent.

Avoidance of massive exposure to *Histoplasma* spores may be accomplished by wearing a mask, wetting down the area, or disinfection with formalin. For example, two epidemics of histoplasmosis occurred following efforts to clear a 5-acre site heavily contaminated with starling droppings. Subsequently, the area was cleared of *H. capsulatum* by disinfection with formalin at a cost of $4,000.

Coccidioidomycosis

Respiratory infection with *Coccidioides immitis* is detected only by a positive coccidioidin (culture filtrate) skin test in about 60 percent of individuals who inhale arthrospores present in the soil in endemic areas of southwestern United States, Mexico, and Central and South America. After an incubation period of about 2 weeks, approximately 40 percent develop an acute, mild self-limited respiratory illness characterized roentgenographically by pneumonitis, hilar lymphadenopathy, and pleural effusion which resolves after several weeks. Manifestations of delayed hypersensitivity appear within 3 weeks in 5 to 20 percent of patients who experience either clinical or subclinical infection. These consist of tender nodular lesions on the anterior surface of the tibia (erythema nodosum) and erythematous wheals and patches on the face, neck, arms, thorax, and back (erythema multiforme). Chronic, progressive disseminated disease occurs with a frequency of about 3 in 1,000 infections; involves the lungs, skin, lymph nodes, bones, joints, and meninges; and results in a fatal outcome in over half of the patients.

In tissues, *C. immitis* occurs as large (20 to 60 μm), round, thick-walled, endospore-filled spherules. The fungus reproduces when the endospores (2 to 5 μm) are released following rupture of the wall of the spherule and develop into new spherules. When cultured on Sabouraud's glucose agar at 24°C, the organism grows as matted white to brown colonies with an abundant cottony aerial mycelium. Microscopically, the mycelium is composed of branching septate hyphae which, as the culture matures, develop into chains of thick-walled, barrel-shaped arthrospores (3 × 4 μm). The arthrospores are highly infectious, and cultures must be handled with extreme care. Screw cap tubes or bottles should be used, and the handling of the cultures should be performed in a biohazard hood.

In nature, the organism is found in the soil in a filamentous, mycelial form. Mature arthrospores easily detach from the mycelium and become airborne. Man acquires infection by inhaling the arthrospores which are deposited in the alveoli and develop into spherules filled with endospores. Upon release of the endospores, new spherules are formed, and the process repeated. As noted above, most infections are localized to the lung and, when clinically manifest, are localized to the lung and, when clinically manifest, are accompanied by pleural effusion. In rare cases, dissemination from the primary pulmonary focus by the lymphatics and the blood may occur within a few weeks and has a grave prognosis which can be confirmed by rising and persistent CF antibodies.

In endemic areas, few individuals escape infection as judged by positive coccidioidin skin tests. New arrivals acquire infection at a rapid rate, up to 50 percent in 1 year and more than 80 percent in 5 years. The disseminated disease occurs more frequently among pregnant women and males than among nonpregnant females and is much more common among Filipino and black men than among white men, perhaps because of enhanced occupational exposure to high concentrations of arthrospores.

Therapy is based on the use of amphotericin B. The drug must be administered intravenously or, in the case of coccidioidal meningitis, intrathecally. The disseminated disease is generally resistant to therapy, but dramatic results have been achieved with amphotericin B, especially in the case of meningitis.

Efforts to prevent infection have not been widely applied but must be directed at avoiding exposure to arthrospores or minimizing exposure in limited areas by planting grass, oiling the ground, or paving high-risk areas in the vicinity of airports.

Blastomycosis

Blastomycosis is a chronic infection caused by the dimorphic fungus *Blastomyces dermatitidis* and characterized by suppurative and granulomatous lesions with a primary focus in the lungs and occasional hematogenous dissemination to the skin, bones, and genitalia. In tissues, the organism is present as a single, thick-walled, spherical yeast (8 to 15 μm) or with a wide septum between the parent and a single bud. When cultured on blood agar at 37°C, the fungus grows slowly over a period of a few weeks and develops waxy colonies which contain yeasts identical to those found in tissues. On Sabouraud's glucose agar at 24°C, the organism grows in the mycelial form, producing white to brown pigmented colonies with cottony aerial hyphae with projecting conidiophores bearing round or oval conidia (5 μm).

The source of the fungus in nature is not known but is assumed to be the soil. Man acquires infection by the respiratory tract and often experiences a subclinical infection but occasionally develops a productive cough, pleural pain, and variable roentgenographic lesions with persistent and increasing infiltration. From the lungs the organism may spread to the skin, bones, and genitalia.

The organism can be demonstrated in KOH-treated preparations of sputum, pus, scrapings, and draining lesions as solitary yeasts or as single budding cells. The thick walls of the yeast are characteristically refractile. Cultures from the patient on Sabouraud's agar at 24°C permit a definitive laboratory diagnosis.

The disease is endemic in the southeastern United States, the Mississippi Valley, and Africa. Clinical manifestations are five to ten times as high in males as in females. In the absence of knowledge concerning the source of human infection and unsatisfactory serological and hypersensitivity tests, little is known concerning the true incidence and mortality associated with blastomycosis.

Amphotericin B is effective in treatment with comparatively low intravenous doses totaling 2 Gm. For milder forms of cutaneous blastomycosis, 2-hydroxystilbamidine has proved useful. However, amphotericin B must be used for the progressive disease, especially when the CNS is involved.

Paracoccidioidomycosis

Paracoccidioidomycosis is a chronic granulomatous infection caused by the dimorphic fungus *Paracoccidioides brasiliensis (Blastomyces brasiliensis)*; characterized by lesions in the oral cavity, lymph nodes, skin, lungs, larynx, and intestine; and limited to Central and South America. Pulmonary manifestations may be primary or secondary but are present in more than 80 percent of the patients. In tissues and when cultured on blood agar at 37°C, the organism appears as a single and multiple budding yeast. On Sabouraud's glucose agar at 24°C the mycelial phase develops slowly forming wrinkled colonies containing hyphae and a few round or oval conidia. Identification of the organism, however, requires the demonstration of multiple budding yeasts on blood agar at 37°C.

In nature, the source of the organism that infects man is not known but may be on plant materials. The portal of entry for most human infections appears to involve the oral mucous membranes, although the lungs represent the primary site of infection in about 20 percent of patients and are secondarily involved in about 60 percent. Invariably, there is lymphadenopathy. In addition, cutaneous, laryngeal, and intestinal lesions are common. From the various primary and secondary sites the lesions may extend or spread hematogenously to involve the liver, spleen, CNS, bones, muscles, adrenals, and heart. Roentgenograms of the lungs usually reveal nodular or infiltrative lesions.

In extensive or disseminated disease CF and precipitin tests using a polysaccharide antigen are almost always positive. Paracoccidioidin skin tests are positive and generally correlate with the CF and precipitin tests when a 1:100 dilution of a culture filtrate is used as the antigen.

Localized and disseminated forms of the disease often persist for years when untreated. The localized disease can be treated effectively with sulfonamides that are excreted slowly (sulfamethoxypyridazine, sulfadimethoxine) or with amphotericin B. Disseminated disease is best treated with amphotericin B if relapses are to be prevented.

Aspergillosis

Aspergillosis is the name applied to a variety of clinical syndromes including otitis externa, allergic asthmatic attacks, pulmonary mycetoma (fungus ball), invasive and necrotizing pneumonitis, endophthalmitis, and disseminated disease frequently involving the brain and kidneys. The causative agents *(Aspergillus fumigatus, A. niger)* are saprophytic fungi that are part of the normal flora of the external auditory canal, oral cavity, and gastrointestinal tract. In tissues, the organism grows as hyphae (4 μm in diameter) with marked branching at 45° angles. Occasionally, when present in the body (external ear, bronchus, pulmonary cavity) in a noninvasive relationship, a second mycelial form is characterized by large conidiophores (5 × 400 μm) which expand terminally into dome-shaped vesicles (20 μm) that produce conidia (3 μm). Similar forms are found on Sabouraud's glucose agar at 24°C in green filamentous colonies. Primary isolation is facilitated by including chloramphenicol in the agar to inhibit bacteria.

Pulmonary aspergillosis and disseminated disease invariably occur in individuals whose resistance is seriously compromised by underlying illness (lymphoreticular malignancy, diabetes, immunodeficiency) or reduced by corticosteroids, immunosuppressive agents, antimicrobial drugs, or alcoholism. Aspergillosis is almost always acquired by the respiratory route. In invasive pulmonary disease the hyphae penetrate the walls of bronchi and bronchioles, causing necrosis and a pyogenic exudate. Disseminated aspergillosis is a suppurative process that primarily attacks the brain and kidneys but may also involve the gastrointestinal tract, heart, and bones.

Laboratory diagnosis is difficult because *Aspergillus* species are widely dispersed in the environment as well as being present as part of the normal flora. Therapy of invasive pulmonary and disseminated aspergillosis is generally unsatisfactory because of the often fulminant nature of the disease and the resistance of the fungi to the best available drug, amphotericin B. When the disease is more chronic, amphotericin B may be beneficial.

RICKETTSIAL PNEUMONIA

Q Fever

Q fever is an acute disease of the reticuloendothelial system caused by an obligate intracellular rickettsial parasite, *Coxiella burnetii,* and characterized clinically by pneumonitis, hepatomegaly, splenomegaly, and rarely by endocarditis. Although chronic disease may occur and the organism had been recovered many years after the initial attack from the lymph nodes of patients undergoing abdominal surgery, Q fever is a self-limited disease with a mortality of less than 1 percent, and recovery is associated with a strong immunity.

Unlike other rickettsial diseases of man (Chaps. 22 and 26), the infection is not transmitted to man by arthropods and there is no rash. In nature, however, the organism is widely distributed in ticks and wild and domestic animals, and the infection is spread among wild animals by ticks and from them to domestic animals by ticks. The human disease primarily occurs as a consequence of inhaling aerosolized particles containing the organism in dried material derived from cattle, sheep, and goats. These animals usually have a mild or subclinical disease, but excrete large quantities of rickettsiae in placental tissues, amniotic fluid, milk, and feces. The organism is unusually resistant to physical and chemical agents, can survive prolonged desiccation, resists ordinary pasteurization (140°F for 30 min.), and remains viable in water and milk for years and in phenol and formaldehyde for days. *Coxiella burnetii*, however, can be killed by the flash method of pasteurization (161°F for 15 sec.). As with the other rickettsiae (Chaps. 2, 22, and 26), *C. burnetii* grows well in the yolk sac of chick embryos and in guinea pigs but does not share common cell wall antigens with *Proteus vulgaris* (Chap. 22) and consequently fails to induce cross-reacting agglutinins (Weil-Felix reaction, Chap. 22).

Following inhalation of a few rickettsiae, the organisms replicate in alveolar phagocytes and in other reticuloendothelial cells throughout the body, especially in the liver and spleen. After an incubation period of 18 to 21 days, there is an abrupt onset of fever, severe headache, chills, and myalgia followed by roentgenographic evidence of pneumonitis together with the appearance of hepatomegaly and splenomegaly. Recovery usually ensues in 1 to 3 weeks but may be complicated by fleeting or continued evidence of endocarditis. In the latter case, a fatal outcome may result.

Because of the hazards involved and the time required to isolate the organism, laboratory diagnosis is established by demonstrating a fourfold or greater rise in CF or agglutinating antibodies. If attempts are made to recover the causative agent in specially equipped laboratories, intraperitoneal inoculation of guinea pigs is usually more sensitive than inoculation of the yolk sac of chick embryos. During the acute phase of the disease the rickettsiae are regularly present in sputum, blood, and urine, with blood being used as the preferred specimen for isolation of the organism.

As with other rickettsial diseases, tetracyclines and chloramphenicol are used in therapy. Practical efforts to control or eliminate the source of *Coxiella burnetii* in cattle, sheep, and goats have not been effected. The main problems are that the disease in these animals is of no economic consequence, and the rickettsiae are so resistant that their destruction would be difficult. Immunization of individuals at high risk (livestock, slaughterhouse, and rendering-plant workers) with a killed vaccine has proved to be valuable. Use of the flash method of pasteurization of milk in endemic areas is essential because human infection can occur following the ingestion of raw or inadequately pasteurized milk containing *C. burnetii.*

CHLAMYDIAL PNEUMONIA

Ornithosis (Psittacosis)

Ornithosis is an acute disease of the reticuloendothelial system caused by an obligate intracellular chlamydial parasite and characterized by pneumonitis, occasionally by splenomegaly, and less commonly by hepatomegaly. The disease varies widely in severity, depending partly upon the source of infection. When contracted from psittacine birds (parrots, parakeets, cockatoos, budgerigars), the clinical course is often severe, may be accompanied by a significant mortality, and may spread from man to man to a limited extent (nurses and doctors in close contact with acutely ill patients). This disease has been termed psittacosis to distinguish it from disease associated with other birds (pigeons, doves, chickens, ducks, pheasants, turkeys) which usually results in a milder disease in man. However, the current tendency is to refer to the disease as ornithosis.

The avian disease is frequently mild and often subclinical, but high concentrations of the organism are expelled into the environment in respiratory secretions and droppings. Human infections follow inhalation of the organism in desiccated aerosolized particles. The organism replicates in alveolar phagocytes, disseminates hematogenously, and then multiplies in reticuloendothelial cells throughout the body. After an incubation period of 1 to 2 weeks, the onset may be abrupt or insidious but is usually associated with a rising fever, an increasingly productive cough, nausea, vomiting, myalgia, roentgenographic evidence of pneumonitis, and in more severe or fatal cases, with splenomegaly, hepatomegaly, delirium, stupor, cyanosis, and anoxia.

Mild cases of ornithosis usually recover in 1 to 2 weeks. In severe cases, the clinical manifestations persist for a few more weeks, convalescence is prolonged, and some patients may experience relapses persisting over a period of many years as proved by isolation of the organism from the sputum or blood.

A laboratory diagnosis can be established by (1) isolation of the organism from the sputum or blood in the yolk sac of chick embryos, HeLa or monkey kidney cell cultures or (2) demonstrating a fourfold increase in CF antibodies in paired acute and convalescent serum samples.

Tetracyclines are the drugs of choice for treatment of ornithosis. The organisms are also sensitive to chloramphenicol and apparently to erythromycin. Many, but not all, strains of the organism respond effectively to penicillin G. The extent of the reservoir in wild birds precludes eradication of the infection, but quarantine regulations have minimized the number of human cases in the United States whenever enforced (Fig. 23-1). In 1972, the United States

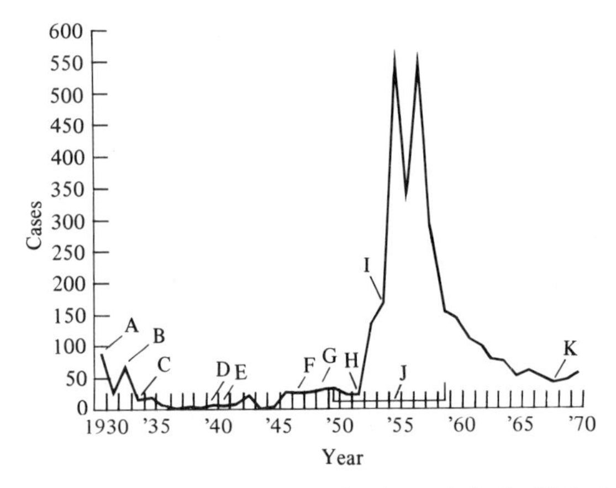

Figure 23-1 Human cases of psittacosis in the United States from 1929 to 1969. *(A)* Public Health Service restrictions placed on the importation of parrots. *(B)* Interstate shipment of psittacine birds prohibited without health certificate; Public Health Service restrictions applied to all psittacine birds. *(C)* Commercial importation and interstate shipment of psittacine birds under 8 months of age prohibited. *(D)* Permitted importation of psittacine birds for commercial purposes, zoological parks, and scientific studies; required laboratory examination for birds for commercial use. *(E)* Recognized in chickens and pigeons. *(F)* Commercial importation of psittacine birds prohibited. *(G)* Recognized in turkeys and ducks. *(H)* Removed all interstate shipment restrictions for psittacine birds from psittacosis-free areas; removed age limit on psittacine birds imported for zoological parks and research institutions. *(I)* Clarified foreign quarantine regulations by defining zoological parks and disposing of excluded birds. *(J)* Many human cases recognized as acquired from commercial poultry. *(K)* Commercial importation of psittacine birds allowed from Public Health Service approved treatment centers after 45 days of chlortetracycline medication. *(United States Department of Health, Education, and Welfare, National Communicable Disease Center, Annual Summary, Psittacosis, 1969, May 1970.)*

Department of Agriculture placed new import restrictions on psittacine birds which require (1) entering or returning birds to be quarantined and to undergo therapy at an approved facility overseas for 45 days and (2) a 30-day postentry isolation period in the United States in approved facilities.

VIRAL PNEUMONIAS

As noted in Chapter 20, pneumonia can be caused by a number of viruses, including influenza viruses, adenoviruses, RS virus, and parainfluenza viruses. In addition, however, pneumonia may be a serious complication of generalized infection with measles, varicella-zoster, smallpox, and cytomegaloviruses. Although the pneumonia may occur in the absence of underlying disease, the resistance of the majority of the patients is compromised by lymphoreticular malignancy, immunodeficiency disease, or the use of immunosuppressive agents.

PNEUMOCYSTIS PNEUMONIA

Pneumocystosis is a progressive pulmonary disease, often fatal, which occurs primarily in patients whose resistance is compromised by immunodeficiency disease, immunosuppressive agents, or lymphoreticular malignancy or in premature and debilitated infants. The causative agent is an obligate intracellular parasite, generally assumed to be a protozoan *(Pneumocystis carinii)*.

In tissues, the parasite often is seen as a group of two to eight round or oval bodies containing a nucleus and cytoplasm located within a cyst (8 to 12 μm), but the individual bodies may occur singly. Pneumocystosis appears to represent the activation of a previous latent infection, but how and when the initial infection occurred are unknown. The onset of the disease is insidious with progressive dyspnea, roentgenographic pneumonitis, increased respiration, and a chronic course which may persist for months or may terminate in asphyxia and cardiac failure in 6 to 10 weeks.

Laboratory diagnosis is often difficult, except when the specimen is obtained by lung biopsy. The organisms are abundant in alveolar exudate. A CF test using antigen prepared from infected lung tissue has proved useful in diagnosing European pneumocystosis but fails to detect antibodies in patients in the United States.

Therapy is reported to be effective when pentamidine isethionate, or the combination of pyrimethamine and sulfadiazine is employed.

BIBLIOGRAPHY

Bach, M. C., Sahyoun, A., Adler, J. L., Schlesinger, R. M., Breman, J., Madras, P., P'eng, F., and Monaco, A. P.: "Influence of Rejection Therapy on Fungal and Nocardial Infections in Renal-Transplant Recipients," *Lancet,* 1:180-184, 1973.

Brodsky, A. L., Gregg, M. B., Lowenstein, M. S., Kaufman, L., and Mallison, G. F.: "Outbreak of Histoplasmosis Associated with the 1970 Earth Day Activities," *Am. J. Med.,* 54:333-342, 1973.

Buechner, H. A., Seabury, J. H., Campbell, C. C., Georg, L. K., Kaufman, L., and Kaplan, W.: "The Current Status of Serologic, Immunologic and Skin Tests in the Diagnosis of Pulmonary Mycoses," *Chest,* 63:259-270, 1973.

Burke, B. A., and Good, R. A.: "*Pneumocystis carinii* Infection," *Medicine,* 52:23-51, 1973.

Doto, I. L., Tosh, F. E., and Farnsworth, S. F.: "Coccidioidin, Histoplasmin, and Tuberculin Sensitivity among School Children in Maricopa County, Arizona," *Am. J. Epidemiol.,* 95:464-474, 1972.

Hughes, W. T., Price, R. A., Kim, H. K., Coburn, T. P., Grigsby, D., and Feldman, S.: "*Pneumocystis carinii* Pneumonitis in Children with Malignancies," *J. Pediatr.,* 82:404-415, 1973.

Kepron, M. W., Schoemperlen, C. B., Hershfield, E. S., Zylak, C. J., and Cherniack, R. M.: "North American Blastomycosis in Central Canada," *Can. Med. Assoc. J.,* 106:243-246, 1972.

Londero, A. T., and Ramos, C. D.: "Paracoccidioidomycosis. A Clinical and Mycologic Study of Forty-one Cases Observed in Santa Maria, RS, Brazil," *Am. J. Med.,* 52:771-775, 1972.

Patterson, R., Fink, J. N., Pruzansky, J. J., Reed, C., Roberts, M., Slavin, R., and Zeiss, C. R.: "Serum Immunoglobulin Levels in Pulmonary Allergic Aspergillosis and Certain Other Lung Diseases with Special Reference to Immunoglobulin E," *Am. J. Med.,* 54:16-22, 1973.

Pierce, A. K., and Sanford, J. P.: "Bacterial Contamination of Aerosols," *Arch. Intern. Med.,* 131: 156-159, 1973.

"Psittacosis" (editorial), *Br. Med. J.,* 1:1-2, 1972.

Richman, D. D., Zamvil, L., and Remington, J. S.: "Recurrent *Pneumocystis carinii* Pneumonia in a Child with Hypogammaglobulinemia," *Am. J. Dis. Child.,* 125:102-103, 1973.

Schacter, J., Sung, M., and Meyer, K. F.: "Potential Danger of Q Fever in a University Hosipital," *J. Infect. Dis.,* 123:301-304, 1971.

Schlenker, J. D., and Barrios, R.: "Gram-negative Pneumonias in Surgical Patients," *Arch. Surg.,* 106:267-272, 1973.

Teres, D., Schiveers, P., Bushnell, L. S., Hedley-Whyte, J., and Feingold, D. S.: "Sources of *Pseudomonas aeruginosa* Infection in a Respiratory/Surgical Intensive-Therapy Unit," *Lancet,* 1:415-417, 1973.

Utz, J. P.: "Chemotherapy of the Systemic Mycoses," *Am. Fam. Physician,* 7:108-114, 1973.

Young, L. S., Armstrong, D., Blevins, A., and Lieberman, P.: "*Nocardia asteroides* Infection Complicating Neoplastic Disease," *Am. J. Med.,* 50:356-367, 1971.

Zehmer, R. B.: "Human Psittacosis in the United States—1970," *J. Infect. Dis,* 124:622-623, 1971.

Chapter 24

Systemic Infections Involving the Central Nervous System

Bernard A. Briody

PERSPECTIVE

Infections of the central nervous system (CNS) of man represent rare and accidental events of little or no consequence in the natural history of the parasite. A multitude of agents have the potential for invading the CNS (Table 24-1). With the exception of rabies and perhaps B virus, the clinical manifestation of CNS involvement occurs in only a small fraction of infected individuals.

In this chapter, emphasis will be given to infections caused by the meningococcus, influenza bacillus, cryptococcus, arboviruses, and enteroviruses (polioviruses, echoviruses, and Coxsackie viruses). In order to gain perspective, how-

Table 24-1 Some of the Infectious Agents Which Produce Disease in the Central Nervous System

Group	Particular causative agents
Bacteria	*Diplococcus pneumoniae, Hemophilus influenzae, Neisseria meningitidis, Staphylococcus aureus,* groups A and B β-hemolytic streptococci, *Escherichia coli, Pseudomonas aeruginosa, Proteus* species, *Enterobacter* species, *Klebsiella pneumoniae, Salmonella* species, *Mycobacterium tuberculosis, Treponema pallidum, Leptospira* species, *Listeria monocytogenes*
Rickettsiae	*Rickettsia prowazekii, Rickettsia rickettsii*
Chlamydiae (bedsoniae)	Lymphogranuloma venereum agent
Viruses	Mumps, poliomyelitis, Coxsackie, varicella-zoster, lymphocytic choriomeningitis, herpesviruses; echoviruses; arthropod-borne encephalitides; B virus; rabies virus
Yeasts	*Cryptococcus neoformans, Candida*
Protozoa	*Plasmodium falciparum, Trypanosoma gambiense, Trypanosoma rhodesiense, Toxoplasma gondii, Naegleria, Hartmannella*
Roundworms	*Trichinella spiralis*

ever, periodic reference will be made to other causative agents. In addition, brief consideration will be given to postvaccinal and postinfectious encephalitis and other noninfectious processes which may simulate CNS infections.

BACTERIAL MENINGITIS

Meningitis is the commonest infection of the CNS. It is an inflammation of membranes covering the CNS and is usually localized to the subarachnoid space. Bacterial meningitis may occur as a primary disease or secondary to trauma or to disease in some other part of the body. It may be acute or chronic, and most cases are sporadic. Epidemics have been initiated primarily by group A strains of the meningococcus, but also by group B and to a lesser extent by group C.

The Causative Agents

It is evident from the data included in Table 24-2 that the relative frequency with which bacterial pathogens produce meningitis varies from time to time in the same area. The more important causative agents certainly include the pneumococcus, influenza bacilli, meningococcus, staphylococci, streptococci, gram-negative enteric bacilli, and tubercle bacilli.

Biologic Properties

Neisseria meningitidis *Neisseria meningitidis*, or the meningococcus, is a strict parasite whose natural habitat is the nasopharynx of man. As indicated by FA procedures, meningococci in the nasopharynx are usually located intracellularly. The organisms are delicate gram-negative intracellular diplococci which lyse spontaneously. Meningococci grow well on

Table 24-2 Causative Agents of Bacterial Meningitis in Boston Hospitals

Bacteria	Percent of infections caused by the bacteria indicated		
	1935	1955	1956–1962
Gram-positive bacteria			
Diplococcus pneumoniae	36	13	30
Staphylococcus aureus	6	14	7
Beta-hemolytic streptococcus	16	1	5
Other streptococci	10	22	2
Other gram-positive bacteria	0	0	1
Total	68	50	45
Gram-negative bacteria			
Hemophilus influenzae	10	4	28
Neisseria meningitidis	8	11	21
Escherichia coli	8	4	3
Other gram-negative bacilli	6	31	3
Total	32	50	55
Total number of cases in the years indicated	50	113	188

Source: Data for the years 1935 and 1955 adapted from M. Finland, W. F. Jones, Jr., and M. W. Barnes, *J.A.M.A.*, 170:2188–2197, 1959 (Copyright 1959, American Medical Association); data for the years 1956–1962 adapted from M. N. Swartz and P. R. Dodge, *N. Engl. J. Med.*, 272:725–731, 1965.

chocolate agar containing vancomycin, colistimethate, and nystatin (Chap. 21) in an atmosphere of 10 percent carbon dioxide. Acid is formed when the organism is grown in media containing glucose and maltose.

In common with all *Neisseria* and certain other bacteria (Chap. 21), meningococci form cytochrome oxidase (indophenol oxidase). *Neisseria meningitidis* is differentiated from nonpathogenic *Neisseria* found in the nasopharynx on the basis of fermentation reactions in glucose, maltose, and sucrose; failure to grow on plain agar, and resistance to vancomycin, colistimethate, and nystatin.

Hemophilus influenzae *Hemophilus influenzae*, or the influenza bacillus, is a strict parasite whose natural habitat is the nasopharynx of man. The organisms are delicate gram-negative encapsulated coccobacilli which lyse readily. In older cultures, pleomorphism is marked. Influenza bacilli grow well aerobically on chocolate agar.

The name *Hemophilus* derives from the fact that the blood supplies two factors, X and V, essential for the growth of the organism. X factor supplies tetrapyrrole compounds necessary for the synthesis of cytochrome, cytochrome oxidase, catalase, and peroxidase. Protoporphyrin, hematin (the iron complex of protoporphyrin), and iron-free porphyrins can serve as a source of X factor. The coenzymes, NAD and NADP (nicotinamide-adenine-dinucleotide and NAD phosphate), function as V factor and play a fundamental role in respiration of the organism. Colonies of influenza bacilli grow much larger around colonies of staphylococci and certain other organisms which synthesize V factor which diffuses into the medium (satellite phenomenon).

Antigenic Structure

Neisseria meningitidis Meningococci are divided into groups A, B, C, and D (formerly designated I, II, II^x, and IV) on the basis of specific polysaccharide or polysaccharide-polypeptide haptens. In the past group A strains have been primarily responsible for epidemics of meningitis. Since 1963, however, group B strains have been responsible for the epidemic cases. Sporadic cases of meningococcal meningitis are usually due to group B and C strains. Cases due to group D strains are rarely encountered. About 15 percent of the isolated strains are nontypable.

Group A and C strains contain capsular haptenic polysaccharides which are responsible for the specific serologic reactions of the bacteria. The interactions can be demonstrated by capsular swelling (quellung or halo reaction) which consists of a ring of precipitate around the capsule in the presence of the homologous antiserum. In group A strains, there is a close correlation between the antipolysaccharide content of serum and protective antibody. No capsule has been demonstrated in group B strains, but a polysaccharide-polypeptide surface hapten has been isolated which confers serological specificity. Antigens contained in group B meningococcal cell walls are highly antigenic for mice and induce protective antibody but are not related to the polysaccharide-polypeptide hapten.

Three other antigens have been found which cross-react with all *Neisseria*. These include the endotoxin, the nucleoprotein, and a polysaccharide C antigen. The endotoxin and the nucleoprotein may be concerned with the pathogenesis of the disease.

Hemophilus influenzae There are six antigenic types of *Hemophilus influenzae* based on the presence of capsular polysaccharides which in activity and chemical structure are similar to pneumococcal polysaccharides. Types a, c, and f are polyhexose or hexosamine phosphates; types d and e are polysaccharides lacking phosphorus and sulfur; type b is a polyribophosphate. The type-specific polysaccharides are responsible for virulence and for the production of protective antibody and react with antibody in capsular swelling, agglutination, and precipitin tests.

Type b *H. influenzae* cross-reacts with pneumococcal types 6, 15A, 29, and 35B. It is by far the most important pathogenic type. The explanation for the distinctive ability of type b *H. influenzae* to produce severe disease with a high incidence of bacteremia and meningitis is unknown.

Two other antigens in *H. influenzae* have been demonstrated. The internal nucleoprotein (P) antigen makes up much of the bacterial mass, is nontoxic, and differs among strains. The M antigen is labile, is located on the surface of the organism, is toxic for animals, and is common to all strains.

Nontypable, nonencapsulated R variants are much more commonly present in the nasopharynx of man than the typable, encapsulated influenza bacilli. The R variants probably are spontaneous mutants of the encapsulated organisms which are selectively favored by the presence of specific capsular antibody which has developed in response to encapsulated strains.

Pathogenesis

As indicated by the list of predisposing factors included in Table 24-3, bacterial meningitis is often preceded by foci of infection elsewhere in the body; by direct inoculation of the organism following head trauma, neurosurgery (craniotomy or laminectomy), and spinal anesthesia; by direct extension of the bacteria through anatomic defects in the cribiform plate and is associated with underlying pathologic processes. It is important to emphasize, however, that in most cases of meningococcal meningitis, in about half of the cases of influenzal meningitis, and in about a quarter of the cases of pneumococcal meningitis it is not known what transforms an asymptomatic infection into meningitis.

Table 24-3 Predisposing Factors in Bacterial Meningitis

Causative agent	Predisposing factors (in order of frequency)
Diplococcus pneumoniae	Acute suppurative otitis media, pneumonia, head trauma (especially skull fracture), anatomical defects (particularly in the cribiform plate leading to cerebrospinal fluid rhinorrhea), underlying pathologic processes (leukemia, lymphoma, diabetes)
Hemophilus influenzae	In children: upper respiratory tract infection, tonsillitis, head trauma, acute suppurative otitis media In adults: anatomic defects, parameningeal focus, defect in antibody synthesis
Neisseria meningitidis	Unknown
Gram-negative enteric bacilli [*Escherichia coli, Pseudomonas aeruginosa, Proteus* species, *Klebsiella pneumoniae, Enterobacter* (*Aerobacter*) *aerogenes*]	In infants: prematurity, birth trauma, prolonged rupture of membranes, maternal infection, hydrocephalus, neurosurgery In children: upper respiratory tract infection, acute suppurative otitis media, head trauma, wound infections, congenital defects, neurosurgery In adults: pyelonephritis, neurosurgery, spinal anesthesia, underlying pathologic processes (brain tumor, lymphoma), empyema
*Streptococcus pyogenes**	In infants: skin and umbilical infections In children and adults: acute suppurative otitis media
Staphylococcus aureus	In infants: skin and umbilical infections In children and adults: neurosurgery, sinusitis, osteomyelitis, endocarditis

* In addition, group B β-hemolytic streptococci are involved.

Meningococcal Infections For the most part infection with the meningococcus remains localized to the nasopharynx of man, and clinical manifestations are usually absent or inconsequential. From this site, the organism may occasionally invade the blood directly and may produce metastatic lesions in the skin, meninges, joints, and less commonly the eyes, ears, lungs, and adrenals. Meningococcemia varies from an acute fulminating illness to a chronic recurrent disease. The most striking feature of meningococcemia is a petechial or purpuric rash which results from thrombosis, extravasation of red blood cells, and inflammatory changes about the capillaries and subterminal vessels in the skin. Acute fulminant infections often give rise to the Waterhouse-Friderichsen syndrome characterized by circulatory collapse, shock, and bilateral hemorrhagic necrosis of the adrenals. The profound shock in fulminating meningococcemia is probably due to the combined action of bacterial endotoxin and tissue anoxia which induces widespread vascular dysfunction rather than to acute adrenal cortical failure. The fundamental vascular lesions are associated with endothelial damage, inflammation of the vessel wall, necrosis, and thrombosis.

Meningitis is the most important and the most characteristic manifestation of infection with the meningococcus. The reasons for extension to the meninges and the mechanism whereby the organisms penetrate the blood-cerebrospinal fluid barrier have not been defined. A petechial or purpuric rash occurs in about half of the cases with meningitis. Most of the characteristic clinical findings are due to meningococcal inflammation and increased intracranial pressure. Meningeal inflammation is responsible for pain in the neck and back, nuchal rigidity, retraction of the head, Kernig's and Brudzinski's signs, hyperesthesia, hyperirritability, and exaggerated reflexes. Severe headache, nausea, vomiting, dilated or irregular pupils, engorgement of the veins of the fundi, choking of the disks, irregular slow pulse, and moderately elevated blood pressure result from increased intracranial pressure. In infants, signs of meningeal irritation are usually much less prominent. The majority of untreated cases progress to a fatal outcome, accompanied by delirium, convulsions, depression, somnolence, stupor, or coma. In patients who recover, the complications may include epilepsy, focal signs of cerebral dysfunction, impaired cranial nerve function, cerebral edema, and subdural effusions.

Infections Caused by Influenza Bacilli Type b is the only type of *H. influenzae* that is a consistent cause of disease. Upper respiratory tract infection, sinusitis, pneumonia, acute laryngotracheitis (croup or epiglottitis), and meningitis may be produced by type b. The acute infectious episodes which frequently recur in chronic bronchitis and chronic pulmonary emphysema (Chap. 20) are often due to influenza bacilli.

In infants and young children who lack protective antibody, type b influenza bacilli may spread from the nasopharynx, enter the blood, and invade the meninges. Occasionally, the organism may spread by direct extension rather than by way of the blood when preceded by upper respiratory tract infection, tonsillitis, otitis media, or head trauma. In children over 6 years of age and in adults, influenzal meningitis is extremely rare and is almost always secondary to anatomic defects, parameningeal foci, or agammaglobulinemia.

In contrast with meningococcal meningitis, a rash does not develop in influenzal meningitis, and the disease tends to progress more slowly over several days. On the other hand, the pathogenesis, pathophysiology, clinical manifestations, and complications of influenzal meningitis are essentially similar to those for meningococcal meningitis.

Laboratory Diagnosis

Cerebrospinal Fluid Characteristics In the typical case of bacterial meningitis, the CSF contains an increased number of neutrophils, reduced sugar levels, and elevated protein levels. As indicated by the data included in Table 24-4, these findings are often helpful to the clinician in suggesting the group of causative agents which might be involved in producing the meningitis.

In bacterial meningitis, the number of neutrophils varies widely, with counts as low as 1 cell per cu mm and as high as 87,000 cells per cu

Table 24-4 Cerebrospinal Fluid Findings in Meningitis Caused by Microorganisms

Causative agents	Average cell count per cu mm	Predominant cell type	Sugar level	Protein content (mg/100 ml)
Bacteria	1,000–10,000	Neutrophil	Reduced	100–800
Yeasts	50–100	Lymphocyte or neutrophil	Reduced	100–500
Viruses	50–500	Lymphocyte	Normal	10–100

mm. In the majority of cases, the cell count ranges between 1,000 and 10,000 per cu mm. On the other hand, 20 percent of patients with meningococcal meningitis may have cell counts of less than 100. There is no relation between the extent of pleocytosis and the prognosis.

Approximately half of the patients with bacterial meningitis have sugar values of 40 mg/100 ml or less, i.e., less than 40 percent of a simultaneous blood sugar. The protein content is elevated in 80 to 90 percent of the cases with the majority of the specimens containing between 100 and 800 mg/100 ml.

Bacteriologic Methods The basic methods for establishing a laboratory diagnosis of bacterial meningitis are the microscopic examination of Gram-stained smears of the centrifuged sediment of CSF and culture of the sediment on chocolate agar in an atmosphere of 10 percent carbon dioxide. Since some of the more important causative agents rapidly undergo autolysis, these procedures must be carried out as soon as possible after withdrawal of the CSF.

As indicated by the results recorded in Table 24-5, the bacteria that commonly cause meningitis can be demonstrated in CSF smears in one-half to three-quarters of the fluids examined and in 87 to 96 percent of the CSF cultures. A positive smear is particularly valuable because, in most cases, it provides the information which permits the immediate institution of chemotherapy with the drug of choice. Cultures are positive in 14 to 38 percent of the CSF specimens which are negative on smear. Even when the smears are positive, cultures should be employed to verify the diagnosis.

Meningococcal Infections In positive CSF smears the majority of meningococci are situated within neutrophils. Their number, however, varies greatly from case to case and in relation to the stage of the disease.

Early in the disease before the CSF is purulent, the proportion of positive cultures is much lower than in later stages. In one study 33, 61, and 96 percent of the cultures were positive when the CSF was clear, slightly turbid, and turbid, respectively. Colonies appearing on chocolate agar in 18 hr. are checked for the presence of typical gram-negative diplococci, for agglutination with specific antisera, for oxidase activity, and for their ability to ferment glucose and maltose.

Accessory methods employed in establishing a laboratory diagnosis of meningococcal infection include attempts to isolate the organism from the blood (5 ml of blood seeded into 45 ml of enriched medium), from the petechial or purpuric rash, and from the nasopharynx (chocolate agar containing vancomycin, colistimethate, and nystatin). Blood cultures and cultures from the rash are useful in cases of meningococcemia without meningitis. Nasopharyngeal cultures may prove positive when CSF cultures are negative and are also valuable in detecting carriers.

A serological diagnosis is achieved either by

Table 24-5 Frequency of Demonstrating the Common Causative Agents of Bacterial Meningitis by Smear and Culture

Causative agent	CSF smear (% positive)	CSF culture (% positive)	Blood culture (% positive)	CSF specimens negative on smear and positive on culture
Diplococcus pneumoniae	77	91	56	14%
Hemophilus influenzae	67*	96	79	16%
Neisseria meningitidis	54	87	33	38%

*An additional 13 percent of the smears were positive but were misinterpreted as proved by culture.
Source: Adapted from M. N. Swartz and P. R. Dodge, *N. Engl. J. Med.*, 272:725–731, 1965.

performing a precipitin or a CF test. In the precipitin test the CSF is examined for the presence of specific antigens by first removing particulate matter by centrifugation and then layering the supernatant fluid with known antiserum. In the CF test the patient's serum is examined for specific antibody by reacting it with known antigens. The CF test is used in cases in which the organisms have been suppressed by treatment.

Infections with Influenza Bacilli In stained smears gram-negative, encapsulated influenza bacilli (almost always type b) are located within neutrophils early in the disease but later are found free in the CSF. Because of their tendency to stain somewhat more darkly at both poles influenza bacilli are sometimes mistaken for pneumococci when the smears are too heavily stained or when they are not sufficiently decolorized. However, this difficulty may be obviated by demonstration of capsular swelling with type-specific *H. influenzae* antibody.

H. influenzae colonies appearing on chocolate agar when stained and examined microscopically reveal gram-negative encapsulated coccobacilli. Following contact with type-specific antiserum, the organisms exhibit capsular swelling. Precipitin reactions and immunofluorescence may also be used to identify the influenza bacillus.

Epidemiology

Meningococcal Infection

Infection versus Disease Meningococcal meningitis is a rare complication of a widely distributed, inapparent, nasopharyngeal infection which occurs sporadically and occasionally in epidemics. Infection is spread by close contact from person to person via airborne droplets. The healthy or asymptomatic carrier state is, thus, the most common outcome of infection. Even at the peak of an epidemic, few carriers develop meningitis. It is, therefore, appropriate to refer to meningococcal epidemics as carrier epidemics. The ratio of infection to disease in both epidemic and interepidemic periods is estimated at 1,000 to 1.

The Carrier State The carrier state represents a complicated situation. From time to time and from place to place, the carrier rate fluctuates widely, depending in part upon the antigenic structure and virulence of the causative strain. In interepidemic periods the carrier rate is less than 10 percent, and the predominant organisms belong to group B. Group C meningococci are less prevalent, and groups A and D are characterized by their rarity. In accordance with these observations, sporadic cases of meningococcal meningitis are due largely to group B and to a lesser extent to group C organisms.

Preceding an epidemic, group A organisms usually become more prevalent, and the carrier rate rises to 20 to 30 percent. At epidemic peaks carrier rates of 40 to 90 percent are the rule. In the past, the majority of epidemics have been caused by group A meningococci, although small outbreaks due to group C have been reported. In the United States since 1963, however, group B organisms have been responsible for the epidemics and for more than 80 percent of the meningococci isolated from carriers. At the epidemic peaks, group B carrier rates of 60 to 70 percent have been found.

Carriers may eliminate the organism quickly in 3 to 4 days, or they may harbor the organisms for several months. In general, those strains which cause epidemics parasitize the nasopharynx for longer periods than strains which do not cause epidemics. For example, epidemic group B strains tend to persist in the nasopharynx, and in a given population group the number of carriers rises cumulatively over a period of time. On the other hand, group C strains are eliminated quickly, and the number of carriers in the same population group remains relatively constant over a period of time.

Correlation of Carrier Rates and Cases of Meningococcal Meningitis Over the years there has been much controversy and confusion regarding the correlation between carrier rates and cases of meningococcal meningitis. The difficulty has arisen largely because the ratio of infection to disease is probably of the order of 1,000 to 1. Consequently, on the basis of chance alone, it is easy to find population groups of 100 or even 1,000 or more with high carrier rates (60 to 70 percent) and no cases of meningococcal meningitis, while other population groups in the same environment with equivalent carrier rates have multiple cases of meningococcal meningitis. Such situations are most readily observed in the military when different companies and battalions in a recruit training center are compared. Thus, with small population groups it is not possible to establish a positive quantitative correlation between meningococcal carrier rates and cases of meningococcal meningitis. On the other hand, if the entire recruit training center comprising several thousand individuals is considered, it has been repeatedly observed that overall carrier rates by month are highest in months of highest incidence of meningococcal meningitis.

Epidemic Characteristics Despite high carrier rates, epidemics of meningococcal meningitis are characterized by a low morbidity and a high case fatality rate. For example, in the state of California between 1913 and 1965, the incidence of meningococcal meningitis fluctuated between 1 and 16.9 per 100,000 per year, and the case fatality rate varied between 11.5 and 74.7 percent. As indicated by the data included in Table 24-6, even more striking contrasts are noted when groups at special risk (military recruits) are compared with the state at large. During 1963 and 1964, 167 cases of meningococcal meningitis occurred in military recruits at Fort Ord, California, and only two cases in an equal number of men in the regular garrison. The susceptibility of military recruits is associated with a number of factors, including their immunological inexperience and their exposure to excessive fatigue and overcrowding. Most cases of meningitis in recruits develop during the first 6 weeks of their training and rarely occur after the eighth week. At Fort Ord 74.2 and 95.7 percent and at the San Diego Naval Training Center in California 96.9 and 100 percent of the cases appeared in 6 to 8 weeks, respectively.

Although meningococcal meningitis is found in all age groups, young children are particularly prone to develop the disease. For example, in the United States in 1964, 48 percent of the cases occurred in children under 5 years of age (19 percent under 1 year of age), 6 percent of the cases developed in the 10- to 14-year-old age group, 20 percent in the 15- to 24-year-old age group (mostly in military recruits), and 26 per-

Table 24-6 Meningococcal Meningitis in the State of California

Year	Monterey County and Fort Ord* (case rate per 100,000)	California (case rate per 100,000)
1959	1.6	1.2
1960	1.6	1.3
1961	5.2	1.4
1962	11.5	2.0
1963	13.3	2.2
1964	23.8	3.2

* Fort Ord is the recruit training center for the Sixth Army area. During 1964, 18.4 percent of the 561 cases in California occurred in Fort Ord.

Source: Adapted from J. W. Brown and P. K. Condit, *Calif. Med.*, 102(3):171–180, 1965; and from *Mortality and Morbidity Weekly Reports*, 13:438–444, 1964.

cent in those 25 years of age or older. Mortality is highest in infants and in the aged.

Infections with Influenza Bacilli Nontypable strains of *H. influenzae* predominate in the nasopharynx of normal persons in most age groups. When typable strains are present, they are quickly replaced by R mutants which fail to stimulate the synthesis of type-specific antigens.

Serious disease in man is almost exclusively caused by type b organisms. Most cases of influenzal meningitis are primary; i.e., they do not develop secondarily to trauma, underlying pathological processes, or other known predisposing factors.

Initial contact with *H. influenzae* type b almost always results in an asymptomatic infection or a mild upper respiratory tract infection which induces the formation of protective antibody. Susceptibility is primarily associated with infants and children who lack protective antibody, but even in this group meningitis occurs sporadically. At a time when one member of a family has type b meningitis, all the siblings and occasionally the parents carry the same organisms without developing serious disease.

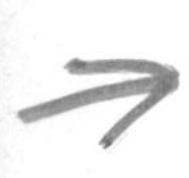

Cases of meningitis due to type b influenza bacilli are rarely seen in those under 6 months or over 6 years of age. Between 60 and 80 percent of the cases develop in those under 2 years of age. In a recent study, 93 percent of the cases occurred in those under 6 years of age, and 97 percent were caused by type b organisms.

Prevention and Control

Chemoprophylaxis for Meningococcal Infections During World War II it was found that chemoprophylaxis with 1 Gm of sulfadiazine per day over a period of months in naval recruits, although intended to prevent streptococcal infections, produced the virtual disappearance of infections due to meningococci. Since then mass chemoprophylaxis with sulfadiazine (1 or 2 Gm daily for 2 days) has been relied upon to control epidemics of meningococcal meningitis among recruits. This method does not eradicate the disease but has been used successfully to abort epidemics whenever the incidence of clinical disease reached a level of 1 case or more per 10,000 recruits per week.

Sulfadiazine-resistant Group B Meningococci In 1963 it became apparent that chemoprophylaxis with sulfadiazine was no longer uniformly successful, since it failed to control epidemics among recruits at the San Diego Naval Training Center and at Fort Ord in California. Investigation revealed that the epidemics were due to sulfadiazine-resistant group B strains of meningococci acquired by the recruits after their arrival at the training centers. Furthermore, even though mass chemoprophylaxis with sulfadiazine was discontinued at Fort Ord, the resistant group B strains persisted and were acquired by new recruits over a period of more than 4 months until the training base was temporarily closed.

Since 1963 sulfadiazine-resistant group B strains of meningococci have spread widely throughout the United States. Studies in 1964 and 1965 have shown that 37 and 31 percent of meningococci recovered from the blood or CSF of civilian and military patients were group B strains which were resistant to 1 mg/100 ml or more of sulfadiazine. No resistant group A strains and only a few resistant group C strains have been identified.

Current Status of Chemoprophylaxis When chemoprophylaxis with penicillin, oxytetracycline, or a combination of penicillin and oxytetracycline was employed for a period of 4 days during an epidemic caused by sulfadiazine-resistant group B meningococci, cases of meningitis due to these organisms continued to occur during the following 2 months. Thus, the evidence available suggests that there is no effective method of short-term chemoprophylaxis for sulfadiazine-resistant group B meningococci. What would have happened if prophylaxis with these antibiotics had been maintained over a period of months is not known. Recent evidence suggests that rifampin or minocycline might prove to be effective in prophylaxis.

The conclusion that mass chemoprophylaxis with sulfadiazine remains the method of choice in aborting epidemics due to group A meningococci has not been challenged. On the other hand, the failure of chemoprophylaxis in group B epidemics indicates the need for caution and for careful surveillance and evaluation of all meningococci isolated from civilian as well as military patients.

Immunization The widespread distribution of sulfonamide-resistant organisms has stimulated greatly renewed interest in the prevention of meningococcal meningitis by immunization. Groups A and C specific polysaccharides have been purified; have been demonstrated to be immunogenic, inducing a brisk bactericidal antibody response in human volunteers; and have been found to be associated with significant protection against infection with groups A and C meningococci. Unfortunately, similar attempts with group B components have been much less promising, but intensive studies are continuing.

Other Control Measures (Meningococcal Meningitis) In the past, prevention and control of meningococcal meningitis have been hampered by failure to develop a satisfactory method of immunization (especially for military recruits) and by the lack of a reliable method for measuring the susceptibility of an individual. The recent failure of chemoprophylaxis in aborting epidemics of meningitis due to group B meningococci has given fresh impetus to investigation of these problems and to the use of older control methods known to reduce the incidence of the disease. As applied to the epidemics at Fort Ord and the San Diego Training Center, these measures included the following:

The input of new recruits was reduced or temporarily halted. Carriers among the training cadre were removed from contact with the recruits.

Additional barracks space was provided so that each recruit had a minimum of 72 sq ft.

New recruits were confined to a specified area.

Contact during training was restricted to a single platoon rather than to a company.

Leaves were canceled during the 8-week training period and prior to transfer to the next duty station.

Treatment Untreated cases of bacterial meningitis almost invariably terminate in death. Although specific serum therapy of meningitis due to meningococci, influenza bacilli, and pneumococci was sound and beneficial, it has been superseded by chemotherapy with sulfonamides and antibiotics. The data included in Table 24-7 indicate the results achieved when optimal chemotherapy and effective supportive care are provided to patients with bacterial meningitis. When the causative agent is known and the

Table 24-7 Mortality of Bacterial Meningitis Treated with the Drug of Choice at Massachusetts General Hospital

Causative agent	Cases	Deaths*	Mortality* (%)
Diplococcus pneumoniae	56	12	21
Hemophilus influenzae	52	4	8
Neisseria meningitidis	39	5	13
Staphylococcus aureus	13	10	77
Streptococcus pyogenes (β-hemolytic streptococci)	9	4	44
Escherichia coli	6	0	0
Pseudomonas aeruginosa	5	3	60

* Excluding deaths within 5 hr. of admission.
Source: Adapted from M. N. Swartz and P. R. Dodge, *N. Engl. J. Med.*, 272:725–731, 1965.

drugs of choice are given without delay, in adequate dosage, and for the necessary period of time, the patient usually shows distinct clinical improvement in 2 to 3 days and is usually afebrile in 3 to 4 days.

Meningococcal Meningitis In view of the prevalence of sulfonamide-resistant group B strains, penicillin is the drug of choice in the treatment of meningococcal meningitis until it can be shown that the organism isolated from the patient is sensitive to the sulfonamides. Penicillin is employed in meningeal doses (12 to 14 million units daily in adults and 3 to 12 million units daily in children) and continued for 12 to 14 days if the meningococcus is resistant to sulfonamides. If the organism is found to be sensitive to sulfonamides, penicillin may be discontinued and the sulfonamide administered. Either sulfadiazine or sulfisoxazole is employed in sufficient dosage to maintain a therapeutic blood level of 10 to 15 mg/100 ml for 10 to 12 days.

Hemophilus influenzae Meningitis A variety of drugs used singly or in combination have produced excellent results in the treatment of meningitis caused by influenza bacilli. These include chloramphenicol alone or in combination with sulfadiazine or sulfisoxazole, ampicillin alone, and streptomycin in combination with sulfadiazine or sulfisoxazole. The drugs are given for a 2-week period to prevent relapse.

Although the initial dose of streptomycin (15 to 50 mg in children and 50 to 75 mg in adults) must be injected intrathecally, it does have the advantage of sterilizing the spinal fluid within 12 hr. in most patients, and within 24 hr. in all patients. Thereafter, streptomycin is given intramuscularly in daily doses of 20 to 40 mg/kg of body weight. When streptomycin is used, another drug (usually a sulfonamide) must be given to prevent the emergence of streptomycin-resistant *H. influenzae.*

Many physicians prefer to use chloramphenicol in combination with a sulfonamide and thus avoid an intrathecal injection. With these drugs *H. influenzae* persists for 24 hr. or more, but the end result in terms of recovery is equivalent to that observed in cases treated with the combination of streptomycin and sulfonamide. When chloramphenicol alone is used, subdural effusions may occur in approximately 10 percent of the patients.

Ampicillin, a broad-spectrum penicillin, because of its efficacy and low toxicity, is more widely employed in the treatment of *H. influenzae* meningitis then any other regimen.

Treatment of Meningitis Caused by Other Bacteria In meningitis due to pneumococci and group A streptococci meningeal doses of penicillin are recommended. For staphylococcal meningitis, nafcillin, a penicillinase-resistant penicillin, is employed unless it is shown that the organism is sensitive to penicillin. Most cases of meningitis due to *E. coli* meningitis respond well to treatment with a combination of chloramphenicol and a sulfonamide. For reasons documented in Chapter 27, however, chloramphenicol and sulfonamides produce serious toxic manifestations in neonates. Consequently, many physicians prefer to treat neonatal meningitis due to *E. coli* with gentamicin or ampicillin when the organism is proved to be sensitive.

Bacterial Meningitis of Unknown Origin Even though stained smears of the CSF fail to reveal the presence of the causative agent, treatment must begin immediately. To delay chemotherapy would needlessly imperil the life of the patient. In selecting the drugs which are to be employed empirically until the cultures are evaluated, the physician must give due consideration to the history, physical examination, the associated infection or disease (if any), and the age of the patient.

Under these conditions a variety of drugs have been utilized in particular patients. For example, on the basis of the most likely pathogens, some physicians use ampicillin and gentamicin in premature and neonatal infants, ampicillin in those between 2 months and 6 years of age, and penicillin G in those over 6 years of age.

It must be emphasized, however, that it is essential to follow the clinical progress, the changes within the CSF, the cultures, and the drug sensitivity of the causative agent so that therapy can be altered if necessary.

BRAIN ABSCESS

Brain abscesses are the most common focal, suppurative intracranial lesions and are etiologically associated with preceding and/or coexisting congenital heart disease, chronic otitis media, paranasal sinusitis, and pulmonary sepsis. In the preantibiotic era, the vast majority of brain abscesses were caused by staphylococci and group A streptococci and were associated with a mortality rate of 30 to 60 percent or more. In the antibiotic era, the causative agents include a variety of bacteria and fungi. Approximately half of all brain abscesses are caused by staphylococci, group A streptococci, aerobic gram-negative enteric bacilli, *H. influenzae*, and *Nocardia*. The other half are caused largely by anaerobic bacteria including peptostreptococci, *Bacteroides* species, peptococci, *Actinomyces*, fusobacteria, and clostridia.

Brain abscesses present a serious diagnostic problem and a critical therapeutic challenge. The keystones for the prevention and control of brain abscesses involve (1) early, intensive, and appropriate therapy of extracranial sepsis, (2) surgical correction of congenital cardiac defects, and (3) most important, early clinical recognition, since the greatest danger is the mass effect of the abscess rather than infection.

The patient with a brain abscess initially seeks medical attention on the basis of headache, fever, and lethargy. If clinical evaluation reveals preceding and/or coexisting pulmonary sepsis, chronic otitis media, paranasal sinusitis, or congenital heart disease, then brain abscess should be suspected. The diagnostic and localizing tests of choice include brain scan, cerebral arteriogram, ventriculogram, and electroencephalogram. Lumbar punctures and roentgenograms of the skull are of much less value.

Brain abscesses develop in patients with chronic otitis media or paranasal sinusitis by retrograde septic thrombophlebitis or less commonly by direct contiguous spread and usually are associated with a solitary abscess. Hematogenous spread from distant sites of infection is characteristic of lung abscesses, pneumonia, empyema, and bronchiectasis and may be associated with multiple abscesses. Other sources of infection which less frequently are associated with brain abscesses include acute endocarditis, septic abortion, dental extractions, and infections of the face, scalp, tonsils, and liver (*Entamoeba histolytica*). In addition, brain abscesses may occur following penetrating cerebral wounds or craniotomy for aneurysm or tumor.

Laboratory diagnosis should be based on the evaluation of blood cultures or clinical specimens obtained from suspected sites of extracranial sepsis, but cultures of CSF are usually negative. The cultures must be designed to permit the recovery of aerobic and anaerobic bacteria, acid-fast bacilli (mycobacteria), and fungi.

Therapy requires intensive antimicrobial therapy, the intravenous use of urea and mannitol to control increased intracranial pressure, and surgical excision when the abscess has been localized. The combination of penicillin and chloramphenicol is frequently used and is effective for most of the causative agents. However, penicillinase-resistant penicillins must be used for the majority of staphylococci, gentamicin and kanamycin for the aerobic gram-negative enteric bacilli, sulfonamides for *Nocardia*, amphotericin B for fungi, metronidazole for amebic abscess, and isoniazid and ethambutol for tubercle bacilli. In the absence of brainstem compression, early recognition, chemotherapy, and surgical excision can reduce the mortality to as low as 10 percent. Neurological deficits, however, may affect 30 percent of the patients who survive.

CRYPTOCOCCAL MENINGITIS

Of all the agents causing systemic mycotic infection, *Cryptococcus neoformans* is the most common cause of mycotic meningitis and is the only species that characteristically produces meningeal involvement. This organism accounted for 24.2 percent of the annual deaths in the United States due to mycotic infection between 1959 and 1968.

Cryptococcus neoformans is a yeast-like, budding fungus (5 to 15 μm in diameter) surrounded both in tissue and on culture by a thick, gelatinous, acidic polysaccharide capsule that is best observed in wet India-ink preparations. The fungus grows readily on Sabouraud's glucose agar and chocolate agar at room temperature and at 37°C. The organism exists throughout the world as a saprophyte in soil and is especially abundant in pigeon nests and excreta. The latter finding is accounted for by the fact that the purine creatinine, present in bird manure, is readily assimilated by *C. neoformans* and not by other species of the genus *Cryptococcus* or by yeasts.

C. neoformans produces disease in animals as well as man. However, like other systemic mycoses, the infection is not transmitted from animals to man or from man to man. The respiratory tract and, to a lesser extent, the skin may serve as the portals of entry for the fungus. Pulmonary and cutaneous lesions may be either primary or secondary manifestations of infection. The primary lesions may heal or may progress to generalized infection. Pulmonary lesions are sometimes confused with tuberculosis or with a neoplastic process. Cutaneous lesions may appear as pustules, ulcers, tumors, or abscesses. Meningeal involvement is invariably found in the late stages of systemic cryptococcosis, occasionally preceded by pulmonary or cutaneous lesions and more rarely by lesions in the visceral organs. The meningitis may be acute or chronic with frequent remissions over a period of several years. The CSF usually shows an increased cell count, an elevated protein content, and a reduced sugar level (Table 24-4).

Approximately 20 percent of the cases of cryptococcosis are associated with serious disorders such as Hodgkin's disease and lymphomas or with serious infections such as tuberculosis or candidiasis. In these patients cryptococcosis probably represents the activation of an existing latent infection rather than a newly acquired exogenous infection. The endogenous nature of cryptococcosis is supported by the finding at autopsy of small subpleural nodules containing *C. neoformans* in patients dying from other causes and by the known ability of steroids, urethane, nitrogen mustard, and folic acid antagonists to activate latent *C. neoformans* infections.

A laboratory diagnosis of cryptococcal meningitis is established by examining the sediment of centrifuged CSF in a wet India-ink preparation, demonstrating the yeast-like cells with their prominent capsules and culturing the specimens on Sabouraud's glucose agar and chocolate agar. A positive urease test is used to distinguish *Cryptococcus* species from *Candida* species and yeasts. Growth at 37°C and mouse pathogenicity distinguish *C. neoformans* from nonpathogenic cryptococci. In other forms of the disease, sputum, pus, and exudates are the materials from which the organism is isolated. Occasionally it may be necessary to establish the diagnosis by demonstrating cryptococcal antigens in the CSF. For this purpose the CF or latex agglutination tests are used.

Treatment of cryptococcal meningitis with amphotericin B is effective, but the nephrotoxicity of the drug must be controlled, and the drug must be given over a prolonged period. Nephrotoxicity is managed by making frequent determinations of the BUN and serum creatinine levels and, when significant elevations occur, by discontinuing the drug until the levels approach normal. The daily dose of the drug is gradually increased from 0.25 mg to a maximum of 1.0 mg/kg of body weight and is given in a liter of 5 percent glucose solution over a period of 6 to 8 hr. Untoward drug reactions other than nephrotoxicity, such as phlebitis, nausea, sweating, fever, and chills, can be reduced by including 10 units of corticotropin or 20 mg of hydrocortisone in each infusion. Because of the frequency of symptomatic remission, treatment must be continued until the cell count, the protein content, and the glucose level of the CSF return to normal values. In most cases this requires about 60 days.

PRIMARY ENCEPHALITIS CAUSED BY ARBOVIRUSES

Primary encephalitis is an acute inflammatory illness in which encephalitic manifestations are an intrinsic part. It is usually caused by viruses, including the arboviruses (arthropod-borne viruses), polioviruses, Coxsackie viruses, echoviruses and mumps, herpes, rabies, and lymphocytic choriomeningitis viruses but may also be due to infection with rickettsiae, chlamydiae, bacteria, fungi, and protozoa.

Approximately one-quarter of the more than 250 arboviruses are known to be associated with disease in man. The clinical patterns of illness vary from an acute benign fever, often accompanied by generalized joint pains and a rash, to a severe and frequently fatal disease with marked hemorrhagic manifestations, to a disease with significant CNS involvement. In this chapter attention will be focused on the few arboviruses which cause encephalitis in man. These include the tick-borne encephalitides (TBE) as well as those spread by mosquitoes and represented by the viruses of Venezuelan equine encephalitis (VEE), eastern equine encephalitis (EEE), western equine encephalitis (WEE), St. Louis encephalitis, Japanese B encephalitis, and California encephalitis. Detailed consideration of arboviruses which commonly produce the acute benign fevers and the hemorrhagic fevers, including yellow fever, will be found in Chapter 25.

Because the arboviruses causing encephalitis are essentially similar, their common properties will be emphasized, and the various aspects of the disease they produce will be considered in general rather than specific terms.

The Causative Agents

Biological Properties The arboviruses are spherical in shape, approximately 30 to 50 nm in diameter, contain RNA and protein, are readily inactivated by ether and sodium deoxycholate due to the presence of essential lipid in the envelope, and rapidly lose infectivity on exposure to pH 3.0.

As the name implies, the viruses multiply in arthropods and are subsequently transmitted to man or other animals through the bite of the hematophagous vectors. The principal arthropod vectors involved are the *Culex* and *Aëdes* species of mosquitoes and the *Ixodes* species of ticks. After a tick becomes infected, the virus is perpetuated in the arthropod by transovarial transmission. Mosquitoes, on the other hand, remain infective only for life and do not pass the infection on to their offspring transovarially.

A vast reservoir of naturally infected animals with viremia serves as the potential source of infection for the infection for the hematophagous vectors. Primarily involved in the viremic reservoir are a variety of birds, rodents, and ungulates. The infected animals frequently develop a prolonged viremia without clinical manifestations, thus providing ample opportunity for infection of the arthropods. Man is purely an accidental and incidental host of no consequence in the cyclic maintenance of the arboviruses causing encephalitis. For a few arboviruses (dengue, urban yellow fever), however, the basic cycle may include man and the vector.

The arboviruses have been experimentally studied most effectively in newborn and adult mice, chick embryos, 12-hr.-old chicks, and a variety of tissue cultures. The viruses are pathogenic for newborn mice following peripheral as well as intracerebral inoculation. With increasing age mice retain their susceptibility to intracerebral inoculation of virus but rapidly develop resistance to peripheral inoculation (except for VEE and TBE). Infected mouse brains, chick embryos, 12-hr.-old chicks, and tissue cultures yield high concentrations of virus (10^8 to 10^{10} PFU/Gm of wet tissue or tissue culture fluid). Viral replication has been studied quantitatively in monolayers of chick and mouse fibroblasts; in chick, duck, hamster, guinea pig, pig, monkey, and human kidney cells; and in HeLa and KB cells.

Arboviruses multiply rapidly in the cytoplasm of the susceptible tissue culture cells and yield high titers in the extracellular fluid (10^{10} PFU/ml) at 12 hr. before any cytopathic effect is evident. Infectious RNA is synthesized at 2½ hr. and reaches a plateau at 3½ hr. Mature virus particles are formed shortly thereafter and are released slowly from the cell for about 36 hr. Cytopathogenicity is demonstrable at 24 hr. and is extensive at 48 hr. During the period when virus is being released from the cell surface, hemadsorption can be demonstrated due to the presence of hemagglutinin in the lipoprotein envelope of the virus.

Antigenic Structure Antigenic classification of the arboviruses is based on the sharing of HA, CF, and neutralizing antigens. Cross-reactions are greatest with HA, less extensive with CF, and least with the neutralizing antigen. Conversely, the greatest degree of antigenic specificity is shown with neutralizing antigen, a lesser degree with CF, and the least with HA. At present, 21 antigenic groups comprising approximately 150 viruses have been recognized. The most important human diseases are caused by groups A, B, and California. VEE, EEE, and WEE are in group A; and St. Louis encephalitis, Japanese B encephalitis, Murray Valley encephalitis, and TBE are in group B. There are subgroups or complexes within groups A and B which are more closely interrelated. For example, St. Louis encephalitis, Japanese B encephalitis, and Murray Valley encephalitis viruses form a subgroup in which extensive sharing of antigens can be demonstrated by neutralization as well as by CF and HA-inhibition (HAI) tests.

In response to clinical infection with arboviruses, HAI and neutralizing antibodies develop rapidly and persist for many years. CF antibody forms slowly (about 10 days after onset) and falls rapidly, rarely persisting for more than 1 or 2 years. Antibody response to inapparent infection, on the other hand, is not especially strong and is not long-lasting.

Pathogenesis

Except for TBE which may be acquired by ingestion of raw or inadequately pasteurized goat's milk and aersol infection of laboratory workers with VEE, arboviruses (including TBE and VEE) are transmitted to man by the bite of an infected arthropod. Although the events occurring during the 1- to 3-week incubation period are not precisely known, the major features of the pathogenesis can be sketched in with reasonable certainty.

The virus is injected through the skin by the arthropod and is transported by the lymphatic channels to the regional lymph nodes. After multiplication in the lymph nodes, small quantities of virus spill over into the bloodstream. In some cases, however, the arthropod may inject the virus directly into the bloodstream, thus bypassing the regional lymph node. The virus is then disseminated to other lymphatic tissue and may multiply in some of the visceral organs. During the brief but more intensive viremia which follows, the virus may localize in the CNS. By the time the incubation period ends with the appearance of encephalitic manifestations, virus has disappeared from the blood but is present in the CNS.

Vascular lesions are prominent with edema, congestion, and hemorrhage occurring throughout the CNS and occasionally in the viscera, but showing great variation in intensity in the individual case. The lesions in the CNS consist primarily of focal areas of neuronal necrosis and neuronophagia accompanied by perivascular infiltration by monocytes, glial cell proliferation and degeneration, and in many cases destruction of medullary fibers, dendrites, and axons.

The severity of the sequelae which result is a direct reflection of the extent of focal necrosis induced by the particular virus. For example, permanent sequelae commonly occur in nonfatal infections with WEE, EEE, Japanese B encephalitis, and Far Eastern TBE but are rarely encountered in St. Louis encephalitis and Central European TBE. This is especially true in infants and young children in whom sequelae are more frequent and more severe than in adults. The sequelae include recurring convulsions, mental retardation and deterioration, muscle weakness, and paralysis. Institutional care of these patients is frequently required, and their chances for long-term survival are poor.

The clinical signs and symptoms vary greatly in intensity, mild cases may resemble viral meningitis, and severe cases may progress rapidly to a fatal outcome. Arbovirus encephalitis usually has an acute onset marked by fever, headache, nausea, vomiting, and evidence of meningeal irritation preceded by restlessness and irritability in infants and children and by mental confusion and drowsiness in adults. Thereafter, convulsions and muscular weakness, pains, tremors, and rigidity may develop quickly and are often accompanied by speech difficulties, photophobia, spasticity, stupor, coma, and delirium. Despite the severity of the clinical manifestations, not only does recovery often occur, but remission is sudden.

Laboratory Diagnosis

A specific diagnosis of arbovirus infection can be established by isolation of the virus or by serological tests. Since virus cannot be recovered from the blood of patients with encephalitis but only from the CNS, attempts at virus isolation are limited to fatal cases, especially those in which death occurs early in the disease when virus is most likely to be found.

Virus may be isolated by inoculating a suspension of the CNS material into tissue cultures, mice, or chick embryos. After preliminary screening by HAI and CF, the virus may be definitely identified by performing a neutralization test which can be most efficiently and economically accomplished in tissue culture.

Most cases of arbovirus encephalitis are confirmed by serological tests. The criteria include any one of the following: a fourfold rise in serum antibody titer between acute and convalescent specimens, a single significant titer of 1:8 or greater of CF antibodies, or a titer of 1:320 or greater of HAI antibodies during an epidemic. Although the CF test has been the more widely used for diagnosis, current recommendations indicate that it should be used in combination with HAI tests. Since HAI antibodies rise early in the first week and since CF antibodies sometimes increase much more slowly, ideally three serum specimens taken at 1, 4, and 10 weeks should be evaluated for HAI and CF antibodies. When both tests are employed, the number of diagnoses can be increased by 15 to 25 percent.

Epidemiology

The Complexity of the Reservoir The ecology of most arboviruses is highly complex and often paradoxical. The complexity arises in part because of the variable distribution, behavior, population dynamics, and movements of the arthropod vectors and their vertebrate hosts as well as meteorological and topographical conditions. Perpetuation of an arbovirus in a given environment requires prolonged and close association between efficient vectors and hosts as well as an effective method for permitting the survival of the virus over the winter *(overwintering).*

Efficient Hosts and Vectors An efficient host is one who responds to arbovirus infection with viremia of sufficient duration and intensity to provide ample opportunity for the female vector to pick up the virus when it takes a blood meal. An efficient vector must prefer to take blood from an efficient host in an environment that will favor extrinsic incubation of the virus (i.e., multiplication of the virus in the vector to the critical level which will permit its transmission to a susceptible host). Furthermore, the population density of both the vector and the host must be high enough to maintain the cycle.

The Arthropod Population As a rule, the female mosquito or tick cannot produce fertile eggs without ingesting blood. Consequently, the number of arthropods in a given environment is directly related to the accessible supply of suitable hosts. The maturation of the eggs is dependent in turn upon such factors as ambient temperature, moisture, rainfall, abundance of vegetation, and susceptibility of the terrain to intermittent flooding.

Animal Hosts A large number of domestic and wild birds infected with VEE, EEE, WEE, St. Louis encephalitis, Japanese B encephalitis, Murray Valley encephalitis, and TBE experience viremia without obvious clinical manifestations. Serious disease occurs only in the case of EEE in pheasants. Subclinical viremic infection of rodents has been established in VEE, EEE, WEE, and TBE, probably occurs in California encephalitis, and possibly occurs with other arboviruses. As the names of the viruses imply, horses frequently develop encephalitis following infection with VEE, EEE, and WEE. Encephalitis also is observed in horses infected with Japanese B encephalitis, but with St. Louis encephalitis subclinical infection is the rule. In addition, stillbirths commonly result when pregnant sows are infected with Japanese B encephalitis, infected goats excrete large quantities of TBE in their milk, and bats exhibit inapparent infection with St. Louis and Japanese B encephalitides.

Human Infection Despite the vast reservoir of arbovirus infection, the particular groups of animals that are primarily responsible for maintaining the cycle is unknown, and the ecological conditions leading to arthropod transmission of the infection to man are often obscure and at best incomplete. Only in those human cases of TBE which follow ingestion of infected goat's milk is the chain of events adequately documented. There may, however, be a close correlation between transmission rates in sentinel birds, infection rates in the vector, virus isolations from nestling birds, and the incidence of encephalitis in man and the horse. For example, in the 1964 epidemics of WEE which occurred in Colorado and Texas and at a time when human and equine cases were reaching a peak, 70 to 92 percent of sentinel chickens showed antibodies against WEE, infection of *Culex tarsalis* mosquitoes with WEE was high, and virus was isolated from more than 22 percent of nestling sparrows.

Present data suggest that birds and rodents are important in perpetuation of the viruses because of the prevalence of infection as well as the intensity and duration of viremia. Man and the horse could not readily support the cycle because of the lower incidence of infection and the limited period and extent of the viremia. There is no evidence to indicate that mosquitoes can pick up infection from one man and transmit the virus to another man.

The Paradoxes The paradoxes encountered in attempting to understand the ecology of arboviruses may be illustrated by recent studies of encephalitis in New Jersey. Human cases of arbovirus encephalitis were reported for the first time in 1959. In that year an epidemic of 31 cases of EEE occurred in Oceanville, Manahawkin, and Forked River. A few miles away in Mays Landing infected birds and mosquitoes were abundant, but neither clinical nor subclinical cases were found. A similar situation obtained in the Great Swamp area near Morristown, but again no human cases were observed. Why, then, is EEE a place disease?

In the periodic epizootics which have occurred in horses and pheasants in New Jersey since 1905, it has been demonstrated that EEE may be a highly restricted place infection. For example, one pheasent pen may be infected and another not infected. In addition, pheasant pens on the ground were infected, whereas those above the ground were not. These findings are hardly compatible with a mosquito-transmitted disease. On the other hand, the observation that pheasants frequently developed the disease after they were seen to carry sick or paralyzed young mice seemed to provide a clue.

The actual isolation of EEE from wild mice and rats during the fall, winter, and spring months suggested a possible explanation. On the other hand, WEE was isolated more frequently from field rodents than was EEE, and serological tests revealed that infection of these animals with WEE was more prevalent than infection with EEE. Antibodies against WEE were present in 6 percent of the rodents tested from September to February, 40 percent during March and April, and 16 percent in May. Despite these findings, however, no human cases of WEE have ever been reported in New Jersey.

Overwintering Overwintering of TBE is readily accounted for by transovarial transmission in the tick, but this may not represent the complete mechanism whereby the virus is maintained throughout the winter. In fact, rodents might play a more important role than ticks in the overwintering of TBE. In the mosquito-transmitted encephalitides, however, the overwintering mechanism is not known. The standard concept holds that the virus is introduced annually by migrating wild birds in whom there is a large reservoir of infection. The demonstration of virus in field rodents throughout the winter and the prevalence of infection in these animals in early spring provide an alternate possibility not only for overwintering but also a means whereby the local nestling population of birds can be infected at an opportune time. Other explanations involving hibernation of infected adult mosquitoes or infected bats appear less plausible.

Epidemic Characteristics

Infection versus Disease Extensive serologic studies over the past several years have amply demonstrated that subclinical infection of man is the rule and encephalitis the exception. The ratio of inapparent to clinical cases has varied between 10 to 1 and 1,000 to 1. Except for EEE, in which there are 10 or 20 infections for every case of encephalitis, the ratio is usually closer to 1,000 to 1.

Attack Rates In those who develop the disease in an epidemic setting attack rates, case fatality rates, and the frequency of sequelae vary widely, depending primarily on the specific virus and the age of the patient. Data from several recent epidemics in the United States will illustrate the extent of variation observed. Since 1955, between 1,900 and 3,200 cases of arbovirus encephalitis have been reported annually. Of the confirmed cases, 72 percent have been caused by St. Louis encephalitis, 21 percent by WEE, 3.5 percent by EEE, and 3 percent by California encephalitis. However, since the first case of California encephalitis was reported in 1963, 11 percent have been produced by California encephalitis. In three of the years since

1955 (1958, 1963, and 1965) WEE has been responsible for the majority of the cases.

The incidence of encephalitis per 100,000 in the epidemic area is highest in WEE and St. Louis encephalitis, less in EEE, and least in California encephalitis. The attack rate in WEE and St. Louis encephalitis is 3 to 50 times higher than in EEE and California encephalitis. In a given epidemic the attack rate may vary from less than 1 per 100,000 to as high as 280 per 100,000. Recent epidemics of WEE and St. Louis encephalitis in Colorado, Kentucky, Illinois, New Jersey, and Texas have shown attack rates between 18 and 190 per 100,000.

The age incidence of encephalitis presents a striking contrast, depending on the causative virus. In EEE, WEE, and California encephalitis, the incidence is highest in young children, the rate being 3 to 15 times the adult rate. In St. Louis encephalitis the incidence is highest in adults, the rate being 5 to 30 times the rate in young children. In Japanese B encephalitis there are two peaks, one in young children and the other in those over 60. The data included in Tables 24-8 and 24-9 illustrate the age incidence of recent outbreaks of St. Louis encephalitis, WEE, EEE, and California encephalitis in the United States.

Table 24-8 Attack Rates per 100,000 Population in Epidemics of St. Louis Encephalitis and Western Equine Encephalitis in the United States

Age group (years)	St. Louis encephalitis	Age group (years)	St. Louis encephalitis	Age group (years)	Western equine encephalitis
0–4	1.9	0–4	7.5	0–1	404
5–14	2.3	5–9	7.6	1–4	161
15–24	11.4	10–14	12.8	5–9	111
25–34	15.1	15–19	16.8	10–19	100
35–44	20.0	20–29	13.7	20–29	146
45–54	41.2	30–39	12.7	30–39	66
55–64	32.6	40–49	15.9	40–59	27
65+	67.8	50–59	20.5	60+	26
		60–69	55.6		
		70+	96.1		
Totals	20.8		17.8		95

Source: *Morbidity Mortality Weekly Reports*, vol. 14, 1965.

Table 24-9 Age Incidence in Epidemics of Eastern Equine Encephalitis and California Encephalitis in the United States

Age group (years)	Cases of eastern equine encephalitis	Cases of California encephalitis	Cases of California encephalitis
0–4	11	6	3
5–9	10	4	5
10–14	2	1	3
15–19	0	0	0
55+	8	0	0
Totals	31	11	11

Source: *Morbidity Mortality Weekly Reports*, vol. 14, 1965.

Case fatality rates are highest in EEE (65 to 70 percent); high in Murray Valley encephalitis, Japanese B encephalitis, and Far Eastern TBE (20 to 30 percent); lower in St. Louis encephalitis, WEE, VEE, and Central European TBE (1 to 10 percent); and minimal in California encephalitis for which only 1 fatal case has been reported. In the 1964 epidemics of St. Louis encephalitis, there were only 9 deaths among 94 cases in New Jersey and 26 deaths among 221 cases in Texas. In the New Jersey outbreak all deaths occurred in those over 55 years of age and 25 of the 26 deaths in the Texas epidemic were in those over 50 years of age, frequently in persons with other underlying illnesses, such as hypertension, arteriosclerotic heart disease, and diabetes. In WEE deaths occur almost exclusively in those under 1 year of age.

Permanent sequelae are especially prone to develop following recovery from EEE, Japanese B encephalitis, Murray Valley encephalitis, and Far Eastern TBE and may occur in any age group. The severity and incidence of sequelae are, however, greatest in those under 5 years of age. WEE sequelae are uncommon in patients over 1 year of age and rare in adults. On the other hand, infection of children under the age of 1 year with WEE is extremely high (Table 24-8) and is marked by a devastating incidence and severity of sequelae. In young infants permanent sequelae may occur in more than half of those infected with WEE. Recovery from infection with St. Louis encephalitis is usually complete. Sequelae are uncommon and are not severe when they do develop. This finding may well be associated with the low incidence of St. Louis encephalitis infection in those under 1 year of age (Table 24-8). No sequelae have been reported in those infected with California encephalitis.

Geographical Distribution The names imply that the arboviruses have a characteristic geographical distribution, which indeed they do. Unfortunately, however, the designations for almost all the viruses have become inappropriate in the light of developing knowledge and are complicated by the finding of essentially identical viruses (called by other names) in many other areas. A few illustrations will suffice to illustrate the problem.

Cases of St. Louis encephalitis have been reported from 29 states, and there is no reason to believe that they may not occur in the other 21 states, with the possible exceptions of Alaska and Hawaii. In addition, the virus is found in Trinidad, Panama, and Jamaica; and serological evidence indicates its presence in Brazil, Colombia, Mexico, and Argentina. In 1964 and 1965 cases of St. Louis encephalitis in the United States were reported from the following 14 states, which are listed in the order of their frequency: Texas, New Jersey, Illinois, Colorado, Kentucky, Pennsylvania, Indiana, Tennessee, Arizona, California, Kansas, Nebraska, Ohio, and Wyoming. Thus, St. Louis encephalitis is hardly an appropriate name for a virus which produces disease over such a wide geographical area.

WEE encephalitis has been found to be more prevalent in the western United States and Canada than in other parts of the two countries. On the other hand, the virus is heavily seeded in the mosquito, bird, and rodent population in New Jersey, Massachusetts, Maryland, Georgia, and Florida which are located along the Eastern coast. Epidemics of EEE have been reported in Massachusetts, New Jersey, Louisiana, the Dominican Republic, and Jamaica. The endemic area spreads from Canada to Argentina. In addition, the virus has been isolated in Czechoslovakia, Poland, the U.S.S.R., the Phillipines, and Thailand.

The only cases of California encephalitis reported in the United States have occurred in Ohio, Indiana, Wisconsin, and Illinois. Virus has, however, been recovered from mosquitoes in California, Florida, and Texas; and serological evidence of infection is widespread. Other viruses, closely related to California encephalitis, have been isolated from South America, Europe, and Africa.

Japanese B encephalitis is not limited to Japan. Epidemics have been recorded in eastern areas of Asia, including China, Korea, Siberia, India, Malaya, and Singapore. The disease is also present in many of the western Pacific islands including Guam, Okinawa, and Taiwan. Murray Valley encephalitis, a virus closely related to Japanese B encephilitis, has produced epidemics in Southern Australia, the coastal areas of Queensland, and New Guinea.

Except for St. Louis encephalitis, in which both urban and rural epidemics occur, infection is more frequent in those engaged in outdoor occupations. For example, a recent serological survey of 637 outdoor workers in Wisconsin showed evidence of infection with California encephalitis, St. Louis encephalitis, and WEE in 25.9, 4.2, and 0.5 percent, respectively. The incidence of infection with California encephalitis was 41 percent in constant outdoor workers, 20 percent in intermittent outdoor workers, and 10.8 percent in summer forest campers. None of the 637 persons had antibody against EEE.

Seasonal Distribution The peak incidence of encephalitis corresponds closely to the period when the arthropod vector is most prevalent. Ordinarily, this is in the late summer and early fall. However, in Far Eastern TBE the peak occurs in the spring and early summer when the principal vector *Ixodes persulcatus* is most abundant. In the United States more than 80 percent of the cases occur in August and September when the mosquito vectors are most prevalent. The epidemics terminate abruptly with the onset of cold weather in October, an environment unfavorable for the vector.

Prevention and Control

Immunization With few exceptions, efforts to prevent or control arbovirus encephalitis have been disappointing. Potent vaccines for human immunization are not available. Even if vaccines were available, the sporadic nature of most outbreaks suggests that they would be of limited value. Effective formalinized chick embryo vaccines have been developed for immunization of horses against EEE and WEE. However, because of the vast reservoir of infection in other hosts and in the vectors, immunization of horses has little effect on the spread of virus in the community. Although the value of these vaccines for man has not been assayed, immunization of laboratory workers and other persons at great risk is recommended.

Formalinized mouse brain vaccines have been used for prevention of Japanese B encephalitis in Japanese school children and for the prevention of TBE in the U.S.S.R. The limited effectiveness of these vaccines and the unfavorable reactions associated with their use indicate the need for further research in developing safer and more potent vaccines. On the other hand, immunization of goats with the existing TBE vaccine appears to be of value in preventing man from acquiring the milk-borne infection.

Arthropod Control Efforts designed to break the biological cycle of arboviruses must be based on the identification of the principal vectors, a detailed knowledge of their general habits and breeding areas, and the consistent application of appropriate control measures over a period of several years. Antimosquito measures include the elimination of breeding places, the use of larvacides, space and residual spraying of insecticides, the use of bed nets, and avoiding exposure. The most effective antitick measures involve avoiding infested areas, wearing protective clothing, and using repellents, especially diethyltoluamide, ether, gasoline, kerosene, or a glowing match. If the ticks are not quickly and effectively removed, *tick paralysis* may develop. This disease is a progressive, ascending, flaccid motor paralysis involving the lower motor neurones of the spinal cord and cranial nerves with destruction of the myelin sheath. The cause is considered to be a toxic substance secreted by the salivary glands of the tick. Although death may occur from respiratory paralysis, most affected persons recover promptly after the removal of the tick.

In highly endemic areas in California and Washington the incidence of WEE has been reduced somewhat as a result of intensive antimosquito measures. Theoretically, it should be possible to control urban epidemics of St. Louis encephalitis with appropriate antimosquito measures because of the domestic habits of the *Culex* vectors. On the other hand, the general habits and extensive breeding areas of the vectors in Japanese B encephalitis, California encephalitis, and TBE suggest that vector control is economically impractical.

Other Control Measures In endemic areas the boiling or pasteurizing of goat's milk is an effective way of preventing infection with Central European TBE by ingestion.

Isolation, disinfection, quarantine, and immunization of contacts are without effect, and no specific treatment is available.

POSTINFECTIOUS AND POSTVACCINAL ENCEPHALITIS

Postinfectious encephalitis is a severe illness with encephalitic manifestations but with a preexisting diagnosed infection. The encephalitis usually develops 4 to 8 days following the onset of the preceding infection which is most frequently caused by mumps, measles, varicella, influenza, or rubella viruses (Table 24-10 and Fig. 24-1). The lesions in the brain and spinal cord are, however, not associated with the presence of any of these viruses. In fatal cases the underlying pathology, irrespective of the etiology of the precipitating infection, involves perivenous infiltration with histiocytes (microglia?) with secondary but prominent demyelination of the white matter.

Postinfectious encephalitis is thought to be an autoimmune disease (Chap. 11) involving a delayed hypersensitive response to antigens in myelinated nervous tissue. Most of the features of the human disease can be reproduced in laboratory animals by autologous or homologous brain and spinal cord tissue injected in combination with Freund's adjuvant (expermental allergic encephalomyelitis).

Except for its severity, the epidemiology of the disease reflects the epidemiology of the precipitating illness. Data from California and Florida indicate that 0.5 to 2.5 percent of reported cases of mumps are followed by encephalitis. Since mumps is the preciptating infection in about 60 percent of the cases of postinfectious encephalitis, it is indeed fortunate that the case fatality rate is so low (about 2 percent). When measles, varicella, influenza, and rubella are the preceding infections, the case fatality rates are much higher (15 to 35 percent).

Table 24-10 Cases of Postinfectious Encephalitis in the United States, from 1960 to 1964

Year	Mumps	Measles	Varicella	Influenza	Rubella
1960	700	299	95	24	0
1961	402	276	75	8	0
1962	358	337	76	40	0
1963	671	239	84	30	0
1964	932	300	106	14	59

Source: Morbidity Mortality Weekly Reports, vol. 14, 1965.

In contrast with mumps, the incidence of encephalitis following infection with measles virus is lower (60 to 70/100,000) and is probably even less with varicella, influenza, and rubella.

The seasonal incidence of postinfectious encephalitis with a peak in the spring and a drop in the late summer is in sharp contrast with the seasonal incidence of arbovirus encephalitis (Fig. 24-1).

The best method of preventing postinfectious encephalitis is to prevent or modify the precipitating illness. This has been readily accom-

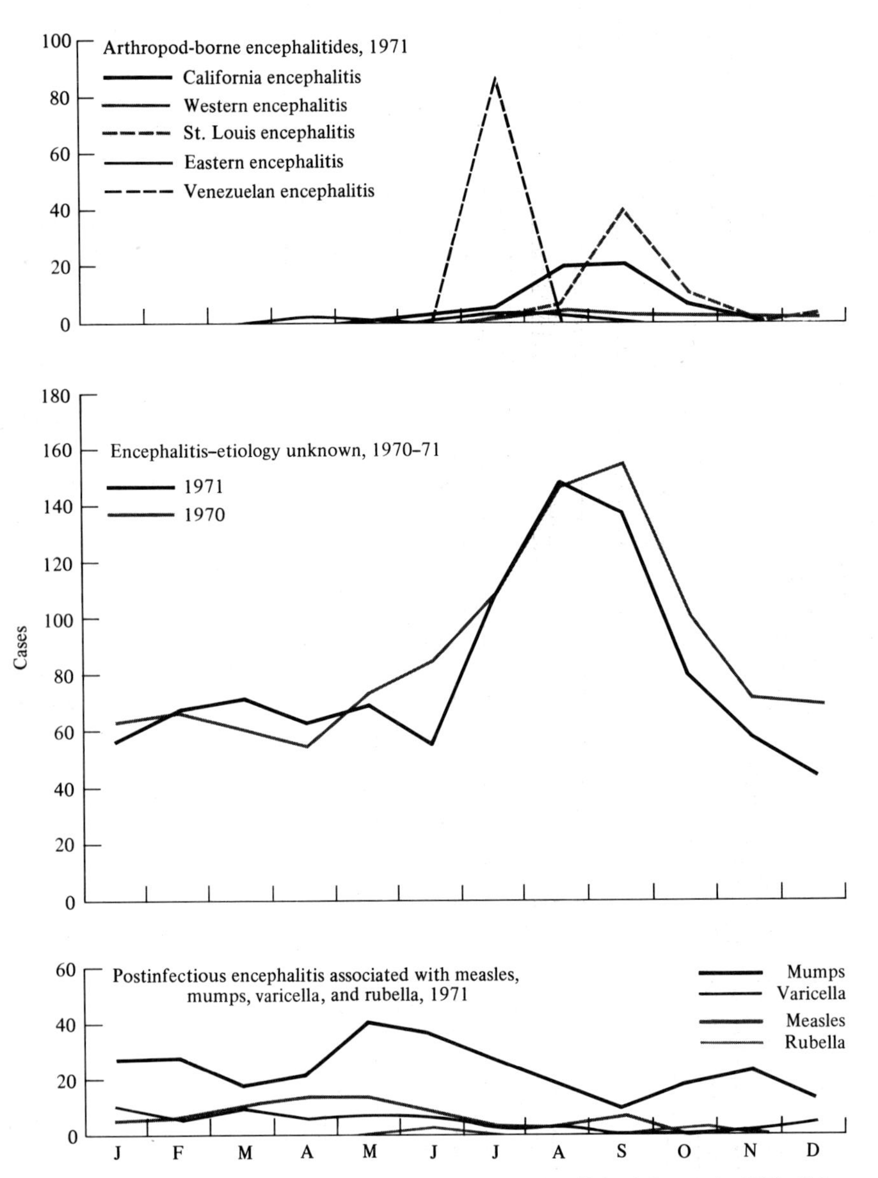

Figure 24-1 National surveillance of encephalitis in the United States in 1971. [*Morbidity Mortality Weekly Report, 20(53):41, 1972.*]

plished in measles by the use of attenuated vaccines and gamma globulin.

Postvaccinal encephalitis is a basically similar disease which develops 10 to 12 days following vaccination for smallpox and 10 to 15 days after rabies vaccination. The incidence of postvaccinal encephalitis is extremely low. There have been only 26 cases in the United States in the last 5 years.

POLIOMYELITIS

Poliovirus is a natural human parasite. Initial contact with the virus usually results in a subclinical infection, occasionally in a minor illness of the respiratory or gastrointestinal tract, and rarely in a disease of the CNS in which motor paralysis may or may not be present. In paralytic poliomyelitis the virus commonly attacks the anterior horn cells of the lumbar and cervical regions of the spinal cord but may also involve the cranial nerves, medulla, autonomic nervous system, cerebral cortex, and posterior columns of the spinal cord.

The Causative Agent

Biological Properties Poliovirus is a member of the enterovirus subgroup of the picornaviruses. The virus is small in size (20 to 30 nm in diameter), icosahedral in shape, has an RNA core and a protein shell, is resistant to acid at pH 3.0, and lacks an envelope containing essential lipid.

Man is the only natural host for poliovirus. The virus is found primarily in the intestinal tract, to a lesser extent in the oropharynx, and only rarely does it invade the CNS. The environment is contaminated largely by healthy carriers who excrete large quantities of virus in their stools for several weeks and who serve as the major source of human infection. The frequent finding of poliovirus in sewage and its occasional isolation from food and flies under unsanitary conditions are due to fecal contamination. In the presence of a rich source of organic matter (feces, sewage) the virus is highly resistant to inactivation by chlorine and other disinfectants.

In aqueous suspensions the virus is destroyed when heated at 55°C for 30 min. However, if the virus is heated in the presence of molar magnesium chloride, there is no loss of infectivity. This property of cationic stabilization of thermal inactivation has been utilized in the preparation of poliovirus vaccines to inactivate the potentially oncogenic SV_{40} virus (Chap. 2) which is frequently present as a contaminant without impairing the infectivity of poliovirus. When added to oral vaccines, magnesium chloride is useful in prolonging the period during which the vaccine can be stored without loss of potency and in eliminating the need to refrigerate vaccine under field conditions.

Poliovirus has been experimentally studied most effectively in primates and in a variety of tissue cultures. Only an occasional strain of the virus will grow in rats and mice following intracerebral or intraspinal inoculation, and one strain has been adapted to multiply in chick embryos. When the virus is fed to chimpanzees, an inapparent infection commonly results with intestinal carriage and excretion of the virus, a short period of viremia, and recovery with the development of neutralizing antibody. Direct inoculation of the virus into the brain or spinal cord of monkeys and chimpanzees causes paralytic disease with characteristic histopathology. Some strains of the virus have the capacity to induce paralytic disease in man, chimpanzees, and monkeys following intramuscular injection.

In tissue culture poliovirus grows in a variety of primary and continuous cell lines of monkey and human origin, including those obtained from kidneys, testes, muscles, and tumors. Infection of tissue cultures with poliovirus results in the production of high concentrations of virus (10^8 to 10^9 or more per milliliter) in fluids that are relatively free of extraneous protein. Assay of the virus and of neutralizing antibody is based on the production of plaques and their inhibition in tissue culture monolayers of monkey kidney or HeLa cells. The development of the plaque method permitted a study of genetic markers and facilitated the selection of attenuated strains for use in oral vaccines.

Poliovirus multiplies rapidly in the cytoplasm of susceptible tissue culture cells. The bulk of infectious RNA and capsid protein is synthesized and integrated in virus-specific, lipid-containing polyribosomes between 2½ and 5½ hr. after infection. After assembly the virus is held within the cell for several hours until the cell bursts, releasing virus.

The Basis of Cellular, Tissue, Organ, and Species Specificity The highly selective susceptibility of cells to poliovirus, and other enteroviruses as well, is determined by protein or lipoprotein receptors located in the plasma membranes. The receptors have two functions: the adsorption of virus and a reorientation of the capsid subunits, leaving the capsid sensitive to proteolytic enzymes, and thus constituting the necessary prelude to the release of viral RNA.

Specific poliovirus receptors are present on the surface of susceptible primate cells and absent on insusceptible nonprimate cells. The virus receptor interaction can, however, be bypassed by exposing the insusceptible cells to infectious RNA from poliovirus or by enclosing poliovirus RNA within the protein capsid of another virus (Coxsackie virus B1) which can react with insusceptible mouse cells. Cells of all warm-blooded species tested are infected by viral RNA. The progeny virus is identical to parental virus in host cell specificity; i.e., it can infect primate cells but cannot infect nonprimate cells of the type in which it replicated.

Tissue and organ specificity in humans and monkeys is also based on receptors. Susceptible primate tissues (brain, spinal cord, intestine) exhibit receptor activity, whereas insusceptible tissue and organs (kidney, heart, lung, skin, muscle) fail to show receptor activity. In this connection, it is interesting to note that the attenuated oral vaccine strain of type 1 poliovirus is bound by intestinal homogenates but not by brain tissue. This observation might partly explain the ability of this oral vaccine strain to multiply in the intestine without causing infection of the CNS, and it implies that receptors in various cells differ from each other.

Nearly all primate cells are susceptible to poliovirus in vitro even though they are not susceptible in the body. For example, direct injection of virus into the kidneys or testes of monkeys does not lead to multiplication, whereas cells from these same tissues after cultivation readily support multiplication of poliovirus. Study of this phenomenon revealed that the cultured cells acquire susceptibility to virus parallel to their acquisition of receptor activity. However, if the cells are cultured in their normal tissue relationship, they fail to produce receptors or to support viral replication. Thus, it would appear that disturbance of normal contact relationships leads to receptor synthesis or unmasking and to viral susceptibility.

Neurovirulence Naturally occurring strains of poliovirus exhibit a wide range of neurovirulence. Although the genetic factors which regulate the neurovirulence of a particular strain of poliovirus are largely unknown, some of the properties associated with highly virulent virus can be described and assayed (Table 24-11). A highly neurovirulent poliovirus causes paralytic disease in chimpanzees and monkeys after peripheral (intramuscular) inoculation, adsorbs

Table 24-11 Properties of Poliovirus with a High Degree of Neurovirulence

Adsorption onto receptors of brainstem and spinal cord cells
Invasiveness (ability to spread) within the CNS
Ability to produce paralytic disease in chimpanzees and monkeys after *intramuscular*, intrathalamic, and intraspinal inoculation
Good growth in tissue cultures at 40°C (rct/40 marker)

onto receptors in the brain stem as well as the spinal cord, progressively invades the CNS, and possesses the rct/40 (reproductive capacity temperature) marker, i.e., grows well in tissue culture at 40°C. Virus of lower virulence produces paralytic disease following intrathalamic and intraspinal inoculation (but not after peripheral inoculation), shows a reduced capacity to adsorb onto receptors in the brain stem, invades the CNS less extensively, and has the rct/40 marker.

Attenuated oral vaccine strains have lost the capacity to produce paralytic disease following intrathalamic inoculation, remain localized after intraspinal inoculation, and are negative for the rct/40 marker.

Antigenic Structure There are three antigenic types of poliovirus, designated types 1, 2, and 3, and each is capable of producing infection and paralytic disease. Infection with type 2 is most prevalent, followed by type 1 and then type 3. Prior to the widespread use of killed and attenuated vaccines, the distribution of paralytic cases was 85, 12, and 3 percent for types 1, 2, and 3, respectively; since the introduction of vaccines, the distribution of paralytic cases has been 80, 1, and 18 percent for types 1, 2, and 3, respectively.

Tissue cultures infected with each type of poliovirus yield particles which exhibit two distinct antigenic specificities. D particles containing D antigen may or may not be infectious, whereas C particles containing C antigen are not infectious. D antigen is associated with particles that contain RNA, evoke neutralizing antibodies, and react predominantly with convalescent phase sera. C antigen is associated with less dense, structurally impaired particles that do not contain RNA, do not evoke neutralizing antibodies, and react predominantly with acute phase sera.

The D and C antigenic configurations are distinct, as indicated by the nonfusion of their specific precipitates in agar, inability to remove each other's antibodies as tested by CF or precipitin tests in agar, and their different behavior as immunizing antigens.

C antigen may be produced from D antigen by heating at 56°C, ultraviolet irradiation, drying, alkaline pH, and treatment with phenol or mercury compounds. C antigen (denatured D antigen) gives CF and precipitin reactions with C antibodies but fails to absorb or react with D antibodies and fails to induce neutralizing antibodies. Consequently, heat-killed vaccines would be of no value in producing immunity to poliovirus infection. The artificially produced C antigen presumably is the result of distortion of protein subunits in the capsid.

Intratypic antigenic differences can be demonstrated but do not greatly affect cross-protection against naturally occurring strains. For example, attenuated oral vaccine strains have some antigenic components which are entirely absent, or are present only in trace amounts, in their virulent parental strains; however, the attentuated strains do not appear to lack any of the protective antigens present in the virulent strains.

Pathogenesis

Subclinical Infection Initial contact with poliovirus almost always results in a subclinical infection characterized by multiplication of the virus in lymphatic tissue, excretion of the virus in oropharyngeal and fecal secretions, viremia, and the development of type-specific neutralizing antibody. The virus is usually transmitted to the oral cavity of a susceptible person by a young child whose fingers contain virus as a result of fecal contamination. Perhaps, occasionally, contaminated oropharyngeal secretions may represent the source of infection.

After entry into the oral cavity poliovirus multiplies in the tonsils and in the Peyer's patches in the ileum (the virus has no difficulty traversing the stomach because it is resistant to acid). In the next 2 to 3 days the virus is released in increasing concentration from the infected cells and is present in the oropharynx and the feces. During this interval the virus invades the deep cervical and the mesenteric lymph nodes and spills over into the blood. The viremia persists for about 3 to 5 days, and virus is present in the oropharynx for about 10 to 12 days and in the feces for 5 weeks or more. Neutralizing antibodies appear about the eighth day.

Minor Illness Occasionally, the infected person may experience a mild respiratory or gastrointestinal illness during the interval when virus is simultaneously present in the pharynx, feces, and blood. The respiratory form may include fever, pharyngeal discomfort, and involvement of lymphatic tissue in the oropharynx or may resemble influenza with aching of muscles, bones, and joints; the gastrointestinal form may involve fever, nausea, vomiting, diarrhea, constipation, and abdominal discomfort. The illness usually subsides in 24 to 48 hr. but may, however, be followed in 3 to 4 days by signs of CNS involvement. A biphasic or dromedary course of the disease occurs in about one-third of paralytic cases in young children but is rarely seen in adults.

CNS Infection In the unlikely event that poliovirus reaches the CNS, the evidence, on balance, indicates that it does so by way of the bloodstream. Infection of the CNS usually occurs 10 to 20 days after ingestion of virus. The virus multiplies in neurones, spreads along nerve fiber pathways within the CNS, and rises abruptly in titer. Clinical manifestations of CNS involvement develop within a few days. The virus persists for a few more days, declines rapidly thereafter, and is rarely detected in the CNS 6 days after onset.

Viral (Aseptic) Meningitis (Nonparalytic Poliomyelitis) Signs of meningeal irritation represent the earliest indication of CNS involvement. These include a stiff neck and back, difficulties of flexion and extension, and abnormalities of the CSF. Most of these patients recover in 3 to 5 days, and the disease is referred to as viral (aseptic) meningitis or nonparalytic poliomyelitis. In a few patients, the CNS may be progressively involved.

Paralytic Poliomyelitis The onset of paralysis is preceded by signs of meningeal irritation and progressive muscle weakness. The location and the degree of paralysis depend on the site and the extent of neuronal lesions. The spinal form of the disease is a result of viral attack on the anterior horn cells (motor neurones) in the cord. In the bulbar form of the disease the virus attacks the cranial nerve nuclei or medullary centers. When both the spinal cord and the brain stem are involved, the designation bulbospinal is used. In rare cases, encephalitis results from diffuse or focal involvement of the brain.

Spinal Poliomyelitis The anterior horn cells of the lumbar and cervical regions of the spinal cord bear the brunt of the damage produced by the virus. Lumbar involvement is the most frequent and results in muscle weakness in the legs and inferior portions of the abdomen and back; cervical lesions are accompanied by weakness in the arms, shoulders, neck, and diaphragm and by the threat of bulbar involvement. Viral attack on the anterior horn cells of the thoracic cord leads to weakness in the muscles of the chest, upper abdomen, and spine and to respiratory difficulty caused by dysfunction of intercostal and other thoracic muscles.

The paralysis is usually asymmetric but varies with the age of the patient. In children under 5 years of age paresis of one leg is common, children between 5 and 15 years show weakness of one arm, or paraplegia; in older children and adults quadriplegia often occurs. The greater severity of the disease in older children and adults is also indicated by the greater frequency of respiratory difficulty and urinary dysfunction.

Bulbar Poliomyelitis The manifestations of bulbar poliomyelitis depend on the areas of the brain stem that are attacked by the virus. Damage to the upper cranial nerve nuclei is associated with disturbances of ocular, facial, masticatory, and vestibular functions; while impairment of swallowing, laryngeal, and lingual functions is the result of damage to the lower cranial nerve nuclei. Paralysis most commonly involves the pharynx, the soft palate, and the vocal cords and may lead to respiratory difficulty due to obstruction of the airway from accumulated secretions. If the medullary respiratory center is attacked, respiratory failure results with irregularity of rhythm, depth, and rate of respiration, followed by hypoxia, cyanosis, and elevated temperature, pulse, and pressure. When the medullary vasomotor center is also damaged, circulatory collapse develops, and the outcome is inevitably fatal.

Predisposing Factors An important unresolved problem in poliomyelitis is the question why the paralytic form of the disease strikes only 1 in every 100 or 1,000 susceptible persons infected with the virus. The established factors that are known to predispose to or be associated with an increased incidence of paralysis account for but a small fraction of the total number of paralytic cases. The risk is greatest during the viremic phase of the disease, but the mechanism is obscure.

Pregnancy increases the risk but not the severity of paralytic poliomyelitis. The increased incidence of paralysis is probably more closely related to the greater exposure of pregnant women to young children who form the main cohort of infection than to hormonal changes associated with pregnancy. The fact that paralysis in pregnancy increases with parity and the number of children in the home tends to support this conclusion. On the other hand, since physical exertion and fatigue during the viremic phase are known to increase the chance of developing paralysis, especially in adults, pregnant women may be more susceptible to paralytic disease on this account.

Tonsillectomy is associated with an increased incidence of bulbar poliomyelitis. If the tonsils are removed within 30 days of the onset of infection, the bulbar form of the disease occurs in the majority of the patients. The explanation is in doubt, but the virus may have an enhanced opportunity to spread along the axons of the peripheral nerves to the brain stem.

Injections of pertussis vaccine and diphtheria or tetanus toxoids 1 to 3 weeks prior to onset of infection with poliovirus lead to an increased incidence of paralysis and a localization of paralysis to the injected arm. Several suggestions have been offered to explain the localization of virus in the cervical area of the spinal cord, but the actual mechanism is unknown.

A speculative explanation in accordance with a number of experimental observations but for which there is no direct evidence can provide a common mechanism for the paralytic form of the disease. The proposed theory holds that the basis for susceptibility to the paralytic form of the disease is the presence of efficient cellular receptors (motor neurones, cranial nerve nuclei, etc.) which can absorb virus during the viremic phase of the disease. Most persons possess neurons which are deficient or totally lacking in receptors and are consequently resistant to the paralytic form of the disease. However, these resistant neurones may be induced to produce the necessary receptors by a variety of stimuli which alter the normal contact relationships of the neurones. These stimuli might include injury, trauma, fatigue, damaged nerve fibers, and hormonal stimulation.

Sequelae The most common sequel of paralytic poliomyelitis is persistence of paralysis. Although complete recovery may occur in patients with slight muscle weakness, a variable degree of residual paralysis persists in most patients. The degree to which muscles recover their function depends on the extent of neuronal damage. When neuronal necrosis is marked, no recovery is possible. With lesser degrees of neuronal damage, partial recovery of muscle function continues for about 2 years. Of the total recovery possible, 60 percent occurs in 3 months, and 80 percent in 6 months.

Signs of myocarditis develop in 10 to 20 percent of patients with paralytic poliomyelitis and are accompanied by electrocardiographic changes.

Disturbances in water and electrolyte balance, major pulmonary atelectases, bacterial pneumonia, and myocardial failure secondary to pulmonary complications are ever-present dangers in patients with respiratory paralysis who require continuous artificial respiration.

Another problem is the threat of urinary tract infection in patients (primarily adults) who require chronic catheterization as a result of bladder dysfunction.

Pathology The major pathological response in paralytic poliomyelitis is the result of viral multiplication in the motor neurones of the spinal cord, medulla, and brain. Neurones attacked by the virus show a graded series of changes, which commence with chromatolysis (decrease in size of Nissl bodies), followed by the disappearance of Nissl bodies, aggregation of nuclear chromatin, decreased nuclear size, and in some cells, the formation of an intranuclear eosinophilic inclusion body. At this stage, there are few inflammatory cells and little edema in the area. Irreversibly injured neurones may be removed by lysis or by neuronophagia by leukocytes and macrophages. Cells that are destroyed by the virus are not replaced, since neurones cannot regenerate.

The inflammatory reaction which accompanies the change in the neurones varies widely in intensity and extent. There is perivascular infiltration with leukocytes, hyperemia, edema, and small hemorrhages. During the acute stage of the disease the inflammatory cells are neutrophils, monocytes, and macrophages. Later in the course of the disease lymphocytes predominate.

Laboratory Diagnosis

A laboratory diagnosis may be established either by isolation and identification of the virus or by demonstrating a rise in neutralizing or CF antibody, preferably by both procedures. Virus is most commonly isolated from stool specimens and less frequently from oropharyngeal secretions. It is present in feces in higher concentration and for a longer period of time than in the oropharynx, but excretion of virus does, however, tend to be intermittent. Consequently, two or more specimens should be tested. Attempts to recover virus from blood during the acute stage of the disease are unrewarding, and virus is not present in the CSF. The specimen to be examined for virus is inoculated onto tissue culture monolayers of monkey kidney or HeLa cells where it produces plaques. Inhibition of plaque formation by type-specific serum identifies the virus and the type.

A serological diagnosis is most readily established by demonstrating a fourfold or greater rise in CF antibody between the acute and convalescent serum specimens. CF antibodies are usually present during the acute phase of the disease, rise sharply during convalesence, and fall rapidly thereafter. Consequently, a high CF titer in a single serum specimen is presumptive evidence of recent infection. Type-specific D antigens are routinely employed in the CF tests because specific rises in antibody are more readily demonstrated with the D antigens than with the C antigens.

It is more difficult, and in about half the cases impossible, to demonstrate a significant rise in type-specific neutralizing antibody. This situation obtains because neutralizing antibody appears early in the course of the infection, often reaches a maximal level during the acute stage of the disease, and persists for many years.

Epidemiology

The Spread of Virus in the Community Preschool children form the main cohort of infection. Their immunological susceptibilty, their unhygienic habits regardless of social class, and the intimacy of their play contacts predispose to ease of transmission. Older children and adults are usually immune, are more careful with their personal hygiene, and are less intimate in their usual interpersonal relationships. The principal pattern of transmission is the spread of virus from young child to young child on the basis of fecal contamination and an intestinal-oral route.

When an infected child brings the virus into the home, almost all susceptible siblings and adults in the household become infected. Seasonal incidence in temperate climates results in part from changes in frequency and degree of play contacts among young children which are maximal in summer. The direct child-to-child pattern may be supplemented in unsanitary populations by indirect transmission through contaminated food and flies.

In areas of poor sanitation paralytic cases are few in number and largely limited to children under 4 years of age. Epidemics are unknown, and protective antibodies are widely distributed in the population in the first few years of life. There is an inverse relationship between the incidence of paralytic poliomyelitis and infant mortality.

Gradually improving sanitary and hygienic practices decrease the opportunities for early infection, thus permitting an increased number of infections in older age groups. Large segments of the population are susceptible, and severe epidemics in older children and young adults occur. With increasing age paralytic disease is more frequent and more severe, and the mortality rate is higher.

Infection Versus Disease The ratio of infections to paralytic cases varies with the virulence of the virus, the antigenic type of the virus, and the age of the host. Type 1 strains are the most paralytogenic; type 2 strains are the most prevalent but the least virulent; type 3 strains are the least likely to be encountered but generally exhibit a high degree of virulence. As indicated by the data included in Table 24-12, type 1 strains are responsible for about 80 percent of paralytic cases, type 3 for 18 percent, and type 2 for 1 percent. Thus, the ratio of infections to paralytic cases is lower for types 1 and 3 than for type 2.

Even in a virus with a high degree of virulence, infection is the rule, and paralytic disease is the exception. The ratio of infections to paralytic cases is usually greater than 1,000 to 1 in young children but may be as low as 75 to 1 in adults.

Mortality When paralytic disease develops, the majority of the patients recover. Overall mortality rates average about 5 percent but may

Table 24-12 Poliovirus Isolations from Paralytic Cases in the United States from 1958 to 1965

Year	Number of specimens examined	Types of viruses identified			Percent due to each type		
		1	2	3	1	2	3
1958	1,479	898	29	194	80.1	2.6	17.3
1959	2,775	1,881	10	228	88.8	0.5	10.8
1960	1,072	603	1	219	73.3	0.1	26.6
1961	481	231	6	145	60.5	1.6	37.9
1962	472	300	8	100	73.5	2.0	24.5
1963	242	160	6	31	81.2	3.0	15.7
1964	77	21	6	24	41.2	11.8	47.0
1965	29	15	6	4	60.0	24.0	16.0
Totals	6,627	4,109	72	945	80.2	1.4	18.4

Source: Adapted from *Morbidity and Mortality Weekly Reports*, 14:442–445, 1966.

be as high as 25 to 75 percent in patients with bulbospinal paralysis. The mortality is lower in children (2 to 4 percent) and higher in adults (10 to 30 percent).

Prevention and Control

Immunization Prevention and control of paralysis and meningitis due to polioviruses are based on active immunization of all children and adults. The development of effective Formalin-inactivated and attenuated vaccines represents an outstanding achievement in preventive medicine. The basic preliminary studies which facilitated the preparation of the vaccines included the demonstration of three specific antigenic types of the virus, the acquisition of more accurate knowledge concerning the pathogensis of the disease, and the finding that polioviruses grow well in tissue cultures of primate cells. Capacity to grow in monkey kidney tissue cultures permitted the production of adequate quantities of virus relatively free of extraneous tissue proteins, the discovery of convenient methods for assaying virus and neutralizing antibody, and the selection of attenuated strains of each of the three antigenic types.

Formalin-inactivated Vaccine (Salk) In the preparation of Salk vaccine each of the three types of virulent poliovirus is grown separately in tissue cultures of monkey kidney cells. The viruses are inactivated by a 1 to 4,000 concentration of formaldehyde at 37°C. After a battery of safety tests to demonstrate that the viruses have lost all infectivity and other tests to indicate that they have retained antigenic potency, the viruses are pooled and ready for use.

A large-scale field trial in 1954 demonstrated that the vaccine was safe and reasonably effective in preventing paralysis. After the vaccine was licensed in 1955, certain lots of the vaccine which contained residual amounts of virulent virus were responsible for producing paralytic disease following intramuscular injection and for producing contact cases. Stricter regulations for production and safety testing of the vaccine were instituted, and no further accidents have occurred. Until 1960, however, many lots of vaccine contained a type 3 component which was poorly antigenic and an extraneous, potentially oncogenic SV_{40} virus derived from the monkey kidney cells. All subsequent lots have shown improved antigenic potency and have been free of SV_{40} virus.

Attenuated Vaccine (Sabin) Attenuated strains of each of the three types of poliovirus are grown separately in tissue cultures of monkey kidney cells and are administered separately or in various combinations after appropriate safety and potency tests. The attenuated vaccine strains were selected on the basis of inability to grow in tissue culture at 40°C (negative rct/40 marker), failure to produce paralytic disease following intrathalamic or intramuscular inoculation in monkeys, and inability to spread within the CNS following intraspinal inoculation in monkeys.

The safety of attenuated oral vaccines is amply confirmed by the fact that hundreds of millions of persons have been vaccinated without proved harmful effects. It has been claimed that there is a minimal risk associated with the use of type 3 oral vaccine in adult males in whom paralysis may develop with a case rate of 1 per 1.5 million. These paralytic cases are said to be compatible when type 3 vaccine strain was ingested within 30 days prior to the onset of paralysis. However, it is important to emphasize that it is impossible to prove a causal association between ingestion of the type 3 vaccine strain and the subsequent development of paralysis in any specific patient.

The Impact of Vaccination A detailed discussion of the many factors involved in determining and evaluating the response of individuals to immunization with Formalin-inactivated and attenuated vaccines and the comparative

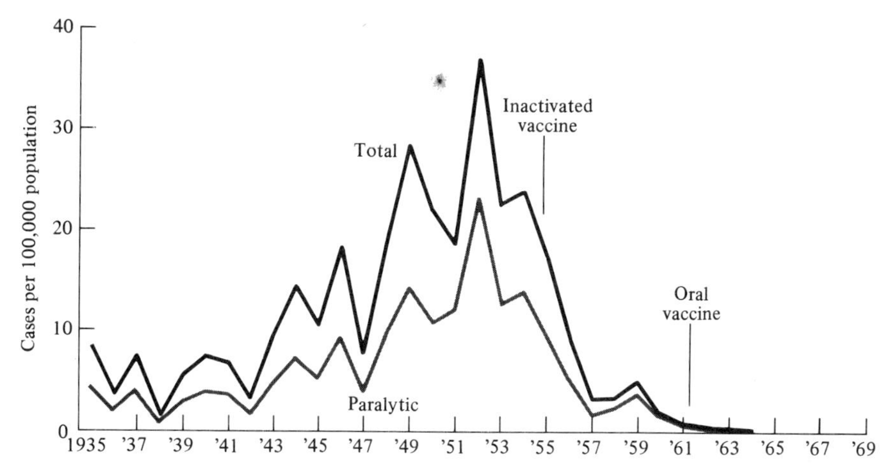

Figure 24-2 The impact of immunization on the incidence of poliomyelitis in the United States. Paralytic cases prior to 1951 are assumed to be 50 percent of the total. Since 1951, cases reported as unspecified were prorated among paralytic and nonparalytic cases. [*Morbidity Mortality Weekly Report, 13(54):42, 1965.*]

merits of the respective vaccines is beyond the scope of this text. However, many aspects of the problem are considered in outline form in Figure 24-2 and in Table 24-13.

Basically, the findings indicate that formalin-inactivated and attenuated vaccines have proved highly effective in the prevention of paralytic poliomyelitis (Fig. 24-2). The attenuated vaccine does, however, have a number of advantages over the Formalin-inactivated vaccine (Table 24-13), and there has been a definite trend toward preference for it over the inactivated vaccine. The principal advantages of attenuated vaccine are listed below.

1 It may be given by mouth instead of by injection. Thus, it is easy to administer in the individual case and in community and national campaigns.
2 It stimulates the production of a high level of protective antibody and a level of intestinal resistance which prevents infection as well as disease.
3 It produces a quicker immune response. Consequently, its use under epidemic conditions halts the epidemic in about 2 weeks.

Current Recommendations for Immunization All persons who have not had attenuated oral vaccine should receive it, preferably in community campaigns involving the use of monovalent vaccines at monthly intervals or the use of monovalent type 1 vaccine followed by types 2 and 3 together. Each administration of vaccine should be given to all persons in the community within a brief period (1 day, if possible). In order to be successful, the mass vaccination must include 80 percent or more of preschool children (the most difficult group to reach) because they are the most susceptible targets in the population and the main cohort of infection. Unless this group is effectively vaccinated, polioviruses will continue to be disseminated throughout the community. The next step is to vaccinate all children born into the community. Immunization of infants is begun at 2 or 3 months of age with monovalent vaccine and continues at monthly or bimonthly intervals.

Treatment A variety of procedures have proved valuable in the treatment of paralytic poliomyelitis, depending on the severity of the disease and the presenting manifestations. These include measures designed to relieve the patient's discomfort and to minimize the possi-

Table 24-13 Comparison of Vaccines Used in the Prevention of Infection and Disease Due to Polioviruses

Property	Formalin-inactivated vaccine (Salk)	Attenuated vaccine (Sabin)
Nature of the antigen	Trivalent (containing each antigenic type)	Monovalent: each type given separately; monovalent type 1 followed by types 2 and 3 given together; trivalent
Route of administration	Intramuscular	Oral
Number of doses required to produce adequate level of protective antibodies in triple negative persons (those who have no detectable antibody to any of the three antigenic types)	Three plus repeated boosters	Three doses if each type given separately; two doses when type 1 followed by types 2 and 3 given together; one dose if three types given together
Time required to produce adequate level of protective antibodies in triple negative persons	10 months or more	7 to 10 days for monovalent (10 weeks for three antigenic types given separately); 6 weeks for monovalent type 1 followed by types 2 and 3 given together; 7 to 10 days for trivalent
Persistence of protective antibody in triple negative subjects in countries with good sanitary and hygienic practices	Type 2 antibody maintained; types 1 and 3 antibodies decrease 25-fold in 3½ years; 30 to 40 percent lack demonstrable antibody	Appears to be equivalent to the response following natural infection and results in lifelong immunity
Effect on disease	Has caused a 90 percent or greater reduction in paralytic poliomyelitis	Has caused the virtual elimination of paralytic poliomyelitis
Effect on infection	Has little effect in preventing natural infection with polioviruses	Prevents infection as well as disease
Viral multiplication in oropharynx	May inhibit viral multiplication, depending on antibody level	Prevents viral multiplication
Viral multiplication in intestine	Does not prevent intestinal infection unless antibody levels exceed titers of 1:1,024, which are rarely achieved and maintained	Regularly prevents intestinal infection, a property that is often unrelated to the antibody level, especially in adults
Circulation of polioviruses in the community	Somewhat diminishes the spread of virus in countries with good sanitary and hygienic practices	Greatly suppresses the dissemination of virus in countries with poor as well as good sanitary and hygienic practices

bility of increasing the degree of paralysis during the acute stage of the disease (bed rest, hot packs, mild analgesics, changing the position of the paralyzed limbs, and gentle and infrequent examination of muscular function). In severely affected patients tracheotomy may be required to prevent lethal obstruction of the airway. When respiratory muscle paralysis develops and vital capacity is halved, artificial respiration with a tank or chest respirator must be given. If the respiratory center is involved, an electrophrenic respirator should be employed. After the acute stage of the disease has passed, physiotherapy is started and is continued daily for as long as 2 years. In the event that considerable residual paralysis persists, surgical rehabilitation should be undertaken. In addition, it is advisable to emphasize that severe paralytic poliomyelitis is often accompanied by emotional, social, and economic problems which can be largely prevented or minimized by the attending physicians and nurses in cooperation with the psychiatrists and the social service agencies.

INFECTIONS CAUSED BY COXSACKIE VIRUSES

Coxsackie viruses are natural human parasites that are members of the enterovirus subgroup of the picorna viruses. Since their original isolation from human feces in 1948 in the town of Coxsackie, New York, the viruses have been frequently recovered from healthy children and from patients with a variety of illnesses.

The Coxsackie A, or group A, viruses usually produce generalized myositis and flaccid paralysis in newborn mice, but only occasionally are they cytopathogenic for tissue cultures. In man some of the Coxsackie A viruses have been implicated in paralysis, meningoencephalitis, viral meningitis, herpangina, vesicular stomatitis with exanthem (hand, foot and mouth disease), acute lymphonodular pharyngitis, fever with lymphadenitis, undifferentiated febrile illness, and the common cold.

The Coxsackie B, or group B, viruses usually induce fat necrosis, focal myositis, and occasionally encephalitis, myocarditis, and pancreatitis in newborn mice. Cytopathogenicity is regularly produced in tissue cultures. All the Coxsackie B viruses have been involved in human disease including paralysis, meningoencephalitis, viral (aseptic) meningitis, neonatal encephalohepatomyocarditis, pericarditis, myocarditis, pleurodynia, orchitis, exanthem, and undifferentiated febrile illness.

The Causative Agent

Biological Properties Like other enteroviruses (polioviruses, echoviruses), the Coxsackie viruses are small in size (20 to 30 nm in diameter), icosahedral in shape, have an RNA core and protein shell, are resistant to acid at pH 3.0, lack an envelope containing essential lipid, and show cationic stabilization of thermal inactivation. Like other enteroviruses, the Coxsackie viruses are found primarily in the human intestinal tract and oropharynx. Healthy carriers excrete large quantities of virus in their stools, which contaminate the environment, serve as the major source of human infection, and account for the finding of virus in sewage.

Unlike polioviruses, the Coxsackie viruses are frequently found in the CSF of patients with viral meningitis; cause fatal disease in newborn mice, hamsters, and ferrets; and rarely produce paralysis in monkeys. Degeneration and destruction of striated muscle (generalized myositis) and flaccid paralysis are produced in newborn mice by all Coxsackie A viruses. Susceptibility of the mice remains high for about the first 72 hr. of life and declines rapidly in 5 to 10 days. A few strains of the virus have been adapted to produce fatal disease in adult mice, and some cause paralysis in monkeys.

Adult mice develop a subclinical infection, during the course of which they form neutralizing antibodies and, with some strains, yield large quantities of virus in the heart rather than in skeletal muscle.

Coxsackie B viruses can produce cytopathogenicity in monkey kidney tissue cultures. Some types of Coxsackie A viruses have been isolated directly in human cell cultures, and others have been adapted to grow in human amnion cells. For primary isolation of Coxsackie A and B viruses, human embryonic kidney cells yield the best results.

Fat necrosis is the outstanding lesion produced by Coxsackie B viruses in newborn mice. Other findings include focal myositis, encephalomalacia, hepatitis, myocarditis, and pancreatitis. Ability to produce myocarditis decreases within a day or so of birth and is not a property of all Coxsackie B viruses. Pancreatitis is a variable finding, is limited to necrosis of acinar epithelial cells, and occurs in newborn and adult mice.

The response of chimpanzees to virus feeding is similar to that observed with polio- and echoviruses. The animals develop an inapparent infection with limited multiplication of virus in the oropharynx, transient viremia, intestinal carriage, the excretion of virus for several weeks, and the formation of neutralizing antibody.

Antigenic Structure There are 24 antigenic types of Coxsackie A viruses, designated types 1 to 24. Coxsackie B viruses consist of six antigenic types, designated types 1 to 6.

The antigenic structure consists of a group-specific precipitating and CF antigen and a type-specific antigen detected by precipitin and neutralization tests. When the type-specific antigen is heated to 56°C for 30 min. it exhibits group-specific reactivity. The change resembles the D to C antigenic shift in poliovirus.

Protective antibodies appear early in the course of human infection, are more readily measured by the plaque neutralization test than by the cytopathogenicity inhibition test, and persist for many years. CF antibodies appear later in the course of the infection, cross-react with a number of types (i.e., show group specificity), and fall to a low level in 6 months.

Coxsackie viruses produce hemagglutinin, and HA-inhibition tests are used for studying antigenic relationships and for laboratory diagnosis of infection.

Intratype Variation Within a given antigenic type, strains of virus (prime strains) have been isolated which are neutralized weakly by antiserum against the prototype virus, whereas antiserum against the prime strain neutralizes the prototype virus to equivalent titer. This one-way versus reciprocal crossing between related strains of the same antigenic type is not uncommon in a number of viruses and bacteria and complicates the evaluation of antigenic relationships and diagnostic serological tests. In many cases the difficulties can be obviated by performing plaque reduction or CF tests which tend to minimize antigenic differences.

Pathogenesis

The Basis of Cellular, Tissue, Organ, and Species Specificity As with the polio- and echoviruses, cellular, tissue, organ, and species specificity of Coxsackie viruses is determined by receptors located in the plasma membrane of susceptible cells. Man possesses a much broader range of target cells with receptors for Coxsackie virus than for polioviruses. Fortunately, however, except for neonates the receptors are rarely located on neurones, heart muscle, and other vital cells. The mucous membranes of the oral cavity, the intestines, and the respiratory tract, the meninges, skeletal muscle, and the skin are the principal targets of the Coxsackie viruses. Under special conditions, however, the brain, spinal cord, myocardium, pericardium, testes, liver, spleen, adrenals, pancreas, lungs, lymph nodes, and parotid may be attacked.

The Response to Infection Initial contact with a Coxsackie virus results in either a subclinical infection or one or more of a wide variety of clinical syndromes (Table 24-14). The manifestations are conditioned largely by the particular virus and the age of the host. In general, Coxsackie B viruses are more pathogenic for man than Coxsackie A viruses, infants and young children are more prone to develop clinical illness, and the few known fatalities are limited to this group. The virus is usually transmitted to the oral cavity of a susceptible person by a young child whose fingers contain virus as a result of fecal contamination. In some cases the virus is known to be transmitted in utero or during parturition and may be transmitted by oropharyngeal secretions.

After entry into the oral cavity Coxsackie viruses multiply in the oropharynx, often producing vesicular (herpangina) or nodular (acute lymphonodular pharyngitis) lesions in 3 to 5 days. Concomitantly, the viruses traverse the stomach without difficulty due to their resistance to acid and multiply extensively in the mucous membranes of the intestine. During this interval the viruses invade deep cervical nodes, producing lymphadenitis and painful stiffness of the neck, invade the mesenteric lymph nodes, and spill over into the blood. The viremia persists for a few days, and virus is disseminated to the meninges (viral meningitis), the skeletal muscles (epidemic myalgia, pleurodynia, or Bornholm disease), or the skin (exanthem, vesicular stomatitis with exanthem or hand, foot, and mouth disease). Virus is usually present in the blood during the incubation period, in the oropharyngeal secretions during the acute stage of the disease, in the feces for 2 to 5 weeks, and in the CSF if meningitis develops.

Less common clinical syndromes may be encountered if the virus has a predilection for the upper respiratory tract (common cold, mild respiratory disease), the testes (orchitis), or the

Table 24-14 Clinical Syndromes Associated with Coxsackie Viruses

Clinical syndrome	Coxsackie A types	Coxsackie B types
Mild paralysis	7, 9	2, 3, 4, 5
Viral meningitis	2, 4, 7, 9, 10	1, 2, 3, 4, 5, 6
Vesicular stomatitis with exanthem	5, 16	
Exanthem	4, 5, 9, 16	1, 3, 5
Vesicular pharyngitis	16, 5, 10	
Herpangina	2, 4, 5, 6, 8, 10	
Acute lymphonodular pharyngitis	10	
Fever with lymphadenitis	4, 5, 6	
Common cold	21, 24	
Pneumonitis of infants	9, 16	5
Undifferentiated febrile illness	2, 4, 5, 6, 7, 8, 9, 10, 16, 21, 24	1, 2, 3, 4, 5, 6
Epidemic myalgia (pleurodynia)		1, 2, 3, 4, 5
Neonatal encephalohepatomyocarditis		1, 2, 3, 4, 5
Pericarditis, myocarditis		1, 2, 3, 4, 5

pericardium (pericarditis which is more frequent in children and pregnant women). If infection with the virus occurs in utero, during parturition or early in neonatal life, the outcome may be disastrous (neonatal myocarditis or encephalohepatomyocarditis). In neonates the virus is widely disseminated, producing acute myocarditis, acute pericarditis, meningitis, encephalitis, paralysis, hepatitis, pancreatitis, and pneumonitis with inevitable death due to cardiac and respiratory involvement. A few of the Coxsackie viruses can cause paralysis in infants and young children, but this occurs only rarely.

In considering the clinical manifestations resulting from infection with Coxsackie viruses it is important to emphasize that not every virus can produce each of the clinical syndromes listed in Table 24-14; on the other hand, a specific virus can cause a number of different clinical syndromes in a particular family or community epidemic. For example, herpangina is produced only by certain Coxsackie A viruses, and epidemic myalgia or pleurodynia is caused by Coxsackie B viruses. On the other hand, any one of the Coxsackie B viruses may cause pleurodynia, aseptic meningitis, orchitis, or any combination of these syndromes in one person or in different individuals infected at the same time.

Herpangina Herpangina is a mild disease of young children caused by any one of eight Coxsackie A viruses. There is an acute febrile onset with temperatures up to 40.5°C, a sore throat (hyperemic pharyngitis), anorexia, and invariably discrete vesicular lesions which quickly rupture, leaving shallow grayish ulcers usually located on the anterior pillars of the fauces. The oral lesions may occasionally be found on the tonsils, pharynx, and soft palate. They are small in size (2 to 5 mm) and number about 5 per patient. The disease is of short duration, and the patient is well again in 2 to 3 days. The oral lesions may, however, persist for a few more days.

Epidemic Myalgia (Pleurodynia or Bornholm Disease) Epidemic myalgia is a frequent manifestation of any one of the Coxsackie B viruses. The disease is characterized by moderate fever (usually less than 40°C) which persists for 4 or 5 days and thoracic and abdominal pain of varying intensity. Pain in the chest (pleurodynia) is most common, especially in adults, is increased by movement, and persists for 2 to 10 days. Abdominal pain is present in about half of the cases, is more common in children, and may occur in the absence of pleurodynia. As noted above, epidemic myalgia is often associated with viral meningitis and orchitis.

Laboratory Diagnosis

A laboratory diagnosis may be established either by isolation and identification of the virus or by demonstrating a rise in neutralizing antibody, preferably by both procedures. The virus is most frequently recovered from feces and oropharyngeal washings, but whenever the clinical manifestations warrant, efforts should be made to recover the virus from the CSF and other tissues.

Recovery of Coxsackie A viruses is best accomplished either by the inoculation of human embryonic kidney cells or by the inoculation of newborn mice by the subcutaneous, intraperitoneal, and intracerebral routes (or a combination of these routes in each newborn mouse). The pathological picture of generalized myositis which is almost always indicative of infection with a Coxsackie A virus can be verified by performing a neutralization test.

Coxsackie B viruses are best isolated in human embryonic kidney tissue cultures in which they produce cytopathogenicity. Identification is based on a neutralization test. In newborn mice Coxsackie B virus produces a pathological picture of fat necrosis, the etiology of which can be confirmed by tissue culture neutralization tests.

Whenever possible, a serological diagnosis is based on a plaque neutralization test in human embryonic kidney tissue cultures by demonstrating a rise in antibody titer between the acute and the convalescent phases of the disease. In some cases, however, it may be necessary to perform a neutralization test in newborn mice with some Coxsackie A viruses.

Epidemiology

The spread of Coxsackie viruses is basically similar to that of the polioviruses and echoviruses. The viruses are found throughout the world, are somewhat cyclic in geographical and temporal distribution, are more readily isolated in summer and early fall in temperate climates, and are recovered more consistently from lower socioeconomic areas than from middle or upper middle class areas. Preschool children form the main cohort of infection and spread the virus vertically and horizontally within the household and the community primarily on the basis of fecal contamination and an intestinal-oral route.

Epidemics are most likely to occur in communities with improving sanitary and hygienic practices which decrease the opportunities for early infection and increase the number of susceptible older children and young adults. This is particularly true of epidemics of viral meningitis and pleurodynia. In areas of poor sanitation virus excretion is three to six times as great, infection in preschool children is widespread, neutralizing antibodies reach the adult level in 6-year-old children, and epidemics of viral meningitis and pleurodynia are less commonly observed.

There is a large reservoir of infection in man, but except for neonatal infections, fatalities are rarely encountered.

Prevention and Control

At present, there are no specific methods for prevention or control of Coxsackie virus infection. In view of the largely self-limited nature of the disease produced by Coxsackie viruses (except in neonates), there has been little demand for a vaccine. However, there may be a future need for effective vaccines against the more pathogenic Coxsackie B, A7, and A9 viruses.

INFECTIONS CAUSED BY ECHOVIRUSES

Enteric cytopathogenic human orphan or echoviruses are natural human parasities that are members of the enterovirus subgroup of the picorna viruses. Since their original isolation from human feces in 1951, the echoviruses have been frequently recovered from healthy children and from patients with a variety of illnesses.

The echoviruses are a common cause of meningitis, attack the skin and the pharynx, occasionally invade the CNS, and may cause diarrhea. Cytopathogenicity is regularly produced in tissue cultures. The viruses are not pathogenic for newborn mice except for some strains of type 9 which after tissue culture passage can produce generalized myositis.

The Causative Agent

Biologic Properties Like other enteroviruses (polioviruses and Coxsackie viruses), the echoviruses are small (20 to 30 nm in diameter), icosahedral, have an RNA core and a protein shell, are resistant to acid at pH 3.0, lack an envelope containing essential lipid, and show cationic stabilization of thermal inactivation. The echoviruses are transient inhabitants of the human intestinal tract and oropharynx. Healthy fecal carriers contaminate the environment and serve as the major source of human infection.

Unlike polioviruses, echoviruses are frequently found in the CSF of patients with meningitis and rarely produce disease in monkeys. Unlike Coxsackie viruses, echoviruses do not produce disease in newborn mice (except for some strains of type 9).

Wistar Institute human diploid (WI-38) tissue cultures are the cells of choice for primary isolation of the virus. Most echoviruses will, however, multiply in human amnion cells, and many will grow in human embryonic lung, skin, muscle, and kidney cells and in monkey kidney cells.

The response of chimpanzees to virus feeding resembles that which is observed with polioviruses and Coxsackie viruses. The animals develop an inapparent infection with limited multiplication of virus in the oropharynx, transient viremia, intestinal carriage, excretion of virus for several weeks, and the formation of neutralizing antibody.

Antigenic Structure There are 33 antigenic types of echoviruses presently recognized, designated types 1 to 33. Antigenic specificity has been established by cross-neutralization, CF, and HA-inhibition tests. As with the Coxsackie viruses, antigenic analysis is complicated by the existence of prime strains but can be circumvented by CF and plaque neutralization tests.

Hemagglutinin Approximately half of the antigenic types of echoviruses cause agglutination of human group O erythrocytes and HA-inhibition is a useful diagnostic procedure. The HA is associated with the infectivity of the virus particle. A purified receptor has been isolated from human red blood cells which in a concentration of 0.2μg inhibits 8 HA units of the virus and irreversibly destroys the infectivity of the virus. Chemically, the receptor is a protein, lipid, carbohydrate complex containing a deoxypolynucleotide, neutral glycolipid, phospholipids, and cholesterol.

Pathogenesis

The Basis of Cellular, Tissue, Organ, and Species Specificity As with polioviruses and Coxsackie viruses, cellular, tissue, organ, and species specificity of echoviruses is determined by receptors located in the plasma membrane of susceptible cells. Man appears to possess a broader range of target cells with receptors for echoviruses than for polioviruses, but the full range and extent of damage produced by echoviruses have been difficult to assay because of the common presence of echoviruses in the feces and pharynx of healthy individuals. There can be no doubt, however, that the virus attacks the mucous membranes of the oral cavity, the intestines, and the respiratory tract, the meninges, and the skin. Accessory targets may include the brain, spinal cord, skeletal muscles, myocardium, pericardium, liver, lymph nodes, and the eyes.

The Response to Infection Initial contact with echovirus commonly results in a subclinical infection with multiplication of virus in the mucous membranes of the oropharynx and the intestinal tract, invasion of lymphatic tissue, a transient viremia, and the excretion of virus in oropharyngeal secretions and feces. Echoviruses may also induce one or more of a variety of clinical syndromes, including meningitis, exanthematous disease, vesicular enanthemata (oral lesions), and gastroenteritis or diarrheal disease (Table 24-15). The virus is usually spread to the oral cavity of a susceptible person by a young child whose fingers contain virus as a result of fecal contamination and perhaps occasionally from oropharyngeal secretions.

After entry into the oral cavity echoviruses multiply in the oropharynx, occasionally producing an enanthem in 2 to 6 days. Concomitantly, the viruses pass through the stomach without difficulty because of their resistance to

Table 24-15 Clinical Syndromes Associated with Echoviruses

Clinical syndrome	Echovirus type
Paralytic disease	1, 2, 4, 6, 7, 9, 11, 16, 18, 30
Encephalitis	2, 3, 4, 6, 7, 9, 11, 14, 18, 19
Viral meningitis	4, 6, 9, 11, 16, 30
Exanthemata	2, 4, 9, 11, 16
Enanthemata	6, 9, 16
Pericarditis	1, 9, 16
Myocarditis	6, 9
Diarrhea	11, 14, 18
Respiratory enteric disease	1, 11, 19, 20
Respiratory disease	1, 3, 6, 11, 19, 20
Ocular disturbances	1, 4, 6, 9, 16, 20
Lymphadenopathy	2, 4, 9, 16, 20
Epidemic myalgia	1, 6, 9

acid, multiply extensively in the mucous membranes of the intestine, and may produce diarrheal disease. During this interval the viruses invade lymphatic tissue, occasionally producing cervical lymphadenopathy, and spill over into the blood. The viremia persists for a few days during which the virus may be disseminated to the meninges (viral meningitis), the skin (exanthematous disease), and less commonly the liver (hepatitis), the myocardium and pericardium (myocarditis and pericarditis), the brain and spinal cord (encephalitis and paralysis), and the skeletal muscles (epidemic myalgia, commonly involving the extremities but occasionally producing pleurodynia).

If the particular virus has a predilection for the mucous membranes of the respiratory tract and the conjunctiva (or perhaps if the virus is introduced by either of these routes), respiratory or ocular disturbances may predominate or be combined with other clinical syndromes (gastroenteritis and exanthem). The upper respiratory tract is involved with clinical syndromes which may resemble the common cold, a febrile pharyngitis, influenza, or pharyngoconjunctival fever. With other echoviruses, photophobia may occur with a frequency of 10 to 25 percent, usually without conjunctivitis.

Many of the echoviruses have not been associated with disease, and others have been isolated only sporadically from patients with a particular clinical syndrome. On the other hand, a number of echoviruses including types 2, 4, 6, 7, 9, 11, 14, and 16 can cause a variety of syndromes in one person or in different individuals infected at the same time. For example, under epidemic conditions echovirus type 9 may produce aseptic meningitis, exanthematous disease, and enanthemata, or any combination of these syndromes.

Laboratory Diagnosis

A laboratory diagnosis of echovirus infection is best established by isolation of the virus in WI-38 tissue cultures in which it produces cytopathogenicity or plaques under agar, identification by a plaque neutralization test, and the demonstration of a rise in neutralizing antibody titer between the acute and the convalescent phases of the disease. Because of the prevalence of echoviruses in the feces and oropharynx of healthy individuals, all three methods should be employed; and whenever possible, the virus should be isolated from the CSF as well as from feces and oropharyngeal secretions.

Epidemiology

The epidemiology of echoviruses is basically similar to that of the polioviruses and Coxsackie viruses. Young children form the main cohort of family-oriented infection and disease. The viruses are worldwide in distribution and exist commonly as transitory infections of the intestinal tract. Excretion of virus in the feces contaminates the environment and serves as the source of infection of susceptible persons. The amount of virus released into the environment is inversely related to age and socioeconomic level and is maximal during summer and early fall in temperate climates.

The ratio of infection to disease has been estimated as 200 to 1. However, echoviruses may be responsible for outbreaks of meningitis which involve 4 to 9 percent of the population in communities with well-developed sanitary and hygienic practices, especially if there are many children and young adults.

Despite the large reservoir of infection in man and the extensive outbreaks of disease in certain population groups, fatalities are rarely encountered, except when neonates are infected.

Prevention and Control

At present, there is no specific method for the prevention and control of echovirus infections. In view of the largely self-limited nature of the disease produced by echoviruses (except in neonates), there has been little demand for a vaccine. However, there may be a need in the future for effective vaccines against the more pathogenic echoviruses, especially types 4, 6, 9, 11, and 16.

VIRAL MENINGITIS (ASEPTIC MENINGITIS)

Viral (aseptic) meningitis is the term applied to an inflammation of the membranes covering the CNS, usually localized to the subarachnoid space (meningitis), in which neither bacteria nor fungi are present (aseptic). Viral meningitis is the most common disease involving the CNS and may be caused by any one of a large number of viruses, most frequently by mumps virus, echoviruses, and Coxsackie B viruses and to a much lesser extent by Coxsackie A, lymphocytic choriomeningitis, and the herpesviruses. Polioviruses were formerly responsible for many cases of viral meningitis (nonparalytic poliomyelitis), but these cases have been eliminated by the development and widespread use of effective vaccines.

The clinical manifestations include fever, headache, a stiff and painful neck and back, and difficulties of flexion and extension. The CSF contains an increased number of cells, predominantly lymphocytes, and elevated protein, but a normal sugar level (Table 24-4).

Invasion of the CNS is preceded by viremia, and the causative agent can be isolated from the CSF during the acute stage of the disease unless the illness is caused by poliovirus. The course of the disease is usually mild with recovery in 7 to 10 days, but fatigue and discomfort may persist for several weeks, especially in adults.

A laboratory diagnosis is best established by isolation of the virus from the CSF in monkey kidney or other appropriate tissue culture and identification of the virus by suitable neutralization or CF tests. In the case of meningitis caused by poliovirus, the virus is recovered from the feces (not the CSF) and is identified by neutralization tests in tissue culture; in addition, a rise in neutralizing antibody titer between the acute and convalescent phases of the disease should be demonstrated.

The epidemiology of the disease reflects the epidemiology of the particular causative agent. Cases of viral meningitis may be sporadic or epidemic with thousands of cases often in combination with other clinical syndromes. Although the etiology of viral meningitis can be established only in the virus laboratory, much can be learned from the close study of the individual case and from epidemiological study of contacts and the community. For example, the presence of parotitis or involvement of the pancreas, ovary, or testis in the case, in household or close contacts, or in the community suggests that the mumps virus might be the causative agent. On the other hand, a Coxsackie B virus might be suspected when pleurodynia is present in contacts or in the community.

The age incidence of viral meningitis is greatest in children and young adults, except for herpesvirus which primarily involves infants and young children. Except when the disease occurs in infants and young children or in the event that paralytic poliomyelitis follows meningitis due to poliovirus, the prognosis is good, and serious sequelae are rare. This is in sharp contrast to the high mortality and severe sequelae encountered with bacterial and fungal meningitis.

PROSPECTIVE

Infections of the CNS still claim more than 3,000 lives in the United States each year. If not for the development and use of effective poliovirus vaccines, the fatalities would be doubled. If any further substantial progress is to be made in reducing the number of deaths caused by CNS infections, it must result from improved methods to prevent and control bacterial meningitis, which is responsible for the majority of the fatalities. However, the prospects of achieving this desirable goal are dim in view of the often fulminating nature of the disease and the unsuspected or serious nature of the predisposing factors which permit the disease to develop. On the other hand, meningococcal vaccines are well along in the developmental stage and may prove valuable. Perhaps an effective vaccine might be prepared for use against *Hemophilus influenzae* type b.

BIBLIOGRAPHY

Baker, C. J., Barrett, F. F., Gordon, R. C., and Yow, M. D.: "Suppurative Meningitis Due to Streptococci of Lancefield Group B: A Study of 33 Infants," *J. Pediatr.,* 82:724-729, 1973.

Barton, L. L., Feigin, R. D., and Lins, R.: "Group B Beta Hemolytic Streptococcal Meningitis in Infants," *J. Pediatr.,* 82:719-723, 1973.

Bottiger, M., Zetterberg, B., and Salenstedt, C.-R.: "Seroimmunity to Poliomyelitis in Sweden after the Use of Inactivated Poliovirus Vaccine for 10 Years," *Bull. W.H.O.,* 46:141-149, 1972.

Feldman, H. A.: "Meningococcal Infections," *Adv. Inter. Med.,* 18:117-140, 1972.

Fraser, D. W., Darby, C. P., Koehler, R. E., Jacobs, C. F., and Feldman, R. A.: "Risk Factors in Bacterial Meningitis: Charleston County, South Carolina," *J. Infect. Dis.,* 127:1-277, 1973.

Gear, J. H. S., and Measroch, V.: "Coxsackievirus Infections of the Newborn," *Progr. Med. Virol.,* 15:42-62, 1973.

Goldfield, M., and Sussman, O.: "The 1959 Outbreak of Eastern Encephalitis in New Jersey: 1. Introduction and Description of Outbreak," *Am. J. Epidemiol.,* 87:1-10, 1968.

———, Taylor, B. F., Welsh, J. N., Altman, R., Black, H. C., Mazzur, S. R., and Bill, J. S.: "The Persistence of Eastern Encephalitis Serologic Reactivity Following Overt and Inapparent Human Infection—An Eight Year Followup," *Am. J. Epidemiol.,* 87:50-57, 1968.

Hoffman, T. A., and Edwards, E. A.: "Group-specific Polysaccharide Antigen and Humoral Antibody Response in Disease Due to *Neisseria meningitidis,*" *J. Infect. Dis.,* 126:636-644, 1972.

Hofman, B.: "Poliomyelitis in the Netherlands 1958-69: The Influence of a Vaccination Programme with Inactivated Poliovaccine," *Bull. W.H.O.,* 46:735-745, 1972.

Horstmann, D. M., Emmons, J., Gimpel, L., Subrahmanyan, T., and Riordan, J. T.: "Enterovirus Surveillance Following a Community-wide Oral Poliovirus Vaccination Program: A Seven-year Study," *Am. J. Epidemiol.,* 97:173-186, 1973.

Kaplan, J. M., McCracken, G. H., and Nelson, J. D.: "Infections in Children Caused by the HB Group of Bacteria," *J. Pediatr.,* 82:398-403, 1973.

Kibrick, S.: "Current Status of Coxsackie and ECHO Viruses in Human Disease," *Progr. Med. Virol.,* 6:27-70, 1964.

Landrigan, P. J., and Witte, J. J.: "Neurologic Disorders Following Live Measles-virus Vaccination," *J.A.M.A.,* 223:1459-1462, 1973.

Lerner, A. M., and Wilson, F. M.: "Virus Myocardiopathy," *Progr. Med. Virol.,* 15:63-91, 1973.

Link, H., Panelius, M., and Salmi, A. A.: "Immunoglobulins and Measles Antibodies in Subacute Sclerosing Panencephalitis," *Arch. Neurol.,* 28:23-30, 1973.

McGowan, J. E., Jr., Bryan, J. A., and Gregg, M. B.: "Surveillance of Arboviral Encephalitis in the United States, 1955-1971," *Am. J. Epidemiol.,* 97:199-207, 1973.

Menlen, V. T., Katz, M., Kackell, Y.-M., Barbanti-Brodano, G., Koprowski, H., and Lennette, E. H.: "Subacute Sclerosing Panencephalitis: In Vitro Characterization of Viruses Isolated from Brain Cells in Culture," *J. Infect. Dis.,* 126:11-17, 1972.

Miller, J. R., and Harter, D. H.: "Acute Viral Encephalitis," *Med. Clin. North Am.,* 56:1393-1404, 1972.

Ogra, P.L., and Karzon, D. T.: "Formation and Function of Poliovirus Antibody in Different Tissues," *Progr. Med. Virol.,* 13:156-193, 1971.

Price, R., Chernick, N. L., Horta-Barbosa, L., and Posner, J. B.: "Herpes Simplex Encephalitis in an Anergic Patient," *Am. J. Med.,* 54:222-228, 1973.

Reeves, W. C.: "Can the War to Contain Infectious Diseases Be Lost?" *Am. J. Trop. Med. Hyg.,* 21: 251-259, 1972.

Samson, D. S., and Clark, K.: "A Current Review of Brain Abscess," *Am. J. Med.,* 54:201-210, 1973.

Sell, S. H., and Karzon, D. T. (eds.): *Hemophilus influenzae; Proceedings of a Conference on Antigen-Antibody Systems, Epidemiology, and Immuno-prophylaxis,* Nashville, Tenn.: Vanderbilt University Press, 1973.

Simpson, D. I.: "Arbovirus Diseases," *Br. Med. Bull.,* 28:10-15, 1972.

Weinstein, L.: "Poliomyelitis—A Persistent Problem," *N. Engl. J. Med.,* 288:370-372, 1973.

Winchester, J. S., and Hambling, M. H.: "Antibodies to Measles, Mumps, and Herpes Simplex Virus in Cerebrospinal Fluid in Acute Infections and Post-infectious Diseases of the Central Nervous System," *J. Med. Microbiol.,* 5:137-143, 1972.

Wyle, F. A., Artenstein, M. S., Brandt, B. L., Tramont, E. C., Kasper, D. L., Altieri, P. L., Berman, S. L., and Lowenthal, J. P.: "Immunologic Response of Man to Group B Meningococcal Polysaccharide Vaccines," *J. Infect. Dis.,* 126:514-522, 1972.

Chapter 25

Infections of the Reticuloendothelial System in Which Man Is the Reservoir

Bernard A. Briody and Zigmund C. Kaminski

PERSPECTIVE

The reticuloendothelial system (RES) is prominently involved as a regular feature of disease caused by a wide spectrum of parasites. Included in this category are such diseases as typhoid (Chap. 18), syphilis (Chap. 21), the exanthemata (Chap. 22), many respiratory pathogens (Chap. 23), and the vast majority of animal diseases transmissible to man (Chap. 26). In this chapter consideration is given to reticuloendothelial infections which either do not show significant dermal, pulmonary, or CNS localization or are not limited to the CNS, as in mumps, trypanosomiasis, or toxoplasmosis. Emphasis is placed on such major diseases as malaria, leishmaniasis, trypanosomiasis, schistosomiasis, hepatitis, yellow fever, mumps, and infectious mononucleosis.

The causative agents involved include viruses, protozoa, helminths, and bacteria. Admittedly, man is not the sole, or even the most important, reservoir of infection in the case of yellow fever or in some forms of leishmaniasis, trypanosomiasis, or toxoplasmosis. On the other hand, there are advantages to considering yellow fever along with other hepatic diseases and including the diseases caused by most of the protozoa in the same chapter. In addition, the causative agents are transmitted by a variety of methods including arthropods, droplet infection, fecal-oral contact, parenteral infection of blood or blood products, ingestion of contaminated meat, larval penetration of the skin, ingestion of eggs, or following placental transfer. Because of this diversity, the diseases are discussed according to their viral, protozoal, helminthic, or bacterial etiology.

Viral Infections

VIRAL HEPATITIS

Viral hepatitis is a common, acute, systemic infectious disease primarily affecting the liver and induced by viruses designated A (infectious hepatitis, IH) and B (serum hepatitis, SH). Diseases caused by A and B viruses are epidemiologically distinct but clinically and pathologically similar. Depending on the virus and the age of the individual, the disease may be *icteric* (with jaundice) or *anicteric* (without jaundice). Many cases of viral hepatitis are recognized only by abnormal liver function tests and, in the case of hepatitis B, by the presence of hepatitis-associated antigen (HAA, or HB Ag) or hepatitis-associated antibody (HB Ab). On the other hand, hepatitis B can be associated with severe disease (chronic active hepatitis, subacute or fulminant hepatic necrosis, cirrhosis, fibrosis, portal hypertension) and an overall mortality rate of approximately 11 percent which reflects the type of hepatitis, the age of the patient, and other underlying illness which the patient may have.

The Causative Agents

The distribution of hepatitis viruses in nature is dependent entirely upon man. Fecal excretion of virus A occurs 2 to 3 weeks before the onset of clinical manifestations, may continue for as long as 1 year after recovery, and is the major source of environmental contamination and infection of susceptible individuals. The resistance of the virus to heat (56°C for 30 min.) and to disinfecting chemicals, including chlorine, permit its survival in sewage, water, and food for prolonged periods. Virus A is found in oysters and clams derived from sewage-polluted waters, apparently as a result of concentration of the virus. Oysters and clams pump as much as 10 gallons of water per day and presumably filter out the virus. Since virus A cannot be propagated in tissue culture or in nonhuman hosts (chimpanzees excepted), precise knowledge of the concentration of the virus found in various tissues is lacking, and serological tests are unavailable.

The important finding of HAA in the blood of patients actively or chronically infected with virus B has greatly expanded knowledge of viral hepatitis. For example, increasingly sensitive methods have been developed for the detection of antigen and antibody and for the identification of some of the carriers of virus B among healthy blood donors. Reliable assay techniques have been provided to follow the apparently successful propagation of virus B in human embryo liver organ cultures. In addition, a noncytopathic assay system using human diploid WI-38 cells has been described. After exposure to HAA, the cells are refractory to infection by Newcastle disease virus. Nonetheless, it is estimated that the best currently available screening techniques for the antigen detect only 20 to 50 percent of virus B carriers.

The presence of HAA in the blood (antigenemia or viremia) occurs 2 to 4 weeks in advance of clinical or biochemical evidence of hepatitis and may persist for several years or more in some patients. An estimated 2 to 10 percent of those infected with virus B become chronic carriers (more than 3 months). Approximately half of the carriers are free of biochemical and histological evidence of hepatitis, but the other half have chronic liver disease which may terminate in cirrhosis. Electron microscopy of negatively stained preparations containing HAA reveal three typical morphological particles: (1) spherical particles, 20 nm in diameter; (2) tubular forms of varying lengths; and (3) spherical double-shelled particles, 42 nm in diameter. The nucleic acid content associated with HAA is low, and the report that it is RNA awaits more definitive clarification. Virus B is even more resistant to heat and disinfecting chemicals than virus A.

Pathogenesis

Viral Hepatitis A Among young children, who form the main cohort of infection, virus A is spread by the direct fecal-oral route. An alternate method of transmission involves fecal contamination of food and water which when ingested often result in epidemics. A variant of this method occurs when raw oysters or clams from sewage-polluted waters are ingested. Less commonly, chimpanzees may acquire the infection from man, excrete the virus in their feces, and in turn, transmit the virus to humans with whom they come in close personal contact. In rare cases, the virus may be transmitted parenterally along with blood or blood products.

Following ingestion, the acid resistance of virus A enables it to traverse the stomach and reach the small intestine. Presumably, the virus infects the mucosal epithelial cells, replicates, and spreads to adjacent cells and via the portal circulation to the liver. About half-way through the incubation period, which averages 30 days, the feces become infective, and the virus persists in the stools for several weeks or months. Serum glutamic pyruvic transaminase and serum glutamic oxaloacetic transaminase levels are usually elevated 7 to 14 days before icterus develops, and virus is present in the blood for several days. During the preicteric stage of the disease there is loss of appetite, fatigue, malaise, abdominal discomfort, fever, and distaste for cigarettes and coffee. With the appearance of icterus the patient feels better, but the liver remains tender and palpable; jaundice persists for 1 to 3 weeks, and recovery usually occurs gradually over a period of 2 to 6 weeks.

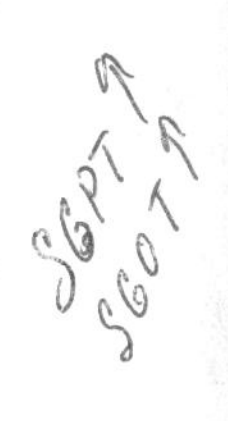

Liver biopsies during the acute stage of the disease reveal an inflammatory reaction consisting of infiltration of lymphocytes, plasma cells, and macrophages in the portal tracts; hypertrophy and hyperplasia of Kupffer cells, which often contain a brown pigment; foci of hepatocyte necrosis distributed within the lobules, and variable bile stasis. Ultrastructurally, the hepatocytes show dilatation of the endoplasmic reticulum and an increased number of lysosomes and mitochondria. After the appearance of icterus and during the recovery process, liver cell regeneration commences with increasing evidence of proliferation and mitotic figures. Jejunal and duodenal biopsies show mononuclear cell infiltration of the villous stroma and lamina propria with shortening or loss of villi and an increased number of goblet cells, changes that may be the result of viral replication in the epithelial cells.

Viral Hepatitis B Although hepatitis B has been transmitted experimentally to children following ingestion of infected serum, naturally occurring cases invariably develop following the peripheral intentional or accidental injection of human blood or blood products. The incubation period usually averages 2 to 4 months, and the disease in most patients is clinically and pathologically similar to hepatitis A. However, about 1 to 5 percent of patients develop chronic aggressive (active) hepatitis (subacute hepatic necrosis) accompanied by persistence of HAA and, ultimately, in most instances cirrhosis. Fulminant hepatic failure is a rare complication of virus B infection and is characterized by massive necrosis of liver cells or sudden severe impairment of hepatic function, an acute onset of progressive and severe mental changes advancing rapidly to stupor and coma with intense jaundice, and a high mortality rate (30 to 80 percent).

The Role of Immune Complexes Although the data are limited, several lines of evidence implicate immune complexes in the pathogenesis of hepatitis B, especially in chronic aggressive hepatitis and fulminant hepatic failure. Hepatitis B often occurs in association with a syndrome resembling serum sickness (urticaria, arthralgia, angioneurotic edema) which seems to be correlated with HAA and depressed levels of complement. Chronic carriers free of hepatitis contain HAA focally distributed within the cytoplasm of hepatocytes and in the blood, but antibody and immune complexes are missing. Patients with chronic aggressive hepatitis have excess HAA in Kupffer cells, sinusoidal endothelial cells, and in infiltrating monocytes. Free antibody cannot be detected in these patients, but immune complexes containing HAA, antibody, and complement are deposited together in the liver. In fulminant hepatic failure, free HAA cannot be found, but excess antibody and immune complexes are present in the liver. Thus, tentatively, it appears that the carrier is healthy when free HAA is the only component found in the liver; but with the appearance of antibody, immune complexes are formed, and hepatic disease results.

Predisposing Factors Previously unexposed individuals appear to be uniformly susceptible to virus B but vary widely in their response, depending upon their age and the presence or absence of underlying disease. For example, chronic aggressive hepatitis and fulminant hepatic failure are more prevalent in patients with mongolism, lepromatous leprosy, diabetes, leukemia, thalassemia, and immunodeficiency; in drug addicts; in those receiving corticosteroids, cytotoxic drugs, and immunosuppressive therapy; in infants born following maternal hepatitis; and in patients exposed to halothane, a general anesthesic. While the overall mortality rate of hepatitis B is 11 percent, in patients under 40 years of age it is only 5.5 percent. Undoubtedly, the increased mortality associated with advancing age reflects the progression of the underlying illness as well as the stress imposed by the hepatitis.

Laboratory Diagnosis

Although a positive hepatic biopsy, elevated transaminase, and a compatible clinical pattern in the absence of HAA strongly suggest the diagnosis of virus A infection, there is no suitable laboratory test.

On the other hand, a battery of tests can be used to detect HAA in the serum of patients or carriers infected with virus B. The tests vary more than 10,000-fold in relative sensitivity and in the time required to complete the test. The methods of detecting HAA employ immunodiffusion, immunoelectroosmophoresis (counterimmunoelectrophoresis or electrophoretic immunoprecipitation), complement fixation, passive hemagglutination and hemagglutination inhibition, radioimmunoassay, electron microscopy and immune electron microscopy, immunofluorescence, immune adherence hemagglutination, and latex agglutination. To date no single test has been employed as a standard. Passive hemagglutination and latex agglutination tests appear to provide greater speed and simplicity than other tests. The same procedures can be adapted for the detection of antibody against HAA.

Hopefully, within a short time, isolation of virus B in human embryo liver organ cultures, WI-38, or other cells will be proved practical. Certainly, information derived from such studies will further expand knowledge concerning hepatitis B, may provide a method for detecting carriers that escape identification by currently available procedures, and may lead to the development of effective vaccines.

Epidemiology

Viral Hepatitis A Children between the ages of 5 and 9 years have the highest attack rates, form the main cohort of infection, and spread the disease by the fecal-oral route largely within the family to 10 to 40 percent of their adult and child contacts. Clinical cases, however, reach a peak in 20- to 25-year-olds (Fig. 25-1). Outside the family the disease is disseminated to the neighborhood as a result of close personal contact with other children who then introduce the infection into their families. As the number of cases increases, the risk of water-borne and food-borne epidemics also rises and reaches epidemic peaks every 3 to 10 years, depending upon the number of susceptible persons available (Fig. 25-2). Infection is prevalent in prisons, mental institutions, camps, travelers in highly endemic areas, and overcrowded localities associated with poor sanitation and a low socioeconomic level. Although formerly higher in rural than in urban areas of New York, recent data show that the disease is twice as prevalent in urban as opposed to rural areas (56.4 compared to 27.2 per 100,000). Among children

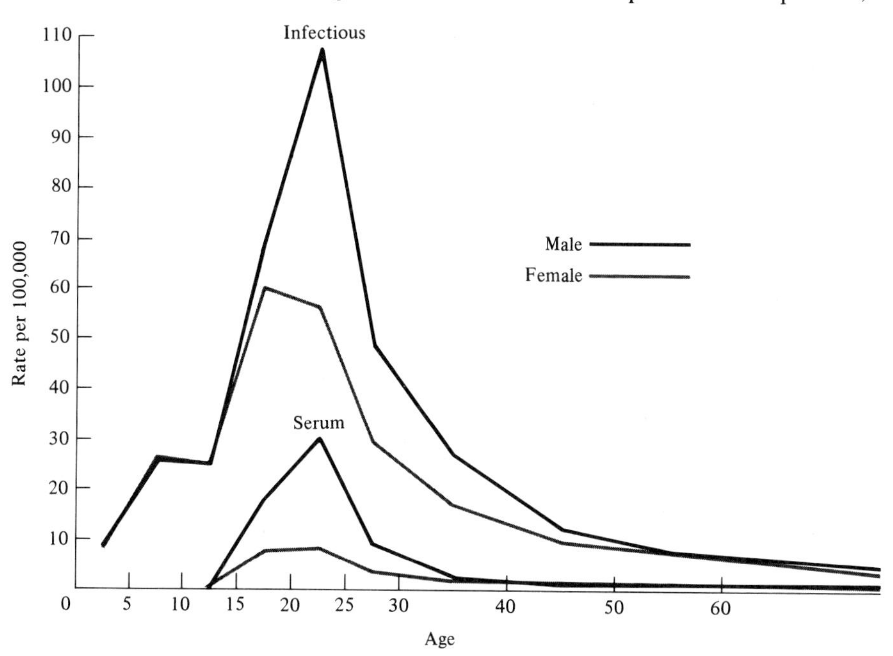

Figure 25-1 Incidence of hepatitis in the United States in 1971 according to sex and age. [*Morbidity Mortality Weekly Report, 20(53):1, 1972.*]

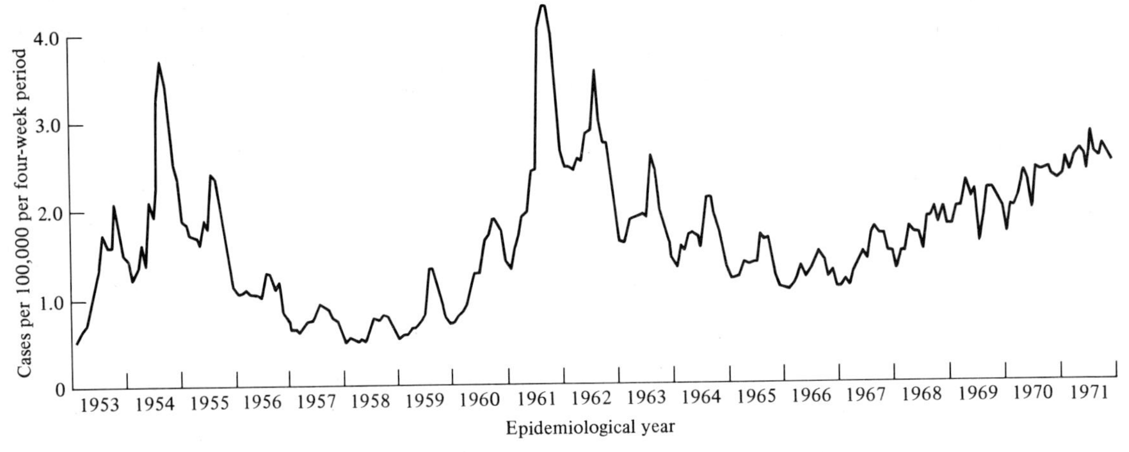

Figure 25-2 Incidence of viral hepatitis in the United States from 1953 to 1971. [*Morbidity Mortality Weekly Report, 20(53):45, 1972.*]

the anicteric/icteric ratio is about 12/1 but approaches 1/1 in adults. The mortality is low (0.1 to 0.4 percent), and the highest incidence occurs during the autumn and winter. When contaminated oysters or clams serve as the common epidemic source, the disease is usually limited to adult males.

Viral Hepatitis B All ages are susceptible to infection following intentional or accidental injection of blood or blood products containing HAA. Pooled plasma is particularly dangerous, and the incidence following blood transfusion is about 0.3 to 0.4 percent but rises rapidly with multiple transfusions. The chronic carrier state in the general population is estimated to be as low as 0.07 percent and as high as 0.1 percent. HAA is present in as many as 20 percent of selected populations (Peruvian Indians), and a prevalence of more than 5 percent is found in diabetics; patients with mongolism, thalassemia, mental retardation; and those requiring chronic renal dialysis in certain countries. Prevalences of 1 to 5 percent are reported to occur in the same patients in other countries, in commercial blood donors, drug addicts, hemophiliacs, and prisoners. Hospitalized patients show a higher incidence of hepatitis B, about five times that in nonhospitalized persons. Hospital personnel, especially those working in renal dialysis units and in clinical pathology laboratories routinely handling blood and blood products, are at special risk. An indication of the prevalence of virus B in hospital personnel is the finding that they comprise 7 percent of hospitalized cases.

The chronic HAA carrier is a major source of hepatitis B infection for those who come in contact with his blood. Persons who are likely to become chronic carriers in addition to those mentioned above include those suffering from genetically inherited, naturally acquired, or induced immunodeficiency. The overall mortality of 11 percent rises with debilitated states and falls in younger healthy persons.

The incidence of hepatitis B appears to be increasing twice as rapidly as hepatitis A. Several lines of evidence indicate that drug abuse is a major factor in the rising incidence of hepatitis B. For example, in the period 1963–1966, 4 percent of hepatitis patients acknowledged narcotic use; whereas in the period 1967–1971, 30 percent used narcotics. In Harlem (New York) where narcotic addiction is prevalent, HAA is

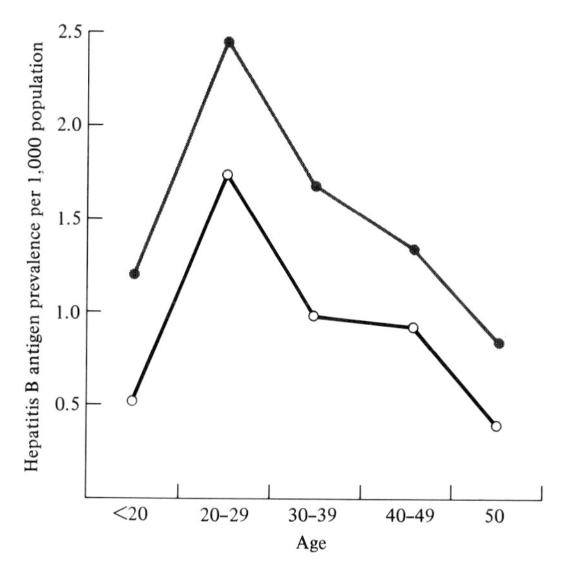

Figure 25-3 Prevalence of hepatitis B antigen among male (●–●) and female (○–○) volunteer blood donors in relation to age. (*W. Szmuness, A. M. Prince, B. Brotman, and R. L. Hirsch, J. Infect. Dis., 127:17–25, 1973.*)

present in 1 percent of the population, as opposed to 0.1 percent elsewhere in the country. In New York City the prevalence among volunteer blood donors averaged 0.215 percent and ranged between 0.171 and 0.326 percent in the different boroughs, as contrasted with 0.101 percent in suburban New York State and 0.093 percent in suburban communities elsewhere. As noted in Figures 25-1 and 25-3, the prevalence of HAA is highest in 20- to 24-year-olds and is higher in males than in females.

Prevention and Control

Viral Hepatitis A The prevalence of hepatitis A can be reduced by sanitary disposal of feces, provision of safe drinking water, and good personal hygiene. Specific protection can be achieved by the use of human gamma globulin prepared from large plasma pools. When administered intramuscularly in doses of 0.02 to 0.06 ml/kg of body weight, human gamma globulin is remarkably effective in interrupting epidemics of viral hepatitis A. Gamma globulin does not prevent infection but leads to (1) mild anicteric or subclinical infection and (2) active immunity superimposed on the passive immunity. In addition, gamma globulin is equally effective in protecting other high-risk groups (household contacts, adults working in mental institutions, travelers to highly endemic countries).

Viral Hepatitis B The prevalence of viral hepatitis B can be reduced by avoiding contact with blood or blood products likely to be contaminated with the virus. With the exception of immunoglobulins and albumin, the virus must be assumed to be present in blood and blood products. Observing the following precautions will lower the incidence of viral hepatitis B.

1 Limit the administration of whole blood or blood products to patients in clear need of such therapy and use the minimal number of units required.
2 Whenever possible, use volunteer as opposed to professional (commercial) blood donors and limit blood donors to persons who (1) have no history of hepatitis; (2) have normal liver function tests; and (3) are free of HAA.
3 Restrict plasma pools to a limited number (1 to 5) of donors who comply with the three requirements listed in item 2.
4 Use a fresh sterile disposable syringe and needle for each patient receiving skin tests, parenteral inoculations, or venipuncture.
5 Sterilize all nondisposable equipment by autoclaving or boiling for 10 min.
6 Instruct health-care personnel (physicians, dentists, nurses, and especially technicians working in hospital hemodialysis units and clinical pathology laboratories) in the importance of taking special precautions to avoid spreading or acquiring infection and provide adequate supervision to insure that the measures are being followed.

Although it has been shown that specific hepatitis B antibody with a potency 50,000 times greater than that contained in standard immune globulin was protective in experimentally infected children, such preparations hardly

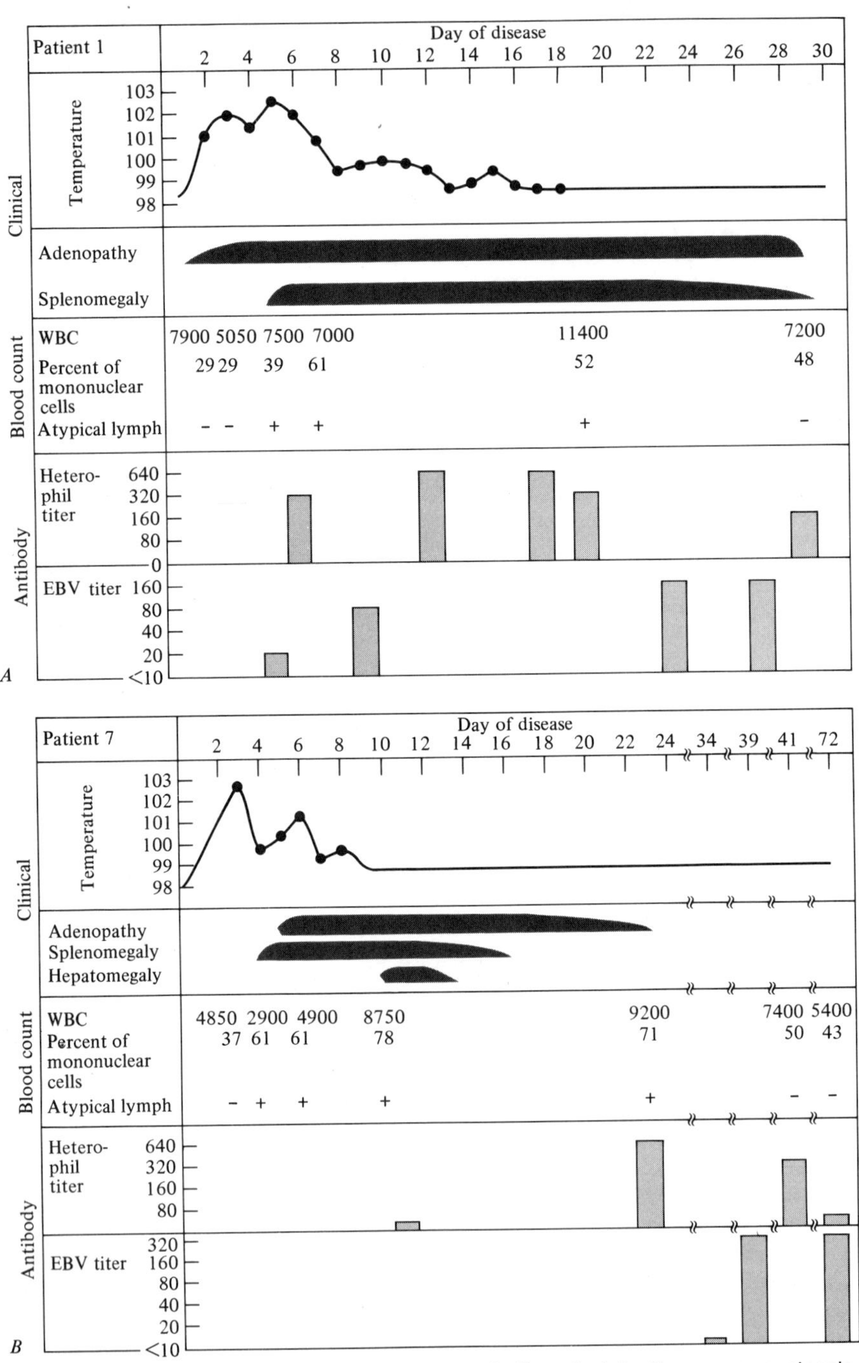

Figure 25-4 Clinical features and laboratory findings in infectious mononucleosis. Time relationships between clinical features, hematological changes, and antibody levels (EB virus and heterophil) in *(A)* a typical case of infectious mononucleosis, *(B)* a patient who had a delayed antibody response (*J. C. Niederman, R. W. McCollum,*

represent a practical method of preventing hepatitis B. The routine administration of immune globulin is not recommended for patients receiving transfusions because its efficacy has not been demonstrated.

Immunization with virus B preparations heated at 98°C for 1 min. appears to be effective in protecting susceptible children against experimental infection. With greater refinement and quantitation utilizing recently developed cell and organ culture methods and serological procedures, perhaps further progress can be anticipated in the development of protective vaccines.

INFECTIOUS MONONUCLEOSIS

Infectious mononucleosis is an acute, usually mild infectious disease of young adults characterized by fever, sore throat, cervical lymphadenopathy, splenomegaly, monocytosis with atypical lymphocytes, abnormal liver function tests, lymphoid and bone marrow hyperplasia, heterophil agglutinins for sheep erythrocytes, antibody against Epstein-Barr (EB) virus, and the appearance of bone marrow cells or peripheral leukocytes that develop into continuous lymphoblastoid cell cultures containing EB virus and EB viral antigens. In young children, subclinical infection is common, and overt disease is infrequent.

Accumulated data have firmly established an etiological relationship of EB virus to infectious mononucleosis. The evidence is based on the observations that (1) EB seronegative individuals become EB seropositive during the course of infectious mononucleosis as indicated by the appearance of immunofluorescent, complement-fixing, and neutralizing antibody; (2) bone marrow cells and peripheral leukocytes obtained from patients with infectious mononucleosis can be cultured as continuous lympho-

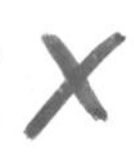

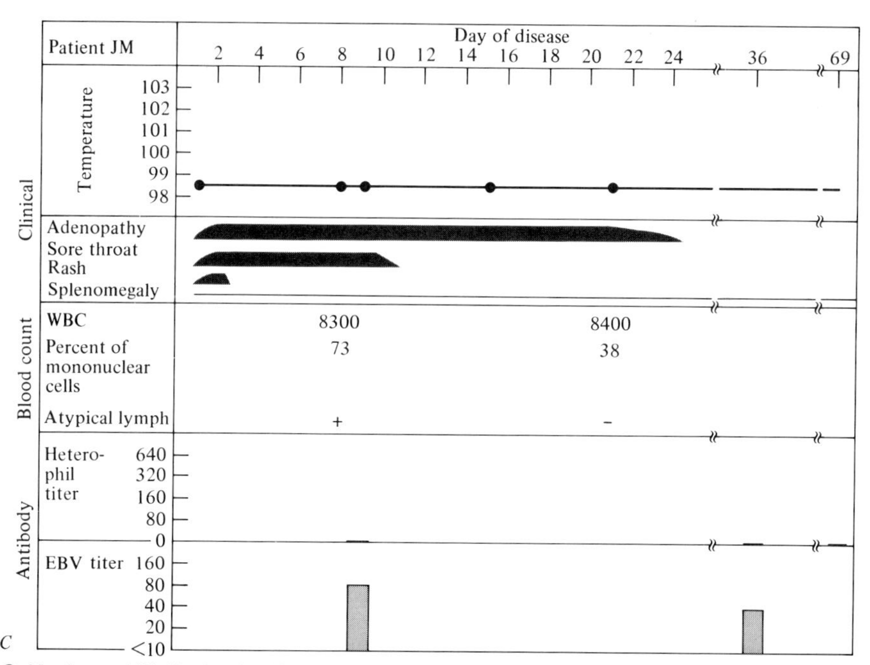

G. Henle, and W. Henle, J.A.M.A., 203:205–209, 1968, Copyright 1968, American Medical Association), (C) a patient with negative heterophil antibody who developed antibody against EB virus (A. S. Evans, J. C. Niederman, and R. W. McCollum, N. Engl. J. Med., 279:1121–1127, 1968).

blastoid cell lines which contain EB virus and EB viral antigens; (3) when EB virus is inadvertently transmitted by blood transfusions, infectious mononucleosis can result if the recipients are EB seronegative; and (4) EB seronegative gibbons injected with EB virus seroconverted and developed tonsillitis after an incubation period of 5 weeks.

The presumed pathogenesis of infectious mononucleosis probably involves transmission of EB virus by droplet infection from an infected patient shortly before or after onset of clinical manifestations or from a person experiencing a subclinical infection (one-third of young infected adults). During the course of an incubation period of 5 weeks, the virus presumably multiplies in the oropharyngeal mucous membrane, passes by way of the lymphatics into the blood, and is widely disseminated throughout the lymphoreticular system. The virus probably replicates in the lymph nodes, spleen, liver, and bone marrow; overflows into the blood; and may cause a rubella-like rash due either to the virus or immune complexes in about 10 percent of patients. Virus may be present in the oropharyngeal secretions as a consequence of replication in both mucosal epithelial cells and lymphocytes, the latter leading to an exudative tonsillitis. Icterus may occur in about 5 percent of patients, but liver function tests are invariably abnormal. Most patients recover uneventfully after an illness of 2 to 3 weeks. Occasionally, however, convalescence may require several months, and rarely, major complications or death may occur following splenic rupture or respiratory paralysis.

The important clinical, hematological, and serological findings are illustrated in Figure 25-4 and vary from patient to patient. There is both a relative and absolute increase in the number of lymphocytes and monocytes, including the presence of atypical lymphocytes which have a basophilic vacuolated or foamy cytoplasm, are actively synthesizing DNA, and show mitotic activity. Heterophil sheep erythrocyte agglutinins develop in about 80 percent of patients, reach a peak about the third week, and disappear in 3 to 6 months. The sheep cell agglutinins remain after absorption of the patient's serum with guinea pig kidney but are removed by bovine erythrocytes and thus can be distinguished from those present in serum sickness or in normal serum. Specific EB antibodies usually appear early in the course of the disease, are known to persist for 13 years or more, and are commonly detected by indirect immunofluorescence or by complement fixation. As noted from the data included in Figure 25-4, the most consistent findings are adenopathy, monocytosis with atypical lymphocytes, and the development of EB antibodies.

Much remains to be learned concerning the epidemiology of infectious mononucleosis, the relationship of EB virus to Burkitt's lymphoma and nasopharyngeal carcinoma (Chap. 2), and the explanation for the high incidence of EB antibody in patients with sarcoidosis, systemic lupus erythematosus, and lepromatous leprosy. However, certain basic epidemiological data are available. Infectious mononucleosis is worldwide in distribution, but infection occurs earlier and is more commonly subclinical in some countries (Philippines, Colombia) than in others (United States, Canada, European countries). In the United States, children usually acquire a mild or subclinical infection, whereas the major-

Table 25-1 Rates of Hospital Admissions of University Students with Infectious Mononucleosis

University	Year	Rate per 100,000
Princeton	1965–1966	1,449
Yale	1965–1966	921
Harvard	1965–1966	608
Wisconsin	1955–1959	450
Nebraska	1965–1966	316

Source: A. S. Evans, J. C. Niederman, and R. W. McCollum, "Seroepidemiologic Studies of Infectious Mononucleosis with EB Virus," *N. Engl. J. Med.*, 279:1121–1127, 1968.

ity of young adults who are infected develop clinical manifestations. Recovery from infection or disease is accompanied by solid immunity and persisting neutralizing antibodies against EB virus. In this country, highest attack rates occur in young adults between 15 and 24 years of age. The disease is especially prevalent among students living in university groups and is associated with high hospital admission rates (Table 25-1). Currently, there are no methods available for prevention and control of the disease.

YELLOW FEVER

Perspective

Even though yellow fever appeared later and disappeared more rapidly than other great historical pestilences (malaria, plague, leprosy, epidemic typhus), it had a dramatic impact on human history for more than 250 years, commencing in the middle of the seventeenth century and coinciding with the movement of slaves from the west coast of Africa to the West Indies. From the Caribbean the disease spread widely and terrorized the highly susceptible urban populations of South, Central, and North America, including the cities of New York and Philadelphia. Along with malaria, yellow fever proved to be a major obstacle in the construction of the Panama Canal. Throughout this period yellow fever took its toll on everyone exposed except the slaves who were subsequently shown to have experienced mild or subclinical immunizing infections during childhood in Africa.

Based on a remarkably comprehensive knowledge of the disease developed within a span of less than 40 years between 1900 and 1937, prevention and control of yellow fever became a reality, thus representing one of the outstanding achievements in the history of medicine. Acting on the conviction of Finlay, who held since 1881 that yellow fever was a mosquito-borne disease, the U. S. Army Commission (Agramonte, Carroll, Lazear, Reed), supplemented by the vector control efforts of Gorgas, began their studies in Havana in 1900 after the conclusion of the Spanish-American War. Within a few years the commission proved largely on the basis of studies in volunteers that:

1. Yellow fever was transmitted by *Aëdes aegypti* mosquitoes.
2. The mosquito became infected only when it took a blood meal from the patient in the first 3 or 4 days of the disease.
3. The mosquito could not transmit the disease to man until about 2 weeks after feeding on a yellow fever patient. 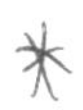
4. The disease could be eliminated from urban areas by controlling the domestic *Aëdes aegypti* mosquitoes.

The last epidemic of yellow fever in the United States occurred in New Orleans in 1905. In the same year Gorgas was sent to the Panama Canal Zone to supervise the successful application of mosquito control measures, and the strategic canal was built shortly thereafter.

Within 10 years after yellow fever was shown to be caused by a virus in 1929, the balance of the data essential for the prevention and control of the disease was accumulated.

1. Monkeys and mice were found to be susceptible to the virus.
2. Serial passage of the virus in mouse brain caused the virus to lose its ability to produce fatal disease in monkeys and in man.
3. Subsequent serial passage of the virus in chick embryo tissue cultures further attenuated the virus and led to the development of the 17 D vaccine, which is used for human immunization.
4. Antibody surveys indicated that in the two major endemic areas (Central Africa and Central America and the Amazon basin) many persons had antibodies without a history of yellow fever.
5. There was a large reservoir of jungle yellow fever in the rain forests of Africa and the jungles of Brazil in nonhuman primates transmitted by *Haemagogus* species of mosquitoes which could initiate epidemics of urban yellow fever (man-*Aëdes aegypti*-man cycle).

Thus, it was amply documented and has since been repeatedly verified that prevention and control of yellow fever require both the eradication of *Aëdes aegypti* mosquitoes and immunization with 17 D vaccine.

Introduction

Yellow fever is an acute, mosquito-transmitted viral disease of man, varying in severity from a mild form to a fatal fulminating hemorrhagic fever. In typically severe cases, the disease develops suddenly and is characterized by a saddleback temperature curve, headache, backache, nausea, vomiting which becomes black (contains altered blood), a slow pulse in relation to the temperature (Faget's sign), progressive neutropenia, intense albuminuria, variable jaundice, low blood pressure, hemorrhages from the gums, stomach, and intestine, coma, and death in 6 or 7 days or rapid and complete recovery commencing on the eighth day. Native populations in endemic areas frequently experience subclinical infection or mild disease.

The Causative Agent

On the basis of cross-reacting hemagglutinin-inhibiting and complement-fixing antibodies (Chap. 24), the causative agent of yellow fever is a member of the group B arboviruses which include dengue (Chap. 22) and St. Louis encephalitis, Japanese B encephalitis, and Murray Valley encephalitis (Chap. 24). As noted above, the virus multiplies in monkeys, mice, chick embryo tissue cultures, and *Aëdes* and *Haemogogus* mosquitoes. The virus is spherical in shape; about 30 nm in diameter; contains RNA, protein, and an envelope with essential lipid; possesses hemagglutinating activity; and is inactivated at pH 3.0.

There is a vast reservoir of yellow fever in the rain forests of Central Africa and the jungles of the Amazon basin in monkeys, *Haemogogus* mosquitoes, and probably also in marsupials. From these areas the virus can spread to villages, towns, and urban areas if the population is unvaccinated and if the density of *Aëdes aegypti* is adequate. In Africa, *Aëdes simpsoni* as well as *Aëdes aegypti* can transmit the disease to man.

Pathogenesis

When an appropriate mosquito takes a blood meal from an infected patient or subhuman primate, the virus replicates in the mosquito over a period of 2 weeks until it reaches the critical concentration required to infect man (extrinsic incubation period). Thereafter, for as long as the mosquito survives, the infection can be transmitted to man when the mosquito takes a blood meal. The virus is injected into the blood by the mosquito and localizes in the lymphoreticular tissues (liver, spleen, bone marrow, lymph nodes) and the kidney. During the course of an incubation period of 4 days the virus replicates extensively in these tissues. As a consequence of the degenerative changes and midzonal necrosis in hepatic lobules and renal tubular damage, clinical manifestations appear, and virus is found in the blood. With the appearance of antibody on the fifth day of the disease, virus disappears from the blood. If the patient fails to survive, death usually occurs in 5 or 6 days. If the patient survives, recovery is rapid and complete, commencing on the eighth day.

Laboratory Diagnosis

A laboratory diagnosis can be established by recovery and identification of the virus or by demonstrating a rise in antibody with paired acute and convalescent phase sera. Because of the probable presence of antibody in blood during the acute phase of the disease, attempts to isolate the virus are improved when the serum is diluted 10 or 100 times prior to inoculating mice intracerebrally. If yellow fever virus is present, the mice will develop encephalitis. Definitive identification of the virus can be made by performing a neutralization test.

Because of the prevalence of other cross-reacting group B arboviruses in yellow fever endemic areas, the use of HA-inhibition and CF tests are of limited value in establishing a diagnosis by these serological procedures. Consequently, it is necessary to perform neutralization tests in mice by mixing varying dilutions of the virus with undiluted acute and convalescent phase sera.

Epidemiology

Despite the extensive reservoir of jungle yellow fever, epidemics of yellow fever in man are rare, thus providing ample testimony to the efficacy of mosquito control measures and immunization. Most recent epidemics have occurred among unvaccinated populations in Ethiopia (100,000 cases in 1961 and 1962), Senegal (2,000 cases in 1965 and 1966), and in West Africa from Mali to Nigeria in 1968 and 1969. The mortality rate varies considerably from epidemic to epidemic and is difficult to determine because of the number of mild and subclinical cases but is generally assumed to be about 5 percent. Why yellow fever has never appeared in Asia is not known, but it is interesting to note that dengue is present in Asia and absent in yellow fever endemic areas and that the two viruses cross-react with each other and exhibit reciprocal interference.

Prevention and Control

The cornerstones of prevention of yellow fever are immunization with the 17 D attenuated vaccine prepared in chick embryos and eradication of the domesticated *Aëdes aegypti* mosquito. Yellow fever is an internationally regulated disease. Travelers to and from endemic areas must be vaccinated at least 10 days before arrival or departure. In addition, most countries require mosquito control of airplanes arriving from endemic areas. Since smallpox is endemic in the same areas as yellow fever, it is common practice to vaccinate simultaneously against both diseases. The results have been highly satisfactory, but on theoretical grounds the U.S.P.H.S. recommends that vaccination against the two diseases be separated by an interval of 1 month. Recent definitive studies, however, have failed to establish a basis for this recommendation when the vaccines were given at intervals of 3, 7, 14, and 28 days.

Prospective

Although the prospects for the elimination of jungle yellow fever are virtually nil, and consequently, spread of disease to man remains a constant threat, there is no reason for apprehension as long as immunization is practiced in endemic areas and vigorous antimosquito measures are employed against *Aëdes aegypti*. The world can and should remain free of human cases of yellow fever.

MUMPS

Mumps is an acute systemic viral disease primarily of children characterized by painful enlargement of the parotid gland, in many cases by involvement of the CNS (meningitis, meningoencephalitis), and occasionally by pancreatitis, labyrinthitis, and arthritis. When mumps develops in the 10 percent of postpubertal individuals who escaped infection during childhood, the disease tends to be more severe and may involve the testes, epididymis, ovaries, heart, kidney, and other tissues. While parotitis is the most constant feature, it is important to recognize that the other clinical manifestations of mumps may develop before, during, after, or in the absence of sialitis.

Despite the potential of mumps virus for widespread involvement of human tissue, most patients recover promptly without sequelae. In fact, about one-third of those infected experience a subclinical infection. Recovery is followed by a strong and persistent immunity to reinfection. The few fatalities that have been recorded are associated with meningoencephalitis, postinfectious encephalitis (Chap. 24), myocarditis, and nephritis.

The Causative Agent

The causative agent is a myxovirus that contains RNA; has helical symmetry, an internal ribonucleoprotein (S antigen) and viral (V) antigen(s) incorporated in an envelope; and is associated with hemagglutinating, hemolytic, and neuraminidase activity. Natural infection is limited to man. Experimentally, the virus can infect monkeys and can be isolated following amniotic inoculation of chick embryos or of monkey or human cell cultures. Because the virus possesses hemagglutinating activity and is released from the surface of the plasma membrane, hemadsorption and hemadsorption-inhibition can be used to detect and identify the virus in cell cultures. There is a single antigenic type of the virus which cross-reacts with parainfluenza and Newcastle disease viruses, but cross-protection between the viruses cannot be demonstrated.

Pathogenesis

Mumps is spread from person to person by droplet infection from patients with the disease or from individuals with subclinical infection. The preponderance of evidence indicates that during the course of an incubation period of 2 to 3½ weeks the virus multiplies throughout the body and can be recovered from the saliva, CSF, urine, blood, and infected tissues. Following penetration of the mucosal epithelium of the upper respiratory tract, the virus replicates and enters the blood by way of the draining lymphatics. Presumably, after replication in the liver and spleen, the virus is disseminated to glandular tissues, CNS, kidney, heart, and other organs. Multiplication of virus in the salivary glands leads to the presence of virus in the oropharyngeal secretions several days before onset to about a week after onset of overt disease. Obstruction of Wharton's and Stensen's ducts as a consequence of edema and debris causes swelling and pain in the parotid glands which is usually bilateral. Lymphocytic pleocytosis in the CSF occurs in more than 50 percent of the patients, but viral meningitis and meningoencephalitis develop only in about 10 percent of patients. Whether the disease involves parotitis, meningoencephalitis, or both, uneventful recovery occurs in 3 to 10 days in more than 99.9 percent of those infected.

Clinical evidence of epididymitis, orchitis, and oophoritis is usually limited to postpubertal individuals. Although the testes may be tender, swollen, and painful and may show atrophy, sterility following mumps has rarely been documented. Similarly, there is no evidence that ovaritis due to mumps virus leads to impaired fertility.

The principal sequel of mumps is deafness which occurs rarely (1 in 15,000 cases) but nonetheless has been a leading cause of hearing loss in children. The mechanism responsible for its development is not known but may be associated with endolymphatic labyrinthitis or acoustic neuritis. Fortunately, this problem should disappear with the use of attenuated mumps vaccine.

Laboratory Diagnosis

Typical mumps with parotitis generally provides an accurate diagnosis, but when mumps occurs in the absence of parotitis, virological or serological criteria must be used to establish the diagnosis. Fortunately, mumps is one of the few viral diseases for which a serological diagnosis can often be made during the acute phase. Simultaneous CF tests performed with S and V antigens early in the disease often reveal S but not V antibodies. Confirmation of these findings is invariably made when serum is obtained and tested 2 to 3 weeks later and a rise in antibody titer demonstrated. Attempts to recover the virus usually involve the use of human or monkey cell cultures because the disease in question might or might not be mumps. Definitive identification of the virus is generally based on CF tests using the V antigen.

Epidemiology

Mumps is worldwide in distribution, is endemically present in most populous areas, shows an increased incidence in winter and spring, and reaches epidemic peaks every 2 to 4 years. About 90 percent of children under 15 years of age have antibody against mumps virus, two-thirds as a result of disease, and one-third following subclinical infection. Prior to 1968 mumps was not a reportable disease in the United States, but in the last 5 years the annual number of cases has varied between approximately 90,000 and 150,000 with less than 50 deaths per year.

Prevention and Control

An attenuated mumps vaccine available since 1968 has proved highly effective in the prevention of mumps in susceptible individuals but has not been widely used. However, in view of the demonstrated efficacy of measles-mumps-rubella combined vaccine when given simultaneously with the third dose of trivalent oral poliomyelitis vaccine early in the second year of life, it is probable that this regimen will become adopted as standard procedure in the future. In the latter event, a sharp drop in the incidence of mumps should occur. Although hyperimmune human antiserum (5 to 10 ml) has been used in susceptible adult males who have been exposed to mumps, evidence that it is protective is not conclusive. General use of mumps vaccine should obviate the need for passive immunoprophylaxis.

PHLEBOTOMUS FEVER

Phlebotomus, or sandfly, fever is an acute but mild disease characterized by an abrupt onset with fever, headache, malaise, and myalgia and, in some patients, by vomiting, conjunctival injection, photophobia, stiffness of the neck and back, giddiness, and arthralgia. Clinically, many patients are diagnosed as having viral meningitis. In most patients, the fever persists for 3 days, and recovery occurs gradually, often accompanied by weakness and giddiness. The causative agent is one of two antigenic types of an arbovirus which is transmitted by the female sandfly, *Phlebotomus papatasii*. The disease is localized to the countries bordering the Mediterranean Sea and to Russia, Iran, Pakistan, and India, endemic areas that correspond to the geographical distribution of the vector between 20 and 45° latitude.

The sandfly is a nocturnal feeder, takes a blood meal, and after an extrinsic incubation period of about a week, can transmit the infection to susceptible individuals. Clinical manifestations develop 3 to 6 days following injection of the virus by the sandfly. Presumably, the virus replicates in the liver and spleen and is present in the blood for a day before onset to 2 days after onset. Primary isolation of the virus is rarely attempted because a prolonged period of adaptation and serial passage is required before the virus produces characteristic pathology or viral antigens. However, a serological diagnosis can be made by demonstrating a rise in CF, HA-inhibiting, or neutralizing antibody using mouse-adapted virus as the antigen.

The prevalence of the disease is greatest when the vector is most abundant in the summer or autumn months. It is suspected that the virus persists over the winter as a result of transovarial transmission. In endemic areas, infection and immunity commonly occur during childhood. Large outbreaks develop when large numbers of susceptible individuals enter the endemic area, as happened during World War II. Prevention of disease in endemic areas is based on the use of residual insecticides in and around living quarters and the application of insect repellents at night. The vector is domesticated, has a short flight range, moves slowly from place to place, and consequently, is easily destroyed by residual insecticides such as DDT sprayed around doors, windows, and walls. Other diseases that are transmitted by sandflies include leishmaniasis and bartonellosis.

CYTOMEGALOVIRUS DISEASE

Human infections with cytomegalovirus, a member of the herpesvirus group, are associated with:

1 One of a number of clinical syndromes often accompanied by chronic and/or latent persistence of the virus and the formation of antibody
2 Latent persistence of the virus and the formation of antibody in the absence of clinical manifestations

The syndromes caused by cytomegalovirus include disseminated disease in infants infected congenitally or in immunosuppressed patients, mononucleosis, and hepatitis.

In utero infection usually occurs as a consequence of primary maternal infection (perhaps associated with a chronic cough and influenza-like illness). Fetal infection may lead to death in utero or, in surviving infants, to devastating rubella-like cerebral, ocular, and auricular abnormalities, hepatosplenomegaly, petechial rashes, thrombocytopenic purpura, low birth weight, pancreatic, pulmonary, and renal inflammation, and mental retardation. Congenitally infected infants may succumb after birth or may survive for many years. Recent studies have established two major additional findings: (1) urinary excretion of cytomegalovirus occurs in 1 to 2 percent of apparently healthy infants, and (2) a proportion of these infants (15 to 20 percent) subsequently develop evidence of CNS damage, including mental retardation. Thus, an apparently mild congenital cytomegalovirus infection may account for a significant component of previously unexplained mental retardation and motor disability.

In patients with lymphoreticular and hematopoietic malignancy, chronic debilitating diseases, or immunodeficiency or in those receiving prolonged therapy with corticosteroids or immunosuppressive agents, cytomegalovirus may induce a spectrum of manifestations varying from pneumonitis to disseminated disease involving the lungs, salivary glands, liver, spleen, kidney, CNS, gastrointestinal tract, pancreas, thyroid, and adrenal glands.

Cytomegalovirus can induce a mononucleosis-like syndrome with fever, numerous atypical lymphocytes, splenomegaly, and abnormal liver function tests that persists for 3 to 6 weeks, but without lymphadenopathy, sore throat, heterophil sheep red blood cell agglutinins, or a rising titer of antibodies to EB virus. The syndrome may develop as a result of natural infection, may occur in 3 to 5 percent of patients undergoing cardiopulmonary bypass perfusion in cardiac surgery, or may follow multiple blood transfusions.

In children, cytomegalovirus frequently causes a mild or subclinical hepatitis. For example, in 20 apparently healthy children excreting the virus in the urine, 17 had abnormal hepatic function tests, 14 had hepatomegaly, and 5 had splenomegaly. In 23 children with unexplained hepatomegaly, 9 were found to be infected with cytomegalovirus.

While the natural history of cytomegalovirus infection remains to be determined, it obviously shares many features with other human herpesviruses (herpes simplex, varicella-zoster, EB virus). Outstanding perhaps is the propensity of these viruses for inducing latent infection or a chronic carrier state in the presence of neutralizing antibody following a primary clinical or subclinical infection. Prior to formulating a theory concerning the natural history of cytomegalovirus infection, it is essential to itemize some of the pertinent basic observations:

1 Early infection is common, as indicated by
 a The detection of the typical cytomegalic (enlarged) cells, 25 to 40 μm in diameter, with intranuclear inclusions (10μm) in 10 to 30 percent of the salivary glands of infants dying from all causes
 b Viruria in 1 to 2 percent of apparently healthy infants, in 35 to 40 percent of institutionalized preschool children, and in 5 to 10 percent of children between 2 and 8 years of age
 c The frequent isolation of virus from the adenoids and gastric washings of healthy children
 d The finding of antibody in as many as 90 percent of selected population groups under 2 years of age (Fig. 25-5)
2 In congenitally infected infants, viruria may persist for 4 to 5 years or more in the presence of antibody.
3 In infected infants, viruria may persist for 2 years or more in the presence of antibody.
4 In young children with antibody, virus can be isolated from saliva and urine for many months.
5 Clinical cases cluster in institutions, families, schools, and hospitals, especially in the presence of congenitally infected infants (symptomatic or asymptomatic).
6 As many as 50 to 60 percent of patients receiving multiple blood transfusions develop serological and/or virological evidence of infection and up to 5 percent show a mononucleosis-like syndrome.
7 Virus has been recovered from the blood of 2 of 35 healthy donors (5.7 percent).
8 Up to 3 percent of pregnant women have viruria, virus can be recovered from the cervix in the last trimester, and rising antibody titers are observed possibly in association with an influenza-like illness with chronic cough.

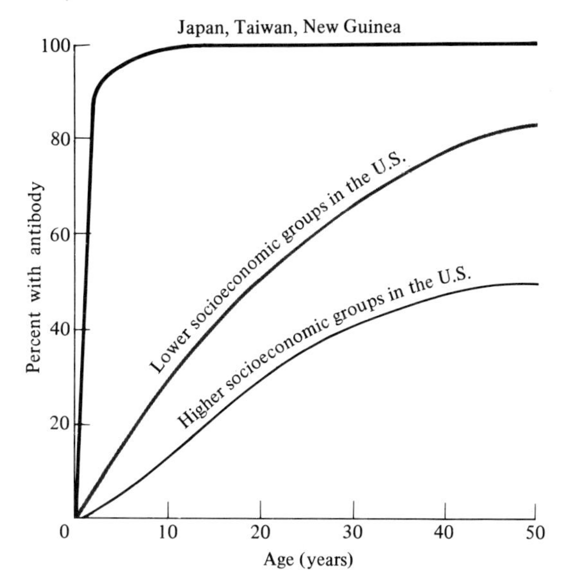

Figure 25-5 Postnatal cytomegalovirus infections as indicated by the formation of antibody.

9 In immunosuppressed and immunodeficient patients, pneumonitis is a common clinical finding, and disseminated disease occasionally ensues. Among renal transplant recipients, 90 percent show evidence of cytomegalovirus infection during life or at autopsy.
10 Virus can be isolated from ill and healthy patients from the saliva, urine, blood, adenoids, gastric washings, cervix, semen, milk, and nasopharyngeal secretions and in disseminated disease from almost every tissue in the body.

The data itemized above suggest that cytomegalovirus is ubiquitously present in the human population and that asymptomatic infants and young children form the main cohort of infection. Ordinarily, the virus is transmitted by close contact with the infected salivary, oral, and nasopharyngeal secretions of an infected infant or child as in primary herpes simplex (Chap. 22). As a matter of fact, the situation depicted in Figure 25-5 could be substituted for herpes simplex. As with herpes simplex, following primary infection which is usually subclinical, cytomegalovirus probably persists indefinitely in a latent form in the presence of neutralizing antibody and may be activated later in life when the function of the immune system is impaired. Individuals who escape infection early in life occasionally may develop the mononucleosis-like syndrome, hepatitis, or respiratory illness upon primary contact with the virus later in life, but generally they experience only a subclinical infection. However, when primary infection occurs during pregnancy, the consequences for the fetus can be devastating.

Isolation and identification of cytomegalovirus can be accomplished by inoculation of cell cultures of human fibroblasts, the demonstration of intranuclear inclusion bodies, and reactivity with CF, neutralizing, or indirect fluorescent antibodies. However, serial passage of the virus is required; and consequently, a laboratory diagnosis is usually established serologically utilizing the CF test. Different isolates of cytomegalovirus share common CF and neutralizing antigens but exhibit incomplete reciprocal cross-neutralization.

Apart from isolation of congenitally infected infants who continuously excrete high concentrations of virus, there are no practical methods for prevention and control of the disease. Accumulated data indicate that there is an increasing and desperate need to develop an effective vaccine that could be used to prevent infections in pregnant women and thereby eliminate congenital infections. In many respects, since more pregnant women are susceptible and more likely to be infected, cytomegalovirus presents a greater threat to the fetus and to infants who survive congenital infection than does rubella virus.

Protozoal Infections

MALARIA

Perspective

Among infectious diseases malaria is without question the greatest scourge that has affected man throughout recorded history. The clinical manifestations are mentioned in the earliest Chinese and Indian medical writings. In the fifth century B.C. Hippocrates differentiated the disease into fever occurring daily (falciparum), on alternate days (vivax), and on every fourth day (malariae) and recognized the association of malaria (bad air) with stagnant, swampy, and marshy areas. The rise and fall of malaria is indelibly woven into the fabric of history, the expansion and contraction of empires, the geopolitical struggles of nations, and the growth and development of many peoples.

It was not until 1898, however, that Bignami, Grassi, and Bastianelli demonstrated that malaria was transmitted from man to man by anopheline mosquitoes. With minimal delay the application of mosquito control methods permitted the construction of the Panama Canal, the reclamation of malarious lands, and the elimination of the disease from many endemic areas. Nonetheless, even in the middle of the twentieth century it was estimated that the annual worldwide morbidity and mortality due to malaria were 300 million and 3 million, respectively.

In 1955 the World Health Organization launched a worldwide malaria eradication program, and by 1960 the disease had been eliminated from 18 countries. The success of the program was accompanied by a sharp reduction in infant and general mortality, a rise in birth rates, and a serious overpopulation problem. Thus, even with its demise, malaria is exerting a strong influence on human history.

Introduction

Malaria is an acute and chronic protozoal disease transmitted from man to man by anopheline mosquitoes and characterized by (1) periodic paroxysmal attacks of chill, fever, and sweating accompanied by headache, myalgia, nausea, and vomiting; (2) splenomegaly; (3) anemia; and (4) a chronic relapsing course. The clinical manifestations primarily reflect the replication of the parasite in the red blood cells, leading to their destruction. In endemic areas, patients with chronic malaria and malnutrition often experience secondary bacterial infections (dysentery, cholera, pneumonia, tuberculosis) which terminate fatally. Under epidemic conditions the case fatality rate may vary between 5 and 25 percent and is usually high in infants and low in adults in endemic areas.

The Causative Agents

Human malaria is caused by one of five sporozoa of the genus *Plasmodium,* with *P. vivax* and *P. falciparum* accounting for 95 percent of infections and *P. malariae, P. ovale,* and *P. knowlesi* accounting for the balance. Sporozoa are unique among the protozoa in that both sexual and asexual life cycles occur. In the case of plasmodia infecting man, the sexual cycle develops in anopheline mosquitoes (the definitive host), and the asexual cycle is found in man (the intermediate host) with the exceptions of *P. malariae,* which can also occur in chimpanzees, and *P. knowlesi,* which is primarily a simian parasite occasionally transmitted to man. Since *P. ovale* induces mild infections rarely encountered except in West Africa and is generally similar to *P. vivax* and since *P. knowlesi* rarely produces disease in man, the ensuing discussion will be limited to *P. vivax, P. falciparum,* and *P. malariae.*

Schizogony Preparatory to taking a blood meal an infected female anopheline mosquito injects the plasmodial parasite in the form of sporozoites along with saliva into the blood vessels of man. Within a few minutes the sporozoites penetrate hepatic parenchymal cells, grow, and undergo several life cycles (asexual) of schizogony, culminating in the release of thousands of merozoites over a period of several days (exoerythrocytic phase). Some of the merozoites persist in the liver (except for *P. falciparum*) and serve as a reservoir which can initiate relapses over a period of years. The merozoites escaping from the ruptured hepatic cells enter the circulation, penetrate red blood cells, transform into trophozoites, and mature into schizonts, each of which produces 6 to 24 merozoites, depending on the species of plasmodia (erythrocytic phase). The fully developed merozoites rupture the red blood cells, are released, and initiate schizogony in uninfected red blood cells. After a variable number of cycles of erythrocytic schizogony, gametocytes appear in the blood, and the parasites (except for *P. falciparum*) replicate in synchrony, giving rise to the periodic paroxysmal attacks of chills, fever, and sweating coincident with the destruction of red blood cells and the release of merozoites.

Sporogony In taking a blood meal from a patient with malaria, the female anopheline mosquito ingests male and female gametocytes. Within the midgut of the mosquito a few flagellated male cells develop and penetrate the female gamete, resulting in a zygote which becomes a motile ookinete that migrates through the gut wall and encysts (oocyst). The oocyst grows and produces a number of sporozoites which are released into the body cavity and migrate into the salivary glands and thence into the saliva. Sporogony (sexual life cycle) varies widely in duration (8 to 35 days), depending upon the plasmodial parasite, the ambient temperature, and the number of gametocytes taken up by the mosquito. The interaction of the asexual and sexual cycles is depicted in the chart on the following page.

Pathogenesis

Many of the features of pathogenesis consequent to the injection of malarial sporozoites by anopheline mosquitoes are included in Table 25-2. A number of interrelated factors influence the course of the disease, including the types of red blood cells that are invaded, the extent of parasitemia, the time required for a cycle of schizogony in the red blood cells, the number of merozoites released during schizogony, the extent of intravascular hemolysis, and the sticky

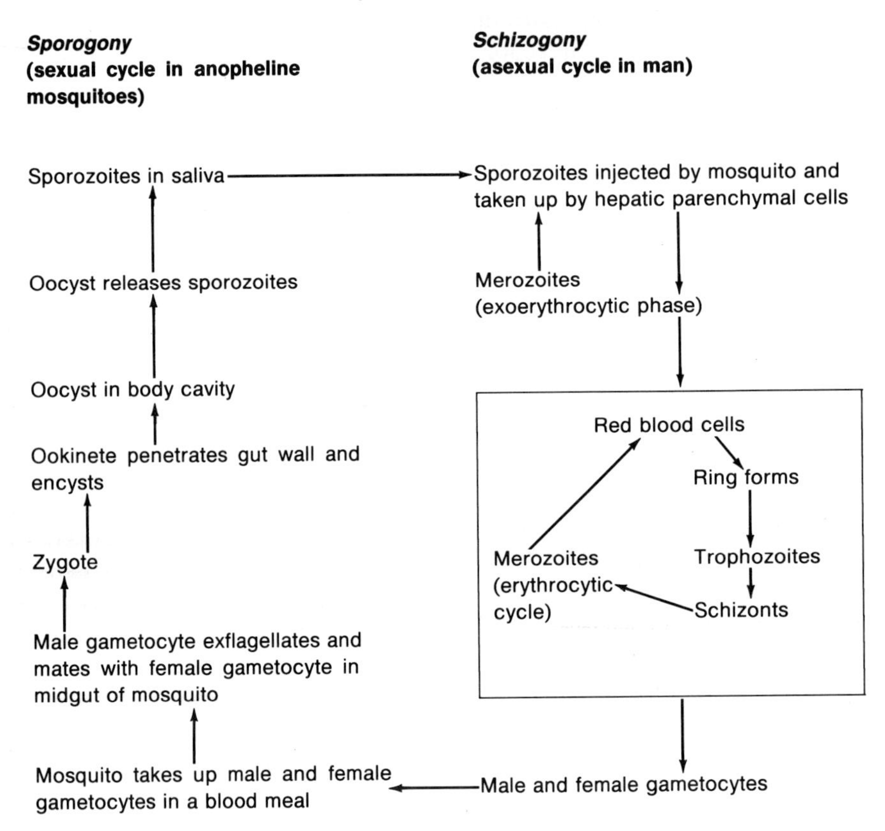

property of red blood cells parasitized by *P. falciparum.*

On the basis of the data included in Table 25-2 plus the sticky property of red blood cells parasitized by *P. falciparum,* the occurrence of schizogony in the visceral circulation, the ability of parasitized cells to localize in any organ (brain, kidney, liver, lungs) and to adhere to each other and to capillary walls, and their predilection for inducing blackwater fever (hemolytic anemia, hemoglobinuria, tubular damage, acute renal failure), it is not surprising that *P. falciparum* infections are more severe than the other forms of malaria and that such infections may terminate fatally. In contrast with *P. vivax* and *P. malariae* infections, however, falciparum malaria is of shorter duration and is not subject to relapse because the hepatic tissue phase is absent.

Laboratory Diagnosis

The laboratory diagnosis of malaria is established by microscopic examination of a Wright- or Giemsa-stained blood smear. The thin film is the same as that in differential blood counting procedures. When parasitemia is low, thick films can often detect the parasite. In this procedure the red blood cells are lysed prior to staining. Identification of the species of plasmodia is based on the findings included in Table 25-2. In falciparum malaria, the demonstration of crescent-shaped gametocytes, multiple ring forms, and the absence of trophozoites and schizonts

Table 25-2 Characteristics of Asexual Malarial (*Plasmodium*) Parasites

Characteristic	*P. vivax*	*P. malariae*	*P. falciparum*
Fever	On alternate days	Every fourth day	Daily
Incubation period	14 to 16 days (up to 12 months)	18 to 42 days (up to years)	9 to 12 days
Time required for red blood cell schizogony cycle	45 to 48 hr.	72 hr.	24 to 48 hr.
Persistence in liver	Present	Present	Absent
Parasitemia per cu mm	20,000	6,000	100,000 to 500,000
Forms seen in blood	All	All	Ring forms and gametocytes
Ring forms	Single	Single	Single or multiple
Trophozoites	Present	Present	Absent
Schizonts	12 to 24 merozoites	6 to 12 merozoites in rosette form	Not seen in peripheral blood (occurs in visceral circulation)
Gametocytes	Large and oval, appear during fever	Large and oval, appear weeks after onset of fever	Crescent-shaped, appear 7 to 10 days after onset of fever
Types of red blood cells infected	Reticulocytes (young red blood cells)	Mature red blood cells	All red blood cells
Size of infected red blood cells	Usually enlarged	Normal or decreased	Normal
Duration of untreated disease	2 to 5 years	1 to 20 years	6 to 18 months

permit the diagnosis. In vivax malaria, the presence of enlarged red blood cells containing Schüffner's dots, all forms of the parasite, and 12 to 24 merozoites in mature schizonts serves to distinguish vivax from malariae and falciparum malaria. Mixed infections are not uncommon in endemic areas. The detection of *Plasmodium falciparum* is important so that therapy can be initiated without delay.

Epidemiology

Although much has been accomplished by the World Health Organization in the control of malaria, an extensive reservoir of the disease persists in large areas of Southeast Asia, Central Africa, and Latin America. Disease is especially severe in infants and young children who are epidemiologically significant because their blood contains a large number of gametocytes. Malnutrition aggravates malaria, tends to occur in the same geographical areas, and leads to serious secondary bacterial infection.

One of the key aspects of malaria is related to the behavior, density, efficiency, distribution, and natural history of the anopheline vector. About 35 species of *Anopheles* can transmit malaria, most of which are rural and tropical in distribution. However, some species prefer human blood, breed in close proximity to human habitation, and consequently are efficient vectors. Perhaps *Anopheles gambiae* is most notorious in this respect, and although indigenous to tropical Africa, this species has proved to be effective in causing epidemics in Brazil after its introduction to that country. Other vectors that prefer human to animal blood include *A. darlingi* in Latin America and *A. culicifacies* in India.

In the United States the chief vectors have been *A. quadrimaculatus* and *A. freeborni*. Historically, the control of malaria in the United States is much more recent than generally realized (Fig. 25-6). Currently, the disease is associated primarily with returning Vietnam veterans (Fig. 25-6), but spread of the disease is usually limited to those injected with merozoites along with narcotics or those receiving blood transfusions. Nonetheless, epidemics have occurred in drug addicts in urban areas. For example, a 1970–1971 epidemic in California involving 48 individuals was traced to a Vietnam veteran who had not taken the prescribed chloroquine-primaquine therapeutic regimen, was addicted to heroin, and initiated a chain reaction among narcotic addicts through the use of contaminated syringes and needles.

Prevention and Control

Immunity Immunity in malaria appears to be cell-mediated and strain-specific and develops only after repeated attacks. For example an individual immune to the indigenous *Plasmodium falciparum* in India would be susceptible to the same species *(P. falciparum)* in Central Africa or Latin America or even in other parts of Southeast Asia.

Therapy The goals of therapy are to (1) prevent schizogony, (2) eliminate the liver phase, and (3) destroy the gametocytes and thereby prevent infection of anopheline mosquitoes. The drugs of choice are chloroquine for schizonts and primaquine for the hepatic phase and the destruction of gametocytes. Chloroquine is a fast-acting schizonticide and should be used as early as possible for the treatment of *P. falciparum* in order to permit a speedy recovery and

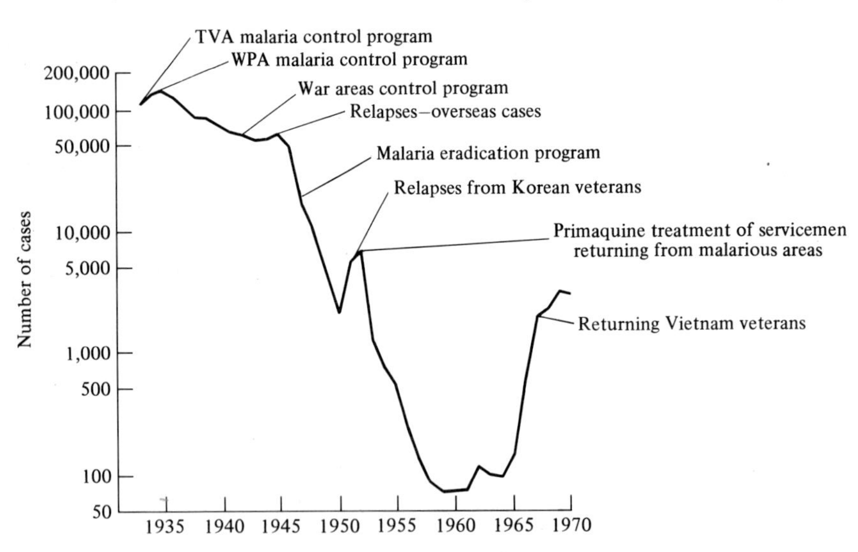

Figure 25-6 Cases of malaria reported in the United States from 1933 to 1971. [*Morbidity Mortality Weekly Report, 20(53):47, 1972.*]

to preclude the development of serious or fatal disease. In vivax and malariae infections primaquine is active against the hepatic stage of the parasite and against all gametocytes. When resistant strains develop, as in *P. falciparum*, alternative drugs are available and should be employed. These include quinine, dimethyldiphenyl sulfone, pyrimethamine, sulfonamides, and trimethoprim. In addition, clindamycin and tetracycline in combination with quinine have proved to be highly effective in therapy of chloroquine-resistant strains of *P. falciparum* encountered in Vietnam.

Control Malaria control programs are based on elimination of mosquitoes, destruction of gametocytes, and chemoprophylaxis. Mosquito control involves the eradication of adult mosquitoes and their breeding locations, residual spraying of dwellings with DDT or other appropriate insecticides, and the use of long-acting repellents such as diethyltoluamide. Destruction of gametocytes is best accomplished through the use of primaquine but should be supplemented with a fast-acting schizonticide such as chloroquine. Chemoprophylaxis with the combination of chloroquine and primaquine should be employed prior to entering and for 2 months after leaving endemic areas. In addition, persons with a history of malaria should be excluded as blood donors.

Prospective

The outstanding success achieved in the World Health Organization malaria eradication campaign must be tempered by the realization that the persisting endemic foci in Southeast Asia, Central Africa, and Latin America are likely to prove more difficult to eliminate than those already destroyed. Nonetheless, the application of available control measures should be able to eliminate the disease from any part of the world.

LEISHMANIASIS AND TRYPANOSOMIASIS

Perspective

Hemoflagellates pathogenic for man cover a broad spectrum of clinical manifestations, syndromes, and diseases, varying widely in severity from a self-limited cutaneous lesion through a destructive and extending mucocutaneous disease to fatal lymphoreticular or lymphoreticular-meningoencephalitic or myocardial disease (Table 25-3). Disease caused by hemoflagellates takes a heavy toll in large areas of Africa and Central and South America, and to a lesser extent in southwestern Asia, and has hampered the economic development of many countries. In many respects, hemoflagellates pathogenic for man induce socioeconomic diseases which could be brought under effective control by elimination or reduction of the arthropod vectors and the animal reservoir and by prompt and vigorous therapy.

The Causative Agents

Hemoflagellates are protozoa that reproduce asexually by binary fission, have 2 to 4 developmental forms in their life cycle (Fig. 25-7), at least one being present in the arthropod vector and at least one is found in man, and are geographically restricted to the distribution of their specific arthropod vectors. As noted in Figure 25-7 and in Table 25-3, the hemoflagellates are found in one of four developmental forms (leishmanial, leptomonad, crithidial, trypanosomal), which consist of a nucleus and kinetoplast plus a flagellum except for the leishmanial form and an undulating membrane in crithidial and trypanosomal forms. On culture at 20 to 25°C on agar containing 10 percent defibrinated rabbit blood, the flagellate leptomonad or crithidial forms develop.

Pathogenesis

Cutaneous leishmaniasis caused by *Leishmania tropica* and transmitted by *Phlebotomus* sand-

Table 25-3 Characteristics of Hemoflagellates Pathogenic for Man

Characteristics	*L. tropica*	*L. brasiliensis*	*L. donovani*	*T. rhodesiense*	*T. gambiense*	*T. cruzi*
Disease	Cutaneous leishmaniasis (oriental sore)	Mucocutaneous leishmaniasis (espundia)	Visceral leishmaniasis (kala azar)	African (Rhodesian) sleeping sickness	African (Gambian) sleeping sickness	American trypanosomiasis (Chagas' disease)
Endemic area	Mediterranean countries, southwestern Asia, central and northeastern Africa	Mexico, Central and South America	Mediterranean countries, southwestern Asia, central and northeastern Africa, Mexico, Central and South America	East Africa (Rhodesia, Zambia, Mozambique, Malawi, Tanzania)	Western and central Africa (Gambia, Liberia, Sierra Leone, Ghana, Congo, Sudan, Uganda)	Mexico, Central and South America
Vector	*Phlebotomus* (sandflies)	*Phlebotomus* (sandflies)	*Phlebotomus* (sandflies)	*Glossina* (tsetse flies) (male and female *Glossina*)	*Glossina* (tsetse flies) (male and female *Glossina*)	*Triatoma* (reduviid bugs)
Form ingested by vector	Leishmanial (intracellular)	Leishmanial (intracellular)	Leishmanial (intracellular)	Trypanosomal	Trypanosomal	Trypanosomal
Extrinsic incubation period	8 to 20 days	8 to 20 days	8 to 20 days	18 to 23 days	18 to 23 days	8 to 20 days
Infective form for man	Leptomonad (in saliva)	Leptomonad (in saliva)	Leptomonad (in saliva)	Trypanosomal (in saliva)	Trypanosomal (in saliva)	Trypanosomal (in feces)
Incubation period	2 to 6 months	2 to 4 weeks	Months to years	2 to 3 weeks	2 to 3 weeks	1 to 2 weeks
Tissue form	Intracellular leishmanial	Intracellular leishmanial	Intracellular leishmanial	Trypanosomal	Trypanosomal	Trypanosomal and intracellular leishmanial
Recovered from	Cutaneous lesion	Skin and mucous membranes, especially oronasal mucosa	Liver, spleen, bone marrow, blood, lymph nodes	Blood, lymph, CSF	Blood, lymph, CSF	Blood (myocardium)

Culture form	Leptomonad	Leptomonad	Leptomonad	Crithidial	Crithidial	Crithidial, trypanosomal
Important reservoir	Man, rodents (gerbils), dogs, forest rodents	Man, forest rodents	Man, dogs, and other canines	Man, antelope, bushbuck, pig	Man (animals ?)	Man, dogs, cats, other animals
Skin test (phenol-killed cultured leptomonas)	+	+	− until after recovery	Not used	Not used	Not used
Formol-gel test	−	−	+ (− after cure)	Not used	Not used	Not used
CF antibodies	−	−	+ (− after cure) (cross-react with trypanosomiasis)	+, but infrequently used	+, but infrequently used	+ (cross-react with leishmaniasis)
Treatment	Pentavalent antimony, sodium gluconate	Pentavalent antimony, sodium gluconate	Pentavalent antimony, sodium gluconate	Suramin sodium (blood) and melarsoprol (CNS)	Suramin sodium (blood) and melarsoprol (CNS)	Unsatisfactory
Alternate treatment	Pentamidine isethionate	Amphotericin B	Amphotericin B	Tryparsamide	Pentamidine isethionate	
Prevention and control	Protective covering for ulcers, vector control (residual spraying at 6-month intervals), rodent control, immunization, mass treatment campaigns	Vector control, prompt treatment, mass treatment campaigns	Vector control, prompt treatment, adequate housing, elimination of diseased dogs	Vector control, treatment of those infected	Vector control, chemoprophylaxis with pentamidine isethionate, treatment of those infected	Vector and animal control, use of solid wall construction in dwellings
Prognosis	Self-limited	Direct extension, secondary infection common	Poor unless treated, cirrhosis, anemia, death from intercurrent infection	Generally fatal, if untreated	25 to 50 percent mortality in untreated cases	About 5 percent mortality in diagnosed cases

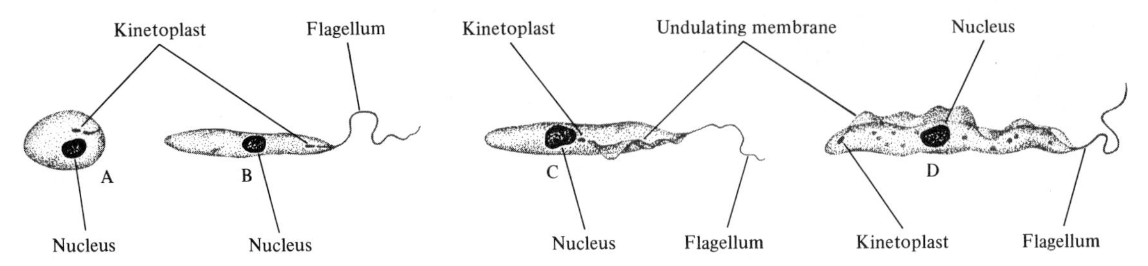

Figure 25-7 Developmental forms of hemoflagellates. *(A)* Intracellular leishmanial form in infected tissue (size about 3 × 1.5 μm). *(B)* Leptomonad form in vector and on culture (size about 15 × 3 μm). *(C) Crithidia* form in vector and on culture (size about 15 to 30 × 2 μm). *(D)* Trypanosomal form in vector and in infected tissue (size about 15 to 30 × 2 μm).

flies is a slowly developing, localized nodular ulcer (s) which heals spontaneously by scar formation in about a year.

Mucocutaneous leishmaniasis caused by *Leishmania brasiliensis* and transmitted by *Phlebotomus* sandflies appears initially as single or multiple papules that usually become nodular, occasionally ulcerate, and in a variable proportion of cases (2 to 20 percent) may spread by direct extension or along lymphatic channels. Generally, the primary lesion heals by scar formation over a period of months or even years but may subsequently reappear and lead to spreading destructive lesions of the oronasal mucosa and supporting cartilagenous tissue. Secondary bacterial infection of these lesions may prove lethal.

Visceral leishmaniasis is a lymphoreticular disease caused by *Leishmania donovani* and transmitted by *Phlebotomus* sandflies. The disease is characterized by fever, lymphadenopathy, hepatosplenomegaly, progressive anemia and leukopenia, hyperglobulinemia (IgG), and secondary bacterial infection which eventually proves fatal. Although acute cases occur, more commonly the disease pursues a chronic and relentless course over a period of years. The leishmania invade and replicate extensively in the phagocytic cells of the spleen, liver, bone marrow, lymph nodes, and the blood.

African sleeping sickness is a lymphoreticular disease which progresses to CNS involvement over a period of months or years. The disease is caused by either *Trypanosoma rhodesiense* or *T. gambiense* and is transmitted by *Glossina* (tsetse flies). Both parasites induce fatal illness with *T. rhodesiense* usually pursuing a more rapid course. Trypanosomes are found in blood, lymph nodes, and CSF. Lymphadenopathy is a prominent feature of the disease, and the presence of trypanosomes in the lymphatic channels causes swelling of the posterior cervical lymph nodes (Winterbottom's sign). CNS involvement usually occurs in 6 to 12 months. Endarteritis and perivascular cuffing are commonly observed, and plasma cells with large eosinophilic inclusions are frequently seen.

American trypanosomiasis is an acute or chronic disease caused by *T. cruzi* and transmitted by *Triatoma* (reduviid bugs). Although the majority of *T. cruzi* infections are mild or subclinical, acute disease in infants and young children is characterized by a lesion at the site of the bite (chagoma) which develops in a few hours and is followed by fever, lymphadenopathy, hepatomegaly, and signs of congestive heart failure. Most patients recover spontaneously (90 percent), but about 5 percent will develop significant myocarditis in the next 30 years. In these patients, a fatal outcome can be anticipated by the age of 45.

Laboratory Diagnosis

The combination of the clinical manifestations, geographical location, and demonstration and/or recovery of the hemoflagellate in blood, the tissue lesions, or on culture usually suffices to establish the diagnosis. It is important to note, however, that the species of *Leishmania* are morphologically indistinguishable from each other, as are the species of *Trypanosoma.* As indicated in Table 25-3, skin tests, the Formol-gel test, and the presence of CF antibodies are also useful. In addition, intraperitoneal inoculation of hamsters is of value in recovering the organism in visceral leishmaniasis and Rhodesian as opposed to Gambian trypanosomiasis; xenodiagnosis or demonstration of trypanosomes in the feces of laboratory-bred triatomid bugs fed on suspected patients is helpful in American trypanosomiasis, and FA tests are being employed more extensively.

Epidemiology, Prevention, and Control

The main epidemiological features of disease caused by hemoflagellates pathogenic for man are included in Table 25-3. Prevention and control are based largely on vector control or protection against vectors by the use of residual insecticides, arthropod repellents, clearing of vegetation, and chemoprophylaxis in Gambian trypanosomiasis; on the control of the animal reservoir whenever possible, as in picrotoxin destruction of gerbils (cutaneous leishmaniasis), and in solid wall construction of dwellings (American trypanosomiasis); and in the prompt detection and vigorous treatment of mucocutaneous leishmaniasis, visceral leishmaniasis, and African trypanosomiasis. Immunization or inoculation of *L. tropica* in covered areas is successfully employed in the Middle East to avoid the cosmetic scarring that is otherwise likely to occur.

Prospective

With the diligent application of available methods for the prevention and control of human pathogenic hemoflagellates, much further progress can be achieved. The leishmania are unique among protozoa in that a solid cell-mediated immunity develops upon recovery from the disease or following therapeutic cure. If a vaccine could be developed against visceral leishmaniasis, its success could be anticipated. Control of American trypanosomiasis, which is the leading cause of cardiovascular death in South America, must await the availability of effective chemotherapy but may not be totally effective because many cases of fatal myocarditis frequently are preceded by subclinical infections.

TOXOPLASMOSIS

Although subclinical immunizing infections of man with *Toxoplasma gondii* predominate, mild or fatal disease may result, with manifestations of fever, headache, myalgia, lymphadenopathy, splenomegaly, hepatitis, pneumonia, myocarditis, encephalitis, and chorioretinitis. In utero infection can result in abortion, prematurity, or stillbirth. Infants who survive may develop a variety of devastating sequelae months or years later, including retinochoroiditis, strabismus, blindness, brain damage (hydrocephaly, microcephaly, cerebral calcification, impaired psychomotor development, mental retardation, epilepsy), deafness, hepatosplenomegaly, and jaundice.

The Causative Agent

Toxoplasma gondii is an obligate intracellular protozoan currently classified with the *Sporozoa.* The postulated life cycle of the parasite is

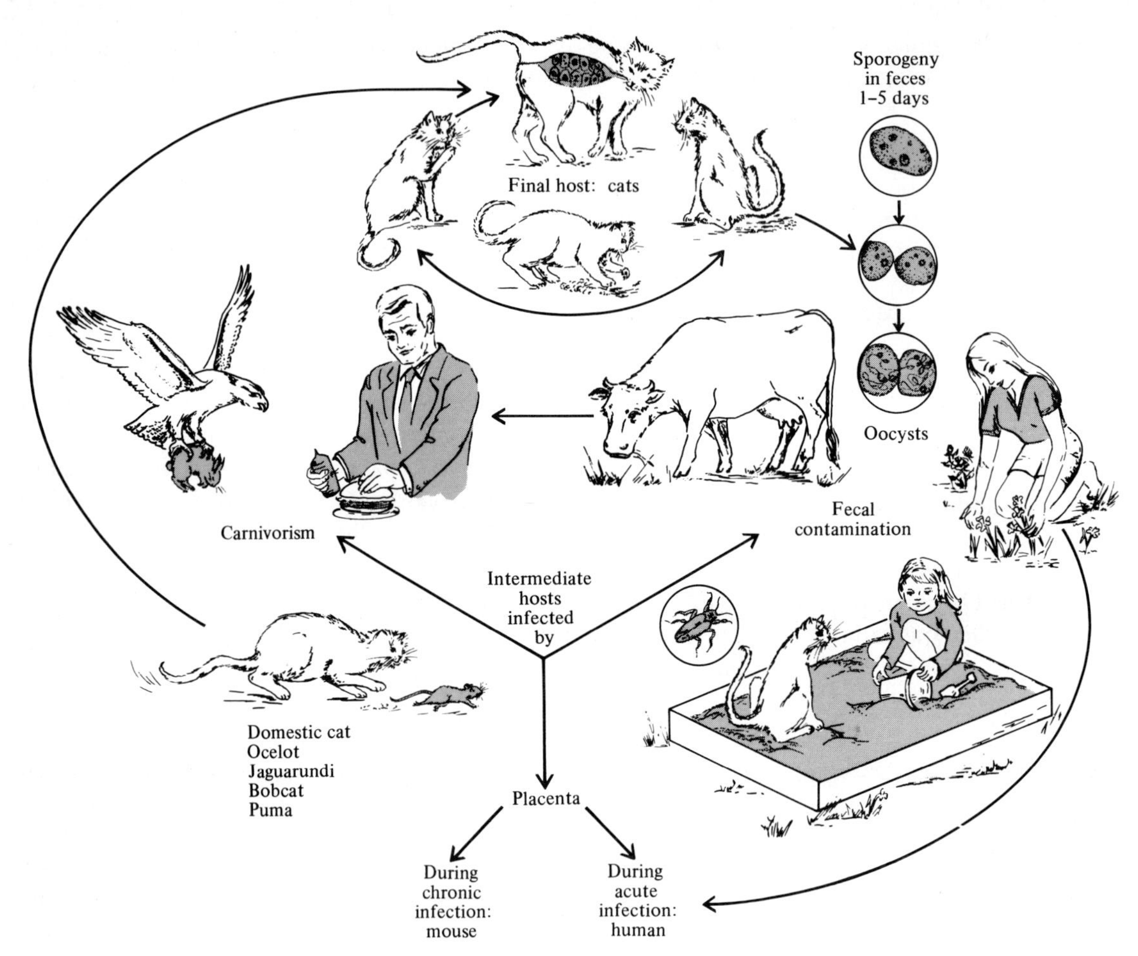

Figure 25-8 Postulated life cycle of *Toxoplasma gondii.* (*J. K. Frenkel and J. P. Dubey, J. Infect. Dis., 126:664-673, 1972.*)

indicated in Figure 25-8. The sexual cycle (sporogeny) presumably occurs in cats (the definitive host) with man serving as an intermediate host. Three forms of the parasite are found in nature. Crescent or oval-shaped trophozoites (7×3 μm) replicate intracellularly in almost every nucleated mammalian cell, are found in infected human tissues and in experimentally infected mice, embryonated eggs, or tissue cultures. Superficially, the trophozoites resemble the intracellular forms of histoplasma (Chap. 23) and leishmania. Tissue cysts (pseudocysts) are large forms (10 to 100 μm) containing numerous viable trophozoites within a cyst wall that may persist for the life of the host. Oocysts (12 μm) are an infective form of the parasite containing the sporozoites and are passed in cat feces. Toxoplasma belong to a single species and exhibit a single antigenic type.

Pathogenesis

Natural infection of man is probably acquired by (1) ingestion of tissue cysts in raw or undercooked meat (pork, lamb, beef), (2) ingestion of oocysts, (3) optic implantation of tissue cysts or oocysts, or (4) in utero transmission. Most human infections presumably follow the ingestion of tissue cysts or oocysts and lead to generalized infection but only occasionally to disease. The probable sequence involves the release of trophozoites from the tissue cysts or oocysts in the small intestine, penetration and replication of the trophozoites in the mucosal epithelial cells and, following their destruction, by hematogenous dissemination and intracellular replication of the trophozoites in many organs and tissues of the body. Tissue cysts frequently develop in the brain, lymphoreticular tissues, and muscle and may persist indefinitely with minimal pathology. Occasionally, however, in immunosuppressed patients breakdown of the cysts may lead to fatal disseminated disease.

Ocular toxoplasmosis is a major cause of granulomatous uveitis, represents localized infection associated with the presence of trophozoites and tissue cysts, tends to recur unpredictably, and subsequently heals with some loss of vision.

Congenital toxoplasmosis usually develops following active but subclinical infection of pregnant women. Infants who survive in utero infection are frequently asymptomatic at birth but over a period of time become progressively disabled by cerebral, optic, and otic sequelae.

Probably one of the more common clinical syndromes encountered in toxoplasmosis is that of an acute but mild mononucleosis-like illness such as that which occurred in a group of medical students who ate inadequately cooked hamburger (Fig. 25-9).

Laboratory Diagnosis

Laboratory diagnosis is based on demonstration of trophozoites or tissue cysts in the lesions, smears prepared from exudates, or in sediments of CSF, blood, and other body fluids. The trophozoites can be recovered following the intraperitoneal inoculation of clinical specimens in mice, embryonated eggs, or tissue cultures.

A serological diagnosis can be established by a variety of procedures including indirect FA, CF, HA-inhibition, dye inhibition, and neutralization tests. The demonstration of a rising titer of antibody is essential in view of the prevalence of antibody in individuals with past infections. Although much of the basic diagnostic and epidemiological data were derived on the basis of CF and dye inhibition tests, the indirect FA test is currently preferred. The dye inhibition test is based on the observation that in the presence of antibody and complement the trophozoites fail to stain with methylene blue.

Epidemiology

Within the past 10 years it has become apparent that man acquires toxoplasmosis primarily by ingestion of raw meat containing tissue cysts or oocysts contained in cat feces. Ocular toxoplasmosis probably results from direct implantation of the parasite by fingers contaminated from handling raw meat, cat feces, or soil contaminated with cat feces. Congenital toxoplasmosis represents an uncommon method of transmission, as does reactivation of latently infected individuals who are immunologically compromised. Many puzzling features remain. For example, the age at which infection occurs and the prevalence of infection varies widely not only in different parts of the world (2 to 90 percent) but in the same country. Perhaps part of the explanation is dependent upon the preference of some groups for raw meat (high incidence) and other groups for thoroughly cooked meat (low incidence).

Prevention and Control

To prevent toxoplasmosis, (1) meat should be thoroughly cooked so that the internal temperature is at least 66°C before eating, and hands

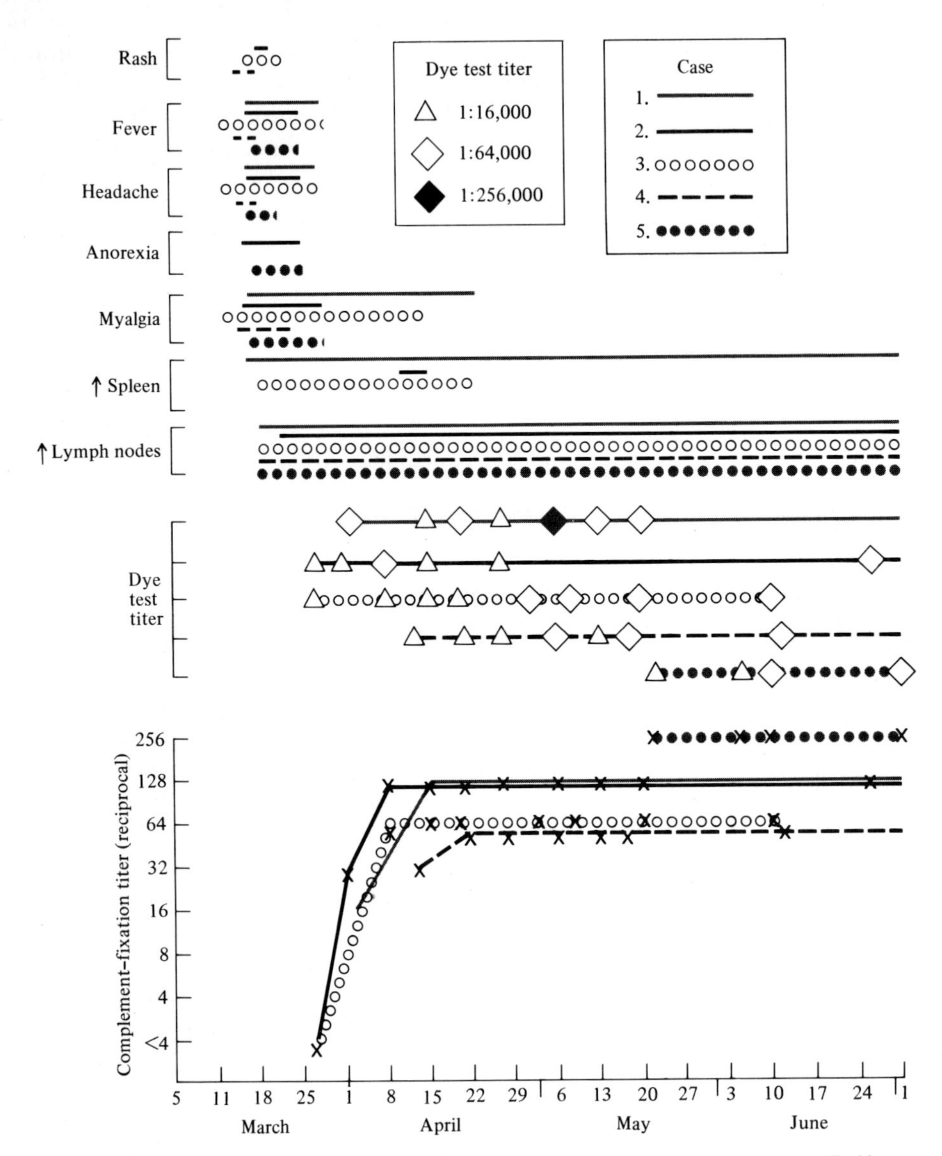

Figure 25-9 Clinical and laboratory findings in an epidemic of toxoplasmosis. (*B. H. Kean, A. C. Kimball, and W. N. Christenson, J.A.M.A., 208:1002–1004, 1969, Copyright 1969, American Medical Association.*)

should be washed with soap and water after handling raw meat; (2) indoor cats should be fed cooked meat and restrained from hunting (rodents, birds); (3) cat feces should be disposed of daily by flushing down the toilet and the litterpans disinfected with boiling water; (4) soil contaminated with cat feces should be avoided, especially preferred deposit areas such as children's sandboxes; (5) pregnant women without antibody should avoid contact with cats whenever possible because of the danger of acquiring infection and transmitting the disease to the fetus.

Therapy is based on the combined use of diaminopyrimidines and sulfonamides, is generally continued for 1 month, and is effective against the trophozoites but apparently not against the tissue cysts. Corticosteroids are usually added to diaminopyrimidines and sulfonamides in the treatment of ocular toxoplasmosis and exert a beneficial effect.

Helminthic Infections

SCHISTOSOMIASIS

Of all helminthic infections, the trematodes parasitizing the blood (schistosomes, bilharzia, or blood flukes) are by far the most important and are second only to malaria as a cause of morbidity, chronic disability, and mortality in the tropics and subtropics wherever the appropriate snails are present to permit the development of the infective cercariae. The severity of schistosomiasis depends primarily upon the location and number of the adult worms, the number of eggs produced, the pattern of egg migration, and the duration of the disease. Clinically, the major manifestations are related to intestinal and hepatic damage (*Schistosoma japonicum* and *S. mansoni*) or to urinary bladder disease *(S. haematobium).*

The Causative Agents

The schistosomes are unique among the flatworms in having separate sexes. As noted in the chart below, the adult worms survive in human venules for 30 years or more, with the female producing a daily quota of eggs and thus providing ample opportunity for contamination of appropriate freshwater snails. The adult worms are small, the male being about 10 × 1 mm and the female 14 × 0.2 mm. The male possesses a ventral groove or gynephoric canal in which the female resides and produces ova. In the case of *S. mansoni* and *S. japonicum,* mating occurs in the liver, and the mated worms migrate to the venules of the small intestine *(S. japonicum)* or the rectosigmoid venules *(S. mansoni)* where the eggs are deposited. The eggs break through the intestinal mucosa and are passed in the feces. In the case of *S. haematobium,* the mating adults establish residence in the venules of the urinary bladder, and the ova are passed in the urine, occasionally in the feces when the adults locate in the intestinal venules.

Pathogenesis

Although there may be a transient dermatitis associated with dermal penetration of cercariae, pathology is primarily associated with the deposition of eggs which commences about 1 to 3 months later (acute stage) and the consequences of granuloma formation (chronic stage). In *S. japonicum* and *S. mansoni* infections, the acute manifestations include fever, abdominal discomfort, diarrhea tinged with blood and mucus, loss of weight, urticaria, and prominent eosinophilia associated with the passage of ova through the intestinal mucosa. In *S. haematobium* infections, the initial clinical manifestations are a mild painless terminal hematuria, occasionally accompanied by cystitis.

In chronic infections, granulomas form in the intestinal mucosa, liver, and urinary bladder, but potentially in any organ. In *S. japonicum* and *S. mansoni* infections, ova are carried via the portal circulation to the liver, granulomas form, and fibrosis ensues; cirrhosis, portal hypertension, and obstruction occur with resulting hepatosplenomegaly and ascites. In the intestines, adhesions develop and rectal prolapse, strictures, or polyps may occur. In *S. haematobium* infections, granulomas in the bladder wall fibrose and calcify, occasionally resulting in hydronephrosis, hydroureter, and renal failure. Disease caused by *S. japonicum* is more severe than that caused by *S. mansoni* because egg production is about ten times greater (3,000 instead of 300 per day). Although disease caused by *S. haematobium* is generally less severe, renal damage and secondary infection eventually present serious problems.

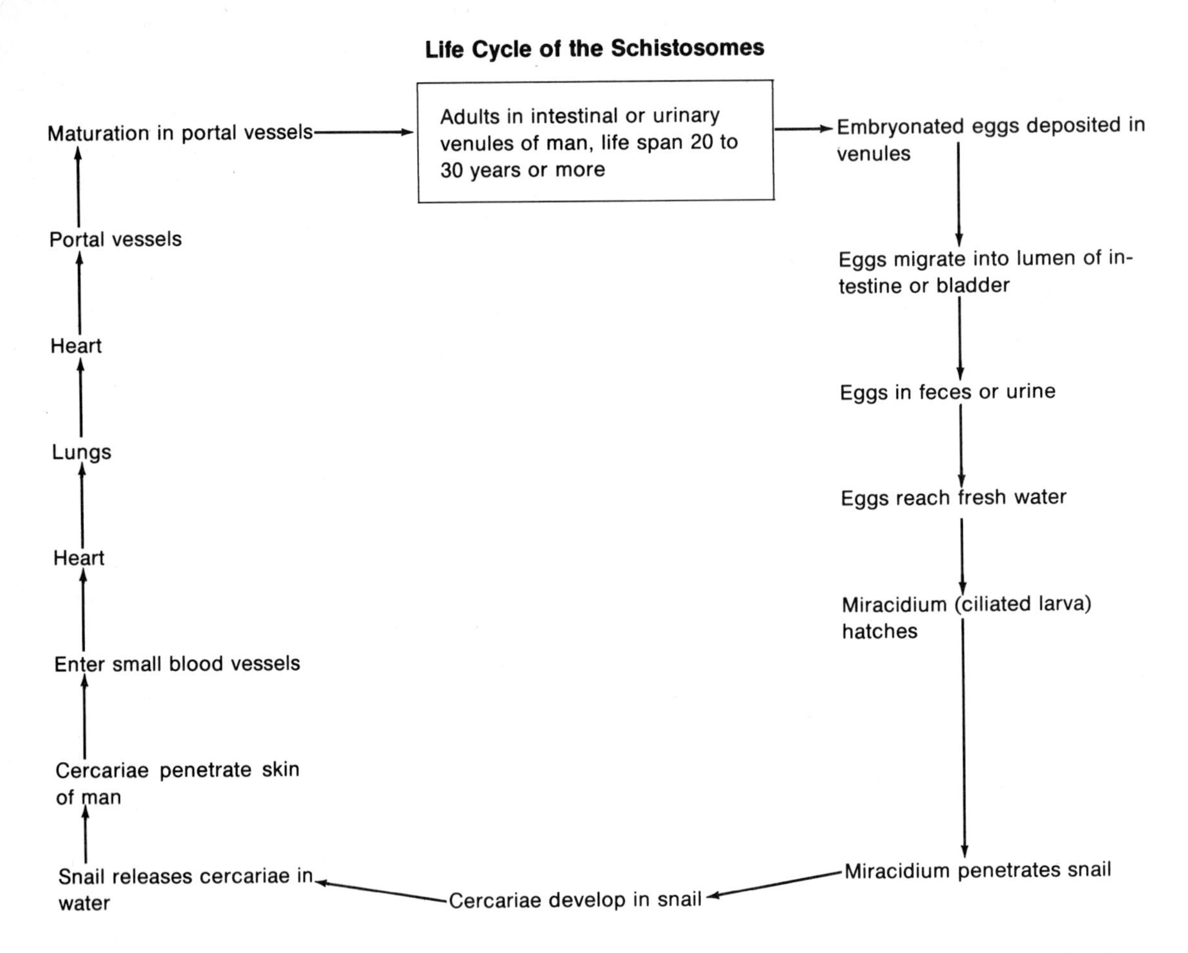

Laboratory Diagnosis

A laboratory diagnosis depends upon the demonstration of the characteristic ova in the stool or urine. The eggs are oval-shaped, approximately 150 × 60 μm, and can be distinguished on the basis of a large lateral spine *(S. mansoni),* a terminal spine *(S. haematobium),* or a short lateral spine *(S. japonicum).* Since ova are passed irregularly, multiple examinations must be performed. When stools are negative, scrapings of the intestinal mucosa or rectal biopsies are often positive.

Epidemiology

Man is the definitive host in *S. mansoni* and *S. haematobium* but is joined by a number of mammals (cattle, pigs, dogs, cats, rodents) in *S. japonicum.* Infection is usually acquired by washing or swimming in cercariae-contaminated fresh water. The geographical distribution of schistosomiasis conforms with that of the intermediate snail host that can support development of the particular cercariae. The endemic area of *S. mansoni* includes Africa, South America, and parts of the West Indies including Puerto Rico. *S. haematobium* is endemic in Africa and the Near East and is hyperendemic in the Nile Valley. *S. japonicum* is found in China, Japan, the Philippines, Taiwan, and other areas of the Far East. The incidence of schistosomiasis in endemic areas varies from about 10 to 90 percent, and more than 100 million persons are estimated to be infected. Untreated schistosomiasis takes a heavy toll in chronic disability; mortality increases with age and is generally associated with cirrhosis and secondary infection.

Prevention and Control

As with most of the helminths, schistosomiasis is a socioeconomic disease. Prevention and control require sanitary disposal of feces and urine, control of the snail population with molluscicides, and education of people living in endemic areas. Therapy is hazardous because the available drugs are toxic. Perhaps antimony pyrocatechin sodium disulfonate and antimony sodium dimercaptosuccinate are preferable because they can be administered intramuscularly, but the patient must be carefully monitored for cardiotoxicity. Attempts have been made to remove the adult schistosomes by extracorporeal filtration by means of a portal-systemic bypass, but even if successful, the procedure is hardly applicable to the 100 million people with schistosomiasis.

DISEASES CAUSED BY FLUKES

Apart from the blood flukes or schistosomes, the adult tissue flukes are flat, leaf-shaped hermaphroditic worms varying in size from 1 mm to 7 cm that can inhabit the lungs, liver, or intestine of man. The major trematodes in addition to the schistosomes include the lung fluke *Paragonimus westermani,* the liver flukes *Fasciola hepatica* and *Clonorchis sinensis,* and the intestinal flukes *Fasciolopsis buski* and *Heterophyes heterophyes.*

The lung, liver, and intestinal flukes are primarily diseases of animals with man being an accidental but occasionally common host, as in clonorchiasis. Except for *Fasciola,* which is cosmopolitan in distribution in sheep and cattle-raising countries, the lung, liver, and intestinal flukes are endemic in the Far East. Disease is generally mild but may involve hemoptysis and pleural pain in the case of the lung fluke, cirrhosis in the liver flukes, and diarrhea and anemia in the intestinal flukes.

Human infection usually follows the ingestion of crustaceans (crab, crayfish) in the case of the lung fluke, raw or uncooked fish in the case of *Clonorchis* and *Heterophyes*, and contaminated vegetation in the case of *Fasciola* and *Fasciolopsis*. Snails are involved in the life cycle of *Paragonimus, Fasciola,* and *Fasciolopsis.* Diagnosis is established by demonstration of the characteristic operculated ova in the feces, except for *Paragonimus,* which is found in sputum. Therapy involves the use of bithionol for *Paragonimus*, chloroquine for *Clonorchis*, and hexylresorcinol for *Fasciolopsis* and *Heterophyes.* Emetine provides symptomatic relief for *Fasciola.* Prevention and control are based primarily upon the sanitary disposal of feces; the proper cooking of crustaceans, fish, and aquatic vegetation; public education; and the treatment of infected individuals.

DISEASES CAUSED BY TISSUE ROUNDWORMS

Included among the tissue roundworms (nematodes) are the filarial worms *(Wuchereria bancrofti, Brugia malayi, Loa loa, Onchocerca volvulus), Dracunculus medinensis, Ancylostoma braziliense, Toxocara canis,* and *Toxocara cati. Onchocerca* was considered with infections of the eye (Chap. 19) and *Dracunculus* and *Ancylostoma* with infections of the skin and subcutaneous tissues (Chap. 16). Consequently, the following discussion is limited to filarial elephantiasis *(Wuchereria bancrofti, Brugia malayi), Loa loa,* and visceral larva migrans (*Toxocara canis,* and *Toxocara cati*).

Filarial Elephantiasis

Microfilariae of *Wuchereria bancrofti* or *Brugia malayi,* the infective larval stage, are transmitted to man following the bite of mosquitoes *(Aëdes, Culex, or Anopheles).* After reaching the circulation by way of the lymphatics, the microfilariae localize, mature, and mate in the lymphatics, releasing microfilariae into the blood. Although a mild illness characterized by fever, lymphadenopathy, orchitis, epididymitis, lymphangitis, edema, and urticaria may occur during the acute state of the disease, most infections are probably subclinical. However, in endemic areas, the population of adult worms builds up over a period of years, leading eventually to lymphatic obstruction and the dramatic manifestations of elephantiasis of the limbs and genitalia. As noted in the chart of the life cycle, microfilariae are taken up by the mosquito and develop into the infective larval stage. Man is the definitive host and the reservoir of infection.

Diagnosis is based on the demonstration of microfilariae in stained smears of blood taken at night because of the nocturnal periodicity of microfilarial release in certain endemic areas. Disease caused by *Brugia malayi* is found in Southeast Asia, whereas infections associated with *Wuchereria bancrofti* occur over a wide geographical area, including Southeast Asia, Africa, the Near East, and parts of the West Indies, Central America, and South America. Although the adult worms cannot be eliminated by chemotherapy, diethylcarbamazine can reduce the worm burden and will kill the microfilariae, thus preventing the infection of mosquitoes. Prevention and control are based primarily on the destruction of mosquitoes and protection against their bites. In endemic areas, antimosquito measures may be combined with mass treatment with diethylcarbamazine to kill the microfilariae.

Loa Loa

Loa loa is a filarial disease occurring in West and Central Africa that develops when *Chrysops* (the deer fly or mango fly) injects microfilariae. The life cycle is basically similar to that of *Wuchereria bancrofti* and *Brugia malayi* except that the adult worms live in the subcutaneous tissues and migrate through the tissues. Infected patients often develop large erythematous swellings (5 to 10 cm) which presumably represent hypersensitivity reactions to the adult worms. Occasionally, the adult worms will move across the cornea and rarely will involve a peripheral nerve. In most cases, the clinical manifestations are mild and transient. Diethylcarbamazine can be used in therapy.

Visceral Larva Migrans

The dog and cat ascarid worms *(Toxocara canis and Toxocara cati)* can produce disease in man associated with the migration of the larvae in the liver, lungs, and occasionally other tissues. Man is an accidental host who acquires infection following the ingestion of embryonated

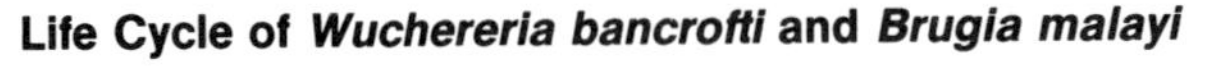

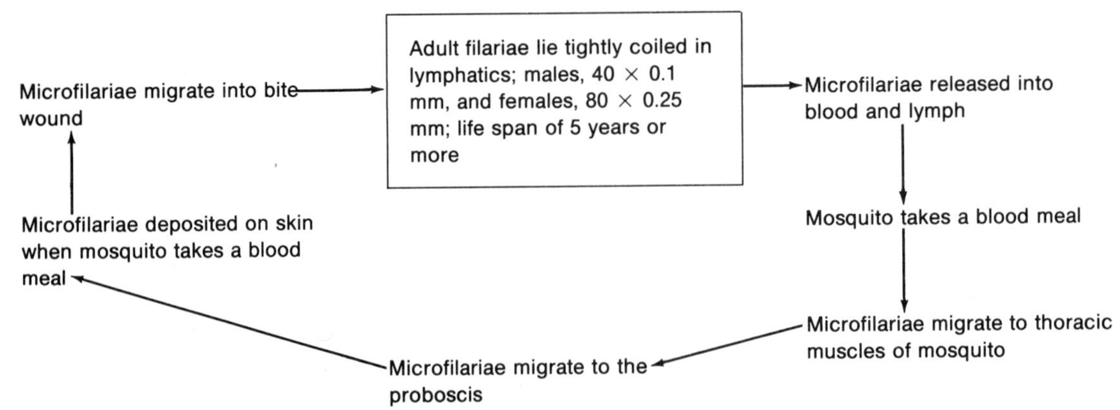

eggs deposited in the soil by dogs and cats. The larvae hatch in the small intestine, penetrate the intestinal mucosa, enter the circulation, are carried to the various tissues, and cause clinical manifestations primarily in the liver and lungs as they migrate over a period of several months before the granulomatous reactions are encapsulated and healed. The severity of the disease is determined largely by the number of eggs ingested which in turn regulates the number of migrating larvae. The diagnosis is suggested by eosinophilia, a persisting febrile illness occasionally associated with hepatomegaly and hyperglobulinemia, and a history of exposure to dogs or cats but can be confirmed only by hepatic biopsy. Thiabendazole can be used in therapy and leads to definite clinical improvement. Prevention and control of visceral larva migrans are based on the periodic deworming of household dogs and cats, the protection of play areas and sandboxes from dog and cat feces, the proper disposal of dog and cat feces, and keeping children from eating dirt likely to be contaminated with dog and cat feces.

Bacterial Infections

LISTERIOSIS

Listeriosis is a bacterial disease caused by *Listeria monocytogenes* and is usually associated with either meningoencephalitis in immunosuppressed patients or intrauterine infection leading to widespread focal necrosis and high mortality. The causative agent is ubiquitously distributed in the environment (animals, water, mud, sewage, fodder), appears as a gram-positive motile rod, produces acid but not gas in numerous carbohydrates, has seven antigenic types, and experimentally can induce conjunctivitis and keratitis following ocular inoculation of rabbits or guniea pigs. Except for in utero infection, the pathogenesis of the disease is unknown. The animal reservoir does not seem to be important in human infections. Penicillin, ampicillin, erythromycin, and tetracyclines have proved effective in therapy. Prevention and control are difficult because most human infections, including those in pregnant women, are subclinical.

MELIOIDOSIS

Melioidosis is a bacterial disease of man caused by *Pseudomonas pseudomallei* and characterized by a broad spectrum of clinical manifestations, varying from pneumonitis to abscess formation to septicemia. Most infections, however, are subclinical, but the organism may persist and become reactivated in debilitated or immunosuppressed patients. The causative agent is found in soil and water in many parts of the world (Southeast Asia, Central and South America, the West Indies), appears as a gram-negative motile rod, has a single antigenic type, and can be identified by passive HA or CF tests. Although infection occurs in wild rodents and domestic animals, human infections appear to be unrelated to animals. Therapy is generally based on the combined use of tetracyclines and sulfonamides and may require a prolonged course.

RELAPSING FEVER

Relapsing fever is an acute, tick- or louse-transmitted, systemic spirochetal disease caused by *Borrelia recurrentis.* There is a large reservoir of infection in animals (rodents, squirrels, prairie dogs, chipmunks) and in ticks who can spread the disease from animal to animal or to man. In man, the disease can be transmitted from man to man by the human body louse, and louse-borne epidemics can develop under stressful conditions (war, famine, crowding, malnutrition) that favor infestation with lice.

The causative agent is a slender (10 to 30 × 0.3 μm), loosely coiled, motile, gram-negative spirochete which has the capacity for antigenic variation during the course of infection and thus can lead to relapses. After an incubation period of 5 to 7 days, during which the organism replicates in lymphoreticular tissues, the spirochete is present in the blood. Clinical manifestations are associated with fever, prostration, intense myalgia and arthralgia, splenomegaly and hepatomegaly, occasionally by jaundice, CNS and respiratory involvement. The illness subsides in less than a week only to relapse after an afebrile period of a week. Additional relapses may occur, especially in the tick-borne disease. The case fatality rate is usually less than 5 percent but in louse-borne epidemics may rise to 30 or 40 percent. The major endemic areas are in Asia, Africa, and South America for the louse-borne disease and in Africa, Asia, and North and South America for the tick-borne disease. Therapy with tetracyclines is effective, and prevention is based on methods for controlling lice (Chap. 22) and ticks (Chap. 24) and the construction of rodent-proof dwellings.

BARTONELLOSIS

Bartonellosis is a serious *Phlebotomus*-transmitted bacterial disease limited to the valleys in the Andes mountains of Peru, Ecuador, and Colombia corresponding to the geographical distribution of the vector. Although the disease varies considerably in severity, it is frequently acute and toxic. After an incubation period of 2 to 3 weeks during which the causative agent, *Bartonella bacilliformis,* grows in the cytoplasm of endothelial cells of blood vessels, the organism reenters the bloodstream, causing a severe hemolytic anemia. The clinical manifestations of this phase of the disease (Oroya fever) include fever, chills, headache, delirium, lymphadenopathy, hepatomegaly, and jaundice along with the hemolytic anemia. If the patient survives the acute phase (40 percent of untreated patients succumb), verruga peruana or nodular, cutaneous, hemangiomas may develop.

The causative agent is a gram-negative motile bacillus that grows at 28°C on semisolid agar containing 10 percent rabbit serum and 0.5 percent rabbit hemoglobin in about 10 days. During the acute phase of the disease numerous organisms can be observed in stained preparations on the surface of red blood cells and in reticuloendothelial cells throughout the body. The high mortality of the disease is associated with enhanced susceptibility to *Salmonella* and malaria infections. Chloramphenicol is the preferred therapy because it will not only be effective against *Bartonella* but in most cases will also inhibit *Salmonella.* Recovery from the acute phase of the disease is usually accompanied by a solid and prolonged immunity interspersed with verruga peruana which may reflect the patient's developing immunity. Prevention is based on the control of the sandfly.

BIBLIOGRAPHY

"African Trypanosomiasis. Report of a Joint FAO/WHO Expert Committee," *W.H.O. Tech. Rep. Ser.,* no. 434, 1969.

Buchman, R. J., Kmiecik, J. E., and LaNoue, A. M.: "Extrapulmonary Melioidosis," *Am. J. Surg.,* 125: 324–327, 1973.

Chin, J., and Morrison, F. R.: "Epidemiology of Viral Hepatitis in California, 1950–1970," *Calif. Med.,* 118(2):24–27, 1973.

Cohen, A. B., Rosenthal, W. S., and Stenger, R. J.: "Autoimmune Response in Experimental Halothane-induced Liver Injury," *Proc. Soc. Exp. Biol.,* 142:817–819, 1973.

"Comparative Studies of American and African Trypanosomiasis. Report of a WHO Scientific Group," *W.H.O. Tech. Rep. Ser.,* no. 411, 1969.

Convit, J., Pinardi, M. E., and Rondon, A. J.: "Diffuse Cutaneous Leishmaniasis: A Disease Due to an Immunological Defect of the Host," *Trans. R. Soc. Trop. Med. Hyg.,* 66:603–610, 1972.

Dorfman, L. J.: "Cytomegalovirus Encephalitis in Adults," *Neurology,* 23:136–144, 1973.

Epstein, M. A.: "Burkitt's Lymphoma and Herpesvirus Saimiri Lymphoma: Comparative Aspects," *J. Natl. Cancer Inst.,* 49:213–217, 1972.

Evans, A. S. "Clinical Syndromes Associated with EB Virus Infection," *Adv. Intern. Med.*, 18:77-93, 1972.

Feigin, R. D.: "Metabolic Changes in Infectious Diseases," *Clin. Pediatr. (Phila.)*, 9:84-93, 1970.

Fine, R. N., Malekzadeh, M., Grushkin, C. M., and Wright, H. T., Jr.: "Cytomegalovirus Syndrome Post-renal Transplantation—Treatment with Cytosine Arabinoside," *Calif. Med.*, 118(3):46-49, 1973.

Gerber, P., Nonoyama, M., Lucas, S., Perlin, E., and Goldstein, L. I.: "Oral Excretion of Epstein-Barr Virus by Healthy Subjects and Patients with Infectious Mononucleosis," *Lancet*, 2:988-989, 1972.

Ghatak, N. R., and Zimmerman, H. M.: "Fine Structure of *Toxoplasma* in the Human Brain," *Arch. Pathol.*, 95:276-283, 1973.

Giglioli, G.: "Changes in the Pattern of Mortality Following the Eradication of Hyperendemic Malaria from a Highly Susceptible Community," *Bull. W.H.O.*, 46:181-202, 1972.

Golubjatnikov, R., Allen, V. D., Steadman, M., Blancarte, M.D.P.O., and Inhorn, S.L.: "Prevalence of Antibodies to Epstein-Barr Virus, Cytomegalovirus and Toxoplasma in a Mexican Highland Community," *Am. J. Epidemiol.*, 97:116-124, 1973.

Gray, J. A.: "Mumps," *Br. Med. J.*, 1:338-340, 1973.

Henle, W., and Henle, G.: "Epstein-Barr Virus and Infectious Mononucleosis," *N. Engl. J. Med.*, 288: 263-264, 1973.

Henson, D., Siegel, S. E., Fuccillo, D. A., Matthew, E., and Levine, A. S.: "Cytomegalovirus Infections during Acute Childhood Leukemia," *J. Infect. Dis.*, 126:469-481, 1972.

Heyneman, D.: "Immunology of Leishmaniasis," *Bull. W.H.O.*, 44:499-514, 1971.

Kean, B. H.: "Clinical Toxoplasmosis—50 Years," *Trans. R. Soc. Trop. Med. Hyg.*, 66:549-567, 1972.

Mahoney, L. E., and Kessel, J. F.: "Treatment Failure in Filariasis Mass Treatment Programmes," *Bull. W.H.O.*, 45:35-42, 1971.

Manson-Bahr, P.E.C.: "Leishmaniasis," *Int. Rev. Trop. Med.*, 4:123-140, 1971.

Marsden, P. D.: "South American Trypanosomiasis (Chagas' Disease)," *Int. Rev. Trop. Med.* 4:97-121, 1971.

"Medical Staff Conference. Malaria," *Calif. Med.*, 118(2):38-45, 1973.

Medoff, G., Kunz, L. J., and Weinberg, A. N.: "Listeriosis in Humans: An Evaluation," *J. Infect. Dis.*, 123:247-250, 1971.

Miller, G., Niederman, J. C., and Andrews, L.-L.: "Infectious Mononucleosis: Prolonged Oropharyngeal Excretion of Epstein-Barr Virus," *N. Engl. J. Med.*, 288:299-232, 1973.

Ogunba, E. O.: "Ecology of Human Loiasis in Nigeria," *Trans. R. Soc. Trop. Med. Hyg.*, 66:748, 1972.

"Parasitology of Malaria. Report of a WHO Scientific Group," *W.H.O. Tech. Rep. Ser.*, no. 433, 1969.

Perine, P. L., Parry, E. H., Vukotich, D., Warrell, D. A., and Bryceson, A. D. M.: "Bleeding in Louse-borne Relapsing Fever: I. Clinical Studies in 37 Patients," *Trans. R. Soc. Trop. Med. Hyg.*, 65:776-781, 1971.

Provost, P. J., Ittensohn, O. L., Villarejos, V. M., Arguedas, J. A. G., and Hilleman, M. R.: "Etiologic Relationship of Marmoset-propagated CR 326 Hepatitis A Virus to Hepatitis in Man," *Proc. Soc. Exp. Biol. Med.*, 142:1257-1267, 1973.

Recavarren, S., and Lumbreras, H.: "Pathogenesis of the Verruga of Carrion's Disease. Ultrastructural Studies," *Am. J. Pathol.*, 66:461-470, 1972.

Rozman, R. S.: "Chemotherapy of Malaria," *Annu. Rev. Pharmacol.*, 13:127-152, 1973.

"Schistosomiasis Control. Report of a WHO Expert Committee," *W.H.O. Tech. Rep. Ser.*, no. 515, 1973.

Shultz, M. G.: "A History of Bartonellosis (Carrion's Disease)," *Am. J. Trop. Med. Hy.*, 17:503-515, 1968.

Southern, P. M., and Sanford, J. P.: "Relapsing Fever: A Clinical and Microbiological Review," *Medicine*, 48:129-149, 1969.

Szmuness, W., Prince, A. M., Brotman, B., and Hirsch, R. L.: "Hepatitis B Antigen and Antibody in Blood Donors: An Epidemiologic Study," *J. Infect. Dis.*, 127:17-25, 1973.

Thompson, P. E.: "The Challenge of Drug-resistant Malaria," *Am. J. Trop. Med.*, 22:139-145, 1973.

"Viral Hepatitis," *Br. Med. Bull.*, 28:103-185, 1972.

"Viral Hepatitis," *W.H.O. Tech. Rep. Ser.*, no. 512, 1973.

Warren, K. S.: "The Immunopathogenesis of Schistosomiasis: A Multidisciplinary Approach," *Trans. R. Soc. Trop. Med. Hyg.*, 66:417-432, 1972.

"WHO Expert Committee on Yellow Fever. Third Report," *W.H.O. Tech. Rep. Ser.*, no. 479, 1971.

Chapter 26

Infectious Diseases of Animals Transmissible to Man

Bernard A. Briody

Bacterial Diseases

PLAGUE

In its biblical and historical connotation, plague is a vividly tragic word that is virtually synonymous with calamity and death. As a disease of man, bubonic plague is described in the Bible (I Samuel 5:6-12; 6:19). In the fourth century B.C., Dionysius indicated that plague was a fatal disease that occurred in Egypt, Libya, and

Syria. During the reign of Justinian in the sixth century, pandemic plague is estimated to have killed 50 percent of the citizens of the Roman empire. In the fourteenth century, the disease became known as the Black Death in tribute to the 25 to 50 million who perished. Numerous pandemics occurred between 1500 and 1720 including the Great Plague of 1665, but thereafter the disease subsided until 1893 and 1894 when the last pandemic began in Hong Kong and continued for the next 25 years. It is estimated that in India alone 10 million people perished of plague between 1898 and 1918, and the disease was disseminated throughout the world, including the United States.

With the recognition of the close association of the household rat *(Rattus rattus)* and the rat flea *(Xenopsylla cheopis)* with human plague and their control, the incidence of plague was sharply reduced throughout much of the world. An uneasy truce, however, exists between plague and man on two accounts: (1) endemic foci of the disease in the rodent population persist in India, other parts of Southeast Asia, and in some areas of Africa and South America (domestic cycle); and (2) there is a wide reservoir of infection in wild rodents (squirrels, chipmunks, prairie dogs, deer mice, voles, gerbils, marmots) not only in the areas indicated above but also in the western portions of North America and Mexico (sylvatic plague).

The Causative Agent

Plague is caused by *Yersinia pestis (Pasteurella pestis),* a short, plump gram-negative bacillus that exhibits bipolar staining, best observed by Wayson or Giemsa stains. The organism grows comparatively slowly on blood agar over a broad temperature range, producing pinpoint colonies in 2 days. Apart from its morphology, the organism can be identified by virulent phage using cultures incubated at 20°C or by serological reactions including the passive HA, FA, and agglutination tests. The primary habitats of the organism are the tissues of domestic and wild rodents and their fleas. Plague bacilli belong to a single antigenic type, possess numerous antigens including the envelope protein which is responsible for the production of protective antibody, and a protein toxin (M. W., 74,000) which is lethal for mice.

Pathogenesis

Bubonic Plague In bubonic plague, the infection is transmitted to man by a flea that had parasitized an infected domestic or wild rodent. Within an incubation period of 2 to 6 days the organism replicates extensively in the draining lymphatics, producing lymphadenitis usually accompanied by lymph node enlargement (bubo) and concomitantly is widely disseminated to and replicates in many tissues and organs, leading to a septicemia. As a consequence of the septicemia, the patient exhibits the classic manifestations of toxicity; prostration; circulatory collapse accompanied by hemorrhagic necrosis in the lymphatics, liver, spleen, lungs, skin, and mucous membranes; and occasionally hemorrhagic pneumonia. Although the plague bacilli are readily recovered from the blood, the concentration of organisms is insufficient to infect fleas. However, if and when pneumonia develops during the course of bubonic plague, the organism is excreted in large quantities in the sputum.

Pneumonic Plague When plague spreads from man to man, it occurs as a consequence of the development of pneumonia in patients with bubonic plague. Such patients are efficient in transmitting the disease from man to man by droplet infection. Pneumonic plague has a shorter incubation period (2 to 4 days) and pursues a more fulminating course with intense toxicity, prostration, dyspnea, bloodstained sputum, cyanosis, and death the usual outcome a few days after onset.

Epidemiology

The basic interaction of the animal reservoirs in relation to human plague is illustrated in the chart below.

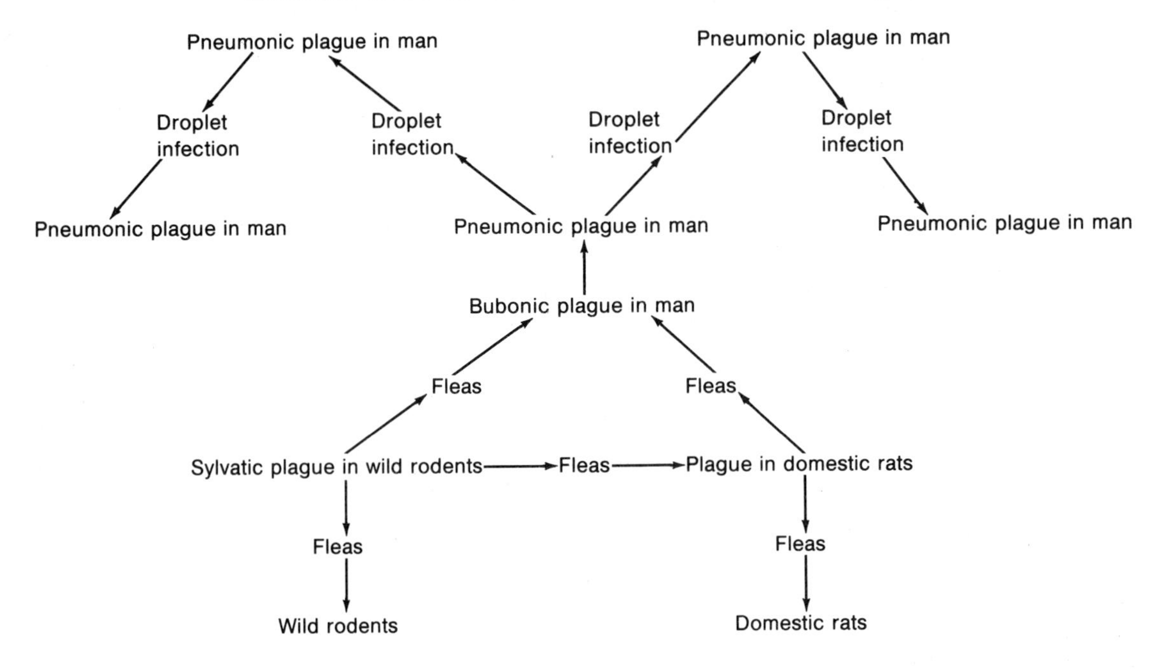

Plague was introduced to California in 1900 by shipboard rats brought from Southeast Asia where a pandemic was raging. About 450 human cases occurred between 1900 and 1907 after which a vigorous campaign succeeded in eliminating the domestic rat as a source of human infection, thus bringing the disease under effective control. Meanwhile, however, enzootic sylvatic plague gradually became established in 15 Western states in squirrels, chipmunks, prairie dogs, and other wild rodents. Since 1908, sylvatic plague has served as the source of human infection in the United States. Between 1908 and 1951 there were 70 cases and 45 deaths, a case fatality rate of 64 percent; while between 1952 and 1972 there were 54 cases with 12 deaths, a case fatality rate of 22 percent. The lower mortality in the last 20 years undoubtedly reflects the efficacy of tetracyclines in therapy.

Under pandemic conditions such as occurred in India between 1898 and 1918, characteristically, three successive epidemic peaks were observed at 3-week intervals in the large gray rat *(Rattus norweigicus)* that lives in sewers and garbage dumps, the domestic black rat *(Rattus rattus)*, and man.

Prevention and Control

Prevention and control are based primarily on rodent and vector control and prompt therapy with tetracyclines, which should be begun as soon as the diagnosis is suspected. In endemic areas, chemoprophylaxis with sulfonamides is effective, especially for contacts, and active immunization with heat-killed vaccine is recommended for persons at high risk.

TULAREMIA

Tularemia is primarily a disease of wild rabbits and is caused by *Francisella tularensis (Pasteur-*

ella tularensis), a gram-negative coccobacillus which requires an enriched medium for growth (glucose-cystine blood agar). There is, however, a large reservoir of infection in other animals (rodents, carnivores, ungulates, birds) and in ticks. Human tularemia is unique in the variety of routes by which man can acquire infection (dermal contact, arthropod transmission, inhalation, ingestion, through conjunctiva) and in the widely disparate virulence of the infecting bacteria.

The causative agent may enter through a break in the skin following contact with an infected animal or as a result of the bite of an arthropod (tick, deer fly or *Chrysops,* lice, mosquitoes), and in about 4 days this leads to the formation of a localized ulcer and regional lymphadenopathy, occasionally accompanied by a caseous and suppurating bubo (ulceroglandular tularemia). Inhalation of the organism may result in a serious necrotizing bronchopneumonia or a tracheobronchitis followed by ingestion of the organism and the typhoidal form of the disease (fever, chills, sweats, severe headache, myalgia, toxemia). Ingestion of the organism may cause ulceroglandular disease (cervical lymphadenopathy and pharyngeal ulceration), pneumonia, or less commonly the typhoidal form of the disease. The oculoglandular type usually involves the formation of an ulcer and lymphadenopathy of the preauricular, submaxillary, and anterior cervical lymph nodes.

The dermal and respiratory routes of infection are the most common and require the fewest number of bacteria (less than 50) to cause disease in man. Ingestion usually requires more than 10 million organisms to cause disease in human volunteers. Although there is but a single antigenic type of *Francisella tularensis,* bacteria acquired from cottontail rabbits or ticks are much more virulent for man than bacteria recovered from hares, moles, beavers, muskrats, squirrels, rats, mice, and birds. The latter less virulent bacteria usually induce mild disease in man regardless of the route of infection, whereas the more virulent organisms can cause a mortality of 5 to 30 percent in untreated ulceroglandular and pneumonic forms of the disease.

Tularemia is endemic in animals in North America and in many parts of Europe and Asia. The more virulent human pathogens are limited to North America, ferment glycerol, and have citrulline ureidase activity. The less virulent organisms also found in North America are glycerol- and citrulline ureidase-negative. Approximately 200 cases are reported annually in the United States.

Diagnosis of human tularemia is best established by recovery of the organism from the ulcer, lymph nodes, sputum, or gastric washings. Primary isolation requires glucose-cystine blood agar and should include cycloheximide and penicillin G to suppress the growth of the normal flora. The organism can be identified by performing agglutination tests with known antitularemia serum. Alternatively, the diagnosis can be established serologically by demonstrating a rise in antibody with paired sera. *Francisella tularensis* cross-reacts with *Brucella* species, since they share common antigens, but this does not present a problem because the antibody titers in the homologous infection are generally five times higher than with the heterologous bacteria. Laboratory cultures must be handled with great care to avoid infection of personnel, and for this reason animal inoculation should be limited to specially equipped laboratories.

Prevention and control are based on vector control and avoiding contact with ill rabbits and other animals. For those exposed to high risk of infection, the attenuated vaccine developed in Russia is safe and effective. Streptomycin is the drug of choice for treatment and has been used effectively in chemoprophylaxis after known exposure. Recovery from the disease is accompanied by a solid and prolonged immunity.

BRUCELLOSIS

Brucellosis is primarily a disease of cattle, goats, swine, sheep, beagles, desert wood rats, and other animals (buffalo, reindeer, deer, moose, hares) and is caused by *Brucella* species of gram-negative coccobacilli. The causative agents have been assigned species names, *B. abortus* (cattle), *B. melitensis* (goats), *B. suis* (swine), *B. ovis* (sheep), *B. canis* (beagles), and *B. neotomae* (desert wood rats). Classically, disease in cattle, goats, swine, and beagles is associated with abortion due to the presence of high placental concentrations of erythritol, a carbohydrate that stimulates the growth of the bacteria. Fortunately, erythritol is not found in human placental tissue.

Most human infections are subclinical and are induced by *B. abortus, B. melitensis,* and *B. suis,* but a variety of clinical manifestations and complications can occur. After contact with sick animals or animal products (raw or unpasteurized milk), the bacteria can enter through a break in the skin, inhalation, or ingestion. During the course of an incubation period of 1 to 5 weeks, the bacteria multiply widely within lymphoreticular cells. The onset of the acute stage of the disease is gradual; is accompanied by fever, headache, myalgia, arthralgia, weakness, chills, and sweats; and is often followed by cervical lymphadenopathy, splenomegaly, and hepatitis. Within 3 months the disease subsides in most patients and is followed by recovery. In about 15 percent of untreated cases, disease continues for a variable period, and in a minority it may persist for as long as 25 years. The most frequent complication is osteomyelitis. Death is uncommon, usually a rate of less than 2 percent, and is most frequently caused by endocarditis.

Diagnosis is established during the acute phase of the disease by recovery of the organism from the blood but is more difficult in the chronic form of the disease, occasionally being isolated from lymph nodes, bone marrow, bile, or liver biopsy. Cultures are performed in enriched broth (trypticase soy) containing 1 percent citrate and incubated in an atmosphere of 10 percent CO_2 for 6 weeks, periodically attempting to subculture on solid media. The three common species infecting man *(B. abortus, B. melitensis, B. suis)* can be distinguished by agglutinin-absorption tests and by their sensitivity to thionine and basic fuchsin dyes. Active brucellosis is also suggested by high agglutinating antibody titers (usually greater than 1:100). *Brucella* species cross-react with the causative agents of cholera and tularemia, but these shared antigens rarely interfere with the specific serological tests.

Brucellosis in man occurs in many countries and continents including the Mediterranean area, Asia, and North and South America. In the United States, the annual incidence in recent years has averaged about 200 cases. Prevention and control of the disease are based primarily upon elimination of the disease in cattle and other animals by detection (positive agglutinin titers), slaughter, and immunization with attenuated vaccines. Pasteurization of milk has also reduced the incidence of the disease. Because of the protected intracellular localization of the bacteria, therapy with tetracyclines must be prolonged, occasionally supplemented with streptomycin, and continued or reinstituted when relapses occur.

ANTHRAX

Anthrax is primarily a disease of cattle, sheep, and other animals (horses, goats, swine, elephants) caused by *Bacillus anthracis,* a large gram-positive, spore-bearing, encapsulated, nonmotile bacillus with squared ends which occurs in long chains on culture and which is pathogenic for mice. Infection of man usually results in disease, the vast majority of cases occurring following the entry of spores through a break in the skin. Occasionally, the disease may develop following inhalation of spores present in animal hides, hair, or bristles and rarely after ingestion of spores. Characteristically, the disease in man appears as a necrotic cutaneous ulcer (malignant pustule) which appears 2 to 5 days after entry of the organism, most commonly on the arm, head, and hand. In 7 to 10 days the ulcer becomes a large (1 to 3 cm) black eschar. The bacilli usually spread to the regional lymph nodes and in about 10 to 20 percent of cases may disseminate widely and rapidly, producing a fatal septicemia with generalized hemorrhage and edema. Inhalation anthrax (woolsorter's disease) is a generally fatal disease even when treated. Death is preceded by profound respiratory distress and ensues within 24 hr. of onset of the acute phase of the disease. Gastrointestinal anthrax also has a high mortality rate (25 to 50 percent); has an acute onset marked by abdominal distress, pain, hematemesis, and occasionally bloody diarrhea; and may progress to shock, cyanosis, and death.

Human disease is found primarily in those countries and regions where endemic anthrax occurs in animals (Asia, Africa, the Middle East). In the United States much progress has been achieved in preventing anthrax in man, most cases resulting from contact with imported animal products containing spores. Only 2 to 5 cases are reported annually in this country.

The causative agent is unique in possessing a high molecular weight capsule composed of polymers of D-glutamic acid which can interfere with phagocytosis of the organism. In addition, the bacilli produce a protective protein antigen which has been separated from the organism and used successfully for immunization of individuals exposed to a high risk of acquiring anthrax.

Prevention and control of the disease are based largely on methods designed to exclude the spores from industrial plants processing animal products and immunization of employees at high risk. Included are such procedures as autoclaving of animal products, regular disinfection and cleaning of equipment and work areas, and instruction of employees in the necessity for personal cleanliness and hygiene, including showering. In areas where anthrax is endemic, immunization of cattle and sheep is helpful, and it is important to destroy infected animals by burning or burying in deep lime pits, since the spores can remain viable in soil for decades, if not indefinitely, and may serve as a source of infection for other animals or man. Penicillin is the drug of choice in treatment and is highly effective in cutaneous anthrax. Because of the danger of septicemia in cutaneous anthrax and the fulminating course of inhalation and gastrointestinal anthrax, penicillin therapy must be initiated as soon as cultures are taken.

LEPTOSPIROSIS

Leptospirosis is primarily a disease of wild and domestic rodents which can lead to natural infection in dogs, swine, cattle, and other animals. Animal infection is characterized by a prolonged renal carrier state during which the organism is excreted in the urine and serves as the major source of human infection. The causative agents are classified as spirochetes of the genus *Leptospira* and have been separated into numerous species on the basis of antigenic specificity, even though all species share common antigens. The principal species include *L. icterohaemorrhagiae, L. canicola, L. pomona, L. grippotyphosa, L. autumnalis, L. australis, L. heb-*

domadis, and *L. pyrogenes. Leptospira* species are slender, tightly coiled motile spirochetes (10 × 0.15 μm) with a terminal hook; they stain poorly but can be visualized by dark-field microscopy and in silver-stained preparations.

Although many human infections are subclinical, disease of varying severity and clinical manifestations can occur. Infection generally develops 1 to 2 weeks following ingestion of water or food contaminated with infected animal urine, but the organism may also enter through breaks in the skin or through the conjunctival or oral membranes. In Weil's disease caused by *L. icterohaemorrhagiae,* the clinical manifestations are severe; include fever, jaundice, hemorrhages, and hepatic and renal failure; and are accompanied by a high mortality rate (10 to 40 percent) invariably due to renal failure. Most of the other species producing disease in man are usually associated with a self-limited illness of varying severity rarely lasting more than 7 days and characterized by fever, prostration, and meningitis, occasionally by a tibial rash, and only rarely by jaundice.

Diagnosis is based on demonstration of the organism in blood smears, culture on semisolid agar containing 10 percent serum and hemoglobin at 30°C, and the appearance of agglutinating antibodies. The disease is found throughout the world, but some species are limited to particular geographical areas. Leptospirosis is an occupational disease of miners, sewer workers, veterinarians, fishermen, and those who work on rice fields, sugar cane fields, or farms, and it occurs in children who swim in stagnant urine-contaminated ponds or who are in close contact with infected dogs. Less than 100 cases are reported annually in the United States. Prevention and control involve the use of protective boots and gloves by workers in hazardous occupations, rodent control, and avoidance of exposure to animal urine. Penicillin, streptomycin, and tetracyclines have been shown to be effective in experimental infections, but their efficacy in the treatment of human leptospirosis has not been established.

RAT-BITE FEVER

Rat-bite fever is an uncommon febrile disease of man characterized by intermittent or relapsing fever, a skin rash, and lymphadenitis and is caused by either one of two bacteria that are part of the normal flora of rodents. *Streptobacillus moniliformis* is a pleomorphic, nonmotile, gram-negative, facultatively anaerobic bacillus that grows slowly on enriched medium containing serum or ascitic fluid when incubated at 37°C in an atmosphere of 10 percent CO_2 and frequently yields L-forms. The organism is a normal inhabitant of the oropharyngeal flora of rodents. The other causative agent, *Spirillum minus,* is a tightly coiled spiral organism which is motile by means of a tuft of flagella at each end but which cannot be cultivated on artificial medium. The organism can be visualized by dark-field microscopy and in Giemsa-stained blood smears both in rodent blood where it is apparently a normal inhabitant and in the blood of infected humans. How the organism reaches the saliva of rodents prior to human transmission is not known.

Human disease caused by *Streptobacillus moniliformis* is usually more severe and is commonly accompanied by migrating polyarthritis. Infections with *Spirillum minus,* although less severe, generally persist for 4 to 8 weeks, and clinical manifestations may continue for several months or even years. During the course of infection agglutinins for *Streptobacillus moniliformis* develop, and the organism can be isolated from blood, joint fluid, or pus. *Spirillum minus* cannot be cultivated but can induce spirillemia in mice known to be free of the organism. Penicillin is effective in therapy of both infections, but tetracyclines may be required if L-forms develop in *Streptobacillus* infections. Rat-bite fever occurs throughout the world wherever rodents have access to human habitations and, thus, is a socioeconomic disease.

GLANDERS

Glanders is an infectious disease of horses caused by *Pseudomonas mallei,* a small, nonmotile gram-negative bacillus that is genetically and antigenically related to *Pseudomonas pseudomallei* (Chap. 25), the causative agent of melioidosis. Rarely, the disease may be acquired by man following contact with infected horses. Most commonly, human infection is associated with entry of the organism through a break in the skin, the formation of a cutaneous ulcer followed by lymphangitis, and septicemia. A similar disease occurs when the organism enters through the oropharyngeal mucous membranes. Inhalation of the bacteria leads to pneumonitis with abscess formation. Before the advent of sulfonamides, human glanders was a serious disease with a high mortality rate. By the persistent slaughter of infected horses, both the equine and human disease have been eliminated from Europe and North America. Endemic foci, however, persist in Asia, Africa, and South America. The organism can be separated from *P. pseudomallei* on the basis of its resistance to specific *P. pseudomallei* phage and its antigenic composition. Diagnosis is based on recovery of the organism on blood agar plates, the appearance of agglutinating antibody, and the development of a positive delayed skin reaction (mallein test).

ERYSIPELOID

Erysipeloid is primarily a disease of animals, especially swine, and is caused by a gram-positive, nonmotile bacillus, *Erysipelothrix insidiosa,* which unlike *Listeria monocytogenes,* fails to induce a progressive ocular infection in rabbits. Human infection with the organism results in a slowly developing, self-limiting migrating dermatosis commonly affecting the face and the scalp which generally clears up in about 3 weeks. Human erysipeloid is acquired by persons who regularly handle meat, poultry, fish, shellfish, or their bones or shells, the organism entering through a break in the skin. Swine do not appear to be involved as a source of human disease. The organism is highly susceptible to penicillin, and the rare patient who might develop endocarditis or arthritis responds effectively to penicillin therapy.

RICKETTSIAL DISEASES

As noted in Chapter 2, rickettsiae are obligate intracellular parasites that generally resemble gram-negative bacteria. With the exception of epidemic typhus (Chap. 22), in which man is the reservoir, rickettsial diseases have a reservoir in rodents (also cattle, sheep, and goats in Q fever; see Chap. 23) and, with the exception of epidemic and murine typhus, in ticks or mites, in which transovarial transmission occurs. Except for Q fever, in which inhalation of rickettsiae is the method of acquiring infection, rickettsiae are transmitted by an arthropod vector. The pathogenesis of rickettsial infections involves widespread multiplication of the organism in the vascular endothelial cells and, with the exception of Q fever, a rash associated with necrosis and thrombosis of capillaries together with perivasculitis (Chap. 22).

Antigenically, rickettsiae can be grouped on the basis of shared CF antigens and their cross-reactions with strains of *Proteus* (Weil-Felix agglutination; see Chap. 22), as indicated in Table 26-1. Within each rickettsial organism, there is a single antigenic type, except for scrub typhus.

Table 26-1 Antigenic Components of Rickettsiae

Disease	Rickettsial CF group antigen			*Proteus* agglutination		
	Typhus	Rocky Mountain spotted fever	Q fever	OX 19	OX 2	OX K
Epidemic typhus	+	−	−	+ + +	+	−
Murine typhus	+	−	−	+ + +	+	−
Rocky Mountain spotted fever and tick typhus	−	+	−	+ to + + +	+ to + + +	−
Rickettsialpox	−	+	−	−	−	−
Q fever	−	−	+	−	−	−
Scrub typhus	−	−	−	−	−	+ + +

MURINE TYPHUS

Murine typhus is a natural infection of rats and mice and is caused by *Rickettsia mooseri;* it is transmitted from rat to rat by the rat flea *(Xenopsylla cheopis)* and occasionally may be transmitted to man by the same vector. After the flea feeds on an acutely ill rat with rickettsemia, the rickettsiae replicate intracellularly and are discharged in the feces for life. While feeding on man, the flea defecates, and the rickettsiae are rubbed into the bite wound. The ensuing disease is essentially similar to epidemic typhus but is much milder, with recovery occurring in 2 weeks. In untreated cases, the mortality is about 2 percent, compared with about 30 percent in epidemic typhus. Like epidemic typhus, the disease is worldwide in distribution. Control is based on rat and vector control. About 25 cases are reported annually in the United States.

THE SPOTTED FEVERS

Rocky Mountain Spotted Fever and Other Tick Typhus Diseases

There is a large group of rickettsial diseases occurring in various parts of the world which are caused by antigenic variants of *Rickettsia rickettsii* and transmitted by ticks, including Rocky Mountain spotted fever (RMSF) in the Western Hemisphere; boutonneuse fever in Africa, Europe, the Middle East, and India; Queensland tick typhus in Australia; and North Asian tick typhus in Siberia and Mongolia. Ticks including *Dermacentor andersoni* (wood tick), *Dermacentor variabilis* (dog tick), and *Amblyomma americanum* (Lone Star tick) function as both reservoir and vector for the cycle in animals as well as for transmitting the disease to man.

Clinically, RMSF is a serious disease which may pursue a rapid and fulminating course, untreated cases having a mortality of about 20 percent, whereas the other tick typhus diseases are much milder, and recovery is the rule. The appellation RMSF is a misnomer, since the majority of cases in the United States occur in the South Atlantic states, and the disease is also found in Canada, Mexico, Colombia, and Brazil.

In view of the potential severity of RMSF, early clinical diagnosis and therapy with chloramphenicol or tetracyclines are essential. Perhaps the earliest and most reliable diagnostic sign is the appearance of the rash on the wrists and ankles prior to the trunk and its regular presence on the palms and soles. The principal clinical features in addition to the rash include fever, an intense and continuous headache, marked muscle tenderness, toxicity, mental confusion, delirium, and coma. Although a killed vaccine is available for those exposed to a high risk of infection, control is based primarily on the use of repellents on clothes and exposed parts of the body and thorough inspection and removal of ticks several times a day. An infected tick must feed for 4 to 6 hr. or more before reactivating the rickettsiae and transmitting the disease to man. Approximately 400 cases are reported annually in the United States.

Rickettsialpox

Rickettsialpox is a natural infection of house mice, rats, and wild rodents caused by *Rickettsia akari* and transmitted by the mouse mite *(Allodermanyssus sanguineus)* both to rodents and to man. The disease occurs in the United States, Russia, Korea, and probably in other parts of the world, including Africa. Human rickettsialpox is a mild disease which usually subsides in 10 days and is characterized by an eschar at the site of the arthropod bite, regional lymphadenopathy, and a rash that occurs on the palms, soles, and oropharyngeal mucosa as well as on the trunk. As noted in Table 26-1, *Proteus* agglutinins do not develop. In the United States, rickettsialpox has occurred in New York, Philadelphia, Boston, Cleveland, and other nearby areas, frequently in association with the accumulation of garbage and trash in large housing developments which favors an increased population of mice. Control should be directed toward the elimination of house mice and their vectors.

SCRUB TYPHUS

Scrub typhus is a natural infection of wild rodents caused by *Rickettsia tsutsugamushi* which is found in Asia, Japan, and the southwest Pacific and is transmitted by larval mites of the genus *Trombicula*. Man becomes infected when he enters an enzootic area and is attacked by the larval mite. Clinically scrub typhus is characterized by an eschar at the site of the arthropod bite, fever, a severe headache, a rash which appears on the trunk and extends to the extremities, and usually signs of CNS involvement (apathy, delirium, muscular twitching). Untreated cases of the disease are associated with a significant mortality which averages about 15 percent but which may vary widely from about 1 to 60 percent, depending upon the virulence of the rickettsiae found in particular geographical areas. The numerous antigenically distinct types of *R. tsutsugamushi* have precluded the development of a vaccine that could be widely used. In endemic areas, control is based on vector control by applying repellents to clothing and exposed skin, by clearing vegetation and applying miticides before establishing campsites, and occasionally, by chemoprophylaxis with chloramphenicol in hyperendemic area for short periods followed by continued treatment for 1 month after departure.

Viral Diseases

Rabies

Although it is evident that rabies is a disease rarely encountered in man, no disease generates greater terror because of the virtual certainty of death once clinical manifestations appear. Rabies is primarily a disease of wild animals, especially carnivores, but can occur in practically any mammalian species. Enzootic rabies occurs in parts of Asia, Africa, Europe, and North and South America and leads to about 1,000 human cases annually, most of which develop in Iran, India, the Philippines, North Africa, and Thailand. Despite an extensive animal reservoir in the United States, only 15 cases of human rabies have been reported in the past 10 years.

The Causative Agent

Rabies virus is classified as a rhabdovirus, contains RNA, exhibits helical symmetry, is bullet-shaped, rounded at one end and flattened at the other, is surrounded by an envelope with projecting spikes, and has a diameter of 70 nm and a length of 175 nm. The host range of rabies virus involves all warm-blooded animals and produces fatal infection except in frugivorous, insectivorous, and vampire bats. In different animals species, virus may be found in varying concentration in the CNS, saliva, urine, lymph, milk, blood, and droppings. When present in impression smears of infected tissues, specific intracytoplasmic inclusions in neurones (Negri bodies) are pathognomonic of rabies. Negri bodies are oval or spherical eosinophilic inclusions 2 to 10 μm in size which contain rabies virus antigens. The virus can be grown in the chick embryo and in tissue cultures of hamster and human origin.

Pathogenesis

After its transmission to man in the saliva of the biting animal (dogs, foxes, skunks, mongooses, vampire bats, jackals, wolves), rabies virus travels from the site of inoculation to the CNS along sensory nerve pathways. The virus replicates in neurones and may then spread along autonomic nerves to various tissues, including the salivary glands. The incubation period is highly variable, usually 1 to 3 months but may be shorter or longer. The sequential clinical manifestations usually include pain at the site of the bite, anxiety, agitation, excessive motor activity, intense painful contraction of pharyngeal muscles which leads to hydrophobia (fear of water), and increasing respiratory, cardiac, and neurologic manifestations accompanied by cyanosis, convulsions or generalized flaccid paralysis, and death. When encephalitis develops, the disease is assumed to be inevitably fatal. A reported recovery of a child with rabies encephalitis has been challenged on diagnostic grounds as an example of postvaccinal rabies encephalitis (Chap. 24). A few cases have been reported to occur following inhalation in persons exploring infected bat caves.

Prevention and Control

Treatment of the Exposed Person Persons bitten by animals should have the wound flushed and washed immediately with soap and water, detergent, or water alone. As early as possible, the wound should be cleansed but not sutured by a physician or under his direction with a 20 percent solution of soap or disinfectant known to inactivate the virus. If warranted, as noted in Table 26-2, antirabies serum or vaccine should be administered.

The results of antirabies prophylaxis (serum and vaccine) are clearly effective in preventing rabies in persons bitten by animals proved to be rabid. It is important, however, to recognize that the incidence of rabies in untreated individuals bitten by rabid animals may be low (5 to 15 percent after dog bites) or high (70 percent after wolf bites). The incidence is apparently determined by the regular or irregular presence of virus in saliva and the concentration of virus present in a particular species.

Prospects for Control The danger of acquiring rabies in man has been dramatically decreased by the rapid application of the measures indicated above and in Table 26-2; by the licensing, restriction, and immunization of dogs; and by efforts to reduce the numbers of wild animals known to be efficient vectors (foxes and skunks in the United States) by monitoring the incidence of rabies and taking measures to limit its spread. Where bat-transmitted rabies is a serious problem, cattle should be immunized. Immunization of man is generally limited to those

Table 26-2 World Health Organization Recommendations after Exposure to Rabies

Nature of exposure	Status of biting animal (whether vaccinated or not) at time of exposure	Status of biting animal (whether vaccinated or not) during observation period of 10 days	Recommended treatment
I No lesions; indirect contact	Rabid	—	None
II Licks			
1 Unabraded skin	Rabid	—	None
2 Abraded skin, scratches, unabraded or abraded mucosa	**a** Healthy	Clinical signs of rabies or proved rabid (laboratory)	Start vaccine at first signs of rabies in the biting animal
	b Signs suggestive of rabies	Healthy	Start vaccine immediately; stop treatment if animal is normal on fifth day after exposure
	c Rabid, escaped, killed, or unknown	—	Start vaccine immediately
III Bites			
1 Mild exposure	**a** Healthy	Clinical signs of rabies or proved rabid (laboratory)	Start vaccine at first signs of rabies in the biting animal
	b Signs suggestive of rabies	Healthy	Start vaccine immediately; stop treatment if animal is normal on fifth day after exposure
	c Rabid, escaped, killed, or unknown	—	Start vaccine immediately
	d Wild (wolf, jackal, fox, bat, etc.)	—	Serum immediately, followed by a course of vaccine
2 Severe exposure (multiple, or face, head, finger, or neck bites)	**a** Healthy	Clinical signs of rabies or proved rabid (laboratory)	Serum immediately; start vaccine at first sign of rabies in the biting animal
	b Signs suggestive of rabies	Healthy	Serum immediately, followed by vaccine; vaccine may be stopped if animal is normal on fifth day after exposure
	c Rabid, escaped, killed, or unknown	—	Serum immediately, followed by vaccine
	d Wild (wolf, jackal, pariah dog, fox, bat, etc.)	—	Serum immediately, followed by vaccine

Source: WHO Expert Committee on Rabies, Fifth Report, *W. H. O. Tech. Rep. Ser.*, no. 321, Geneva 1966.

exposed to high risk (veterinarians, speliologists, animal caretakers, forest workers) and involves the use of the inactivated duck embryo vaccine. An experimental attenuated rabies vaccine developed by passing the virus in WI-38 human diploid cells is highly antigenic and nonpathogenic in monkeys and may prove useful in the future.

On the other hand, the prospects are dim for the elimination of rabies in the wild animal reservoir that extends over much of the globe. The tragic effects of human rabies can, however, be limited by following the recommendations included in Table 26-2.

LYMPHOCYTIC CHORIOMENINGITIS

Lymphocytic choriomeningitis (LCM) is primarily an infection of mice, dogs, monkeys, and guinea pigs which may occasionally be transmitted to man, presumably following inhalation of the virus in dried urine or feces of house mice. Apparently, human infection is reasonably common, perhaps involving 10 percent of the population, but disease is much less frequent. Clinically, the disease is generally recognized as a self-limited meningitis and only rarely as a more severe meningoencephalomyelitis. Subcutaneous inoculation of volunteers was followed by fever which appeared in 2 days and persisted up to 3 weeks, accompanied by an influenza-like illness, meningitis in half of the patients, and recovery of the virus in the blood and cerebrospinal fluid. It is estimated that LCM may be responsible for 5 to 10 percent of sporadic (nonepidemic) cases of viral meningitis.

LCM is an enveloped RNA virus (50 nm) which possesses RNA-containing granules that resemble ribosomes and consequently has been classified as an arenavirus. LCM shares common antigens and is morphologically identical with arthropod viruses of the Tacaribe complex. The latter include a virus isolated from bats in Trinidad (Tacaribe), viruses that cause hemorrhagic fever in man and appear to have a reservoir in rodents (Junin virus in Argentina and Machupo virus in Bolivia), disseminated Lassa fever in Nigeria, and the Marburg virus of vervet monkeys which has caused a serious and fatal disease in laboratory workers in Germany and Yugoslavia. One of the fascinating properties of congenital and neonatal LCM infections of mice is that the mice excrete the virus for the balance of their lives, i.e., until they develop what appears to be an immune complex disease involving the CNS which terminates fatally when the mice become 1 year of age. Thus, LCM may serve as an animal model for the slow virus diseases of man which include kuru, Creutzfeldt-Jakob disease, and subacute sclerosing panencephalitis, the latter representing the slow destruction of the CNS by measles virus.

Diagnosis of LCM in man can be based on the demonstration of a rise in CF or neutralizing antibody which usually appears after the patient has recovered (3 and 7 weeks, respectively). Alternatively, the virus can be isolated in mice, chick embryos, or tissue cultures and identified by CF reactions. Prevention and control depend on the avoidance of contact with mice and their excreta and their elimination from the home.

HEMORRHAGIC FEVERS

A number of arboviruses and arenaviruses can induce disease in man which is characterized primarily by fever and hemorrhages in the gastrointestinal tract, kidneys, lungs, and brain, occasionally accompanied by shock, encephalitis, and a significant mortality (5 to 50 percent). Included among the causative agents are dengue, a group B arbovirus (Chap. 22), viruses of the Russian spring-summer encephalitis complex of group B arboviruses (Omsk hemorrhagic fever, Kyasanur Forest disease) that are transmitted by ticks and have a reservoir in field rodents, ungrouped arboviruses (Crimean hemorrhagic fever, Central Asian hemorrhagic fever) spread by ticks and presumably having a reservoir in cattle, the Junin and Machupo arenaviruses (see LCM above) which have a reservoir in field rodents, and hemorrhagic nephrosonephritis caused by an unknown virus. Generally, except for dengue, the diseases characteristically occur either in Eastern Europe and Asia or in Argentina and Bolivia. As the vectors, reservoirs, and names imply, human disease tends to occur in rural or forest areas. At present, prevention and control are limited to vector control in the diseases transmitted by ticks. Except for hemorrhagic nephrosonephritis, diagnosis can be established by demonstrating a rise in CF or neutralizing antibody. Alternatively, the virus can be recovered from a variety of clinical specimens (blood, throat washings, urine, spinal fluid) in infant mice or tissue culture and identified by CF or neutralization tests.

COLORADO TICK FEVER

Colorado tick fever is primarily a disease of ground squirrels and is caused by a double-stranded RNA virus (orbivirus) with icosahedral symmetry and transmitted by ticks from animal to animal, and occasionally from ticks to man. Human disease typically presents a biphasic fever curve interspersed with an afebrile period of 2 to 3 days followed by uneventful recovery. During the febrile periods the patient experiences severe pain in the back and extremities, headache, nausea, malaise, and leukopenia. The onset occurs about 5 days after the tick bite and persists for about 1 week. Virus can be recovered from the blood by inoculation of embryonated eggs, infant mice, or cell cultures and identified by FA, CF, or neutralization tests. Alternatively, the diagnosis can be established by demonstrating a rise in FA, CF, or neutralizing antibody. Colorado tick fever has been reported to occur in 10 western states of the United States, and serological evidence of infection has been found in western Canada. Tick control measures represent the most practical approach to prevention of the disease in endemic areas.

RIFT VALLEY FEVER

Rift Valley fever is primarily a disease of sheep occurring in Africa and is probably caused by an arbovirus. Human disease is essentially similar to Colorado tick fever and presumably is transmitted by an arthropod, possibly a mosquito. The virus has a diameter of about 30 nm, contains RNA, can be recovered from the blood by inoculating mice or tissue cultures, and can be identified by CF, HA-inhibition, or neutralization tests. Alternatively, the diagnosis can be established by demonstrating a rise in CF, HA-inhibiting, or neutralizing antibody. The vector has not been identified, but since sheep can be protected if they are screened at night, the arthropod is known to be a nocturnal feeder, perhaps a mosquito.

COWPOX AND MONKEYPOX

As the names imply, cowpox and monkeypox are natural diseases of cattle and monkeys and are caused by poxviruses which are closely related to smallpox and vaccinia (Chap. 22). In humans who have not been vaccinated against smallpox, cowpox may be acquired by man during milking, usually resulting in a local lesion on the hand combined with fever and lymphadenitis and healing in a few weeks. An outbreak of monkeypox in man occurred in 1970 in Liberia, Sierra Leone, and the Congo among people living in an endemic area of monkeypox. The patients experienced a typical smallpox-like disease but recovered uneventfully, and the disease did not spread from man to man.

BIBLIOGRAPHY

Adams, W. H., Emmons, R. W., and Brooks, J. E.: "The Changing Ecolory of Murine (Endemic) Typhus in Southern California," *Am. J. Trop. Med.,* 19:311-318, 1970.

Bentley, E. W.: "A Review of Anticoagulant Rodenticides in Current Use," *Bull. W.H.O.,* 47:275-280, 1972.

Brooks, G. F., and Buchanan, T. M.: "Tularemia in the United States: Epidemiologic Aspects in the 1960s and Follow-up of the Outbreak of Tularemia in Vermont," *J. Infect. Dis.,* 121:357-359, 1970.

Butter, T.: "A Clinical Study of Bubonic Plague: Observations of the 1970 Vietnam Epidemic with Emphasis on Coagulation Studies, Skin Histology and Electrocardiograms," *Am. J. Med.,* 53:268-276, 1972.

Cadigan, F. C., Jr., Andre, R. G., Bolton, M., Gan, E., and Walker, J. S.: "The Effect of Habitat on the Prevalence of Human Scrub Typhus in Malaysia," *Trans. R. Soc. Trop. Med. Hyg.,* 66:582-587, 1972.

Cho, C. T., and Wenner, H. A.: "Monkeypox Virus," *Bacteriol. Rev.,* 37:1-18, 1973.

Claflin, J. L., and Larson, C. L.: "Infection-Immunity in Tularemia: Specificity of Cellular Immunity," *Infect. Immun.,* 5:311-318, 1972.

Cole, J. S., Stoll, R. W., and Bulger, R. J.: "Rat-bite Fever: Report of Three Cases," *Ann. Intern. Med.,* 71:979-981, 1969.

Davies, D. G., and Harvey, R. W. S.: "Anthrax Infection in Bone Meal from Various Countries of Origin," *J. Hyg. (Camb.),* 70:455-458, 1972.

Elsner, B., Schwarz, E., Mando, O. G., Maiztegui, J., and Vilches, A.: "Pathology of 12 Fatal Cases of Argentine Hemorrhagic Fever," *Am. J. Trop. Med.,* 22:229-236, 1973.

Gan, E., Cadigan, F. C., Jr., and Walker, J. S.: "Filter Paper Collection of Blood for Use in a Screening and Diagnostic Test for Scrub Typhus Using the IFAT," *Trans. R. Soc. Trop. Med. Hyg.,* 66: 588-593, 1972.

Greenberg, M.: "Rickettsialpox in New York City," *Am. J. Med.,* 4:866-874, 1947.

Hattwick, M. A. W.: "Rocky Mountain Spotted Fever in the United States, 1920-1970," *J. Infect. Dis.,* 124:112-114, 1971.

Henderson, G. E., Gary, G. W., Jr., Kissling, R. E., Frame, J. D., and Carey, D. E.: "Lassa Fever: Virological and Serological Studies," *Trans. R. Soc. Trop. Med. Hyg.,* 66:409-416, 1972.

Howe, C., and Miller, W. R.: "Human Glanders: Report of Six Cases," *Ann. Intern. Med.,* 26:93-115, 1947.

Iwasaki, Y., Wiktor, T. J., and Koprowski, H.: "Early Events of Rabies Virus Replication in Tissue Cultures: An Electron Microscope Study," *Lab. Invest.,* 28:142-148, 1973.

"Joint FAO/WHO Expert Committee on Brucellosis. Fifth Report," *W.H.O. Tech. Rep. Ser.,* no. 464, 1971.

Lamb, R.: "Anthrax," *Br. Med. J.,* 1:157-160, 1973.

Lewis, G. E., Jr., and Anderson, J. K.: "The Incidence of *Brucella canis* Antibodies in Sera of Military Recruits," *Am. J. Public Health,* 63:204-205, 1973.

Linnemann, C. C., Jr., Jansen, P., and Schiff, G. M.: "Rocky Mountain Spotted Fever in Clermont County, Ohio: Description of an Endemic Focus," *Am. J. Epidemiol.,* 97:125-130, 1973.

Macrae, A. D.: "Rabies," *Br. Med. J.,* 1:604-606, 1973.

McCracken, A. W., Mauney, C. U., Huber, T. W., and McCloskey, R. V.: "Endocarditis Caused by *Erysipelothrix insidiosa,*" *Am. J. Clin. Pathol.,* 59: 219-222, 1973.

Miller, R. P., and Bates, J. H.: "Pleuropulmonary Tularemia. A Review of 29 Patients," *Am. Rev. Resp. Dis.,* 99:31-41, 1969.

Murphy, F. A., Bauer, S. P., Harrison, A. K., and Winn, W. C., Jr.: "Comparative Pathogenesis of Rabies and Rabies-like Viruses: Viral Infection and Transit from Inoculation Site to the Central Nervous System," *Lab. Invest.,* 28:361-376, 1973.

Notkins, A. L., and Koprowski, H.: "How the Immune Response to a Virus Can Cause Disease," *Sci. Am.,* 228(1):22-31, 1973.

Palmer, D. L., Kisch, A. L., Williams, R. C., Jr., and Reed, W. P.: "Clinical Features of Plague in the United States: The 1969–1970 Epidemic," *J. Infect. Dis.,* 124:367–371, 1971.

Smadel, J. E.: "Influence of Antibiotics on Immunological Response in Scrub Typhus," *Am. J. Med.,* 17:246–258, 1954.

Spruance, S. L., and Bailey, A.: "Colorado Tick Fever. A Review of 115 Laboratory Confirmed Cases," *Arch. Intern. Med.,* 131:288–293, 1973.

Turner, L. H.: "Leptospirosis," *Br. Med. J.,* 1:537–540, 1973.

Velimirovic, B.: "Plague in South-East Asia: A Brief Historical Summary and Present Geographical Distribution," *Trans. R. Soc. Trop. Med. Hyg.,* 66: 479–504, 1972.

Walker, J. S., Remmele, N. S., Carter, R. C., Mitten, J. Q., Schuh, L. G., Stephen, E. L., and Klein, F.: "The Clinical Aspects of Rift Valley Fever Virus in Household Pets. I Susceptibility of the Dog," *J. Infect. Dis.,* 121:9–18, 1970.

Warkel, R. L., Rinaldi, C. F., Bancroft, W. H., Cardiff, R. D., Holmes, G. E., and Wilsnack, R. E.: "Fatal Acute Meningoencephalitis Due to Lymphocytic Choriomeningitis Virus," *Neurology,* 23:198–203, 1973.

Wiktor, T. J., Gyorgy, E., Schlumberger, H. D., Sokol, F., and Koprowski, H.: "Antigenic Properties of Rabies Virus Components," *J. Immunol.,* 110: 269–276, 1973.

Williams, E.: "Brucellosis," *Br. Med. J.,* 1:791–793, 1973.

Chapter 27

Chemotherapy of Infectious Disease

Bernard A. Briody

The response of an infected patient to antimicrobial therapy is the result of a series of complex interactions involving the parasite, the host, and the drug. Pertinent components that influence the chemotherapy of infectious disease include the mechanism of drug action and resistance (Chap. 4), the operation of factors that determine pathogenicity (Chap. 5), the structural and functional integrity of the host (Chap. 6), and the immune response of the host to the parasite (Chaps. 7 to 11). The intents of the ensuing discussion are (1) to formulate a rational approach to chemotherapy of infectious disease in the light of the nature and severity of the disease, the integrity of the host, the properties of the antimicrobial agent, and the complications that can occur; (2) to evaluate the indications for combined therapy and for chemoprophylaxis; and (3) to identify the shifting etiology and the changing patterns of infectious disease.

NATURE AND SEVERITY OF THE DISEASE

Selection of the Drug

In most instances the selection of the appropriate antimicrobial agent requires the isolation and identification of the causative agent and the determination of its sensitivity to the drug. In other cases, antibiotic sensitivity tests are superfluous, as in pneumococcal, group A streptococcal, and gonococcal infections. Frequently the physician can await the laboratory diagnosis and antibiotic sensitivity results before prescribing the antimicrobial agent (urinary tract infections). In life-threatening infections, however, the physician must base his decision on the results of a Gram stain and, after taking the necessary cultures, must initiate therapy without delay and follow the response of the patient, changing the therapy when indicated by either the condition of the patient or the results of cultural and sensitivity tests (meningitis).

Sensitivity tests performed on the etiological agent must be based on the use of drug concentrations ordinarily attainable in blood with the particular antimicrobial agent without causing toxcity. However, the physician must take into account special situations in which the drug may not penetrate the blood-brain or blood-CSF barriers or in which it may be concentrated, as in urine. For example, if the patient has meningitis and the drug of choice is penicillin, the physician can compensate for relative inability to penetrate the CSF by employing meningeal doses (20 million units per day for 10 days or more), thus establishing an effective concentration gradient. However, if the drug of choice is streptomycin, it must be injected intrathecally in view of the toxicity that would be encountered if an attempt were made to develop a similar concentration gradient.

Nature of the Disease

Even when an identical causative agent of uniform sensitivity to a particular antimicrobial drug is responsible for the infection, the concentration of the drug and the duration of its administration required to effect a cure will depend on the nature of the disease process. For example, therapy of pneumococcal pneumonia, empyema, and endocarditis ordinarily involves daily doses of 1, 6, and 20 million units of penicillin for 1, 2, and 2 weeks, respectively. In alveolar exudates, pneumococci are readily accessible to penicillin and phagocytes; whereas in empyema the bacteria are protected from the phagocytes, and the penicillin that diffuses into the pleural fluid is partially bound by the pus and necrotic debris. In endocarditis, the bacteria are inaccessible to the phagocytes because of their location inside a network of fibrin and platelets.

In acute diseases (streptococcal pharyngitis, pneumococcal pneumonia, gonorrhea), the response to therapy is characteristically prompt, recovery is rapid, and relapses rarely develop. In chronic diseases (tuberculosis, leprosy, typhoid, brucellosis, and chlamydial, fungal, protozoal, and some viral and rickettsial infections), the causative agent survives for prolonged periods in the host, recovery is slow, relapses are anticipated, and treatment must be extended for many weeks or months. In the majority of these chronic diseases, the causative agent replicates intracellularly, making it inaccessible to phagocytes and to many antimicrobial agents. For example, the intracellular concentration of streptomycin is 5 percent of the extracellular concentration. In chronic diseases, the tissue reaction often impedes the ability of phagocytes to make contact with the parasite as in tuberculosis, abscesses due to staphylococci and other parasites, osteomyelitis, granulomatous diseases, endocarditis, renal, biliary and pulmonary disease proximal to obstruction, and tissue cyst formation in toxoplasmosis. In some acute diseases, the direct transfer of viruses from cell to cell by fusion of virus and cell membranes as in herpes simplex, varicella, measles, parainfluenza, and respiratory syncytial infections, precludes intervention by antibody and phagocytes. In acute meningococcal meningitis and gonorrhea, the ability to survive and replicate intracellularly is a critical factor in pathogenicity and creates a difficult problem for the phagocytes and for the antimicrobial agent to inhibit or kill the susceptible parasite.

In addition to antimicrobial therapy, surgical debridement, excision, drainage, or repair is a prerequisite for effective resolution of the infection in a number of situations. Examples include gas gangrene; brain, abdominal, and metastatic abscesses; osteomyelitis; renal, biliary, and pulmonary infections proximal to obstruction; and fungal growths on cardiac valves or in the pulmonary tract. Even though the causative agent is susceptible to the prescribed antimicrobial therapy, failure to take appropriate surgical action may lead to repeated relapses, direct or hematogenous extension of the infection, permanently disabling complications, and sequelae or death which could otherwise be avoided.

Severity of the Disease

The severity of the disease often dictates the use of a cidal instead of a static drug and its administration by the intravenous, intrathecal, or intrapleural route. Bacterial meningitis, bacterial endocarditis, and patients with septicemia, hypotension, bleeding diathesis, or impaired host defenses can be cited as examples for which cidal drugs are indicated. Even though the primary disease may not be severe, as in streptococcal pharyngitis, therapy with a cidal drug (penicillin) is mandatory in order to prevent the immunologically damaging sequel of rheumatic carditis. In other cases in which antimicrobial drugs are accessory therapeutic procedures, as in diphtheria, tetanus, and gas gangrene, a cidal drug (penicillin) is indicated in order to halt the synthesis of toxin as rapidly as possible.

The early initiation of therapy is critical in many serious diseases if a fatal outcome is to be avoided. Included in this category are such diseases as pneumococcal bacteremia, fulminant meningococcemia, gram-negative septicemia, anthrax septicemia, pneumonic plague, and Rocky Mountain spotted fever. Death may occur in the presence of a microbiological cure because of the irreversible pathology that developed before therapy was initiated.

THE CONDITION OF THE HOST

Whenever the structural and functional integrity of the host is compromised by genetic, developmental, or acquired defects, therapy of infectious disease is often a complicated, hazardous, demanding, and at times an impossible task for the physician. Successful treatment may be effected relatively simply and permanently by removal of a foreign body or obstruction or by surgical repair of the defect. In other cases, the acute episode may be resolved by temporary withdrawal of the precipitating factor (corticosteroids, antimetabolites, cytotoxic drugs, immunosuppressive agents), but the underlying disease remains, and future infections can be expected when use of the precipitating agent is resumed, as in most situations it must be. In uncontrolled diabetes, correction of the metabolic disturbance must accompany antimicrobial therapy. Agammaglobulinemic patients can be treated with pooled human immunoglobulins. Patients with genetic defects in C3, C4, or C5 components of complement can be treated with appropriate purified component (s). Individuals with cell-mediated defects in immunity are prime targets for progressive intracellular infections that may be temporarily held in check by heroic measures, but they inevitably succumb to one of the continuing series of infections to which they are susceptible.

The major points to be emphasized are that (1) host participation is normally a critical factor in recovery from infectious disease, (2) in the compromised host, a cidal drug must be used whenever possible, and (3) whenever practical, the underlying defect must be corrected if antimicrobial therapy is to be effective or if repeated infections are to be prevented.

PROPERTIES OF THE ANTIMICROBIAL AGENT

While the absorption, distribution, metabolism, excretion, and toxicity of antimicrobial drugs are the proper sphere of textbooks of pharmacology, there are several facets of drug action that are pertinent to their efficacy in therapy of infectious disease. As noted earlier, whether a drug is static or cidal can exert a marked influence on the outcome of certain infections. Static drugs are dependent on the immune response of the host for the elimination of the parasite. Consequently, their use in diseases in which immune phagocytosis is precluded or ineffective may be associated with relapses (endocarditis, intracellular infections) or progression of the disease (in compromised hosts). The cidal antimicrobial drugs include the penicillins, cephalosporins, aminoglycosides (streptomycin, kanamycin, neomycin, gentamicin), polymyxins, vancomycin, ristocetin, bacitracin, and cycloserine. Static chemotherapeutic agents include the sulfonamides, chloramphenicol, tetracyclines, erythromycin, lincomycin, clindamycin, rifampin, and the urinary antiseptics (Mandelamine, nalidixic acid, nitrofurans).

Other key aspects of antimicrobial drug activity are based on the ability of the agent to come in contact with the parasite in effective concentration. For example, many antimicrobial agents (penicillin, streptomycin) penetrate poorly into the CSF or pleural spaces, others (nitrofurantoin) do not produce effective concentrations at any other site except the urinary tract, sulfonamides are antagonized by pus and necrotic debris, streptomycin is unable to penetrate cells as effectively as extracellular fluids, some drugs (aminoglycosides, erythromycin) are inactive in acidic urine, and others (Mandelamine) are only effective in acidic urine.

COMPLICATIONS

Biologic Complications

The principal complications associated with the use of antimicrobial agents may be classified as biologic, immunologic, and pharmacologic. The major biologic problems involve the emergence of antibiotic-resistant parasites (Chaps. 3, 4, and 18), the alteration of the normal microbial flora leading to superinfection with drug-resistant microorganisms, and the persistence of the causative agent followed by relapse of the disease. Careful monitoring of the patient, selection of the most appropriate drug and its use in adequate dosage for a sufficient period of time, and when necessary, combined therapy can obviate the emergence of resistant forms of the causative agent in the majority of cases. Awareness of the common situations under which resistant mutants present a problem should alert the physician to the need for special care, e.g., in chronic infections, in many of which the parasite is located intracellularly or in which the tissue reaction precludes the effective intervention of phagocytes. Included in this category are endocarditis, pyelonephritis, tuberculosis, typhoid, brucellosis, tularemia, leprosy, and chlamydial, rickettsial, and protozoal infections.

The alteration of the normal microbial flora by antibiotics has many consequences (Chap. 6), including enhanced susceptibility to infection with pathogens and especially infection with drug-resistant members of the normal flora (superinfection). Superinfection is most commonly caused by staphylococci, gram-negative enteric bacilli, and the fungi *Candida* and *Aspergillus,* all members of the indigenous flora that are resistant to many or most of the available antimicrobial drugs. The initial sites of superinfection are mucous membranes supplied with an abundant microbial flora (oral cavity, upper respiratory tract, gastrointestinal tract, vagina), but the infection may spread to involve the lower respiratory tract or may lead to disseminated disease. It is estimated that about 2 percent of patients treated with antibiotic agents develop superinfections. Although superinfections occur with all antimicrobial agents, the incidence is greater with broad-spectrum agents, such as the tetracyclines. While the patient's own microbial flora represents the major source of the superinfecting parasite, it is important to recognize that in the hospital environment the patient may acquire antibiotic-resistant microorganisms, which are ordinarily considered part of the normal human flora, from other patients or from hospital personnel.

Immunologic Complications

Hypersensitivity reactions (types I, II, III, and IV; see Chap. 8) are common complications associated with the use of antimicrobial drugs. The reactions vary widely in type and severity. For example, the hypersensitivity may be manifest by fever, skin rashes, serum sickness, Arthus reactions, hemolytic anemia, autoimmune disease, or severe or fatal anaphylactic reactions. Fortunately, skin rashes are the most frequently encountered manifestation of hypersensitivity to many antimicrobial drugs (sulfonamides, streptomycin, penicillins) and should alert the physician to the potential danger of continued or future use of the agents. There are no suitable skin tests to detect hypersensitivity in advance of treatment, and the manifestations may develop in a few minutes or not for as long as a month later. The appearance of drug-induced fever is another convenient danger signal for the physician who must be alert to the possibility and avoid continued use or increased dosage of the drug. Generally, the drug-induced fever occurs after the patient has become afebrile and is recovering from infection. Most fatal anaphylactic reactions caused by antimicrobial agents occur in atopic patients.

Apparently, patients with certain diseases are particularly prone to develop skin rashes. For example, when patients with infectious mononucleosis were treated (for whatever reason) with ampicillin or penicillin G, 80 and 40 percent, respectively, developed skin rashes. Unfortunately, many aspects of drug-induced hypersensitivity reactions remain poorly understood. For example, why do patients with infectious mononucleosis show such a high incidence of skin rashes? What will be their response when reexposed to the drug? Are they prime candidates for severe allergic reactions?

Pharmacologic Complications

The toxic manifestations of most antimicrobial drugs are well documented, diverse, and vary widely in severity. For example, when exposed to tetracyclines in utero or during the first few years of life, children may develop mottling and discoloration of the teeth. If exposed in utero or to premature or newborn infants, chloramphenicol (750 mg/kg of body weight per day) can induce the gray syndrome which is characterized by lethargy, a gray cyanosis, circulatory collapse, and death associated with the accumulation of chloramphenicol in the blood due to the immaturity of the glucuronyltransferase system. Other important examples of drug-induced damage include ototoxicity and nephrotoxicity of the aminoglycosides, reversible anemia and the rare but more severe genetically determined pancytopenia of chloramphenicol, and serious renal, neural, and cardiac toxicity of amphotericin B.

When given in full therapeutic dosage, some antimicrobial agents (chloramphenicol, amphotericin B) are so toxic for man that they must be administered under carefully controlled hospital conditions. Particular attention must be given to the use of antimicrobial drugs in patients with impaired renal function. For example, the following drugs are highly toxic and should be avoided: sulfonamides, tetracyclines, streptomycin, cephaloridine, and the urinary antiseptics (Mandelamine, nalidixic acid, nitrofurans). Kanamycin, gentamicin, polymyxins, and vancomycin are potentially toxic, and dosage must be reduced. Penicillins, cephalothin, erythromycin, lincomycin, and chloramphenicol are relatively safe and can be used in normal or slightly reduced dosage.

COMBINED THERAPY

The primary indications for prescribing combinations of antimicrobial drugs are (1) to prevent, delay, or reduce the emergence of resistant mutants; (2) to achieve the eradication of the causative agent which cannot be accomplished by a single antimicrobial agent; (3) to provide an effective drug for different, but probable, causative agents in the case of life-threatening infections until a definite microbiologic diagnosis is established; and (4) to treat mixed infections in which the causative agents are sensitive to different antimicrobials. Apart from a few specific infectious diseases, the use of drugs in combination cannot be justified. For this reason, it is necessary to delineate those infections in which combined therapy is beneficial.

The outstanding examples of combined therapy are for all practical purposes limited to tuberculosis, enterococcal endocarditis, brucellosis, tularemia, and malaria. In tuberculosis, combined therapy prevents the emergence of resistant mutants. In enterococcal endocarditis, brucellosis, and tularemia, the combined drugs prevent the emergence of resistant mutants and achieve the eradication of the causative agent; these results cannot be accomplished by either of the individual drugs. In malaria, the two drugs act on different forms of the parasite, chloroquine acting as a schizonticide and primaquine functioning as a gameticide and also destroying the hepatic tissue phase. Mixed infections are relatively uncommon but may be encountered in wound infections, chronic pyelonephritis, bronchiectasis, and peritonitis. The main indications for preliminary combined therapy in life-threatening infections are meningitis and septicemia.

Unfortunately, the use of drugs in combination is far more widespread than is warranted by their demonstrated efficacy. In many cases, the in vivo effects are frankly antagonistic, as in the combination of penicillin and tetracycline in the treatment of pneumococcal meningitis. Furthermore, in the majority of instances, in vitro indications of synergistic action of two drugs cannot be demonstrated in vivo.

CHEMOPROPHYLAXIS

Antimicrobial drugs can be employed effectively in chemoprophylaxis either before or after infection in many specific infectious diseases but have been used indiscriminately in many diseases in which their value is inconclusive or known to be ineffective. Chemoprophylaxis is of proved value in many or all cases in the following situations: sulfonamides or penicillin in the prevention of group A streptococcal infections and rheumatic fever recurrences; penicillin in the prevention of congenital syphilis, acute gonococcal urethritis, gonococcal ophthalmitis, diphtheria in contacts, anthrax in patients exposed to spores; penicillin in the prevention of group A streptococcal infections and glomerulonephritis under epidemic conditions when given prior to exposure; tetracyclines in those exposed to pneumonic plague; isoniazid in tuberculosis; chloroquine or other antimalarial agents in the suppression of malaria followed by primaquine upon leaving the endemic area; tetracyclines in scrub typhus; pentamidine isethionate in gambian trypanosomiasis; N-methylisothiosemicarbazone in smallpox; neomycin in patients with hepatic coma; sulfonamides in type A meningococcal meningitis; neomycin in enteropathogenic *E. coli* infections; mass chemoprophylaxis with effective drugs under epidemic conditions in the nonvenereal treponematoses, bacillary dysentery, type A meningococcal meningitis, diphtheria, and other diseases; penicillin and streptomycin in patients with damaged heart valves who are undergoing abdominal or genitourinary surgery.

Chemoprophylaxis is of questionable value in burned patients and patients with cystic fibrosis, chronic pulmonary disease, glomerulonephritis, endocarditis, trachoma, and wounds. Chemoprophylaxis is ineffective and in many instances harmful in the case of surgical procedures, compromised hosts, measles, influenza, and pneumonia.

THE CHANGING PATTERNS OF INFECTIOUS DISEASE

With the advent of antimicrobial drugs many significant changes have occurred in the spectrum of infectious agents. While the mortality formerly associated with acute bacterial infections caused by a limited number of pyogenic pathogens has been sharply curtailed, and while the life span has been correspondingly lengthened, there has been little, if any, alteration in morbidity of infectious disease. On the other hand, there has been a significant shift in the etiology of infectious disease caused by organisms of limited virulence for normal tissues, organisms that are part of the resident flora of the skin and mucous membranes, and organisms which are characteristically resistant to many or most antimicrobial drugs. The major culprits are staphylococci, gram-negative enteric bacilli, and fungi such as *Candida* and *Aspergillus,* but they are joined by an extensive group of other bacteria and fungi. The parasites that have come into prominence typically invade the tissues of hosts whose resistance is impaired by lymphoreticular and other malignancies; advanced atherosclerosis; underlying metabolic, pulmonary, renal, and cardiac disease; or immunosuppressive agents used in therapy of noninfectious disease. The shift from exogenous pathogens sensitive to antimicrobial agents to endogenous microorganisms resistant to antimicrobial agents reflects both the success of therapy in acute bacterial infections and the marked progress in the management of the noninfectious, chronic, and previously fatal diseases, leading to older individuals who are more susceptible to infection by their own microbial flora.

BIBLIOGRAPHY

Altemeier, W. A., Culbertson, W. R., Fullen, W. D., and Shook, C. D.: "Intra-abdominal Abscesses," *Am. J. Surg.,* 125:70-79, 1973.

Bennett, W. M., Singer, I., and Coggins, C. H.: "Guide to Drug Usage in Adult Patients with Impaired Renal Function," *J.A.M.A.,* 223:991-997, 1973.

"Boston Collaborative Drug Surveillance Program. Ampicillin Rashes. Collaborative Study," *Arch. Dermatol.,* 107:74-76, 1973.

Burke, J. F.: "Preventive Antibiotic Management in Surgery," *Annu. Rev. Med.,* 24:289-294, 1973.

Chisholm, G. D., Waterworth, P. M., Calnan, J. S., and Garrod, L. P.: "Concentration of Antibacterial Agents in Interstitial Tissue Fluid," *Br. Med. J.,* 1:569-573, 1973.

Chusid, M. J., and Atkins, E.: "Studies on the Mechanism of Penicillin-induced Fever," *J. Exp. Med.,* 136:227-240, 1972.

Davis, R. E., and Jackson, J. M.: "Trimethoprim/Sulfamethoxazole and Folate Metabolism," *Pathology,* 5:23-29, 1973.

Durack, D. T., and Petersdorf, R. G.: "Chemotherapy of Experimental Streptococcal Endocarditis: I. Comparison of Commonly Recommended Prophylactic Regimens," *J. Clin. Invest.,* 52:592-598, 1973.

Kerns, D. L., Shira, J. E., Go, S., Summers, R. J., Schwab, J. A., and Plunket, D. C.: "Ampicillin Rash in Children. Relationship to Penicillin Allergy and Infectious Mononucleosis," *Am. J. Dis. Child.,* 125:187-190, 1973.

Levine, A. S., Siegel, S. E., Schreiber, A. D. Hauser, J., Preisler, H., Goldstein, I. M., Seidler, F., Simon, R., Perry, S., Bennett, J. E., and Henderson E. S.: "Protected Environments and Prophylactic Antibiotics: A Prospective Controlled Study of Their Utility in the Therapy of Acute Leukemia," *N. Engl. J. Med.,* 288:477-483, 1973.

Morrison, J. C., Coxwell, W. L., Kennedy, B. S., Schreier, P. C., Wiser, W. L., and Fish, S. A.: "The Use of Prophylactic Antibiotics in Patients Undergoing Cesarean Section," *Surg. Gynecol. Obstet.,* 136:425-428, 1973.

Riley, H. D., Jr.: "Drug Interactions: Part IV. Interactions among Antimicrobial and Nonantimicrobial Agents," *Pediatrics,* 50:954-955, 1972.

Rudolph, A. H., and Price, E. V.: "Penicillin Reactions among Patients in Venereal Disease Clinics: A National Survey," *J.A.M.A.,* 223:499-501, 1973.

Sparling, P. F., Wiesner, P. J., Holmes, K. K., and Kass, E. H.: "Treatment of Gonorrhea," *J. Infect. Dis.,* 127:578-580, 1973.

Stewart, G. T.: "Allergy to Penicillin and Related Antibiotics: Antigenic and Immunochemical Mechanism," *Annu. Rev. Pharmacol.,* 13:309-324, 1973.

Turck, M.: "Therapeutic Principles in the Treatment of Urinary Tract Infections and Pyelonephritis," *Adv. Intern. Med.,* 18:141-152, 1972.

Index